Handbook of Local Anesthesia

Handbook of Local Anesthesia

Editor: Monica Chase

AMERICAN
MEDICAL PUBLISHERS
www.americanmedicalpublishers.com

AMERICAN
MEDICAL PUBLISHERS
www.americanmedicalpublishers.com

Cataloging-in-Publication Data

Handbook of local anesthesia / edited by Monica Chase.
p. cm.
Includes bibliographical references and index.
ISBN 978-1-63927-535-9
1. Local anesthesia. 2. Conduction anesthesia. 3. Anesthesia. 4. Anesthesiology. I. Chase, Monica.
RD84 .H36 2022
617.964--dc23

American Medical Publishers,
41 Flatbush Avenue,
1st Floor, New York,
NY 11217, USA

ISBN 978-1-63927-535-9 (Hardback)

Contents

Preface

I am honored to present to you this unique book which encompasses the most up-to-date data in the field. I was extremely pleased to get this opportunity of editing the work of experts from across the globe. I have also written papers in this field and researched the various aspects revolving around the progress of the discipline. I have tried to unify my knowledge along with that of stalwarts from every corner of the world, to produce a text which not only benefits the readers but also facilitates the growth of the field.

The technique used to cause the absence of sensation in a certain body part is referred to as local anesthesia. It can be used for minor procedures as it does not cause unconsciousness, just local insensitivity to pain. Local anesthesia helps patients to go through surgical and dental procedures with reduced or no pain and distress. It can also be used to decrease the effects of non-surgical pain. The local anesthetic drug is used to cause reversible local anesthesia as well as a loss of nociception. The effects of local anesthesia particularly depend on the nerve pathways it uses. Loss of pain sensation known as analgesia and loss of muscle power termed as paralysis are the major effects caused by it. This book outlines the processes and applications of local anesthesia in detail. It presents researches and studies performed by experts across the globe. This book will provide comprehensive knowledge to the readers.

Finally, I would like to thank all the contributing authors for their valuable time and contributions. This book would not have been possible without their efforts. I would also like to thank my friends and family for their constant support.

Editor

1

Lipid Emulsion for Local Anesthetic Systemic Toxicity

Sarah Ciechanowicz and Vinod Patil

Department of Anaesthesia, BHR University Hospitals NHS Trust, Romford, London RM7 0AG, UK

Correspondence should be addressed to Vinod Patil, vinodpatil@doctors.org.uk

Academic Editor: James B. Eisenkraft

The accidental overdose of local anesthetics may prove fatal. The commonly used amide local anesthetics have varying adverse effects on the myocardium, and beyond a certain dose all are capable of causing death. Local anesthetics are the most frequently used drugs amongst anesthetists and although uncommon, local anaesthetic systemic toxicity accounts for a high proportion of mortality, with local anaesthetic-induced cardiac arrest particularly resistant to standard resuscitation methods. Over the last decade, there has been convincing evidence of intravenous lipid emulsions as a rescue in local anesthetic-cardiotoxicity, and anesthetic organisations, over the globe have developed guidelines on the use of this drug. Despite this, awareness amongst practitioners appears to be lacking. All who use local anesthetics in their practice should have an appreciation of patients at high risk of toxicity, early symptoms and signs of toxicity, preventative measures when using local anesthetics, and the initial management of systemic toxicity with intravenous lipid emulsion. In this paper we intend to discuss the pharmacology and pathophysiology of local anesthetics and toxicity, and the rationale for lipid emulsion therapy.

1. Introduction

Local anesthetics (LAs) can be defined as drugs that reversibly block transmission of a nerve impulse, without affecting consciousness. Medical use of local anesthetic agents began some years after the isolation of cocaine from Peruvian coca in the 1860s. Chance discovery in 1884 by Freud while using cocaine to wean a morphine addict lead Koller to use cocaine successfully in ophthalmic surgery as a topical anesthetic. Halsted and Hall took more invasive steps by directly injecting cocaine into oral cavity nerves in order to produce anesthesia for removal of a wisdom tooth [1].

However, the euphoria, subsequent addiction, and cases of mortality from the clinical use of the natural ester cocaine created a drive to the development of the less toxic newer amino esters. Einhorn's synthesis of procaine in 1905 was to dominate LA use for the next forty years, but with amino esters slow onset of action and allergen potential, the hypoallergenic amino amides gradually came into force with lignocaine appearing in 1948 and is still the most commonly used LA in dentistry.

Amino amides mepivacaine, prilocaine, and bupivacaine were all developed by 1963 and all have roles in modern dentistry. In 1969, articaine was synthesized by chemist Muschaweck, and with its potency and safety profile is now the most common LA for dental procedures in most of Europe [2].

Despite these efforts, all of the amide LAs harbor varying levels of cardiovascular (CVS) and central nervous system (CNS) toxicity that is still a major complication seen today. Methods of administration have also progressed since August Bier first practiced intravenous regional anesthesia in 1908, allowing a whole limb to be anesthetized with the aid of a tourniquet and LA [3].

Simultaneously, plexus anesthesia came about in the early 1900s with brachial plexus blocks for upper limb surgeries, these peripheral techniques more refined in recent decades to prolong blocks via continuous infusion regional anesthesia using catheters and pumps [4].

The use of LA in neuraxial anesthesia is another significant development that began with James Corning's experiment in 1885 of spinal anesthesia on a dog [5], but it was not used clinically until 1899 by August Bier [6]. Lumbar epidural anesthesia came about later in 1921 by Spanish military surgeon Fidel Pages. It was popularized by the Italian surgeon Dogliotti in the 1930s [7].

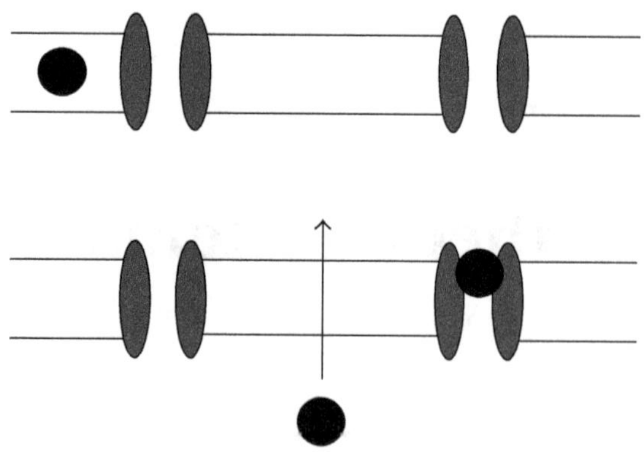

FIGURE 1: Mechanism of action of local anesthetics. Unionized LA enters nerve axon and becomes ionized to block sodium channels. LA also has direct effects by expanding the cell membrane to increase fluidity.

The idea of continuous infusion of epidural anesthesia, however, was not started until use of caudal blocks for emergency caesareans in 1942 [8], and in more recent decades the introduction of small flexible catheters has improved safety, delivery, and duration of epidural anesthesia.

2. Mechanism of Action

The physicochemical properties of LAs determine their properties as anesthetic agents. They have three structural groups, an aromatic ring, connecting group (ester or amide), and an ionizable amino group. This lipid-soluble hydrophobic aromatic group and a charged, hydrophilic amide group enables them to exert their effects by two mechanisms: in their uncharged (unionized) state they lipid soluble and able to traverse the lipid bilayer of the neuronal cell membrane, to then gain a hydrogen ion and become ionized making them able to bind intracellularly to voltage-gated sodium channels, rendering the channel reversibly inactive, and so unable to allow for sodium entry to generate and propagate the action potential [9] (see Figure 1). Binding can also occur to the closed sodium channel to retain its inactive state. Secondly, LAs have direct effects on the lipid bilayer, disrupting impulses by incorporating into the cell membrane, causing expansion [10, 11]. The sensitivity of nerve fibers depends upon their axonal diameter and degree of myelination with small, myelinated fibers more susceptible. Generally the small pain and temperature fibers (C unmyelinated, A-δ myelinated) are blocked first with the larger touch and pressure (A-Υ, A-β) fibres next, and large muscle tone and postural A-α fibres last. It is thought that the prolonged action potential of smaller fibres provides more time for LA entry, and more frequently stimulated nerves show increased susceptibility from a high degree of open channels. The story does not end there, however, in addition to blocking sodium channels, newer amino amide ropivacaine has been found to bind to human cardiac potassium channels (hKv 1.5) to block repolarization of the membrane [12]. A number of anesthetics, including bupivacaine and ropivacaine, have also been shown to block L-type Ca^{2+} channels in rat

TABLE 1: Pharmacology of common local anesthetics. Potency is relative. Potency: toxicity ratio is a useful evaluation to consider, articaine has the best ratio making it clinically efficacious as well as safe. %PB = protein binding.

	Potency	Pot : Tox	LWPC	Onset	pKa	$t^{1/2}$ (min)	%PB
Bupivacaine	8	2	27.5	Slow	8.1	162	95.6
Articaine	3	3.3	17	Fast	7.8	20	94
Lignocaine	2	2	2.9	Fast	7.9	96	64.3
Mepivacaine	2	2.2	19.3	Fast	7.8	114	78
Prilocaine	2	2.7	0.9	Fast	7.7	93	55
Ropivacaine	4	2.25	2.9	Mod	8.1	96	94

cerebrocortical membranes. From a systemic viewpoint, LAs may improve pain by inhibiting local inflammatory response to injury by decreasing inflammatory cytokine release from neutrophils.

3. Clinical Pharmacology

Potency is decided by the lipid solubility of the agent and can be expressed as a lipid : water partition coefficient (LWPC), the ratio of the amount of agent in each phase. High coefficients increase lipophilic properties and allows for ease of passage into the cell membrane thus facilitating potency. Onset of action is determined by the ionization constant or pKa value, which determines the proportion of ionized to unionized form of the agent at a given pH. Agents with a pKa value closer to the physiological pH permit more LA in the unionized, lipid soluble form to enter the cell. So factors that alter tissue pH also affect the proportion of LA in the unionized form and hence can slow onset of action in an acidic, infected wound. Table 1 demonstrates these properties in some common anesthetic agents.

4. Pharmacokinetics and Metabolism

The primary aim of local anesthetic administration is to saturate the targeted nerves while causing minimal systemic absorption. Infiltration of skin, subcutaneous tissues, intrathecal, and epidural spaces will result in varying absorption into the systemic circulation depending on the surface area for absorption and vascularity of the area. Intercostal muscles and epidural administration being particularly susceptible, and in dentistry the gingiva of the maxillary alveolar ridge is prone to inducing rapid systemic absorption. Lignocaine has a vasodilatatory effect and so is often mixed with adrenaline or phenylephrine to reduce vascular absorption and hence prolong action and reduce the risk of systemic toxicity. Conversely, cocaine is a potent vasoconstrictor.

High protein binding of the LA to plasma protein alpha 1-glycoprotein will protect it from metabolism and hence prolong its duration of action. All amino esters except for cocaine are rapidly degraded by circulating plasma esterases, and excreted in the urine. The amide prilocaine is also metabolized extrahepatically. All other amides such as lignocaine and bupivacaine are more slowly metabolized by the liver and hence are of higher risk of accumulation.

5. Local Anesthetic Systemic Toxicity

5.1. Incidence. Before 1981, epidural use for labor analgesia had reported LA systemic toxicity (LAST) in 100 per 10,000 cases [13].

Improvements in regional techniques and precautions have greatly improved the safety profile over the past 30 years, including the withdrawal of higher concentration 0.75% bupivacaine preparations for obstetrics. Although incidence of bupivacaine cardiotoxicity has declined since 1980 it still poses a potentially fatal risk for patients. Epidemiological reports have been clinically diverse and with different outcome measures used, but overall rate of systemic toxicity has been reported in France to be 0–20 per 10,000 in 2002 and is greatly dependent on the site of peripheral nerve block [14]. A study by Brown in 1995 showed seizures associated with interscalene and supraclavicular brachial plexus blocks to be as high as 79 in 10,000 [15].

For example, dentists administer thousands of local anesthetic injections every day with few adverse events. However, LAST can occur even with the most experienced practitioner. Human error misjudging dose, anatomy, patient factors, or bad luck can contribute to the unintended development of serious systemic complications. Lignocaine is the most common LA used in dentistry and has been reported to cause systemic toxicity [16, 17]. Articaine, even with its excellent safety profile, may cause systemic intoxication if unintentional intravascular injection is performed during a block: it has been reported that the rate of intravenous injection for inferior alveolar nerve block is as high as 15.3% [18], which can occur due to the high vascularization of the oral mucosa.

5.2. Clinical Manifestations. The signs of LAST are an extension of pharmacological action. The classic description is of a progressive "biphasic" effect on the CNS and then CVS, two areas highly sensitive to changes in tissue electrophysiology. CNS excitation (agitation, auditory change and metallic taste) progresses to seizures or CNS depression (drowsiness, coma, and respiratory arrest). This is followed by CVS excitation (tachycardia, ventricular arrhythmia, and hypertension) then depression (bradycardia, conduction block, asystole, and cardiac depression) [19].

Of particular importance is the nature of this collapse, with high incidence of LA-cardiac arrest being resistant to standard resuscitative measures.

However, a recent review of 93 published case reports of LAST found that over 40% of presentations did not fit this classic description [20]. This includes the simultaneous presentation of CNS and CVS signs, and cases with only CVS effects manifest. CVS-only effects were seen in 4 out of 10 cases under general anesthesia or form of sedation, and were more likely to show delayed onset of signs.

Regarding CNS symptoms, the prodromal features, for example, perioral numbness, dizziness, confusion, obtundation, and dysarthria totaled only 18% of symptom frequency, with seizures seen in 68% of cases and loss of consciousness and agitation also frequent. Half of CVS signs were arrhythmias, with bradycardia/asystole seen in 27%.

They reported that timing is variable, for single injections although most onset of LAST occurred "rapidly," at 50 seconds or less in half of cases, 25% were delayed by 5 minutes or more. Interestingly, all instances of LAST during continuous infusions were substantially delayed, often by a number of days after initiation.

5.3. Toxic Plasma Levels. Systemic toxicity from local anesthetic overdose occurs due to accidental intravascular injection, absorption from tissue depot, or repeated doses without balanced elimination. The concentration of bupivacaine present in the aqueous portion of plasma is directly related to the myocardial tissue absorption, and hence cardiotoxicity [21]. The degree of toxicity is therefore dependent on plasma levels of LA; with highly aerobic tissues vulnerable to hypoxia being most vulnerable, that is, myocardium, lungs and central nervous system. For regional blocks, the plasma levels of lignocaine are typically 3–5 mcg/mL, with toxic plasma levels seen at 6–10 mcg/mL.

5.4. Risk Factors. Intuitively, one would speculate that the plasma levels of a given dose of drug would have strong correlation to the weight or body mass index of the individual. In the case of LAs, this is largely true in children, but in adults we see that the methods of administration, nature of the drug preparation, and the physiological status of the patient have far greater association. A poorly vascular injection site of the block, vasoconstrictor activity of the LA, and concurrent use of adrenaline would slow systemic absorption, hence reducing plasma levels, but physiologically, impairment of hepatic and renal function involved in metabolism and elimination can have a profound effect to maintain plasma levels.

Accidental intravascular injection is the major cause of systemic toxicity, for example, regional anesthesia of the neck (interscalene block, cervical plexus block, and stellate ganglion block) can cause direct intra-arterial injection and cause rapid toxicity from early entry to the cerebral circulation. Epidural anesthesia holds a risk of intravenous injection into the engorged epidural venous plexus of the parturient [22], and the oral mucosa is also highly vascular. Regarding site of injection, rapid absorption occurs via infiltration of highly vascular tissues such as intercostal muscles, the oral mucosa, and the epidural space. High cardiac output states also promote systemic uptake by maintaining the gradient for diffusion.

Choice of agent also has clear implications for toxicity. Longer-acting amide LAs such as bupivacaine improve analgesia after surgery and have use in cutaneous infiltration, regional nerve blocks, epidural anesthesia, and spinal anesthesia. However, bupivacaine is more cardiotoxic than shorter-acting lignocaine, with smaller doses often resulting in cardiotoxic symptoms without prior CNS effects

[23]. Addition of vasoconstrictors such as epinephrine can dramatically slow the absorption of LAs from the site of injection, improving their safety and prolonging the anesthesia, which is why higher doses of some agents are possible with a vasoconstrictor additive.

Patient physiological factors also have influence on the LA toxicity threshold. Rosen studied the effect of both lignocaine and bupivacaine in anesthetised sheep and found that acidosis, hypoxia, and hypercarbia potentiated cardiotoxic effect [24]. In this sense the elderly are a prime example of risk of imbalance between absorption and metabolism of LA.

Reduction of hepatic blood flow by drugs or hypotension will decrease the hepatic clearance of amide LAs, and having reduced cardiac output and poor renal or hepatic function leads to prolonged absorption and drug accumulation, respectively. This has implications with use of the recent continuous infusion anesthesia for postoperative orthopedics and acute pain [4, 25]. In addition, use of postoperative pain pumps in plastic surgery can involve bupivacaine combined with epinephrine, which can extend the halflife of bupivacaine from 3.5 hours to 5–7 hours [26].

On top of this, underlying cardiac pathology of ischemic heart disease, conduction blocks, and cardiac failure will additionally render the elderly more vulnerable to toxic CVS effects. The majority of the cases of LAST seen in dentistry occur in children, as due to their small size, dose- to- weight ratio is more difficult to calculate and so overdose is more likely. It is also more likely to progress in adversity because a high number of blocks are done with the child anesthetized. The early signs of paraesthesia and mental state changes would not be detected [26]. Conversely, some studies show that newborns and children can actually tolerate higher plasma levels of bupivacaine compared to adults [27, 28]. Kiuchi et al. [29] reports that 2-week old rats (equivalent to 3-year old children) exhibit a lethal dose 4 times higher than 16-week-old animals, and that this difference can be seen as less profound cardiac depression. They speculate this to be due to a difference in calcium regulation at the intracellular sarcoplasmic reticulum. However, in clinical practice, Bosenberg et al. [30] have reported the use of 3 mg/kg of ropivacaine in children without observing symptoms of systemic toxicity or plasma levels of ropivacaine in the range of potential risk for systemic toxicity.

In pregnancy, the higher cardiac output will speed up absorption and with reduced plasma proteins this will increase the free fraction of LA in the plasma. Plasma protein levels can also vary in different pathological states and there is a reduction seen postoperatively, in chronic diseases such as cancer, also old age, smoking increases the unbound free fraction of agent available to bind to cardiac myocytes and cause toxicity. Lerman et al. [31] have shown that alpha-1 glycoprotein plasma levels are low in newborns and toddlers but the clinical significance of this reduction is not clear.

Drug interactions are an important patient factor to consider when determining risk of cardiotoxicity. Amide local anesthetics are metabolized by the liver and specifically the cytochrome p450 system that has potential for drug interactions by competitive metabolism and up, or down-regulation of the system by chronic exposure to certain drugs. Cimetidine inhibits the cytochrome p450 system and can allow the accumulation of plasma levels of LAs. Drugs altering plasma esterase activity have the potential to decrease hydrolysis of the lesser-used ester LAs. Increased vigilance is also necessary in patients taking digoxin, calcium antagonists, or beta-blockers [32].

Table 2: Factors affecting LA toxicity.

Site of injection	Drug	Patient factors
Surface area	Potency	Age
Vascularity	Dose *(volume × concentration)*	Genetics
	Vasoactivity	Cardiac pathology
	± vasoconstrictor	Pregnancy
		Drug interactions
		Acidosis
		Hypoxia
		Hypercarbia

There is debate as to whether general anesthesia provides some protection from toxicity, the effect of general anesthesia in sheep caused plasma LA concentrations to increase due to cardiovascular depression, leading to slower efflux from visceral to nonvisceral organs; however, less severe CNS effects and cardiovascular arrhythmias occurred in these sheep [33, 34]. The clinical significance of this is not yet established. For a summary of LAST risk factors see Table 2.

5.5. Ion Channels and the Lipid Bilayer. As there are such a myriad of ion channels and processes affected by LAs there is a risk of the culpable mechanism of cardiotoxicity being missed [35]. The pathophysiology of LAs are thought to be an extension of their uses, blocking cardiac voltage-gated sodium channels, preventing myocyte depolarization, blocking repolarization via potassium channels, and blocking the sarcoplasmic reticulum voltage-dependent calcium channels to limit the rise of intracellular calcium available for excitation-contraction coupling [35, 36]. Mio et al. describe a loss of sensitivity of rat ventricular muscle myofilaments to calcium a basis for the loss of calcium-activated tension in trabeculae following access of LA. Furthermore, myocyte ATP is reduced, thus limiting the energy available for coupling of actin-myosin cross-bridge cycles [37]. Work on ion channel involvement is extensive but is not necessarily consistent with cardiotoxicity seen from different agents. Studies on biometric membranes support the notion of increasing lipid membrane fluidity to confer potency of agent and cardiotoxicity [11].

Animal studies and case reports indicate a difference in cardiotoxicity between short-acting agent lignocaine and the longer-acting bupivacaine. For both agents there is dose-dependent cardiac depression but the greater toxicity potential of bupivacaine is disproportionate and does not correlate entirely with potency of inhibition of cardiac sodium channels. This difference could rely on an alternative mechanism of toxicity for bupivacaine, and we see this clinically in case reports of bupivacaine showing a more significant CVS toxicity than CNS, with arrhythmia and cardiac arrest often occurring without seizures. There appears to be a more potent mechanism occurring at the myocardium, in animal studies lignocaine induces dramatic hemodynamic depression while bupivacaine markedly impairs *both* electrophysiologic and haemodynamic variables [38]. To examine more specifically, Reiz and Nath [39] directly injected lignocaine or bupivacaine into the coronary circulation of dogs and found that the difference in depression of contractility was proportional to their relative potencies, 1 : 4. However, the effect on cardiac conduction was 1 : 16 with recovery of the EKG taking longer for bupivacaine at a ratio of 1 : 8, confirming that the major difference in cardiotoxicity between long-acting and shorter-acting agents is their influence on conduction through the cardiac axis. Clarkson and Hondeghem suggest that bupivacaine has this pronounced effect due to the strength of binding to inactive sodium channels [40].

5.6. Cardiac Mitochondria. In light of work on the mitochondrial pathogenesis of local anesthetic cardiotoxicity and information from studies and a case report [41] of a child with carnitine deficiency, mitochondrial abnormalities also seem to confer increased susceptibility [42]. Bupivacaine-induced myopathies have led to rat and human cell studies to demonstrate structural alterations in muscle, the sarcomere, and calcium homeostasis by LAs. High bupivacaine concentrations caused abnormal mitochondrial autophagy with reduction in mitochondrial content, inhibition of ATP production by action on mitochondrial ATP-synthase, and inhibition of oxidative phosphorylation [43]. In cardiac tissue, in vivo and vitro studies on rat hearts demonstrate bupivacaine and ropivacaine's ability to uncouple oxidative phosphorylation at complex I in the mitochondria [44], and block the enzyme carnitine acylcarnitine transferase used for transporting acylcarnitines across the mitochondrial membrane in fatty acids during aerobic metabolism [45, 46]. Importantly, inhibition of the respiratory chain complexes was prevented by antioxidant treatment and reversed following removal of the anesthetic thereby suggesting an oxidant-mediated feedback mechanism reinforcing the primary inhibitory action of the anesthetic. Recent developments implicate the mitochondrial phospholipid cardiolipin, involved in respiration, to be the major determinant of LA cardiotoxicity, established by means of theoretic and structural biological methods [47].

5.7. Vasoactivity. Secondly to these direct effects on the myocardium, a signif-icant cause of hypotension is due to peripheral vasodilatation from direct action on the vasculature. Bupivacaine and levobupivacaine cause vasodilatation at clinical doses, but lower doses appear to cause vasoconstriction [45]. Direct cardiac depression of bupivacaine has been studied in vivo to demonstrate a deleterious double-whammy on the cardiac output via negative inotropic effects and increasing afterload, which appears to be mediated by $\alpha 1$ adrenoceptors [48]. Ropivicaine and levobupivacaine are far less toxic in this sense.

Thirdly, a mechanism of toxicity appears to be inhibition of autonomic reflexes. There is evidence for inhibition of the baroreceptor reflex in rats [49], and Pickering et al. show bupivacaine to be selectively toxic to the brainstem area for control of cardiac sympathetic outflow, the nucleus tractus solitarius, without effecting respiration, leading to hypotension and dysrhythmias [50]. Lida et al. reveal a differing influence of bupivacaine and ropivacaine on dog spinal pial vessel diameter, with ropivacaine causing vasoconstriction and bupivacaine vasodilatation [51]. Laser doppler imaging studies on human skin has revealed nitric oxide (NO) to be responsible for the vasodilatatory effect of local anaesthetics, however, NO does not appear to be involved when the blood vessel is uninnervated such as the in vitro umbilical artery [52, 53].

6. Lipid Emulsion Therapy

20% lipid infusion is the first safe intravenous lipid emulsion (ILE) used in medicine and has been around since 1962 for its use in parenteral nutrition. The commercial preparation Intralipid 20% is manufactured by Fresenius Kabi, 1 liter consists of 200 g purified soybean oil, 12 g purified egg phospholipids, and 22 g anhydrous glycerol, and it is a source of omega-3 and -6 essential fatty acids with total energy content 8.4 MJ (2,000 kCal). ILEs use in LAST came about from an unexpected finding by Weinberg in 1998. Following a case report of a carnitine-deficient patient showing increased susceptibility to bupivacaine cardiotoxicity, he postulated the impaired fatty acid oxidation was the etiology and in seminal work, preloaded rats with ILE prior to bupivacaine in hope to establish this. The result was quite the opposite, with an increase in the mean lethal dose (LD50) by 50% [54]. He later went further to demonstrate the efficacy of ILE by rescuing dogs from bupivacaine-induced cardiac arrest [55]. ILE therapy for treatment of LAST is now well established, following a crop of over 19 peer-reviewed case reports appearing since Rosenblatt's successful application of ILE to clinical practice in 2006 [56], and supports the use of ILE for bupivacaine, levobupivacaine, and ropivacaine cardiotoxicity [56–61]. This year we also saw a successful case report from seemingly intractable lignocaine-induced cardiac arrest [62].

This evidence strongly supports the use of ILE in the resuscitation of LAST and because of this efficacy, ILE is has been incorporated into safety guidelines for management of LA-induced cardiotoxicity in the UK since 2007 and in the US since 2008 [63, 64]. In 2010, the American Society of Regional Anesthesia and Pain Medicine (ASRA) published its practice advisory on LAST [65], highlighting the importance of airway management and early cardiopulmonary resuscitation with addition of ILE therapy. In 2010 the American Heart Association incorporated lipid emulsion for LAST-cardiac arrest in the special situations section of the ACLS guidelines [66].

6.1. Mechanism. The current agreed hypothesis for ILE's efficacy in treating cardiotoxicty, although not well defined but supported by in vitro studies, is the formation of a "lipid sink"; that is, an expanded intravascular lipid phase that acts to absorb the offending circulating lipophilic toxin, hence

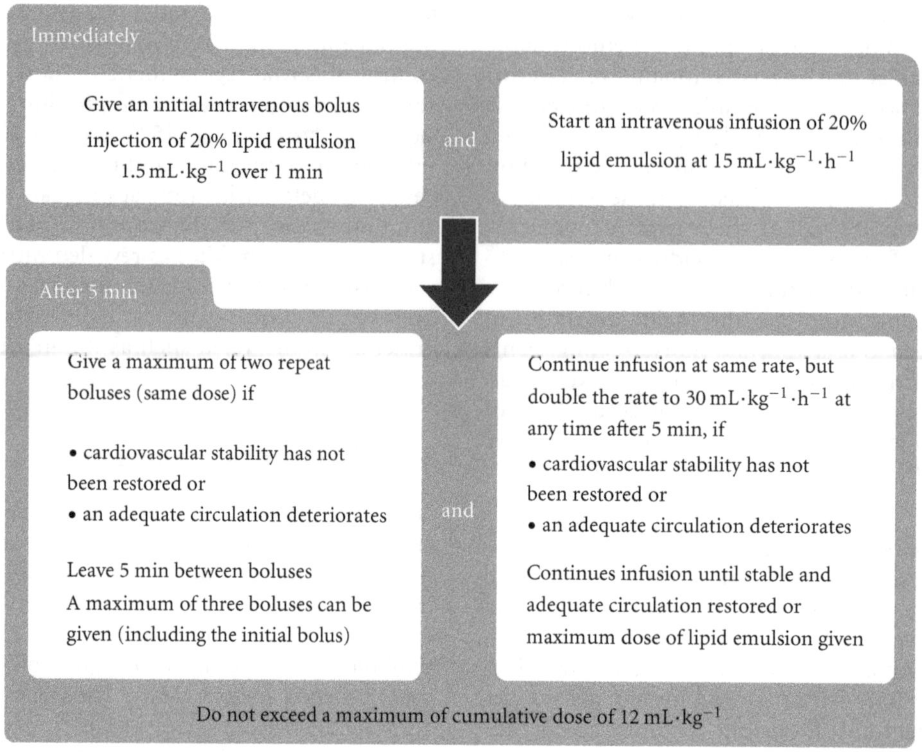

FIGURE 2: AAGBI local anaesthetic toxicity guideline 2010 (with permission) [63].

reducing the unbound free toxin available to bind to the myocardium. The effect of ILE has been disputed to be no more than a haemodilution effect from the volume administered, especially pronounced in rat models [67]. However, convincing evidence from rat studies by Weinberg show ILE to reduce the aqueous plasma bupivacaine concentration three-times greater than that predicted by haemodilution alone [68], and subsequently ILE therapy has shown clear superiority over adrenaline and/or vasopressin in rats that is directly linked to reduced myocardial tissue content and improved cardiac function [21]. Influences on metabolism also seem to confer the success of ILE; there is evidence of increased washout of bupivacaine in rat hearts in the presence of ILE [69]. ILE could be acting as a direct energy source to the myocardium, countering the deleterious effect of LAs on fatty acid delivery by acting as a lipid provider, the fatty acid substrate necessary to enrich mitochondrial respiration in the heart and hence ATP production, thus improving the cardiac output [70]. A further mechanism advocated is that of action of raised triglyceride on cardiac calcium channels to increase myocardial calcium concentration, hence enhancing cardiac function [71]. In addition to its use in LAST, but beyond the scope of this review, is a discussion about the more recent but no less significant discovery of ILE in treatment of cardiotoxicity from a range of other lipophilic drugs including chlorpromazine, beta-blockers, calcium channel antagonists, and bupropion [61].

6.2. Regimen. The AAGBI recommended ILE or Intralipid regimen following cardiac arrest from LAST involves a large initial intravenous bolus injection of 20% lipid emulsion at 1.5 mL/kg over 1 minute; followed by an infusion of 15 mL/kg/h. Cardiopulmonary resuscitation should be continued throughout. In the absence of return of spontaneous circulation or deterioration after 5 minutes, two further boluses (1.5 mL/kg) may be given at 5-minute intervals. The intravenous infusion rate should also be doubled to 30 mL/kg/hr. A maximum of three boluses can be given, and a cumulative dose of 12 mL/kg should not be exceeded (Figure 2). The ASRA guidelines differ in that only one additional bolus is recommended, and the infusion should continue for 10 minutes after haemodynamic stability is reached, with a maximum dose of 10 mL/kg over 30 minutes [72].

Initial case reports show ILE to often succeed after standard resuscitation has failed and led to the suggestion of ILE as a "last resort" in severe resuscitation resistant LAST. However, there is growing evidence to support its use early in the management with successful case reports supporting the immediate use in cardiac arrest [73–76].

Development of optimal dosing regimens for different patient groups in on the horizon, this year ILE has been recommended for use in obstetrics [77]. Support for ILE in pediatric LAST can be seen from a recent case report of ropivacaine and lignocaine-induced toxicity in a 13-year-old girl after lumbar plexus block [57]. Ventricular tachycardia was impressively converted to sinus rhythm after a bolus of 3 mL/kg of lipid emulsion was given over 3 minutes. This is encouraging to read and also poses the question as to whether we need to develop optimal dosing regimens for

TABLE 3: Safe doses of common LAs.

	Maximum safe dose (mg/kg)
Bupivacaine	2.0
Levobupivacaine	2.5–3.0
Articaine	7.0
Lignocaine	4.0
with epinephrine	7.0
Mepivacaine	7.0
Prilocaine	6.0
Ropivacaine	3.0-4.0

children. There exists debate about the use of vasopressors with ILE for treatment of LAST, and what combination, if any, is beneficial [78]. Weinberg shows greater survival with ILE alone than with epinephrine and/or vasopressin in rodent models, and combination of ILE and epinephrine worsened outcomes by impairing cardiac function and metabolic indices [79], possibly by worsening coronary perfusion. This is mirrored in the study use of epinephrine and/or vasopressin in cardiac arrest in humans that resulted in early survival but later demise [80, 81]. So perhaps only small doses of epinephrine, if any, are advisable in the treatment of LAST and vasopressin-vasoconstriction is likely to worsen the LA-induced cardiac failure. Further studies are needed to clarify the use of vasopressors in LA-induced cardiac arrest, but at present it is not advised to deviate from standard resuscitation guidelines, with the addition of ILE therapy.

Of interest, the commercial preparation Intralipid may not be the most effective emulsion formulation to use clinically, as described by electrophoresis studies comparing it with liposome vesicle dispersions. The dispersion preparations had increased interaction with local anesthetics compared to standard Intralipid [82], so when financially viable it should be considered for clinical use. There is also discussion of the specific importance of omega-3 fatty acids [83].

7. Prevention of Toxicity

Prevention is better than cure, and although no single preventative measure can eliminate the risk of developing LAST, they do provide improved safety. Regarding site of injection, care must be taken to avoid intravascular injection and awareness of tissues prone to rapid uptake, such as the head and neck, is useful. Since the introduction of the measures to prevent inadvertent intravascular injection that began with the epinephrine test dose for labor epidurals by Moore and Batra in 1981 [84], the incidence of LAST has fallen 10–100 fold [85]. The following methods, although singularly unproven, likely promote safety.

(i) Incremental injection of 3–5 mL aliquots with pause of one circulation time between each, although it increases risk of needle migration. Note circulation time greater in the lower limb.

(ii) Aspirate needle prior to each injection (but 2% false negatives).

(iii) For large volumes, first use intravascular marker, for example, epinephrine 10–15 mcg/mL in adults and 0.5 mcg/kg in children and observe any CVS response.

Although these methods are useful for avoiding intravascular injection, they do not predict the possibility of rapid tissue absorption from the site. To this end, it is important not to exceed the safe dose of local anesthetic involved [86]. The cardiotoxic potential of the amide local anesthetics can be expressed as a maximum safe dose for administration (Table 3). However, for procedures such as tumescent liposuction, the relative avascularity of subcutaneous fat and epinephrine-induced vasoconstriction account for slow lignocaine absorption, and this allows for doses of lignocaine as high as 18 mg/kg to be administered safely.

7.1. MLAC and Protocols. The minimum local analgesic concentration (MLAC) of local anesthetics is a clinical model introduced in 1995 to compare the relative potencies of epidural bupivacaine and lignocaine in laboring women. Trials follow up and down sequential allocation of the effective concentration of local anesthetic that produces effective analgesia in 50% of subjects (EC50), to provide an equivalent of the volatile anesthetic "MAC" value [87]. Adoption of this model has allowed for lowest adequate dose regimens and determination of the LA sparing efficacy of adjunct analgesics in obstetrics [88].

7.2. US-Guided Regional Anesthesia. Ultrasound (US) can be used to guide the accurate placement of the needle for LA injection over soft tissues, avoiding intravascular injection and damage to surrounding structures and allowing smaller volumes of LA to be used, as direct application to the nerve is more likely. However, systematic review of the Cochrane database finds no difference in the success rate or duration of analgesia between landmark/peripheral nerve stimulator techniques and US-guided blocks, with larger and higher-quality studies lacking [89]. A reduction in incidence of LAST from US has also not yet been proven [90], and there is debate as to whether the reduced volume blocks actually compromise postoperative analgesia [91].

7.3. Newer Agents. Stereoisomerism contributes to the differing potency of local anesthetics. Molecules with an asymmetric carbon atom exist in three-dimensional forms that are mirror images (enantiomers and stereoisomers), distinguished by how they rotate polarized light. The terms R and S are used for the two different enantiomers, and an equimolar amount of both R and S constitutes a racemic mixture. Racemic bupivacaine has been in use for decades but is not without its safety concerns. The relatively high toxicity of bupivacaine had led for it to be the main agent implicated in toxicity research. Ropivacaine and levobupivacaine are S-enantiomer pipecoloxylidines that have improved safety profiles compared to racemic bupivacaine. A recent study by Tsuchiya et al. investigating the interaction of racemic bupivacaine and R+ and S-enantiomers of bupivacaine and ropivacaine with biomimetic membranes of chiral lipids demonstrated the greater interaction of the R+ enantiomers, with S-Ropivacaine presenting least influence of all. This is consistent with reported clinical cardiotoxicity of the agents and also supports the hypothesis of potency of increasing the lipid bilayer membrane fluidity [11]. For regional blocks involving sites of high vascularity, the use of alternative long-acting amide levoenantiomers may be vindicated to further reduce the risk to patients, and this has already been suggested in dentistry for interior alveolar nerve blocks [92]. However, a median effective dose study shows ropivacaine and levobupivacaine to, respectively, have 35% and 3% reduced analgesic potency to racemic bupivacaine, and so decisions to use these safer agents must be balanced against a loss of clinical efficacy [93].

7.4. Surgeon's Awareness. Where LA is provided by nonanesthetists, misdiagnosis and underreporting of LA-associated complications is likely [94]. This includes offices, outpatients, and small surgical centers, and so the true incidence of LAST in these settings is unclear. There are, however, case reports of significant morbidity following LA use in such areas [95–98]. The importance of surgeon's knowledge of safe use of LAs and management of complications is signified by the reported incidence of five deaths from suspected lignocaine systemic toxicity or related complication following tumescent liposuction in New York between 1993–1998 [99–102]. It is of interest to note that this procedure is still very popular today and commonly performed without the presence of an anesthesiologist. Also concerning is a recent survey in the UK by Collins that suggests only half of hospital surgeons know how to calculate the correct dose of local anesthetic being used and fewer than 25% of nonanesthetic doctors knew the recommended safe doses. Only 7% of nonanesthetic doctors knew the correct treatment to be intralipid and only 3% knew the initial dose [103]. These finding highlight the importance of education, which is of particular significance to practitioners who regularly use LAs without the presence of an anesthesiologist.

8. Summary

Vigilance is required when performing procedures that have a potential for systemic toxicity. There are numerous examples of local anesthetic systemic complications in the literature, many in the hands of nonanesthesiologists. We see that strategies to reduce the risk of LAST can never eliminate its risk. Although uncommon, the consequences can be fatal. Advances in ILE therapy and understanding is providing a life-saving rescue in the most dreaded situations faced by practitioners, and further progress will likely improve on our safe use of LAs in the future. Rapid identification of toxicity and a good recall of the ILE therapy regimen can save lives, but we need to expand awareness to practitioners in remote locations such as outpatients, offices, and especially those who work without an anesthesiologist. We encourage these facilities to put together a "rescue kit" in a specified location with the current guidelines readily available. LAs are used more frequently by surgeons and dentists than anesthesiologists, and on that note we feel that the respective colleges should also develop guidelines for management of LAST incorporating lipid emulsion therapy.

References

[1] H. Ws, "Practical comments on the use and abuse of cocaine; suggested by its invariably successful employment in more than a thousand minor surgical operations," *New York Medical Journal*, vol. 42, pp. 294–295, 1885.

[2] N. Nizharadze, M. Mamaladze, N. Chipashvili, and D. Vadachkoria, "Articaine—the best choice of local anesthetic in contemporary dentistry," *Georgian Medical News*, no. 190, pp. 15–23, 2011.

[3] M. Bannister, "Bier's block," *Anaesthesia*, vol. 52, no. 7, p. 713, 1997.

[4] J. E. Chelly, D. Ghisi, and A. Fanelli, "Continuous peripheral nerve blocks in acute pain management," *The British Journal of Anaesthesia*, vol. 105, supplement 1, pp. i86–i96, 2010.

[5] J. L. Corning, "Spinal anaesthesia and local medication of the cord," *New York Medical Journal*, vol. 42, pp. 483–485, 1885.

[6] A. Bier, "Experiments regarding the cocainization of the spinal cord," *Deutsche Zeitschrift für Chirurgie*, vol. 51, pp. 361–369, 1899.

[7] J. C. Diz, A. Franco, D. R. Bacon, J. Rupreht, and J. Alvarez, "The history of anesthesia," in *Proceedings of the 5th International Symposium on the History of Anesthesia*, Elsevier, Santiago, Spain, September 2001.

[8] R. A. Hingson and W. B. Edwards, "Comprehensive review of continuous caudal analgesia for anesthetists," *Reprinted from Anesthesiology*, vol. 4, no. 2, pp. 181–196, 1943.

[9] J. M. Ritchie, B. Ritchie, and P. Greengard, "The active structure of local anesthetics," *Journal of Pharmacology and Experimental Therapeutics*, vol. 150, no. 1, pp. 152–159, 1965.

[10] H. Tsuchiya, T. Ueno, M. Mizogami, and K. Takakura, "Local anesthetics structure-dependently interact with anionic phospholipid membranes to modify the fluidity," *Chemico-Biological Interactions*, vol. 183, no. 1, pp. 19–24, 2010.

[11] H. Tsuchiya, T. Ueno, and M. Mizogami, "Stereostructure-based differences in the interactions of cardiotoxic local anesthetics with cholesterol-containing biomimetic membranes," *Bioorganic & Medicinal Chemistry*, vol. 19, no. 11, pp. 3410–3415, 2011.

[12] C. Valenzuela, E. Delpón, L. Franqueza, P. Gay, D. J. Snyders, and J. Tamargo, "Effects of ropivacaine on a potassium channel (hKv1.5) cloned from human ventricle," *Anesthesiology*, vol. 86, no. 3, pp. 718–728, 1997.

[13] N. B. Kenepp and B. B. Gutsche, "Inadvertent intravascular injections during lumbar epidural anesthesia," *Anesthesiology*, vol. 54, no. 2, pp. 172–173, 1981.

[14] Y. Auroy, D. Benhamou, L. Bargues et al., "Major complications of regional anesthesia in France: the SOS regional anesthesia hotline service," *Anesthesiology*, vol. 97, no. 5, pp. 1274–1280, 2002.

[15] D. L. Brown, D. M. Ransom, J. A. Hall, C. H. Leicht, D. R. Schroeder, and K. P. Offord, "Regional anesthesia and local anesthetic-induced systemic toxicity: seizure frequency and accompanying cardiovascular changes," *Anesthesia and Analgesia*, vol. 81, no. 2, pp. 321–328, 1995.

[16] P. Mehra, A. Caiazzo, and P. Maloney, "Lidocaine toxicity," *Anesthesia Progress*, vol. 45, no. 1, pp. 38–41, 1998.

[17] B. E. Virts, "Local anesthesia toxicity review," *Pediatric Dentistry*, vol. 21, no. 6, p. 375, 1999.

[18] A. T. Zenouz, M. Mahdipour, S. Pourshahidi, P. Amini, and M. Vatankhah, "The incidence of intravascular needle entrance during inferior alveolar nerve block injection," *Journal of Dental Research, Dental Clinics, Dental Prospects*, vol. 2, no. 1, 2008.

[19] J. E. Heavner, "Cardiac toxicity of local anesthetics in the intact isolated heart model: a review," *Regional Anesthesia and Pain Medicine*, vol. 27, no. 6, pp. 545–555, 2002.

[20] G. Di Gregorio, J. M. Neal, R. W. Rosenquist, and G. L. Weinberg, "Clinical presentation of local anesthetic systemic toxicity: a review of published cases, 1979 to 2009," *Regional Anesthesia and Pain Medicine*, vol. 35, no. 2, pp. 181–187, 2010.

[21] G. Weinberg, B. Lin, S. Zheng et al., "Partitioning effect in lipid resuscitation: further evidence for the lipid sink," *Critical Care Medicine*, vol. 38, no. 11, pp. 2268–2269, 2010.

[22] A. H. Tahir, J. Adriani, and M. Naraghi, "Acute systemic toxicity from bupivacaine during epidural anesthesia in obstetric patients," *Southern Medical Journal*, vol. 68, no. 11, pp. 1377–1380, 1975.

[23] G. A. Albright, "Cardiac arrest following regional anesthesia with etidocaine or bupivacaine," *Anesthesiology*, vol. 51, no. 4, pp. 285–287, 1979.

[24] M. A. Rosen, J. W. Thigpen, and S. M. Shnider, "Bupivacaine-induced cardiotoxicity in hypoxic and acidotic sheep," *Anesthesia and Analgesia*, vol. 64, no. 11, pp. 1089–1096, 1985.

[25] J. D. Swenson, G. S. Cheng, D. A. Axelrod, and J. J. Davis, "Ambulatory anesthesia and regional catheters: when and how," *Anesthesiology Clinics*, vol. 28, no. 2, pp. 267–280, 2010.

[26] S. S. Liu, J. M. Richman, R. C. Thirlby, and C. L. Wu, "Efficacy of continuous wound catheters delivering local anesthetic for postoperative analgesia: a quantitative and qualitative systematic review of randomized controlled trials," *Journal of the American College of Surgeons*, vol. 203, no. 6, pp. 914–932, 2006.

[27] C. B. Berde, "Toxicity of local anesthetics in infants and children," *Journal of Pediatrics*, vol. 122, no. 5, pp. S14–S20, 1993.

[28] P. De Negri, G. Ivani, T. Tirri, and A. C. Del Piano, "New local anesthetics for pediatric anesthesia," *Current Opinion in Anaesthesiology*, vol. 18, no. 3, pp. 289–292, 2005.

[29] M. G. Kiuchi, G. Zapata-Sudo, M. M. Trachez, D. Ririe, and R. T. Sudo, "The influence of age on bupivacaine cardiotoxicity," *Anesthesia and Analgesia*, vol. 112, no. 3, pp. 574–580, 2011.

[30] A. T. Bosenberg, J. Thomas, T. Lopez, G. Huledal, L. Jeppsson, and L. E. Larsson, "Plasma concentrations of ropivacaine following a single-shot caudal block of 1, 2 or 3 mg/kg in children," *Acta Anaesthesiologica Scandinavica*, vol. 45, no. 10, pp. 1276–1280, 2001.

[31] J. Lerman, H. A. Strong, K. M. LeDez, J. Swartz, M. J. Rieder, and F. A. Burrows, "Effects of age on the serum concentration of α1-acid glycoprotein and the binding of lidocaine in pediatric patients," *Clinical Pharmacology and Therapeutics*, vol. 46, no. 2, pp. 219–225, 1989.

[32] M. Naguib, M. M. Magboul, A. H. Samarkandi, and M. Attia, "Adverse effects and drug interactions associated with local and regional anaesthesia," *Drug Safety*, vol. 18, no. 4, pp. 221–250, 1998.

[33] S. E. Copeland, L. A. Ladd, X. Q. Gu, and L. E. Mather, "The effects of general anesthesia on the central nervous and cardiovascular system toxicity of local anesthetics," *Anesthesia and Analgesia*, vol. 106, no. 5, pp. 1429–1439, 2008.

[34] S. E. Copeland, L. A. Ladd, X. Q. Gu, and L. E. Mather, "The effects of general anesthesia on whole body and regional pharmacokinetics of local anesthetics at toxic doses," *Anesthesia and Analgesia*, vol. 106, no. 5, pp. 1440–1449, 2008.

[35] J. F. Butterworth, "Models and mechanisms of local anesthetic cardiac toxicity: a review," *Regional Anesthesia and Pain Medicine*, vol. 35, no. 2, pp. 167–176, 2010.

[36] Y. Mio, N. Fukuda, Y. Kusakari, Y. Amaki, Y. Tanifuji, and S. Kurihara, "Comparative effects of bupivacaine and ropivacaine on intracellular calcium transients and tension in ferret ventricular muscle," *Anesthesiology*, vol. 101, no. 4, pp. 888–894, 2004.

[37] Y. Mio, N. Fukuda, Y. Kusakari, Y. Tanifuji, and S. Kurihara, "Bupivacaine attenuates contractility by decreasing sensitivity of myofilaments to Ca2+ in rat ventricular muscle," *Anesthesiology*, vol. 97, no. 5, pp. 1168–1177, 2002.

[38] P. Bruelle, J. Y. Lefrant, J. E. De La Coussaye et al., "Comparative electrophysiologic and hemodynamic effects of several amide local anesthetic drugs in anesthetized dogs," *Anesthesia and Analgesia*, vol. 82, no. 3, pp. 648–656, 1996.

[39] S. Reiz and S. Nath, "Cardiotoxicity of local anaesthetic agents," *The British Journal of Anaesthesia*, vol. 58, no. 7, pp. 736–746, 1986.

[40] C. W. Clarkson and L. M. Hondeghem, "Mechanism for bupivacaine depression of cardiac conduction: fast block of sodium channels during the action potential with slow recovery from block during diastole," *Anesthesiology*, vol. 62, no. 4, pp. 396–405, 1985.

[41] G. K. Wong, D. T. Joo, and C. McDonnell, "Lipid resuscitation in a carnitine deficient child following intravascular migration of an epidural catheter," *Anaesthesia*, vol. 65, no. 2, pp. 192–195, 2010.

[42] G. K. Wong and M. W. Crawford, "Carnitine deficiency increases susceptibility to bupivacaine-induced cardiotoxicity in rats," *Anesthesiology*, vol. 114, no. 6, pp. 1417–1424, 2011.

[43] K. Nouette-Gaulain, C. Jose, X. Capdevila, and R. Rossignol, "From analgesia to myopathy: when local anesthetics impair the mitochondrion," *International Journal of Biochemistry and Cell Biology*, vol. 43, no. 1, pp. 14–19, 2011.

[44] D. W. Maughan, "Kinetics and energetics of the crossbridge cycle," *Heart Failure Reviews*, vol. 10, no. 3, pp. 175–185, 2005.

[45] D. J. Newton, G. A. McLeod, F. Khan, and J. J. F. Belch, "Vasoactive characteristics of bupivacaine and levobupivacaine with and without adjuvant epinephrine in peripheral human skin," *The British Journal of Anaesthesia*, vol. 94, no. 5, pp. 662–667, 2005.

[46] G. L. Weinberg, J. W. Palmer, T. R. VadeBoncouer, M. B. Zuechner, G. Edelman, and C. L. Hoppel, "Bupivacaine inhibits acylcarnitine exchange in cardiac mitochondria," *Anesthesiology*, vol. 92, no. 2, pp. 523–528, 2000.

[47] X. Shen, F. Wang, S. Xu et al., "Is cardiolipin the target of local anesthetic cardiotoxicity?" *Revista Brasileira de Anestesiologia*, vol. 60, no. 4, pp. 445–454, 2010.

[48] C. F. Royse and A. G. Royse, "The myocardial and vascular effects of bupivacaine, levobupivacaine, and ropivacaine using pressure volume loops," *Anesthesia and Analgesia*, vol. 101, no. 3, pp. 679–687, 2005.

[49] K. S. K. Chang, D. R. Morrow, K. Kuzume, and M. C. Andresen, "Bupivacaine inhibits baroreflex control of heart

rate in conscious rats," *Anesthesiology*, vol. 92, no. 1, pp. 197–207, 2000.

[50] A. E. Pickering, H. Waki, P. M. Headley, and J. F. R. Paton, "Investigation of systemic bupivacaine toxicity using the in situ perfused working heart-brainstem preparation of the rat," *Anesthesiology*, vol. 97, no. 6, pp. 1550–1556, 2002.

[51] H. Lida, Y. Watanabe, S. Dohi, and T. Ishiyama, "Direct effects of ropivacaine and bupivacaine on spinal pial vessels in canine. Assessment with closed spinal window technique," *Anesthesiology*, vol. 87, no. 1, pp. 75–81, 1997.

[52] H. Bariskaner, S. Tuncer, A. Taner, and N. Dogan, "Effects of bupivacaine and ropivacaine on the isolated human umbilical artery," *International Journal of Obstetric Anesthesia*, vol. 12, no. 4, pp. 261–265, 2003.

[53] K. L. Rossner, E. Natke, M. Liu-Barnett, and K. J. Freese, "A proposed mechanism of bupivacaine-induced contraction of human umbilical artery smooth muscle cells," *International Journal of Obstetric Anesthesia*, vol. 8, no. 1, pp. 24–29, 1999.

[54] G. L. Weinberg, T. VadeBoncouer, G. A. Ramaraju, M. F. Garcia-Amaro, and M. J. Cwik, "Pretreatment or resuscitation with a lipid infusion shifts the dose-response to bupivacaine-induced asystole in rats," *Anesthesiology*, vol. 88, no. 4, pp. 1071–1075, 1998.

[55] G. Weinberg, R. Ripper, D. L. Feinstein, and W. Hoffman, "Lipid emulsion infusion rescues dogs from bupivacaine-induced cardiac toxicity," *Regional Anesthesia and Pain Medicine*, vol. 28, no. 3, pp. 198–202, 2003.

[56] M. A. Rosenblatt, M. Abel, G. W. Fischer, C. J. Itzkovich, and J. B. Eisenkraft, "Successful use of a 20% lipid emulsion to resuscitate a patient after a presumed bupivacaine-related cardiac arrest," *Anesthesiology*, vol. 105, no. 1, pp. 217–218, 2006.

[57] H. Ludot, J. Y. Tharin, M. Belouadah, J. X. Mazoit, and J. M. Malinovsky, "Successful resuscitation after ropivacaine and lidocaine-induced ventricular arrhythmia following posterior lumbar plexus block in a child," *Anesthesia and Analgesia*, vol. 106, no. 5, pp. 1572–1574, 2008.

[58] G. Foxall, R. Mccahon, J. Lamb, J. G. Hardman, and N. M. Bedforth, "Levobupivacaine-induced seizures and cardiovascular collapse treated with Intralipid," *Anaesthesia*, vol. 62, no. 5, pp. 516–518, 2007.

[59] R. J. Litz, T. Roessel, A. R. Heller, and S. N. Stehr, "Reversal of central nervous system and cardiac toxicity after local anesthetic intoxication by lipid emulsion injection," *Anesthesia and Analgesia*, vol. 106, no. 5, pp. 1575–1577, 2008.

[60] J. A. Warren, R. B. Thoma, A. Georgescu, and S. J. Shah, "Intravenous lipid infusion in the successful resuscitation of local anesthetic-induced cardiovascular collapse after supraclavicular brachial plexus block," *Anesthesia and Analgesia*, vol. 106, no. 5, pp. 1578–1580, 2008.

[61] G. Cave, M. Harvey, and A. Graudins, "Intravenous lipid emulsion as antidote: a summary of published human experience," *Emergency Medicine Australasia*, vol. 23, no. 2, pp. 123–141, 2011.

[62] S. K. Dix, G. F. Rosner, M. Nayar et al., "Intractable cardiac arrest due to lidocaine toxicity successfully resuscitated with lipid emulsion," *Critical Care Medicine*, vol. 39, no. 4, pp. 872–874, 2011.

[63] AAGBI, *Management of Severe Local Anaesthetic Toxicity*, AAGBI Safety Guideline, 2010, http://www.aagbi.org/publications/guidelines/docs/la_toxicity_2010.pdf.

[64] A. Gabrielli, M. O'Connor, and G. A. Maccioli, "Anesthesia advanced circulatory life support," in *Committee on Critical Care Medicine*, The American Societyof Critical Care Anesthesiologists & The American Society of Anesthesiologists, 2008.

[65] J. M. Neal, C. M. Bernards, J. F. Butterworth et al., "ASRA practice advisory on local anesthetic systemic toxicity," *Regional Anesthesia and Pain Medicine*, vol. 35, no. 2, pp. 152–161, 2010.

[66] T. L. Vanden Hoek, L. J. Morrison, M. Shuster et al., "Part 12: cardiac arrest in special situations: 2010 American Heart Association guidelines for cardiopulmonary Resuscitation and emergency cardiovascular care," *Circulation*, vol. 122, supplement 3, pp. S829–S861, 2010.

[67] Y. A. Zausig, B. M. Graf, and W. Zink, "Is it "lipid sink," hemodilution, or both?" *Critical Care Medicine*, vol. 37, no. 10, p. 2863, 2009.

[68] G. L. Weinberg, G. Di Gregorio, R. Ripper et al., "Resuscitation with lipid versus epinephrine in a rat model of bupivacaine overdose," *Anesthesiology*, vol. 108, no. 5, pp. 907–913, 2008.

[69] G. L. Weinberg, R. Ripper, P. Murphy et al., "Lipid infusion accelerates removal of bupivacaine and recovery from bupivacaine toxicity in the isolated rat heart," *Regional Anesthesia and Pain Medicine*, vol. 31, no. 4, pp. 296–303, 2006.

[70] L. R. Silveira, S. M. Hirabara, L. C. Alberici et al., "Effect of lipid infusion on metabolism and force of rat skeletal muscles during intense contractions," *Cellular Physiology and Biochemistry*, vol. 20, no. 1–4, pp. 213–226, 2007.

[71] M. Coat, J. P. Pennec, M. Guillouet, C. C. Arvieux, and G. Gueret, "Haemodynamic effects of intralipid after local anaesthetics intoxication may be due to a direct effect of fatty acids on myocardial voltage-dependent calcium channels," *Annales Francaises d'Anesthesie et de Reanimation*, vol. 29, no. 9, p. 661, 2010.

[72] G. L. Weinberg, "Treatment of local anesthetic systemic toxicity (LAST)," *Regional Anesthesia and Pain Medicine*, vol. 35, no. 2, pp. 188–193, 2010.

[73] G. L. Weinberg, "Intravenous lipid emulsion: why wait to save a life?" *Emergency Medicine Australasia*, vol. 23, no. 2, pp. 113–115, 2011.

[74] S. Markowitz and J. M. Neal, "Immediate lipid emulsion therapy in the successful treatment of bupivacaine systemic toxicity," *Regional Anesthesia and Pain Medicine*, vol. 34, no. 3, p. 276, 2009.

[75] H. Charbonneau, T. A. P. Marcou, J. X. Mazoit, P. J. Zetlaoui, and D. Benhamou, "Early use of lipid emulsion to treat incipient mepivacaine intoxication," *Regional Anesthesia and Pain Medicine*, vol. 34, no. 3, pp. 277–278, 2009.

[76] D. H. Sonsino and M. Fischler, "Immediate intravenous lipid infusion in the successful resuscitation of ropivacaine-induced cardiac arrest after infraclavicular brachial plexus block," *Regional Anesthesia and Pain Medicine*, vol. 34, no. 3, pp. 276–277, 2009.

[77] S. Bern and G. Weinberg, "Local anesthetic toxicity and lipid resuscitation in pregnancy," *Current Opinion in Anaesthesiology*, vol. 24, no. 3, pp. 262–267, 2011.

[78] D. B. Hiller, G. D. Gregorio, R. Ripper et al., "Epinephrine impairs lipid resuscitation from bupivacaine overdose: a threshold effect," *Anesthesiology*, vol. 111, no. 3, pp. 498–505, 2009.

[79] G. Di Gregorio, D. Schwartz, R. Ripper et al., "Lipid emulsion is superior to vasopressin in a rodent model of resuscitation from toxin-induced cardiac arrest," *Critical Care Medicine*, vol. 37, no. 3, pp. 993–999, 2009.

[80] P. Y. Gueugniaud, J. S. David, E. Chanzy et al., "Vasopressin and epinephrine vs. epinephrine alone in cardiopulmonary resuscitation," *The New England Journal of Medicine*, vol. 359, no. 1, pp. 21–30, 2008.

[81] S. D. Hicks, D. D. Salcido, E. S. Logue et al., "Lipid emulsion combined with epinephrine and vasopressin does not improve survival in a swine model of bupivacaine-induced cardiac arrest," *Anesthesiology*, vol. 111, no. 1, pp. 138–146, 2009.

[82] J. Lokajova, J. Laine, E. Puukilainen, M. Ritala, J. M. Holopainen, and S. K. Wiedmer, "Liposomes for entrapping local anesthetics: a liposome electrokinetic chromatographic study," *Electrophoresis*, vol. 31, no. 9, pp. 1540–1549, 2010.

[83] A. R. Heller and T. Koch, "Local anesthetic systemic toxicity-concept: inclusion of omega-3 fatty acids may reduce adverse effects," *Regional Anesthesia and Pain Medicine*, vol. 36, no. 3, pp. 309–310, 2011.

[84] D. C. Moore and M. S. Batra, "The components of an effective test dose prior to epidural block," *Anesthesiology*, vol. 55, no. 6, pp. 693–696, 1981.

[85] M. F. Mulroy and M. R. Hejtmanek, "Prevention of local anesthetic systemic toxicity," *Regional Anesthesia and Pain Medicine*, vol. 35, no. 2, pp. 177–180, 2010.

[86] P. H. Rosenberg, B. T. Veering, and W. F. Urmey, "Maximum recommended doses of local anesthetics: a multifactorial concept," *Regional Anesthesia and Pain Medicine*, vol. 29, no. 6, pp. 564–575, 2004.

[87] M. O. Columb and G. Lyons, "Determination of the minimum local analgesic concentrations of epidural bupivacaine and lidocaine in labor," *Anesthesia and Analgesia*, vol. 81, no. 4, pp. 833–837, 1995.

[88] I. Gall and M. Columb, "Minimum local analgesic concentration of local anaesthetics," *Continuing Education in Anaesthesia, Critical Care and Pain*, vol. 10, no. 4, pp. 114–116, 2010.

[89] K. J. Walker, K. McGrattan, K. Aas-Eng, and A. F. Smith, "Ultrasound guidance for peripheral nerve blockade," *Cochrane Database of Systematic Reviews*, no. 4, p. CD006459, 2009.

[90] J. M. Neal, "Ultrasound-guided regional anesthesia and patient safety: an evidence-based analysis," *Regional Anesthesia and Pain Medicine*, vol. 35, no. 2, pp. S59–S67, 2010.

[91] M. J. Fredrickson, R. White, and T. K. Danesh-Clough, "Low-volume ultrasound-guided nerve block provides inferior postoperative analgesia compared to a higher-volume landmark technique," *Regional Anesthesia and Pain Medicine*, vol. 36, no. 4, pp. 393–398, 2011.

[92] F. P. Branco, J. Ranali, G. M. B. Ambrosano, and M. C. Volpato, "A double-blind comparison of 0.5% bupivacaine with 1:200,000 epinephrine and 0.5% levobupivacaine with 1:200,000 epinephrine for the inferior alveolar nerve block," *Oral Surgery, Oral Medicine, Oral Pathology, Oral Radiology and Endodontology*, vol. 101, no. 4, pp. 442–447, 2006.

[93] Y. Y. Lee, W. D. Ngan Kee, S. Y. Fong, J. T. C. Liu, and T. Gin, "The median effective dose of bupivacaine, levobupivacaine, and ropivacaine after intrathecal injection in lower limb surgery," *Anesthesia and Analgesia*, vol. 109, no. 4, pp. 1331–1334, 2009.

[94] W. Gl, http://www.lipidrescue.org/.

[95] E. Dorf, A. F. Kuntz, J. Kelsey, and C. P. Holstege, "Lidocaine-induced altered mental status and seizure after hematoma block," *Journal of Emergency Medicine*, vol. 31, no. 3, pp. 251–253, 2006.

[96] D. E. Marra, D. Yip, E. F. Fincher, and R. L. Moy, "Systemic toxicity from topically applied lidocaine in conjunction with fractional photothermolysis," *Archives of Dermatology*, vol. 142, no. 8, pp. 1024–1026, 2006.

[97] M. J. Donald and S. Derbyshire, "Lignocaine toxicity; a complication of local anaesthesia administered in the community," *Emergency Medicine Journal*, vol. 21, no. 2, pp. 249–250, 2004.

[98] M. Smith, W. Wolfram, and R. Rose, "Toxicity—seizures in an infant caused by (or related to) oral viscous lidocaine use," *Journal of Emergency Medicine*, vol. 10, no. 5, pp. 587–590, 1992.

[99] M. A. Martínez, S. Ballesteros, L. J. Segura, and M. García, "Reporting a fatality during tumescent liposuction," *Forensic Science International*, vol. 178, no. 1, pp. e11–e16, 2008.

[100] J. A. Klein and N. Kassarjdian, "Lidocaine toxicity with tumescent liposuction. A case report of probable drug interactions," *Dermatologic Surgery*, vol. 23, no. 12, pp. 1169–1174, 1997.

[101] R. Seigne, "Lignocaine toxicity—a surgical surprise," *Anaesthesia*, vol. 52, no. 1, p. 91, 1997.

[102] R. B. Rao, S. F. Ely, and R. S. Hoffman, "Deaths related to liposuction," *The New England Journal of Medicine*, vol. 340, no. 19, pp. 1471–1475, 1999.

[103] J. Collins, "Awareness of local anaesthetic toxicity issues among hospital staff," *Anaesthesia*, vol. 65, no. 9, pp. 960–961, 2010.

2

New Formulations of Local Anaesthetics

Edward A. Shipton

Department of Anaesthesia, University of Otago, Christchurch 8042, New Zealand

Correspondence should be addressed to Edward A. Shipton, shiptonea@xtra.co.nz

Academic Editor: James B. Eisenkraft

Part 1 comments on the types of local anaesthetics (LAs); it provides a better understanding of the mechanisms of action of LAs, and their pharmacokinetics and toxicity. It reviews the newer LAs such as levobupivacaine, ropivacaine, and articaine, and examines the newer structurally different LAs. The addition of adjuvants such as adrenaline, bicarbonate, clonidine, and corticosteroids is explored. Comment is made on the delivery of topical LAs via bioadhesive plasters and gels and controlled-release local anaesthetic matrices. Encapulation matrices such as liposomes, microemulsions, microspheres and nanospheres, hydrogels and liquid polymers are discussed as well. New innovations pertaining to LA formulations have indeed led to prolonged action and to novel delivery approaches.

1. Introduction

Local anaesthetics (LAs) are used clinically for anaesthesia and analgesia either following surgery or for management of other acute and chronic pain conditions; they only last a few hours. Part 1 of this paper deals with the newer LAs, more recent LA formulations, a better understanding of the mechanisms of action of LAs, and their pharmacokinetics and toxicity.

Local anaesthesia for a prolonged period of days is best provided using catheter techniques [1] with disposable pumps [2] or multiple injections [3]. Most attempts to prolong LA action have so far only doubled or tripled the plain drug effect time, using adjuncts to LA agents of readily available agents. These include opioids and clonidine that delay local anaesthetic clearance from their site of action [4] and dexamethasone that prolongs peripheral nerve and plexus blocks [5].

2. Types of Local Anaesthetics

Lignocaine is perhaps most commonly used or known local anaesthetic agent; it is used either in local or regional anaesthesia, or in epidural or spinal blockade; it has a number of uses in anaesthesia and pain medicine. However, it is also given parenterally in the management of neuropathic pain states. EMLA, a eutectic mixture of lignocaine and prilocaine, is an effective topical anaesthetic in preventing pain associated with needle procedures [6].

Local anaesthetics can be classified into two groups based on the nature of the link, namely, amides [–NH–CO–] and esters [–O–CO–] (Figures 1 and 2). The amide group is the most commonly used clinically; it includes lignocaine, prilocaine, levobupivacaine, bupivacaine, mepivacaine, and ropivacaine.

The ester group is weak bases, solubilised for injection as strong conjugate acidic hydrochloride salts (pH 3–6); it includes cocaine, procaine, chloroprocaine, and amethocaine (Figure 3) [3, 7]. Benzocaine and butamben are ester-type local anaesthetics mostly used in topical and mucous formulations. Anaphylaxis to local anaesthetics is very uncommon and has decreased in frequency because of the decreasing use of the ester group of local anaesthetics [8]. Most allergic reactions are due to the common metabolic product of the ester local anaesthetic, para-amino benzoic acid [8]. Cross-reactivity among esters is common. Allergic reactions to amide local anaesthetics remain anecdotal. Ingredients included in local anaesthetic solutions such as antioxidants or preservatives including metabisulphite or parabens (also metabolised to para-amino benzoic acid) may also elicit allergic or adverse reactions [8]. Local anaesthetics (without preservatives or adrenaline) may be skin tested.

3. Pharmacokinetics of Local Anaesthetics

Injectable local anaesthetics are subject to absorption; a large fraction of the injected drug is removed by the systemic circulation and distributed to distant organs according to their vascular density [9]. Highly vascular organs (brain, heart, lung, liver, and kidneys) are exposed to unmetabolised local anaesthetic at peak concentration. The local anaesthetic is taken up within each organ according to its tissue-plasma partition coefficient. Most absorbed local anaesthetic is cleared from the liver. Hepatic clearance is a function of the hepatic extraction ratio and hepatic blood flow. The hepatic extraction ratio, in turn, is dependent on the ratio of free to protein-bound drug. Local anaesthetics bind tightly to plasma proteins greatly limiting the free fraction of available drug. Only the free or unbound fraction that is bioactive. Like most weak bases, local anaesthetics bind mainly to alpha-1-acid glycoprotein. Lignocaine, being moderately protein-bound, has a high hepatic extraction ratio (70–75% per pass) [9]. Clearance is therefore flow-limited and is reduced by factors that limit hepatic blood flow. Conversely, bupivacaine and ropivacaine, being highly protein-bound, are cleared <50% per pass; hence, their clearance depends on free drug concentration [9]. Low cardiac output states may not greatly affect the plasma concentration of the highly protein-bound agents, as their clearance is not flow limited. Intrinsic hepatic disease may alter clearance by altering plasma protein content and degree of protein binding, by decreasing the enzyme activity of the liver, and by reducing hepatic blood flow. Patients with liver disease may have single-shot blocks with normal doses. Doses for continuous infusion and repeat blocks need to be significantly reduced (10–50% relative to the degree of dysfunction) due to the risk of accumulation of the primary compound and its metabolites [10]. Patients with mild or controlled cardiac failure may not need a dose reduction for single-shot blocks. Doses of ropivacaine and bupivacaine for continuous infusion and repeat blocks need to be reduced, as their metabolites will be eliminated slowly. In patients with renal dysfunction, reduced clearance and faster absorption of local anaesthetic lead to an elevation in plasma concentration [10]. Clearance of both bupivacaine and ropivacaine has been shown to be reduced in uraemic patients [9, 10]. The clearance of one of the main metabolites of ropivacaine, 2,6-pipecoloxylidide (PPX), is also decreased in uraemic patients [9].

4. Newer Local Anaesthetics

4.1. Levobupivacaine. In recent years, levobupivacaine, the pure S (−) enantiomer of bupivacaine, emerged as a safer alternative for regional anaesthesia than its racemic parent (Figure 4). In common to all local anaesthetics, levobupivacaine reversibly blocks the transmission of action potential in sensory, motor, and sympathetic nervous fibres by inhibiting the passage of sodium through voltage-sensitive ion channels in the neuronal membrane. Various factors such as site of administration, duration of continuous infusion, and/or addition of agents with vasomotor effect may influence the degree of systemic uptake of levobupivacaine.

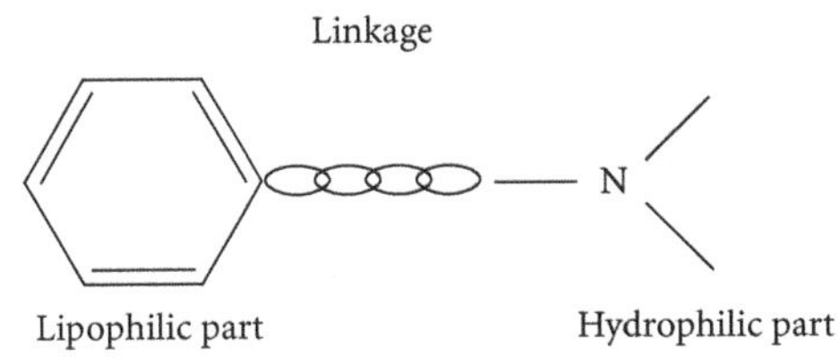

FIGURE 1: Structure of all local anaesthetics.

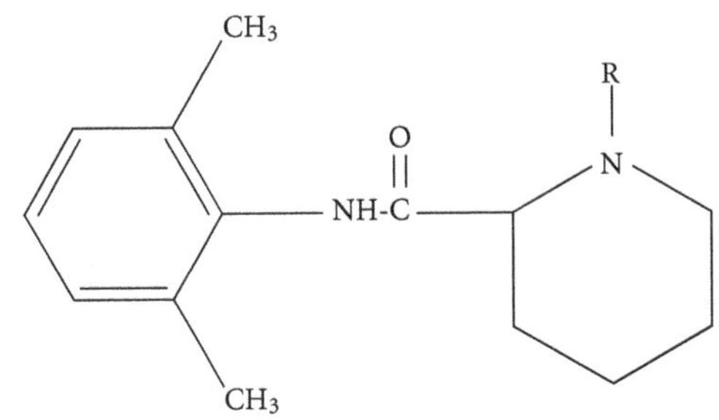

	Ropivacaine	Bupivacaine	Mepivacaine
R =	C_3H_6	C_4H_9	CH_3

FIGURE 2: Amide local anaesthetics.

In pharmacodynamic studies, levobupivacaine demonstrated less affinity and depressant effects on myocardial and central nervous vital centres and a superior pharmacokinetic profile [11]. Clinically, levobupivacaine is well tolerated in a variety of regional anaesthesia techniques both after bolus administration and continuous postoperative infusion.

The incidence of adverse events with levobupivacaine was similar to that after bupivacaine in comparative trials. These include hypotension, nausea, postoperative pain, fever, vomiting, pruritus, back pain, headache, constipation, dizziness, and foetal distress [11]. The early clinical presentation of toxicity after levobupivacaine appears to consist of central nervous symptoms (disorientation, drowsiness, slurred speech), which may culminate with tonic-clonic seizures in some cases. Reports of toxicity with levobupivacaine are scarce; occasional toxic symptoms are usually reversible with minimal treatment with no fatal outcome [11].

Surgical sensory block of similar characteristics and recovery over equal dose ranges of levobupivacaine and bupivacaine has been confirmed in surgical patients [11]. The onset of motor block is slower with levobupivacaine, and its quality follows the rank of order bupivacaine > levobupivacaine > ropivacaine [11]. The regression of motor block was significantly more rapid after levobupivacaine and ropivacaine than bupivacaine; this may be advantageous for early ambulation after day-case surgery.

The effective dose of epidural levobupivacaine for continuous postoperative analgesia approaches 15 mg/hour [11]. The addition of adjunctive agents (adrenaline, opioids, or clonidine) to levobupivacaine in epidural anaesthesia and analgesia may increase the duration and quality of analgesia and further decrease the risk of toxicity. Traditionally, the dose of levobupivacaine used for spinal anaesthesia is 15 mg

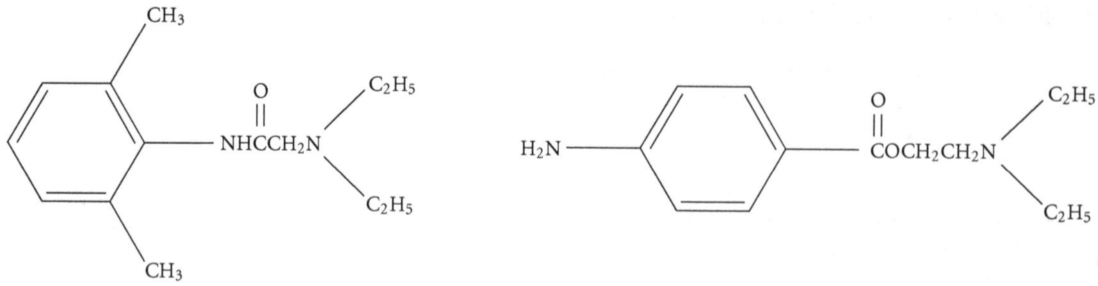

Lignocaine Procaine

FIGURE 3: Amide local anaesthetic (lignocaine) and ester local anaesthetic (procaine).

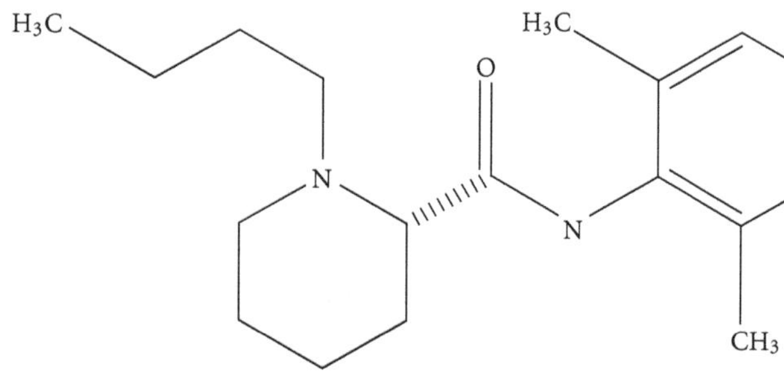

FIGURE 4: Structure of levobupivacaine.

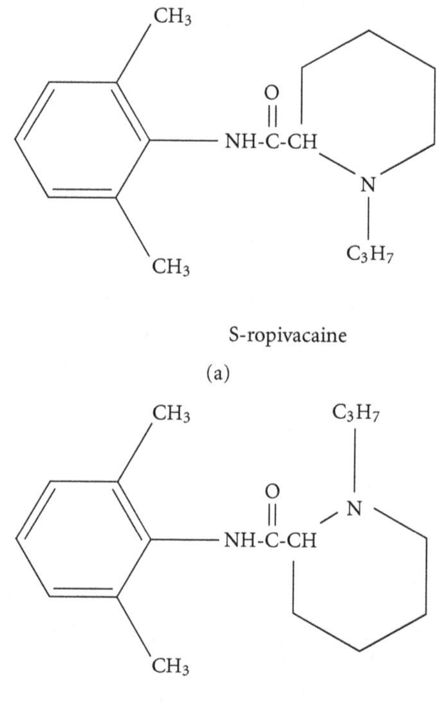

S-ropivacaine

(a)

R-ropivacaine

(b)

FIGURE 5: Structure of S and R enantiomers of ropivacaine (marketed as the S enantiomer).

[11]. Smaller doses (5–10 mg) have been used in ambulatory surgery and allow a more rapid recovery and subsequent discharge home.

Current evidence suggests a potency hierarchy of bupivacaine > levobupivacaine > ropivacaine for epidurals in labour [11]. Using an epidural bolus of 10 mL levobupivacaine 0.2%–0.25% followed by epidural infusions or top-ups of low concentrations levobupivacaine (0.1%–0.125%) provides the same good-quality labour analgesia as bupivacaine, but possibly with less motor block [11]. A combined spinal-epidural technique with intrathecal levobupivacaine 1.2–2.5 mg combined with a small dose of opioid (e.g., fentanyl 12.5–25 μg) provides excellent prolonged sensory block with minimum motor blockade [11].

In brachial plexus nerve blocks, a sensory and motor block of similar onset (6–10 min) and duration (14–16 hours) follows the administration of an equal dose of levobupivacaine 0.5% or bupivacaine 0.5% [11]. Continuing the administration of levobupivacaine via a peripheral nerve block continuous catheter is associated with excellent postoperative analgesia as demonstrated by a significant decline in the postoperative systemic opioids requirements.

4.2. Ropivacaine. Ropivacaine is a long-acting, enantiomerically pure (S-enantiomer) amide local anaesthetic regional anaesthetic with an efficacy broadly similar to that of bupivacaine (Figure 5). However, it may be a preferred option because of its reduced central nervous system (CNS) and cardiotoxic potential and its lower propensity for motor block [12]. It has a high pKa and low lipid solubility that block nerve fibres involved in pain transmission (A delta and C fibres) to a greater degree than those controlling motor function (A beta fibres). The drug is less cardiotoxic than equal concentrations of racemic bupivacaine but more so than lignocaine; it has a significantly higher threshold for CNS toxicity than racemic bupivacaine. Extensive clinical data have shown that epidural ropivacaine 0.2% is effective for the initiation and maintenance of labour analgesia, and provides pain relief after abdominal or orthopaedic surgery especially when given in conjunction with opioids [12]. Ropivacaine had an adverse event profile similar to that of bupivacaine in clinical trials. Comparative data suggest that higher concentrations of ropivacaine (0.75%) may be needed to provide the same sensory and motor blockade as bupivacaine 0.5% [12]. Brachial plexus anaesthesia was broadly similar to that achieved with equivalent volumes of bupivacaine 0.5%, although the time to onset of sensory block tended to be faster and the duration of motor block shorter with ropivacaine [12].

4.3. Articaine. Articaine is a relatively new local anaesthetic used now in dentistry in many countries. It is an amide type local anaesthetic, and, instead of benzene ring, it contains a thiophene ring that increases its lipid solubility. Unlike other local anaesthetics, articaine is exceptional in that it contains an additional ester group that is rapidly metabolised by plasma esterase to articainic acid [13]. As a result, its half-life, about 20 minutes, is also very short compared to other local anaesthetics. Thus, it can rapidly be cleared from the systemic circulation through kidney, minimising adverse effects [13]. Advantages are low lipid solubility, high plasma protein binding rate, fast metabolism, fast elimination half time, and low blood levels [14]. Articaine seems to be the local anaesthetic of first choice in tissues with suppurative inflammation, for adults, children (over 4 years old), elderly, pregnant women, breastfeeding women, and patients suffering from hepatic disorders and renal function impairment [14]. Articaine solutions must not be used in persons who are allergic or hypersensitive to sulphite, due to the content of sodium metabisulphite as the vasoconstrictor's antioxidant in it.

4.4. Newer Structurally Different Local Anaesthetics. Another group of potent LAs includes the basic esters of phenylcarbamic acid [15]. Basic esters of alkoxy-substituted phenylcarbamic acid have shown high LA potency, while maintaining a relatively safe toxicity profile [15]. The most potent phenylcarbamic anaesthetics exceed the potency of the most common clinically used local anaesthetics by 100–300 times [15]. Their potency uniquely increases with the decreasing pH of the external medium. This is of importance when using LAs in inflamed tissues, where the action of common LAs is often problematic. Further study of their action is required.

5. Mechanisms of Action of Local Anaesthetics

Local anaesthetics directly block transmission of pain from nociceptive afferents. Local anaesthetic agents are applied directly, and their efficacy results from action on the nerve where the inward Na^+ current is blocked at the sodium ionophore during depolarisation. LAs not only block Na^+ channels but Ca^{2+} and K^+ channels [16–18], transient receptor potential vanniloid-1 receptors [19], and other ligand-gated receptors as well. Local anaesthetics also disrupt the coupling between certain G proteins and their associated receptors [20]. Through this action, LAs exert potent anti-inflammatory effects, particularly on neutrophil priming reactions [21]. Local anaesthetics inhibit local inflammatory response to injury that can sensitise nociceptive receptors and contribute to pain and hyperalgesia. Studies have observed that local anaesthetics reduce the release of inflammatory mediators from neutrophils, reduce neutrophil adhesion to the endothelium, reduce formation of free oxygen radicals, and decrease oedema formation [22]. There are, in addition, a variety of other antithrombotic and neuroprotective actions of intravenous LAs [20] that are independent of Na^+ channel blockade but may account for many of the improvements in pain after surgery [16, 22]. Local anaesthetics can alleviate some types of neuropathic pain, and part of this effect may be related to sensitisation of the antinociceptive pain pathways that occur in the neuropathic pain state; spinal glial cells have been shown to play some part in this as well [23].

Lignocaine seems to have some modulatory effect on the NMDA receptor [24]. Intravenous application of lignocaine in a rat model of acute and neuropathic pain demonstrated antinociception in both pain models [25]. Several studies have previously shown that lignocaine at antiarrhythmic doses or lower doses demonstrates neuroprotective effects [24]. A randomised, double blinded, placebo controlled study of neuroprotection with lignocaine in cardiac surgery showed a potential protective effect of lower lignocaine doses in nondiabetic patients. LAs have long been known to inhibit the growth of different species in vitro [24]. The antibacterial activity of various LAs and additives used in epidural infusions has been tested [26]. Bupivacaine was shown to have the most efficient activity against microorganisms [26]. LAs have been used to enhance bowel function recovery after surgery or trauma. Twenty-two patients scheduled for elective bowel surgery randomised into two groups were given intravenous lignocaine or placebo to assess differences in surgical pain, length of postsurgical ileus, and hospital stay [27]. The lignocaine group showed less pain after 24 hours, a faster return of bowel movements, and an earlier discharge from hospital. LAs stimulate the activity of natural killer cells during the perioperative period [24]. Perioperative lignocaine has been found to improve immediate postoperative pain management and reduce surgery-induced immune alterations [28]. The long-term effect of anaesthesia/analgesia provided by LAs on cancer recurrence needs further investigation.

6. Local Anaesthetic Toxicity

Toxicity primarily involves the central nervous system followed by the cardiovascular system. More potent agents (bupivacaine, levobupivacaine, ropivacaine) produce cardiotoxic effects at lower blood concentrations and doses than less potent LA agents (lignocaine) [29]. The (+)-(*R*)-enantiomers bind with greater affinity to cardiac Na^+ channels than the (−)-(*S*)-enantiomers do. LA agents cause marked but reversible lesions to skeletal muscle tissue [3]. Myotoxicity seems to be explained by mitochondrial bioenergetics alteration. In the animal model, this toxic effect was significantly more severe in young rats [30]. The nitric oxide pathway is involved in the development of tachyphylaxis [31]. In addition, there is a growing amount of evidence that intra-articular administration of bupivacaine is chondrotoxic especially at a higher concentration and with prolonged exposure [24].

A lipid emulsion infusion alongside cardiopulmonary resuscitation appears to be an effective treatment for cardiac toxicity induced by lipophilic medications [32]. The practice advisory on LA systemic toxicity of the American Society of Regional Anesthesia and Pain Medicine suggests that 20% lipid emulsion initially be administered as a bolus of 1.5 mL/kg over a minute [33]. Following completion of the bolus, a continuous infusion of 0.25 mL/kg/min should be started [33, 34]. If the patient does not respond to the initial bolus, one to two additional boluses may be administered. The rate of the infusion may be increased to 0.5 mL/kg if there is persistent hypotension. The infusion should be continued until 10 minutes after the patient regains haemodynamic stability [33, 34]. Given the difficulties of performing clinical trials, further laboratory investigation and clinical correlation are needed to better define its role in resuscitation. Another potential treatment is the use of pegylated anionic liposomes to reduce free drug concentration of LA [35]. In summary, LA cardiotoxicity primarily arises from a blockade of sodium channels. As for treatment, in addition to ventilation, oxygenation, and chest compressions, lipid emulsion therapy should be a primary element in the treatment [36].

6.1. Prevention of Local Anaesthetic Toxicity. There is no single measure that can prevent LA toxicity in clinical practice. The lowest effective dose of local anaesthetic should be used (dose = product of volume × concentration). LAs should be injected incrementally through a catheter [33]. The needle or catheter should be carefully aspirated before each injection with close observation when injecting LA. More dilute LAs should be used. The use of ultrasound guidance may reduce the frequency of intravascular injection. Intravascular injection of adrenaline 10–15 microgram/mL in adults produces a >10 beat heart rate increase or a >15-mm Hg systolic blood pressure increase in the absence of beta-blockade, active labour, advanced age, or general/neuraxial anaesthesia [33]. Intravascular injection of adrenaline 0.5 microgram/mL in children produces a >15-mm Hg increase in systolic blood pressure [33]. All these measures have improved morbidity and mortality following LA use.

7. Adjuvants

Adrenaline induces vasoconstriction, reducing local anaesthetic clearance from the site of action, thus prolonging the duration of action. Solutions such as 1 : 200000 or 1 : 400000 are commonly used [37].

The addition of bicarbonate raises the pH of LA solution thereby increasing the proportion of unionised LA available to cross the neuronal phospholipid membrane, increasing speed of onset. The recommended dose is 1 mL of 8.4% of sodium bicarbonate per 10 mL of LA. The stability of LAs with added bicarbonate is not well studied; such mixtures cannot be recommended for continuous perineural infusions [37].

Clonidine is an alpha-2 receptor agonist whose effect may be mediated by inhibiting action potentials. Its effect is dose dependent, increasing the duration of anaesthesia and analgesia when used with intermediate acting LAs [37].

Corticosteroids have been shown to specifically inhibit C-fibre transmission [38]. Dexamethasone prolongs peripheral nerve and plexus blocks [5]. It prolongs analgesia from interscalene blocks using ropivacaine or bupivacaine [39], and prolongs the duration of analgesia after supraclavicular brachial plexus blockade using mepivacaine [40].

8. Topical Local Anaesthetics

Topical delivery systems for LA are characteristically composed by a diversity of formulations (viscosity inducing agents, preservatives, permeation enhancers, emollients,) and presentations such as semisolid (gel, creams, ointments), liquid (emulsions, dispersions), and solid (patches) pharmaceutical forms [41]. The proposed formulations aim to reduce the LA concentration used, increase its permeability and absorption, keep the LA at the target site for longer and decrease the clearance, and limit local and systemic toxicity [41].

8.1. Bioadhesive Plaster and Gels. Different topical local anaesthetics have varying effects on skin blood flow and vascular reactivity. The vasoactive properties of 70 mg lignocaine/70 mg tetracaine medicated plaster (Rapydan), a new topical local anaesthetic, were compared with those of tetracaine base (4.0% w/w or Ametop) and 2.5% lignocaine/2.5% prilocaine (EMLA) creams in 20 healthy volunteers [42]. The tetracaine base produced a greater degree of vasodilatation than that seen after the application of a lignocaine/tetracaine medicated plaster [42]. The eutectic patch will be discussed further on.

In the laboratory, the anaesthetic action of the formulated mepivacaine gel containing enhancer and vasoconstrictor was evaluated with the tail-flick analgesimeter [43]. Among the enhancers used, polyoxyethylene 2-oleyl ether showed the greatest enhancement of permeation. The vasoconstrictor tetrahydrozoline showed prolonged and increased local anaesthetic action compared to the control used [43]. Mepivacaine gel is not available commercially for use in humans. Mepivacaine's spinal use was largely abandoned in the late 1990s due to a relatively high incidence of transient neurological symptoms with concentrated mepivacaine solutions [44].

8.2. Controlled-Release Local Anaesthetic Matrix. An absorbable, controlled-release lignocaine matrix delivery system has been developed; it is a suspension of a water-insoluble particulate and a hydrophobic carrier containing 16% lignocaine (w/w) (Xybrex) [45]. It can block the rat sciatic nerve for 1-2 days and suppress postincisional pain [16].

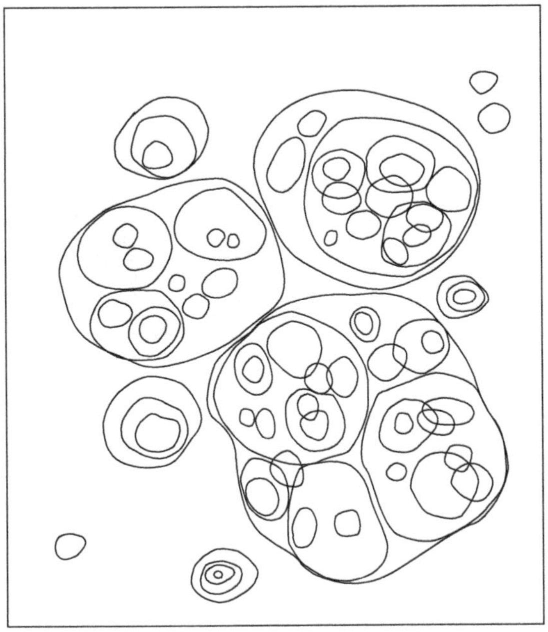

Figure 6: Liposomes.

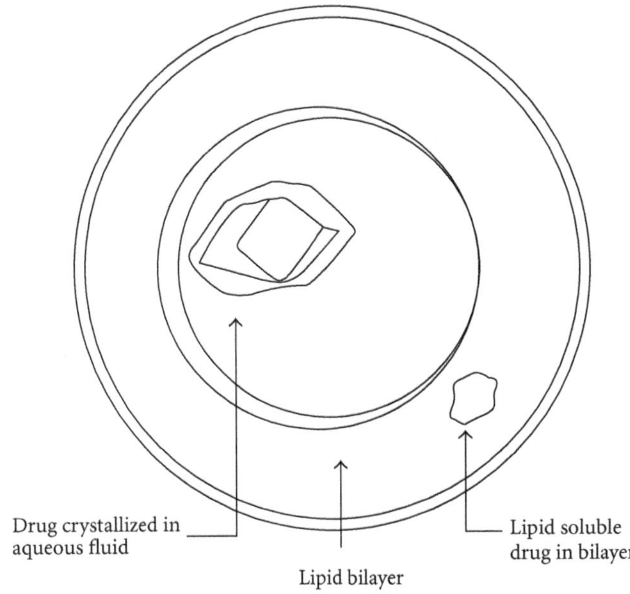

Figure 7: Liposome for drug delivery.

9. Encapsulation Matrices

A rapidly growing research topic is the use of vesicular carriers such as liposomes, niosomes, ethosomes (soft lipid vesicles), and elastic and deformable vesicles to provide an efficient dermal delivery system [46]. Encapsulation of local anaesthetic agents allows large doses to be released slowly and provides analgesia over a prolonged period without toxicity [47]. Encapsulating agents include liposomes [48], lipospheres [49], cyclodextrins [50], and microparticles [51]. Following injection of a depot of the formulation, much of the LA agent is bound or carried inside another agent and is not immediately available. The duration of the analgesia depends on the release rate of the LA agent from the carrier agent. Several properties such as hydrophobicity and internal membrane pH affect encapsulated drug release rates [3]. Some synergistic agents such as dexamethasone and clonidine encapsulated with the main effective agent have been formulated; these increased the anaesthesia time for several days [3, 52].

9.1. Liposomes. Liposomes act as reservoirs for drugs. Lipid vesicles are sealed sacs containing a lipid bilayer, usually phospholipids (Figure 6). There are three types of liposomes, namely, multilamellar vesicles, small unilamellar vesicles, and large unilamellar vesicles [3]. Lipid-soluble drugs can be carried in the bilayer itself; liposomes may contain one or more bilayers. Alternatively, aqueous drugs can be carried inside the aqueous compartment contained inside the bilayer [53].

Liposomes supply both a lipophilic region and an aqueous "milieu interior" in one system making them suitable for hydrophobic, aliphatic, and hydrophilic drugs (Figure 7) [54]. They are biocompatible due to their biodegradability and low toxicity. Liposomes help to reduce exposure of sensitive tissues to toxic drugs. They can be administered by a variety of routes (topical, intramuscular, subcutaneous, pulmonary, nasal, oral, and intravenous) [54]. Their route of administration and their lipid composition size can manipulate their pharmacokinetics and in vivo distribution. Following a single injection at the time of surgery, they remain in subcutaneous tissues (around the surgical incision) around a neural plexus or in the epidural space for a much longer period of time compared to the free drug [54].

Liposomes suffer lack of reliability and reproducibility during manufacture owing to oxidation and hydrolysis, which results in leaking of the encapsulated drug [3, 55]. Liposome metabolite compounds have been found to be neurotoxic. The mechanism for this may be lethicin fatty acid oxidation. Also, uncontrolled leakage of drug may occur following breakdown of the liposomes. Ideally, desirable attributes should include prolonged analgesic action; no neurotoxicity; sterility; physical and chemical stability giving a long shelf life; absence of unwanted side products (e.g., residues of organic solvents in bilayer); a reproducible production process [54].

Liposomal formulations of various anaesthetics allow an increase in clinical efficacy in comparison with the plain drugs [56]. Recently, classical liposomes have evolved to "highly deformable" liposomes, endowed with enhanced skin penetration ability and drug skin delivery [57]. "Highly deformable" liposomes consist of phospholipids and an edge activator that is often a single chain surfactant which destabilises the liposomal lipid bilayers, increasing their elasticity and flexibility [58]. Several studies have demonstrated the penetration across the skin of liposomal vesicles to be directly related with their deformability. The high adaptability of such elastic vesicles enable them to squeeze between the cells of the stratum corneum to penetrate intact to the deep layers of the skin; this gives an effect comparable to that of a subcutaneous injection [59].

Limitations of encapsulated local anaesthetic agents include neurotoxicity, myotoxicity, tachyphylaxis, motor block, and viscosity [3]. Many formulations including polymer and liposome carriers have facilitated prolonged local anaesthetic action for several days, although few clinical studies have been performed. Many routes of drug administration have been described, including central neuraxial administration and peripheral nerve administration [3].

Grant et al. [60] described safe and prolonged analgesia for 48 hours following local anaesthetic infiltration of 2% liposomal lignocaine. Boogaerts et al. [61] demonstrated a twofold increase in the duration of the analgesia following epidural administration of liposomal bupivacaine in patients following abdominal surgery. For intraoral topical anaesthesia, liposome-encapsulated 2% ropivacaine gel was as effective as 20% benzocaine gel in reducing pain during needle insertion and inducing soft-tissue anaesthesia; neither, however, was able to induce pulpal anaesthesia [62]. In a recent randomised single-blinded, placebo-controlled (2.5% lignocaine/2.5% prilocaine) cross-over study, liposomal-encapsulated ropivacaine formulations (1%, 2%) did not reduce the pain of insertion of a needle into the palatal mucosa [63]. Another blinded cross-over study in volunteers undergoing intraoral injections at four different sessions evaluated the injection discomfort comparing 2% and 3% liposome-encapsulated mepivacaine with 2% mepivacaine with 1 : 100,000 adrenaline and 3% mepivacaine [64]. The encapsulation of mepivacaine was found to increase the duration of anaesthesia and reduce the injection discomfort caused by these vasoconstrictor-associated formulations [64].

The entrapment of hydrophobic drugs in the aqueous core of liposomes as soluble inclusion complexes with cyclodextrins has been proposed to avoid the use of organic solvents, giving rise to drug-in cyclodextrin-in liposome systems [65]. The main types of cyclodextrin are α-, β-, and γ-cyclodextrins, comprising six to eight sugar units in the ring. This combined approach that simultaneously exploits the cyclodextrin solubilising power towards the drugs and the liposome carrier function through the skin has recently been demonstrated by using both classic [66] and deformable liposomes [67]. The use of this double-loading technique by preparing liposomes loaded with the plain drug in the lipophilic phase and its cyclodextrin complex in the aqueous phase of the vesicles gives rise to a fast onset action and a prolonged effect [68]. The composition vesicles containing the cationic surfactant allowed a significant ($P < 0.05$) improvement of the drug anaesthetic effect in terms of intensity and duration of action [68].

9.2. Microemulsions. Microemulsions have penetration-enhancing properties. Local anaesthetics encapsulated in microemulsions result in fast transdermal penetration and effect [39, 69]. Microemulsions contain a large amount of surfactants and cosurfactants that have the potential to cause haemolysis or histopathological changes [69].

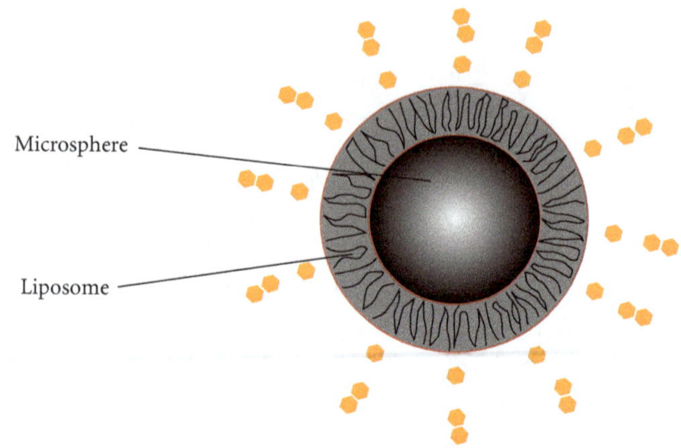

FIGURE 8: Microspheres (or nanospheres) within liposome.

9.3. Poly(lactic-co-glycolic acid) Microspheres and Nanospheres. The most commonly used micro- and nanoscale vehicles for drug encapsulation and delivery are microspheres and nanospheres. They are usually prepared from biodegradable synthetic hydrophobic materials such as homo- or copolymers of polylactic and polyglycolic acids [70].

Microparticles are perfect for drug delivery as they remain at the depot site for long periods allowing slow prolonged release of the encapsulated drug [3]. Particle size and the thickness of thin, free films are factors in drug release. The lipospheres are stable structures consisting of a solid hydrophobic fat core such as triglycerides or fatty acid derivatives, estabilised by a monolayer of phospholipids (Figure 8) [3].

More recently, a nanoliposphere has been developed that does not gelify and is suitable for injection [3, 71]. When poly(dL-lactic acid) microspheres were embedded into poloxamer 407-based hydrogel, this microsphere-gel system containing lignocaine was easy to inject. In addition, it proved degradable [3]. Clinically, in human intercostal blockade studies, dexamethasone added to microcapsules containing bupivacaine showed longer duration of anaesthesia affect compared with microcapsules without dexamethasone [3].

9.4. Hyaluronic Acid-Based Hydrogels. Hyaluronic acid is a nonimmunogenic naturally occurring mucopolysaccharide used as a viscous carrier solution to prolong LA action [3]. However, addition of cross-linked hyaluronic acid doubled the length of action of bupivacaine compared with the noncross-linked hyaluronic acid. It is in an easily injectable liquid form.

9.5. Calcium Phosphate Apatite Loaded with Bupivacaine. Synthetic calcium-deficient apatites are structurally similar to biological apatites; they are chemical precursors of biphasic calcium phosphates. Biphasic calcium phosphates are mixtures of hydroxyapatite and beta-tricalcium phosphate and are widely used as bone substitutes in human surgery [72]. In Wistar male rats, bupivacaine has been loaded on to calcium-deficient apatites using isostatic compaction [72]. This was able to release local anaesthetic in a manner that prevented or limited postoperative pain following bone surgery [72].

9.6. Controlled-Release Local Anaesthetic Matrix. As previously mentioned, the absorbable, controlled-release, local anaesthetic delivery system containing 16% (w/w) lignocaine (Xybrex) is capable of providing up to several days of reversible rat sciatic nerve block in a dose- (mass-) dependent fashion [73]. Two sets of lignocaine-containing drug delivery matrices (OSB-L and OST-R) have been used in subfascial sciatic nerve blocks in rats as well. The OSB-L formulations consisted of four different concentrations of lignocaine ranging from 1.875% to 15% (w/w). These are denoted as OSB-1.875L, OSB-3.75L, OSB-7.5L, and OSB- 15L [73]. The OST-R formulations consisted of four different concentrations of the drug release rate modifier, ranging from 5% to 20% (w/w) in 5% increments, with lignocaine concentration kept constant at 16% (w/w). These formulations are denoted OST-5R, OST-10R, OST-15R, and OST-20R [73]. All OSB-L formulations produced complete and reversible, dose-dependent blockade of nociceptive and motor functions [73]. Blockade by OST-R formulations varied with the concentration of the release rate modifier. All formulations gave complete, reversible blocks of both functions; importantly, their durations did not change monotonically with increasing concentrations of the release rate modifier [73]. Implants of slow-release lignocaine formulations are most effective against postincisional pain when placed at the ipsilateral nerve innervating the area of incision [74]. No human studies of its use have been published as yet.

9.7. Injectable Liquid Polymers. There are three types of polymers for encapsulation, namely, nondegradable polymers, synthetic polymers, natural biodegradables (that degrade to nontoxic products that are completely eliminated from the body), and drug-conjugated polymers (where a drug is attached to water-soluble polymer by a cleavable bond) [3]. The drug-polymer conjugate can be directly targeted to the site of specific action. The use of a 15% bupivacaine lactic acid-*co*-castor oil copolymer prolonged the in vivo effect to 96-hour sensory block [75].

Injectable polymers are simple and reliable to prepare; simple mixing combines the local anaesthetic. The main disadvantage is the prolonged time these polymer carriers dwell in the injection site, far beyond the time of the effect of the local anaesthetic agent [3]. The safety and tissue compatibility of biodegradable pasty polymers have been tested and found to be safe with no systemic tissue damage or polymer-related lesions [3, 76].

9.8. Films. One of the key areas of intense research is therefore to achieve an optimal and desirable controlled and sustained drug release from the use of biodegradable films. The buccal route has some unique compelling benefits making it worth trying; such benefits include avoiding first pass effect, easy accessibility, and better patient compliance. Adhesion of buccal adhesive drug delivery devices to mucosal membranes leads to an increased drug concentration gradient at the absorption site and therefore improved bioavailability of systemically delivered drugs [77]. Various bioadhesive mucosal dosage forms have been developed as films. An ideal buccal film should be flexible, elastic, and soft, with accepted size and thickness, yet adequately strong to withstand breakage due to stress from mouth activities. It must also possess good bioadhesive strength so that it can be retained in the mouth for a desired duration [78]. It should be nonirritant, not cause teeth discoloration, resistant to metabolism, and be capable of releasing a drug at appropriate rate. Buccal films were developed using carbopol 971P as a mucoadhesive polymer and glycerol as a plasticizer. In testing, a buccal mucoadhesive film using lignocaine and its hydrochloride salt as a model drug found that drug concentration affected the mucoadhesive properties of the films [79].

A slow-release lignocaine sheet has been produced and has been used for sciatic nerve block in the rat model of postoperative pain. Single treatment of this controlled-release lignocaine inhibited hyperalgesia and c-fos expression in the spinal cord dorsal horn for one week without inducing inflammation of the sciatic nerve [80]. Bioadhesive films containing benzocaine have been tested in the rat model for benzocaine local delivery [81]. Tail-flick tests have shown the duration of benzocaine-induced analgesia to be significantly prolonged with the films compared to commercial creams [81].

10. Conclusion

Local anaesthetics are widely used to manage acute, chronic, and cancer pain, for anaesthesia, and for diagnostic purposes. Local anaesthetics may have similar chemical structures, but differing pharmacokinetic properties and spectra of pharmacodynamic effects. This influences the selection of agents for use in various clinical situations [82]. New innovations pertaining to LA formulations lead to prolonged action or to novel delivery approaches. Decades after the introduction of local anaesthetics for analgesia/anaesthesia, new properties may still be discovered. New applications of this class of drugs may still be anticipated. The use of regional anaesthesia may affect cancer recurrence rates following surgical resection of tumours via immunomodulation [79]. The preservation of the body's immune processes by local anaesthetics needs to be further studied.The development of new effective delivery systems should suitably modulate the release rate of these drugs, extend their anaesthetic effect, and enhance their localisation; this should reduce problems of systemic toxicity. Part 2 of this paper will deal with new techniques for the delivery of topical and injectable local anaesthetics.

Disclosure

No benefits in any form have been or will be received from a commercial party related directly or indirectly to the subject of this paper.

Conflict of Interests

The author declares that there is no conflict of interests.

References

[1] S. A. Grant, K. C. Nielsen, R. A. Greengrass, S. M. Steele, and S. M. Klein, "Continuous peripheral nerve block for ambulatory surgery," *Regional Anesthesia and Pain Medicine*, vol. 26, no. 3, pp. 209–214, 2001.

[2] S. M. Klein, S. A. Grant, R. A. Greengrass et al., "Interscalene brachial plexus block with a continuous catheter insertion system and a disposable infusion pump," *Anesthesia and Analgesia*, vol. 91, no. 6, pp. 1473–1478, 2000.

[3] C. F. Weiniger, M. Golovanevski, M. Sokolsky-Papkov, and A. J. Domb, "Review of prolonged local anesthetic action," *Expert Opinion on Drug Delivery*, vol. 7, no. 6, pp. 737–752, 2010.

[4] P. S. Hodgson, J. M. Neal, J. E. Pollock, and S. S. Liu, "The neurotoxicity of drugs given intrathecally (Spinal)," *Anesthesia and Analgesia*, vol. 88, no. 4, pp. 797–809, 1999.

[5] P. A. Vieira, I. Pulai, G. C. Tsao, P. Manikantan, B. Kelle, and N. R. Connelly, "Dexamethasone with bupivacaine increases duration of analgesia in ultrasound-guided interscalene brachial plexus blockade," *European Journal of Anaesthesiology*, vol. 27, no. 3, pp. 285–288, 2010.

[6] J. A. Lander, B. J. Weltman, and S. S. So, "EMLA and amethocaine for reduction of children's pain associated with needle insertion," *Cochrane Database of Systematic Reviews (Online)*, vol. 3, Article ID CD004236, 2006.

[7] M. O. Columb and K. MacLennan, "Local anaesthetic agents," *Anaesthesia and Intensive Care Medicine*, vol. 8, no. 4, pp. 159–162, 2007.

[8] P. Dewachter, C. Mouton-Faivre, and C. W. Emala, "Anaphylaxis and anesthesia: controversies and new insights," *Anesthesiology*, vol. 111, no. 5, pp. 1141–1150, 2009.

[9] D. Dillane and B. T. Finucane, "Local anesthetic systemic toxicity," *Canadian Journal of Anesthesia*, vol. 57, no. 4, pp. 368–380, 2010.

[10] P. H. Rosenberg, B. T. Veering, and W. F. Urmey, "Maximum recommended doses of local anesthetics: a multifactorial concept," *Regional Anesthesia and Pain Medicine*, vol. 29, no. 6, pp. 564–575, 2004.

[11] C. L. Burlacu and D. J. Buggy, "Update on local anesthetics: focus on levobupivacaine," *Therapeutics and Clinical Risk Management*, vol. 4, no. 2, pp. 381–392, 2008.

[12] K. J. McClellan and D. Faulds, "Ropivacaine: an update of its use in regional anaesthesia," *Drugs*, vol. 60, no. 5, pp. 1065–1093, 2000.

[13] E. H. Mojumdar and A. P. Lyubartsev, "Molecular dynamics simulations of local anesthetic articaine in a lipid bilayer," *Biophysical Chemistry*, vol. 153, no. 1, pp. 27–35, 2010.

[14] N. Nizharadze, M. Mamaladze, N. Chipashvili, and D. Vadachkoria, "Articaine—the best choice of local anesthetic in contemporary dentistry," *Georgian Medical News*, no. 190, pp. 15–23, 2011.

[15] V. Vegh, J. Cizmarik, and K. Hahnenkamp, "Is there a place for local anesthetics structurally different from classical amid or ester local anesthetics?" *Current Opinion in Anaesthesiology*, vol. 19, no. 5, pp. 509–515, 2006.

[16] C. F. Wang, C. Pancaro, P. Gerner, and G. Strichartz, "Prolonged suppression of postincisional pain by a slow-release formulation of lidocaine," *Anesthesiology*, vol. 114, no. 1, pp. 135–149, 2011.

[17] X. Guo, N. A. Castle, D. M. Chernoff, and G. R. Strichartz, "Comparative inhibition of voltage-gated cation channels by local anesthetics," *Annals of the New York Academy of Sciences*, vol. 625, pp. 181–199, 1991.

[18] Z. Xiong and G. R. Strichartz, "Inhibition by local anesthetics of Ca^{2+} channels in rat anterior pituitary cells," *European Journal of Pharmacology*, vol. 363, no. 1, pp. 81–90, 1998.

[19] K. Hirota, D. Smart, and D. G. Lambert, "The effects of local and intravenous anesthetics on recombinant rat VR1 vanilloid receptors," *Anesthesia and Analgesia*, vol. 96, no. 6, pp. 1656–1660, 2003.

[20] M. W. Hollmann, D. Strumper, S. Herroeder, and M. E. Durieux, "Receptors, G proteins, and their interactions," *Anesthesiology*, vol. 103, no. 5, pp. 1066–1078, 2005.

[21] M. W. Hollmann, A. Gross, N. Jelacin, and M. E. Durieux, "Local anesthetic effects on priming and activation of human neutrophils," *Anesthesiology*, vol. 95, no. 1, pp. 113–122, 2001.

[22] A. Kaba, S. R. Laurent, B. J. Detroz et al., "Intravenous lidocaine infusion facilitates acute rehabilitation after laparoscopic colectomy," *Anesthesiology*, vol. 106, no. 1, pp. 11–18, 2007.

[23] I. Power, "An update on analgesics," *British Journal of Anaesthesia*, vol. 107, no. 1, pp. 19–24, 2011.

[24] A. Borgeat and J. Aguirre, "Update on local anesthetics," *Current Opinion in Anaesthesiology*, vol. 23, no. 4, pp. 466–471, 2010.

[25] U. Muth-Selbach, H. Hermanns, J. U. Stegmann et al., "Antinociceptive effects of systemic lidocaine: involvement of the spinal glycinergic system," *European Journal of Pharmacology*, vol. 613, no. 1–3, pp. 68–73, 2009.

[26] M. W. Coghlan, M. J. Davies, C. Hoy, L. Joyce, R. Kilner, and M. J. Waters, "Antibacterial activity of epidural infusions," *Anaesthesia and Intensive Care*, vol. 37, no. 1, pp. 66–69, 2009.

[27] K. P. Harvey, J. D. Adair, M. Isho, and R. Robinson, "Can intravenous lidocaine decrease postsurgical ileus and shorten hospital stay in elective bowel surgery? A pilot study and literature review," *American Journal of Surgery*, vol. 198, no. 2, pp. 231–236, 2009.

[28] I. Z. Yardeni, B. Beilin, E. Mayburd, Y. Levinson, and H. Bessler, "The effect of perioperative intravenous lidocaine on postoperative pain and immune function," *Anesthesia and Analgesia*, vol. 109, no. 5, pp. 1464–1469, 2009.

[29] C. W. Clarkson and L. M. Hondeghem, "Mechanism for bupivacaine depression of cardiac conduction: fast block of sodium channels during the action potential with slow recovery from block during diastole," *Anesthesiology*, vol. 62, no. 4, pp. 396–405, 1985.

[30] K. Nouette-Gaulain, C. Dadure, D. Morau et al., "Age-dependent bupivacaine-induced muscle toxicity during continuous peripheral nerve block in rats," *Anesthesiology*, vol. 111, no. 5, pp. 1120–1127, 2009.

[31] R. T. Wilder, M. G. Sholas, and C. B. Berde, "N(G)-nitro-L-arginine methyl ester (L-NAME) prevents tachyphylaxis to local anesthetics in a dose-dependent manner," *Anesthesia and Analgesia*, vol. 83, no. 6, pp. 1251–1255, 1996.

[32] G. Weinberg, R. Ripper, D. L. Feinstein, and W. Hoffman, "Lipid emulsion infusion rescues dogs from bupivacaine-induced cardiac toxicity," *Regional Anesthesia and Pain Medicine*, vol. 28, no. 3, pp. 198–202, 2003.

[33] J. M. Neal, C. M. Bernards, J. F. Butterworth et al., "ASRA practice advisory on local anesthetic systemic toxicity," *Regional Anesthesia and Pain Medicine*, vol. 35, no. 2, pp. 152–161, 2010.

[34] P. Toledo, "The role of lipid emulsion during advanced cardiac life support for local anesthetic toxicity," *International Journal of Obstetric Anesthesia*, vol. 20, no. 1, pp. 60–63, 2011.

[35] B. A. Howell and A. Chauhan, "Bupivacaine binding to pegylated liposomes," *Anesthesia and Analgesia*, vol. 109, no. 2, pp. 678–682, 2009.

[36] J. W. Wolfe and J. F. Butterworth, "Local anesthetic systemic toxicity: update on mechanisms and treatment," *Current Opinion in Anaesthesiology*, vol. 24, no. 5, pp. 561–566, 2011.

[37] W. C. Culp Jr. and W. C. Culp, "Practical application of local anesthetics," *Journal of Vascular and Interventional Radiology*, vol. 22, no. 2, pp. 111–118, 2011.

[38] B. A. Williams, B. B. Murinson, B. R. Grable, and S. L. Orebaugh, "Future considerations for pharmacologic adjuvants in single-injection peripheral nerve blocks for patients with diabetes mellitus," *Regional Anesthesia and Pain Medicine*, vol. 34, no. 5, pp. 445–457, 2009.

[39] K. C. Cummings, D. E. Napierkowski, I. Parra-Sanchez et al., "Effect of dexamethasone on the duration of interscalene nerve blocks with ropivacaine or bupivacaine," *British Journal of Anaesthesia*, vol. 107, no. 3, pp. 446–453, 2011.

[40] S. J. Parrington, D. O'Donnell, V. W. S. Chan et al., "Dexamethasone added to mepivacaine prolongs the duration of analgesia after supraclavicular brachial plexus blockade," *Regional Anesthesia and Pain Medicine*, vol. 35, no. 5, pp. 422–426, 2010.

[41] E. de Paula, C. M. S. Cereda, G. R. Tofoli, M. Franz-Montan, L. F. Fraceto, and D. R. De Araújo, "Drug delivery systems for local anesthetics," *Recent Patents on Drug Delivery and Formulation*, vol. 4, no. 1, pp. 23–34, 2010.

[42] M. D. Wiles, S. A. Dobson, and I. K. Moppett, "The effect of a new topical local anaesthetic delivery system on forearm skin blood flow reactivity," *Anaesthesia*, vol. 65, no. 2, pp. 178–183, 2010.

[43] C.-W. Cho, J.-S. Choi, and S.-C. Shin, "Enhanced local anesthetic action of mepivacaine from the bioadhesive gels," *Pakistan Journal of Pharmaceutical Sciences*, vol. 24, no. 1, pp. 87–93, 2011.

[44] J. G. Förster and P. H. Rosenberg, "Revival of old local anesthetics for spinal anesthesia in ambulatory surgery," *Current Opinion in Anaesthesiology*, vol. 24, no. 6, pp. 633–637, 2011.

[45] C. F. Wang, A. G. Djalali, A. Gandhi et al., "An absorbable local anesthetic matrix provides several days of functional sciatic nerve blockade," *Anesthesia and Analgesia*, vol. 108, no. 3, pp. 1027–1033, 2009.

[46] C. Sinico and A. M. Fadda, "Vesicular carriers for dermal drug delivery," *Expert Opinion on Drug Delivery*, vol. 6, no. 8, pp. 813–825, 2009.

[47] A. Shikanov, A. J. Domb, and C. F. Weiniger, "Long acting local anesthetic-polymer formulation to prolong the effect of analgesia," *Journal of Controlled Release*, vol. 117, no. 1, pp. 97–103, 2007.

[48] J. G. Boogaerts, N. D. Lafont, S. Carlino et al., "Biodistribution of liposome-associated bupivacaine after extradural administration to rabbits," *British Journal of Anaesthesia*, vol. 75, no. 3, pp. 319–325, 1995.

[49] M. D. Blanco, M. V. Bernardo, C. Gómez, E. Muñiz, and J. M. Teijón, "Bupivacaine-loaded comatrix formed by albumin microspheres included in a poly(lactide-co-glycolide) film: in vivo biocompatibility and drug release studies," *Biomaterials*, vol. 20, no. 20, pp. 1919–1924, 1999.

[50] G. Dollo, D. O. Thompson, P. Le Corre, F. Chevanne, and R. Le Verge, "Inclusion complexation of amide-typed local anesthetics with β-cyclodextrin and its derivatives. III. Biopharmaceutics of bupivacaine-SBE7-βCD complex following percutaneous sciatic nerve administration in rabbits," *International Journal of Pharmaceutics*, vol. 164, no. 1-2, pp. 11–19, 1998.

[51] J. Curley, J. Castillo, J. Hotz et al., "Prolonged regional nerve blockade: injectable biodegradable bupivacaine/polyester microspheres," *Anesthesiology*, vol. 84, no. 6, pp. 1401–1410, 1996.

[52] C. Dräger, D. Benziger, F. Gao, and C. B. Berde, "Prolonged intercostal nerve blockade in sheep using controlled-release of bupivacaine and dexamethasone from polymer microspheres," *Anesthesiology*, vol. 89, no. 4, pp. 969–979, 1998.

[53] T. Lian and R. J. Y. Ho, "Trends and developments in liposome drug delivery systems," *Journal of Pharmaceutical Sciences*, vol. 90, no. 6, pp. 667–680, 2001.

[54] S. A. Grant, "The Holy Grail: long-acting local anaesthetics and liposomes," *Best Practice and Research: Clinical Anaesthesiology*, vol. 16, no. 2, pp. 345–352, 2002.

[55] G. J. Grant, Y. Barenholz, B. Piskoun, M. Bansinath, H. Turndorf, and E. M. Bolotin, "DRV liposomal bupivacaine: preparation, characterization, and in vivo evaluation in mice," *Pharmaceutical Research*, vol. 18, no. 3, pp. 336–343, 2001.

[56] P. Mura, F. Maestrelli, M. L. González-Rodríguez, I. Michelacci, C. Ghelardini, and A. M. Rabasco, "Development, characterization and in vivo evaluation of benzocaine-loaded liposomes," *European Journal of Pharmaceutics and Biopharmaceutics*, vol. 67, no. 1, pp. 86–95, 2007.

[57] G. Cevc, A. Schätzlein, and H. Richardsen, "Ultradeformable lipid vesicles can penetrate the skin and other semi-permeable barriers unfragmented. Evidence from double label CLSM experiments and direct size measurements," *Biochimica et Biophysica Acta*, vol. 1564, no. 1, pp. 21–30, 2002.

[58] M. M. A. Elsayed, O. Y. Abdallah, V. F. Naggar, and N. M. Khalafallah, "Lipid vesicles for skin delivery of drugs: reviewing three decades of research," *International Journal of Pharmaceutics*, vol. 332, no. 1-2, pp. 1–16, 2007.

[59] G. M. El Maghraby, B. W. Barry, and A. C. Williams, "Liposomes and skin: from drug delivery to model membranes," *European Journal of Pharmaceutical Sciences*, vol. 34, no. 4-5, pp. 203–222, 2008.

[60] G. J. Grant, Y. Barenholz, E. M. Bolotin et al., "A novel liposomal bupivacaine formulation to produce ultralong-acting analgesia," *Anesthesiology*, vol. 101, no. 1, pp. 133–137, 2004.

[61] J. G. Boogaerts, N. D. Lafont, A. G. Declercq et al., "Epidural administration of liposome-associated bupivacaine for the management of postsurgical pain: a first study," *Journal of Clinical Anesthesia*, vol. 6, no. 4, pp. 315–320, 1994.

[62] M. Franz-Montan, E. De Paula, F. C. Groppo, A. L. R. Silva, J. Ranali, and M. C. Volpato, "Liposome-encapsulated ropivacaine for intraoral topical anesthesia," *Oral Surgery, Oral Medicine, Oral Pathology, Oral Radiology and Endodontology*, vol. 110, no. 6, pp. 800–804, 2010.

[63] M. Franz-Montan, E. de Paula, F. C. Groppo, A. L. R. Silva, J. Ranali, and M. C. Volpato, "Liposomal delivery system for topical anaesthesia of the palatal mucosa," *British Journal of Oral and Maxillofacial Surgery*. In press.

[64] G. R. Tofoli, C. M. S. Cereda, F. C. Groppo et al., "Efficacy of liposome-encapsulated mepivacaine for infiltrative anesthesia in volunteers," *Journal of Liposome Research*, vol. 21, no. 1, pp. 88–94, 2011.

[65] F. Maestrelli, M. L. González-Rodríguez, A. M. Rabasco, C. Ghelardini, and P. Mura, "New "drug-in cyclodextrin-in deformable liposomes" formulations to improve the therapeutic efficacy of local anaesthetics," *International Journal of Pharmaceutics*, vol. 395, no. 1-2, pp. 222–231, 2010.

[66] M. C. B. Lira, M. S. Ferraz, D. G. V. C. da Silva et al., "Inclusion complex of usnic acid with β-cyclodextrin: characterization and nanoencapsulation into liposomes," *Journal of Inclusion Phenomena and Macrocyclic Chemistry*, vol. 64, no. 3-4, pp. 215–224, 2009.

[67] A. Gillet, A. Grammenos, P. Compère, B. Evrard, and G. Piel, "Development of a new topical system: drug-in-cyclodextrin-in-deformable liposome," *International Journal of Pharmaceutics*, vol. 380, no. 1-2, pp. 174–180, 2009.

[68] M. Bragagni, F. Maestrelli, N. Mennini, C. Ghelardini, and P. Mura, "Liposomal formulations of prilocaine: effect of complexation with hydroxypropyl-ß-cyclodextrin on drug anesthetic efficacy," *Journal of Liposome Research*, vol. 20, no. 4, pp. 315–322, 2010.

[69] C. X. He, Z. G. He, and J. Q. Gao, "Microemulsions as drug delivery systems to improve the solubility and the bioavailability of poorly water-soluble drugs," *Expert Opinion on Drug Delivery*, vol. 7, no. 4, pp. 445–460, 2010.

[70] P. Le Corre, J. H. Rytting, V. Gajan, F. Chevanne, and R. Le Verge, "In vitro controlled release kinetics of local anaesthetics from poly(D,L-lactide) and poly(lactide-co-glycolide) microspheres," *Journal of Microencapsulation*, vol. 14, no. 2, pp. 243–255, 1997.

[71] J. Pietkiewicz, M. Sznitowska, and M. Placzek, "The expulsion of lipophilic drugs from the cores of solid lipid microspheres in diluted suspensions and in concentrates," *International Journal of Pharmaceutics*, vol. 310, no. 1-2, pp. 64–71, 2006.

[72] E. Verron, O. Gauthier, P. Janvier et al., "Analgesic properties of calcium phosphate apatite loaded with bupivacaine on postoperative pain," *Journal of Biomedical Materials Research B*, vol. 94, no. 1, pp. 89–96, 2010.

[73] P. Gerner, C. F. Wang, B. S. Lee et al., "The relationship between functional sciatic nerve block duration and the rate of release of lidocaine from a controlled-release matrix," *Anesthesia and Analgesia*, vol. 111, no. 1, pp. 221–229, 2010.

[74] C. F. Wang, C. Pancaro, P. Gerner, and G. Strichartz, "Prolonged suppression of postincisional pain by a slow-release formulation of lidocaine," *Anesthesiology*, vol. 114, no. 1, pp. 135–149, 2011.

[75] M. Sokolsky-Papkov, L. Golovanevski, A. J. Domb, and C. F. Weiniger, "Prolonged local anesthetic action through slow release from poly(lactic acid co castor oil)," *Pharmaceutical Research*, vol. 26, no. 1, pp. 32–39, 2009.

[76] B. Vaisman, M. Motiei, A. Nyska, and A. J. Domb, "Biocompatibility and safety evaluation of a ricinoleic acid-based poly(ester-anhydride) copolymer after implantation in rats," *Journal of Biomedical Materials Research A*, vol. 92, no. 2, pp. 419–431, 2010.

[77] Y. Sudhakar, K. Kuotsu, and A. K. Bandyopadhyay, "Buccal bioadhesive drug delivery—a promising option for orally less efficient drugs," *Journal of Controlled Release*, vol. 114, no. 1, pp. 15–40, 2006.

[78] A. K. Singla, M. Chawla, and A. Singh, "Potential applications of carbomer in oral mucoadhesive controlled drug delivery system: a review," *Drug Development and Industrial Pharmacy*, vol. 26, no. 9, pp. 913–924, 2000.

[79] R. Abu-Huwaij, S. Assaf, M. Salem, and A. Sallam, "Mucoadhesive dosage form of lidocaine hydrochloride: I. Mucoadhesive and physicochemical characterization," *Drug Development and Industrial Pharmacy*, vol. 33, no. 8, pp. 855–864, 2007.

[80] M. Tobe, H. Obata, T. Suto et al., "Long-term effect of sciatic nerve block with slow-release lidocaine in a rat model of postoperative pain," *Anesthesiology*, vol. 112, no. 6, pp. 1473–1481, 2010.

[81] D. R. De Araujo, C. Padula, C. M. S. Cereda et al., "Bioadhesive films containing benzocaine: correlation between in vitro permeation and in vivo local anesthetic effect," *Pharmaceutical Research*, vol. 27, no. 8, pp. 1677–1686, 2010.

[82] J. E. Heavner, "Local anesthetics," *Current Opinion in Anaesthesiology*, vol. 20, no. 4, pp. 336–342, 2007.

3

Interaction of Local Anesthetics with Biomembranes Consisting of Phospholipids and Cholesterol: Mechanistic and Clinical Implications for Anesthetic and Cardiotoxic Effects

Hironori Tsuchiya[1] and Maki Mizogami[2]

[1] *Department of Dental Basic Education, Asahi University School of Dentistry, 1851 Hozumi, Mizuho, Gifu 501-0296, Japan*
[2] *Department of Anesthesiology and Reanimatology, University of Fukui Faculty of Medical Sciences, 23-3 Matsuokashimoaizuki, Eiheiji-cho, Yoshida-gun, Fukui 910-1193, Japan*

Correspondence should be addressed to Hironori Tsuchiya; hiro@dent.asahi-u.ac.jp

Academic Editor: Yukio Hayashi

Despite a long history in medical and dental application, the molecular mechanism and precise site of action are still arguable for local anesthetics. Their effects are considered to be induced by acting on functional proteins, on membrane lipids, or on both. Local anesthetics primarily interact with sodium channels embedded in cell membranes to reduce the excitability of nerve cells and cardiomyocytes or produce a malfunction of the cardiovascular system. However, the membrane protein-interacting theory cannot explain all of the pharmacological and toxicological features of local anesthetics. The administered drug molecules must diffuse through the lipid barriers of nerve sheaths and penetrate into or across the lipid bilayers of cell membranes to reach the acting site on transmembrane proteins. Amphiphilic local anesthetics interact hydrophobically and electrostatically with lipid bilayers and modify their physicochemical property, with the direct inhibition of membrane functions, and with the resultant alteration of the membrane lipid environments surrounding transmembrane proteins and the subsequent protein conformational change, leading to the inhibition of channel functions. We review recent studies on the interaction of local anesthetics with biomembranes consisting of phospholipids and cholesterol. Understanding the membrane interactivity of local anesthetics would provide novel insights into their anesthetic and cardiotoxic effects.

1. Introduction

Local anesthetics clinically used so far have the common chemical structure that is composed of three portions: the hydrophobic moiety consisting of an aromatic ring, the intermediate chain, and the hydrophilic moiety consisting of an amino terminus. The aromatic residue confers lipid solubility on a drug molecule, whereas the ionizable amino group confers, water solubility. The intermediate portion provides the spatial separation between hydrophobic and hydrophilic end and structurally classifies local anesthetics into amide type and ester type (Figure 1).

Because of the presence of substituted amino groups, local anesthetics are referred to as the bases with p*K*a values ranging from 7.7 to 8.1 at 37°C for the amide type and from 8.4 to 8.9 at 37°C for the ester type [1], so they exist in uncharged and positively charged form. After injected, local anesthetics show an in vivo equilibrium between the uncharged and the charged fraction of molecules. According to the Henderson-Hasselbalch equation, the percentage of uncharged molecules depends on the p*K*a and medium pH (Figure 2). The pharmacokinetics and the mode of action of local anesthetics are closely related to their interaction with membrane lipids. Uncharged molecules can predominantly diffuse through the lipid barriers of nerve sheaths and penetrate into and across the lipid bilayers of cell membranes to reach the acting sites. The pH-dependent effects of local anesthetics have been discussed in association with the pH changes in inflammation, ischemia, and several diseases [2–4].

It is generally recognized that local anesthetics primarily affect sodium channels in sensory nerve fibers and cardiomyocytes [5]. Blocking peripheral nerves to induce local

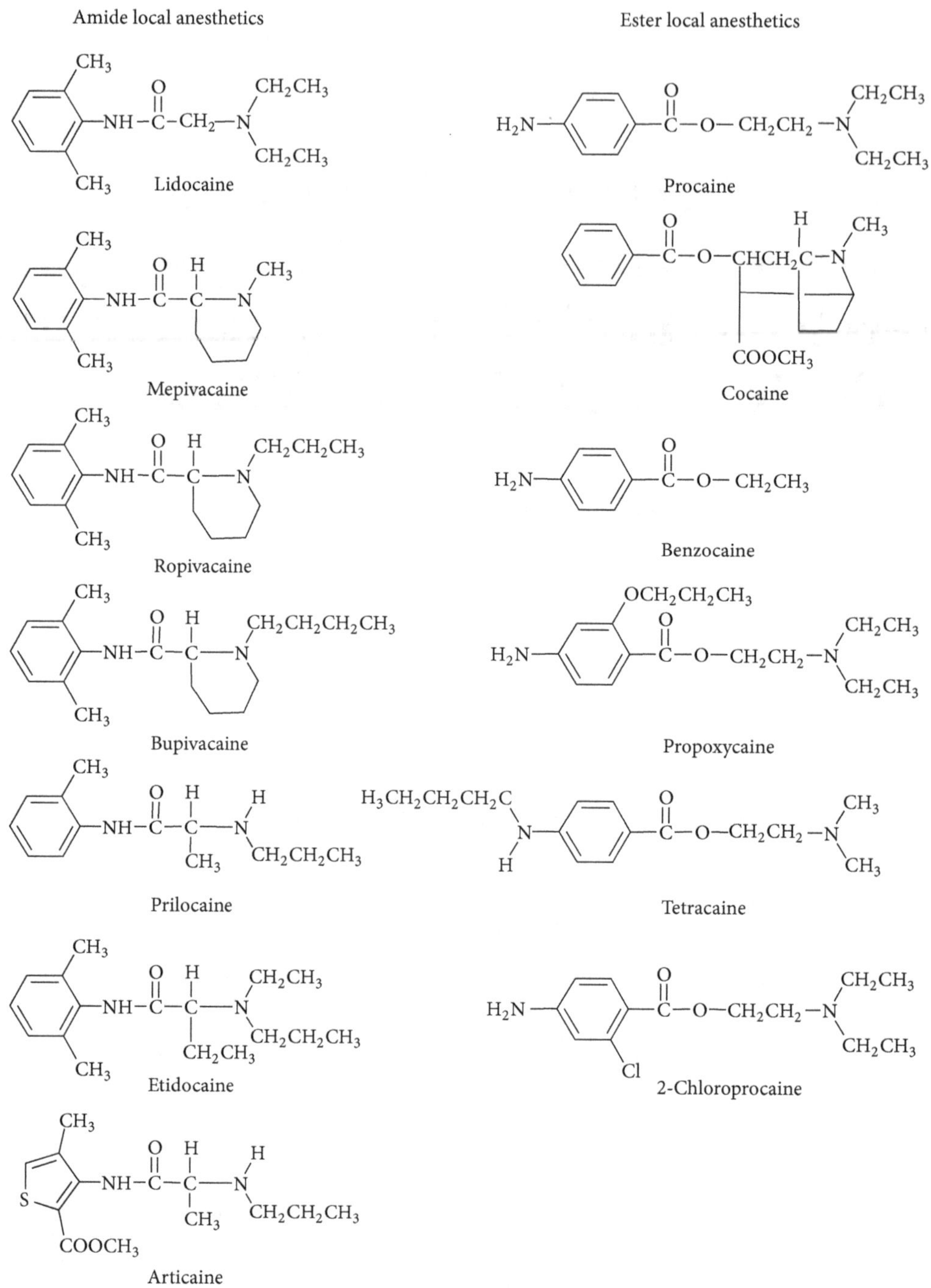

FIGURE 1: Representative amide and ester local anesthetics.

anesthesia is achieved at the relatively high concentrations of drugs in local areas. At lower concentrations, certain local anesthetics also show more subtle effects on hearts, which are clinically important as an antiarrhythmic agent. In addition, lidocaine administered systemically may be useful for reducing the excitability of nociceptive sensory neurons [6].

Local anesthetics block the conduction of nerve impulses by affecting the influx of ions through transmembrane channels. Proposed mechanistic theories include the action on membrane-embedded ion channels, membrane-associated enzymes, membrane lipids, and water. In the protein-interacting theory, local anesthetics are presumed to inhibit the generation and conduction of action potentials in nerve cells and cardiomyocytes by binding to the intracellular site of voltage-gated sodium channels embedded in membrane lipid bilayers (Figure 3). Local anesthetics specifically bind to the D4-S6 region of the α-subunit of neural sodium channels. Since this site is intracellular or cell interior, drug molecules are absolutely required to be in uncharged hydrophobic form for accessing there.

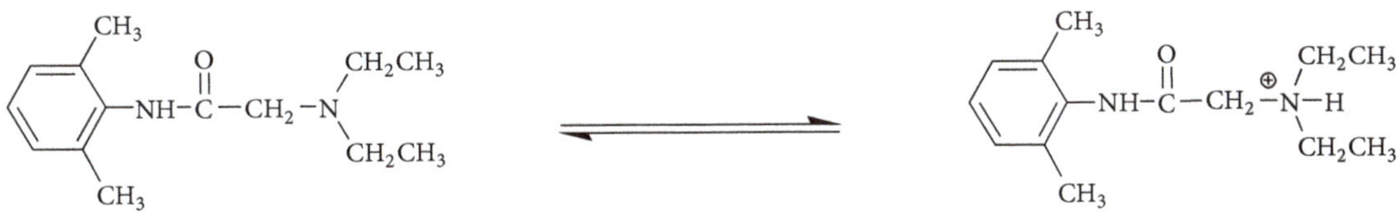

Uncharged (nonionized) lidocaine

Charged (ionized) cationic lidocaine

Log_{10} [uncharged drug]/[charged drug] = pH − p*Ka*

For lidocaine with the p*Ka* of 7.8 at tissue pH of 7.4,
[uncharged lidocaine molecule]/[charged lidocaine molecule] = 0.4

For procaine with the p*Ka* of 8.9 at tissue pH of 7.4,
[uncharged lidocaine molecule]/[charged lidocaine molecule] = 0.03

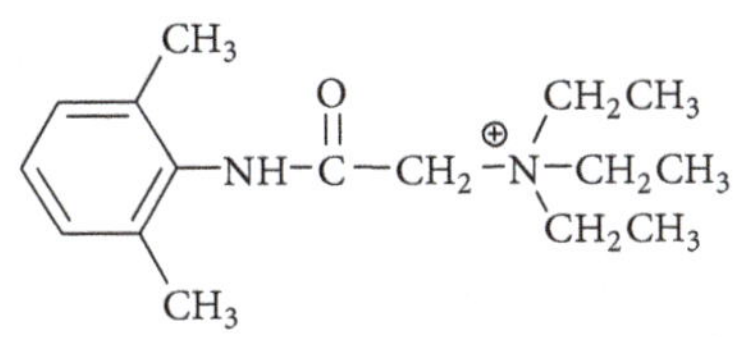

QX-314 (*N*-ethyl lidocaine)

FIGURE 2: Uncharged and charged local anesthetics and permanently charged derivative.

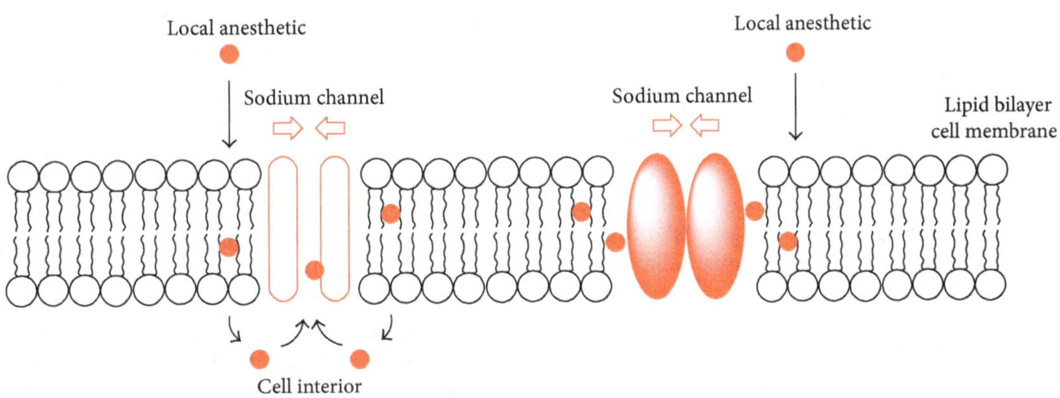

FIGURE 3: Channel protein-interacting and membrane lipid-interacting local anesthetics.

Drugs acting on proteinous channels, receptors, and enzymes also have the ability to act on lipid bilayers and modify membrane physicochemical properties [7]. Local anesthetics interact with membrane lipids to change fluidity, order, microviscosity, and permeability of membranes [8] and also influence the electrostatic potential across lipid bilayers, which may affect the functions of voltage-gated ion channels [7, 9]. They are presumed to act on lipid bilayers, with the resultant alteration of the membrane lipid environments surrounding transmembrane proteins and the subsequent change of protein conformation, thereby influencing the channel activity (Figure 3). Considering the diversity in their chemical structures, a specific single acting site within ion channels has been suggested to be unlikely for all of local anesthetics [10]. Local anesthetics affect various functional membrane proteins such as potassium ion channel, calcium ion channel, acetylcholine receptor, adrenergic receptor, GABA_A receptor, γ-aminobutyric acid receptor, glycine receptor, adenylate cyclase, phospholipase A_2, and Na,K-ATPase [11–13]. Such broad spectra are interpretable by the fundamental action on a target common to local anesthetics, membrane lipids [14]. A wide range of pharmacological and toxicological properties of local anesthetics cannot be ascribed to binding to a single protein target alone [7], so it is reasonable to assume that the interaction of local anesthetics with lipid bilayer biomembranes contributes, at least partly but significantly, to their anesthetic and toxic effects. It has been recently suggested that the responsibility of membrane lipids for and the role of specific membrane component(s) in anesthetic mechanisms should be reverified [15].

2. Drug and Membrane Interaction

2.1. Membrane Preparation. Because biological membranes are a very complex system, biomimetic model membranes

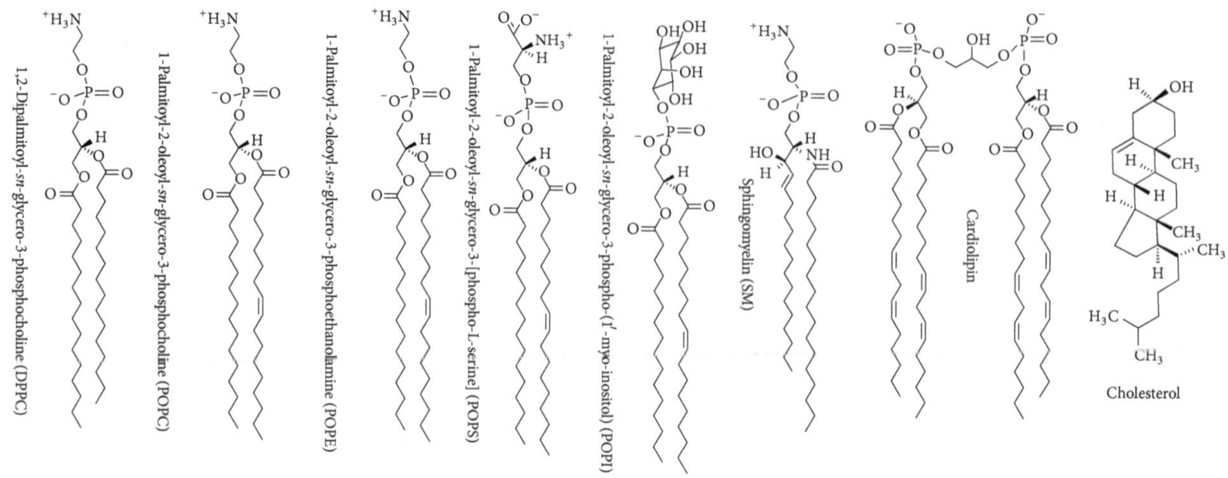

Figure 4: Membrane lipid components.

consisting of lipids have been employed more frequently than natural biomembranes for studying the drug and membrane interaction [16]. The advantages of using protein-free lipid membranes are that one can easily manipulate the reaction condition and the membrane lipid composition, focus only on the interaction between drugs and membrane lipids, avoid the interference from other membrane components, and quantitatively evaluate the membrane response to drugs. Model membranes with the lipid bilayer structure can be prepared to mimic cellular and plasma membranes of interest by adjusting their lipid compositions. One of biomimetic model membranes widely used is a liposome, the vesicle with concentric lipid layers in which an aqueous volume is entirely enclosed by membranous lipids. A unilamellar vesicle is characterized by a single lipid bilayer consisting of inner and outer leaflet.

The major phospholipids constituting biological membranes are glycerophospholipids with the content of 40–60 mol% in total lipid fraction. They consist of a glycerol backbone on which two fatty acids are commonly esterified at the stereospecifically numbered *sn*-1 and *sn*-2 position. The third carbon atom of a glycerol backbone supports the polar head group composed of choline, ethanolamine, serine, inositol, and so forth, which are linked to a negatively charged phosphate group. Representative lipids used for preparing biomimetic membranes are shown in Figure 4. The most abundant steroid in biological membranes is cholesterol that comprises four fused cycles in the *trans*-configuration, a hydroxyl group at the 3-position, a double bond between the carbon 5 and 6, and an iso-octyl lateral chain at the 17-position. Liposomal membranes are prepared by the aqueous dispersion of these authentic lipids (either a single component or a mixture of several lipids) or lipids extracted from cells.

2.2. Membrane Interactivity Analysis. The drug and membrane interaction can be analyzed by different techniques such as electron spin resonance, differential scanning calorimetry, nuclear magnetic resonance, X-ray diffraction, and fluorometry. Of spectroscopic and biophysical methods, fluorescence polarization has been most frequently used to determine the change in membrane fluidity, which is usable as an index for quantitatively evaluating the membrane interactivity of drugs. The term "membrane fluidity" may mean a combination of different kinds of membrane component mobility like the flexibility of membrane phospholipid acyl chains, the lateral or transverse diffusion of molecules in lipid bilayers, and the membrane lipid phase transition.

The polarization of fluorescence emitted by a membrane-incorporated fluorophore reflects its mobility in the surrounding membrane lipid environments. Fluorescence polarization is measured by excitation performed with monochromatic light that is vertically polarized and the emission intensity detected through an analyzer oriented parallel or perpendicular to the direction of polarization of the excitation light. A variety of fluorophores such as 1,6-diphenyl-1,3,5-hexatriene (DPH), 1-(4-trimethylammoniumphenyl)-6-phenyl-1,3,5-hexatriene (TMA-DPH), *N*-phenyl-1-naphthylamine (PNA), and *n*-(9-anthroyloxy)stearic acid (n = 2, 6, 9 and 12, *n*-AS) are usable for measuring fluorescence polarization. These probes penetrate into membranes to align with phospholipid acyl chains and locate in different membrane regions based on their chemical structures and lipid-interacting properties, indicating the fluidity of the membrane region specific to each individual probe. They are subject to the rotational restriction imparted by lipid bilayer rigidity or order. Drugs interact with lipid bilayers to produce more fluid (less rigid) or disordered membranes, which facilitate the probe rotation to emit the absorbed light in all directions, resulting in a decrease in fluorescence polarization. On the contrary, more rigid (less fluid) or ordered membranes produced by drugs disturb the probe rotation to emit the absorbed light in all directions, resulting in an increase in fluorescence polarization. Compared with controls, decreased and increased polarization means an increase of membrane fluidity (membrane fluidization) and a decrease in membrane fluidity (membrane rigidification), respectively.

3. Local Anesthetic Membrane Interaction

Yun et al. [17] investigated the effects of lidocaine, bupivacaine, prilocaine, and procaine on synaptosomes isolated from bovine cerebral cortex and liposomes prepared with extracted lipids by measuring the fluorescence polarization with 2-AS and 12-AS. They showed that these local anesthetics increased the membrane fluidity by preferentially acting on the hydrocarbon interior. Tsuchiya et al. [18, 19] reported that lidocaine, prilocaine, bupivacaine, ropivacaine, and mepivacaine interacted with liposomal membranes to increase the membrane fluidity by measuring DPH, TMA-DPH, and PNA fluorescence polarization. They also revealed that the interactivity with lipid bilayer membranes is to a great extent consistent with the local anesthetic potency [20]. Local anesthetics are speculated to interact with lipid bilayers to rearrange the intermolecular hydrogen-bonded network among phospholipid molecules in association with the liberation of hydrated water molecules on membranes and also alter the orientation of the P–N dipole of phospholipid molecules, resulting in an increase in membrane fluidity [17]. However, the membrane lipid-interacting theory has been criticized as to whether local anesthetics can affect biomembranes at clinically relevant concentrations, whether local anesthetic molecules in charged form can interact with lipid bilayers, and whether local anesthetics like bupivacaine and ropivacaine can stereostructure-specifically act on lipid membranes to show the potency different between stereoisomers. These subjects are discussed in Sections 4, 5, 6, and 8.

4. Membrane Interaction at Clinically Relevant Concentrations

The concentrations of lidocaine typically used in the clinical setting for dentistry are 1–3% (w/v) [14]. At 0.03–0.08 times these concentrations, Tsuchiya and Mizogami [20] applied lidocaine to liposomal membranes consisting of 100 mol% DPPC or POPC and found that lidocaine increases the membrane fluidity by determining DPH fluorescence polarization decreases. At 0.03–0.25 times lower concentrations of usually administered 0.125–0.75% (w/v) [21], Mizogami et al. [19, 20] revealed that bupivacaine and ropivacaine interact with nerve cell-mimetic membranes to increase the membrane fluidity, resulting in decreases in DPH, PNA, and TMA-DPH fluorescence polarization. The interaction of local anesthetics with nerve cell membranes at clinically relevant concentrations is supported by the fact that membrane-interactive agents including local anesthetics are more effective in modifying the physicochemical property of biological membranes than artificial model membranes [17].

Önyüksel et al. [22] reported that bupivacaine enhanced the carboxyfluorescein release from liposomes with increasing the cardiolipin content in liposomal membranes. Tsuchiya et al. [23] found that bupivacaine increases the fluidity of 2.5–12.5 mol% cardiolipin-containing membranes to decrease DPH fluorescence polarization at 10–50 μM, which corresponded to the blood concentrations for free bupivacaine to produce the cardiac collapse and depress the myocardial function. When dogs were administered with bupivacaine of the cumulative dose of 21.7 ± 2.6 mg/kg, the mean plasma concentration of free and total bupivacaine at cardiovascular collapse was 20 and 63 μM, respectively [24]. The dose of bupivacaine of 7.2–8.8 mg/kg caused the arrhythmias of dogs, in which the mean concentration of free and total bupivacaine in plasma reached 4 and 17 μM, respectively [25]. In the range of these cardiotoxic concentrations, bupivacaine is able to interact with cardiolipin-containing biomembranes and significantly change the membrane fluidity.

The membrane effects were frequently investigated by measuring fluorescence polarization with DPH in previous studies [19, 20, 23]. The degrees of local anesthetics-induced changes in DPH polarization correspond to the functional changes of lipid bilayer membranes and membrane-embedded proteins [23, 26, 27], possibly producing the pharmacologic and toxic effects of local anesthetics.

Membrane-acting drugs accumulate in lipid bilayers and their local membrane concentrations are much higher than their concentrations in the bulk aqueous phase to show the intramembrane concentrations being hundreds of times higher than the aqueous concentrations [28]. Their concentrations in lipid bilayer membranes are consistent with the properties of local anesthetics to interact with biomembranes and modify the membrane fluidity at clinically relevant concentrations. While general anesthetics interact with biomembranes as well as local anesthetics do, they show the water-membrane interfacial concentrations much higher than the concentrations in bulk hexane [29]. Kopeć et al. [7] speculated that the drug dosage necessary to effect a protein-mediated response may be higher than that needed for a membrane-mediated mechanism, so clinical dosages for targeting membranes may be lower. They also suggested that the drug membrane concentration is few orders of magnitude higher than typically found in plasma.

5. Membrane Interactivity Depending on Lipid Components

5.1. Lidocaine Derivative QX-314. One reason the membrane lipid-interacting theory is controversial is the general recognition that the pharmacological activity of charged drugs is negligible when they are applied extracellularly. QX-314 (*N*-(2,6-dimethylphenylcarbamoylmethyl)triethylammonium chloride, *N*-ethyl lidocaine) is a quaternary derivative of lidocaine whose structural difference is only an *N*-ethyl group but renders its parent structure permanently charged and water soluble (see Figure 2 for QX-314 structure). In contrast to lidocaine, this cationic agent shows only very slow penetration into membrane lipid bilayers and cannot readily cross lipid barriers [30]. In previous experiments, extracellularly applied QX-314 was not effective in blocking action potentials, whereas the intracellular application of QX-314 exerted the significant effects. Surprisingly, however, Lim et al. [31] recently reported that extracellularly applied QX-314 produced the long-lasting local anesthesia with a slow onset in guinea pigs and mice, challenging the conventional notion that charged molecular species are inactive when administered from the external side of cells [32].

Tsuchiya and Mizogami [20] compared the interactivity of lidocaine and QX-314 with biomimetic model membranes by measuring DPH fluorescence polarization. Lidocaine increased the membrane fluidity of liposomes consisting of 100 mol% DPPC and POPC, but not QX-314. These comparative results agree with previous reports that charged local anesthetics were ineffective on cell membranes when applied extracellularly [32]. On the other hand, QX-314 was revealed to decrease the DPH polarization values of both nerve cell-mimetic membranes and liposomal membranes consisting of POPS, 1-palmitoyl-2-oleoyl-*sn*-glycero-3-phosphate (POPA), 1-palmitoyl-2-oleoyl-*sn*-glycero-3-[phospho-*rac*-(1-glycerol)] (POPG), or cardiolipin and to show almost the same membrane-fluidizing effect as lidocaine [20]. Membrane lipid components and their compositions are very likely to determine whether the charged molecules of local anesthetics can modify membrane physicochemical properties or not.

5.2. Interaction with Specific Phospholipids. A zwitterion is a neutral molecule with positive and negative electrical charge within the molecule. The major membrane phospholipids are zwitterions with the polar head groups consisting of anionic phosphate and cationic quaternary ammonium centers (Figure 4). When comparing phospholipid species, QX-314 was not effective in changing the fluidity of biomimetic membranes consisting of zwitterionic phospholipids such as DPPC, POPC, and POPE [20]. POPS has an additional carboxyl group, neither POPA nor POPC has an ammonium group, and cardiolipin has two phosphate groups. QX-314 significantly decreased the DPH polarization values of biomimetic membranes containing these anionic phospholipids to produce the membrane fluidization as well as lidocaine [20]. Amphiphilic drugs like local anesthetics cause not only the hydrophobic interaction with phospholipid aliphatic acyl chains but also the electrostatic interaction with phospholipid polar head groups. The difference between anionic and zwitterionic phospholipid membranes suggests the electrostatic interaction between positively charged anesthetic molecules and negatively chargeable phospholipid head groups. The interaction of local anesthetics with specific membrane phospholipids also provides a mechanistic clue to explain their structure-dependent cardiotoxicity as described in Section 7.2.

6. Change of Membrane Interactivity

6.1. Anesthetic Efficacy Reduced by Inflammation. Inflammatory diseases alter the pharmacodynamics and pharmacokinetics of various drugs, resulting in a decrease in their beneficial effects and/or an increase in their adverse effects [33, 34]. Such an alteration by inflammation is well known in clinical dentistry, where the local anesthetic failure or the difficulty to obtain satisfactory analgesia commonly occurs in the situations of pulpitis and apical periodontitis [2]. The anesthetic efficacy of lidocaine, mepivacaine, and articaine injections is remarkably reduced in the teeth with pulpitis [35, 36]. The presence of inflammation in dental pulp was reported to cause the inferior alveolar nerve block to fail in approximately 30–45% of cases [37].

6.2. Verification of Conventional Acidosis Theory. Acidic metabolites like lactic acid are increasingly produced and concentrated in inflamed tissues, thereby inducing the acidosis that lowers the tissue pH at least the order of 0.5–1.0 pH unit [38, 39]. The p*Ka* values of almost all of local anesthetics in dental use are larger than 7.5 at 37°C [1], so a greater proportion of administered drugs exist as positively charged molecules in and near inflammatory lesions. Because cationic molecules are much less in membrane permeability and membrane interactivity under acidic conditions, the local anesthetic effects should be remarkably decreased, leading to the mechanistic theory that the local anesthetic efficacy is reduced by inflammatory tissue acidosis. This acidosis theory has been conventionally accepted due to its theoretical simplicity and understandability and most frequently cited for explaining the reduction of local anesthetic efficacy. However, even the fundamental subject as to whether local anesthetics decreasingly interact with lipid bilayers under acidic conditions has not been experimentally confirmed.

Tsuchiya et al. [40, 41] compared the membrane effects of local anesthetics with lowering the reaction pH and varying the composition of membrane lipids. When liposomal membranes consisting of 100 mol% DPPC were treated at pH 5.9–7.4 with lidocaine, prilocaine, and bupivacaine of 0.05–0.2% (w/v), all of the tested local anesthetics increased the membrane fluidity in 15 minutes almost corresponding to their onset time. Compared with pH 7.4, however, their membrane effects were significantly decreased at pH 6.4 that is almost comparable to inflamed tissue conditions [38]. Such a pH dependence in DPPC membranes supports the acidosis theory.

On the other hand, lidocaine, prilocaine, and bupivacaine of 0.05–0.2% (w/v) were revealed to interact even at pH 6.4 with nerve cell-mimetic membranes prepared with POPC, POPE, POPS, SM, and cholesterol, resulting in a significant increase in the membrane fluidity [40, 41]. Their membrane-fluidizing effects under acidic conditions are in conflict with the conventional acidosis theory. Local anesthetics showed less fluidizing effects at pH 6.4 on liposomal membranes consisting of DPPC, POPC, POPE and SM, whereas their effects on POPS liposomal membranes were significantly greater at pH 6.4, contradicting the relative decrease of uncharged molecules, but correlating to the relative increase of charged molecules. Phospholipid DPPC, POPC, POPE, and SM are zwitterionic, but POPS is acidic. Under acidic conditions, the cationic moieties of local anesthetics are likely to electrostatically interact with the anionic head groups of acidic phospholipids, resulting in the modification of membrane fluidity. Therefore, the tissue acidosis is not necessarily related to the local anesthetic efficacy reduced by inflammation.

Punnia-Moorthy [38] revealed that inflamed tissues lower only the order of 0.5 pH unit. In animal experiments, the tissues were found to rapidly buffer the excess acidity after acidic solution infiltrations and such a pH-buffering ability was more potent in inflamed tissues [42]. These pathophysiological features are also unfavorable for the conventional mechanism based on tissue acidosis.

6.3. Possible Mechanism Alternative to Acidosis. Peroxynitrite has been implicated in the pathogenesis of various diseases including inflammation. Inflammatory cells produce peroxynitrite by the reaction between nitric oxide and superoxide anion, both of which are present in inflamed tissues. Peroxynitrite is also known to react with lidocaine and bupivacaine [43, 44]. Ueno et al. [41] focused on inflammatory peroxynitrite responsible for the local anesthetic failure of inflamed tissues. They treated nerve cell-mimetic membranes with lidocaine, prilocaine, and bupivacaine of 0.05–0.2% (w/v) together with 50 μM peroxynitrite at pH 7.4 and 6.4. The following DPH fluorescence polarization measurements showed that the membrane-fluidizing effects of local anesthetics were inhibited by the peroxynitrite treatment. Such inhibitions are causable by peroxynitrite directly acting on anesthetic molecules [45] and indirectly on membrane lipids [46].

Since local anesthetic solutions are injected relatively near to acutely inflamed tissues in dental anesthesia [14], peroxynitrite could interfere with the maxillary and mandibular nerve block by local anesthetics. Inflammation possibly produces hyperexcitability or hyperalgesia [47, 48]. The absorption of local anesthetics into the circulatory system to remove them from the administered site is promoted in inflammatory lesions [42]. In addition to these pathophysiological changes, inflammatory peroxynitrite is responsible for reducing the efficacy of topical and infiltration anesthesia.

7. Membrane Interaction Associated with Cardiotoxicity

7.1. Adverse Effects of Local Anesthetics. The administration of local anesthetics is accompanied by the potential risk that is rare but could be fatal complication. The adverse effects of local anesthetics include systemic and local toxic reactions and allergic reactions mostly related to ester-type drugs. The systemic toxicity occurs in the cardiovascular and central nervous system, while the local toxicity may lead to neurotoxicity, transient neurological symptom, or myotoxicity [49]. The cardiovascular system toxicity of commonly used amide local anesthetics has been clinically of much interest since the report of cardiotoxic effects of bupivacaine and etidocaine [50].

Local anesthetics, especially bupivacaine, cause cardiac disorders that consist of the initial depression of intraventricular conduction followed by reentrant arrhythmia. Great concerns over their cardiotoxicity include profound bradycardia, arrhythmia, myocardial depression, and eventually cardiovascular collapse, which are induced when the drug concentrations in blood are elevated by an accidental intravenous injection and an absolute overdose. Although bupivacaine has been widely used for cutaneous infiltration, regional nerve block, epidural anesthesia, and spinal anesthesia in surgery and obstetrics, this long-acting agent is greater in toxicity compared with shorter-acting amide local anesthetics. The rank order of cardiotoxic potency has been estimated to be bupivacaine > ropivacaine > lidocaine > prilocaine [51]. However, the detailed mechanism(s) for structure-specific or structure-dependent cardiotoxicity has not been clear.

7.2. Interaction with Membrane Cardiolipin. Although myocardial ion channels are referred to as the primary target of local anesthetics, another site of toxic action is assumed to contribute to the cardiotoxicity discrimination between structurally different drugs. Besides binding to ion channels, local anesthetics act on membrane lipids to modify permeability, fluidity, lipid packing order, and lipid phase transition of biomembranes [22, 23, 52]. The inhibitory effects of anesthetic agents on ionic current generations also require the molecular interplay of ion channel proteins and membrane lipids [53].

As cardiotoxic drugs affect the permeability of mitochondrial membranes, local anesthetics also act on lipid bilayers and increase the membrane permeability with the potency correlating to the seriousness of cardiotoxicity. Önyüksel et al. [22] reported that bupivacaine concentration-dependently increased at 100–400 μM the release of carboxyfluorescein from 7.5 mol% cardiolipin-containing liposomes composed of egg yolk phosphatidylcholine and cholesterol, although it showed no significant effects on the membrane permeability of liposomes devoid of cardiolipin. Tsuchiya et al. [23] found that bupivacaine, ropivacaine, lidocaine, and prilocaine increase at 10–300 μM the fluidity of biomimetic membranes with the potency being cardiolipin- ≫ POPA- > POPG- > POPS-containing membranes and that their membrane effects were increased with elevating the anionic phospholipid content in membranes. They also revealed that local anesthetics interact with biomimetic membranes containing 2.5–12.5 mol% cardiolipin to show the rank order of membrane fluidization being bupivacaine ≫ ropivacaine > lidocaine > prilocaine, which agrees with their relative cardiotoxicity.

Since local anesthetics predominantly exist as positively charged molecules at physiological pH, they should electrostatically interact with anionic phospholipids. With respect to the polar head structure, DOPG and POPA have one phosphate group, whereas cardiolipin has two phosphate groups. In the comparative study of anionic phospholipid membranes [23], the relative DPH polarization change induced by bupivacaine was 1.00, 0.40, and 0.49 for 10 mol% cardiolipin-, 10 mol% POPG-, and 10 mol% POPA-containing membranes, respectively, which is consistent with the structural constitution of a cardiolipin polar head group. Cardiolipin is localized in the mitochondrial membranes of cardiomyocytes to play an important role in heart functions, energy metabolism, and membrane dynamics [54]. A relation is presumed between the interaction with mitochondrial membrane cardiolipin and the induction of cardiotoxic effects.

Groban et al. [24] reported that when open-chest dogs were received the incremental infusions of local anesthetics, free and total plasma concentrations at the cardiovascular collapse were 10–38 and 39–100 μM for bupivacaine, 36–142 and 64–163 μM for ropivacaine, and 162–754 and 276–847 μM for lidocaine. While dosing dogs with bupivacaine 7.2–8.8 mg/kg caused cardiac arrhythmia, the plasma concentrations of free and total bupivacaine reached 4 and 17 μM, respectively [25]. In the range of cardiotoxic concentrations, bupivacaine interacts with 2.5–12.5 mol% cardiolipin-containing membranes more intensively and induce the greater membrane fluidization compared with other local anesthetics [23].

Bupivacaine is more hydrophobic than ropivacaine, lidocaine, and prilocaine [18]. The high hydrophobicity of bupivacaine is linked to its strong attraction to myocardial sodium channels, slow dissociation from sodium channels, and access to mitochondrial membranes [55]. The rank order of interactivity with cardiolipin-containing membranes is also correlated to that of cardiotoxicity being bupivacaine > ropivacaine > lidocaine > prilocaine. Since bupivacaine can readily reach mitochondrial membranes even when applied on the outside of cells, the interaction with cardiomyocyte mitochondrial membranes would be responsible for the structure-specific cardiotoxic effects of local anesthetics. A crucial role of anionic phospholipids like cardiolipin in the interaction between local anesthetics and membrane lipids may also lead to the therapeutic possibility for local anesthetic cardiotoxicity [56] as described in Section 7.3.

7.3. Treatment of Cardiotoxicity with Lipid Emulsion. Although newly introduced ropivacaine and levobupivacaine are less toxic, they still cause the life-threatening events, so the cardiotoxicity of long-acting local anesthetics remains an important problem. The property of local anesthetics to hydrophobically interact with or selectively bind to membrane lipids may provide a novel strategy for treating their cardiotoxicity. Weinberg et al. [57] reported that the treatment with a lipid infusion shifted the dose response to bupivacaine-induced asystole of rats and dogs to increase the bupivacaine lethal doses. Since then, the rapid infusion of lipid emulsions has been performed to treat the local anesthetic systemic toxicity in animal models and humans [58–60]. The successful resuscitation of local anesthetic-induced cardiovascular collapse was achieved by an intravenous lipid infusion [61], whereas the failure of a lipid emulsion to reverse local anesthetic-induced neurotoxicity is found in the literature [62].

For entrapping cardiotoxic drug molecules, the commonly used lipid emulsions are composed mainly of soy bean and egg phospholipids with triglycerides of varying chain lengths. There are several lipid emulsions available such as Intralipid, Medialipide, Structolipid, and so forth [63]. Although many case reports support the use of an intravenous lipid infusion for the cardiotoxicity of bupivacaine, levobupivacaine, and ropivacaine, the mode of action of this treatment is not fully apparent. One of proposed mechanisms is the "lipid sink" theory, in which the more hydrophobic (lipid soluble) are drug molecules, the greater are their bindings to lipid emulsions, enabling the emulsions to act like a sink that drains cardiotoxic local anesthetics from plasma [60, 63]. This theory is supported by the comparative emulsification degrees of bupivacaine, levobupivacaine, and ropivacaine in the decreasing order, which correlate to the cardiotoxic intensities [64]. The Association of Anesthetists of Great Britain and Ireland released the guidelines for using a lipid rescue therapy [65].

7.4. Cardiotoxicity Enhanced by Ischemia. Ischemia potentiates the cardiotoxic effects of local anesthetics and hastens the onset of fibrillation induced by local anesthetics. The electrical ventricular fibrillation thresholds of bupivacaine and ropivacaine were decreased during myocardial ischemia [66]. Pacini et al. [67] revealed that the effect of lidocaine on sheep Purkinje fibers is greater under simulated ischemia than that in normal conditions. Freysz et al. [68] also reported that the risk of cardiac disorders in bupivacaine anesthesia was increased by ischemia. However, the detailed mechanism remains unclear for the local anesthetic cardiotoxicity altered by ischemia. Myocardial ischemia is characterized by a significant lowering of tissue pH to 6.5 or less [69]. Since local anesthetics show greater cardiotoxic, not anesthetic, effects in the presence of acidosis [70], their enhanced cardiotoxicity may be related to ischemic acidic conditions. While local anesthetics block sodium channels to decrease the excitability of myocardia and cause the cardiac malfunction, it has been controversial whether their blocking potency is reduced or enhanced at acidic pH. Tan and Saint [4] reported that the block of cardiac sodium channels by lidocaine was decreased by lowering the pH.

In the comparative study of Tsuchiya et al. [71], bupivacaine and lidocaine of cardiotoxically relevant concentrations interacted with liposomal membranes consisting of 100 mol% DPPC and peripheral nerve cell-mimetic membranes to increase the membrane fluidity, and their membrane effects were decreased by lowering the pH from 7.4 to 5.9. In contrast, the fluidizing effects of bupivacaine and lidocaine on mitochondria-mimetic membranes were reversely increased at pH 5.9–6.4 compared with those at pH 7.4. Such increases under acidic conditions were greater in the biomimetic membranes that contained the substantial amounts of cardiolipin and phosphatidylserine. Positively charged bupivacaine and lidocaine are presumed to interact with the negatively charged head groups of phospholipids, thereby increasing their membrane effects at acidic pH. The interactivity with cardiolipin-containing mitochondrial membranes, which is enhanced by lowering the pH, is associated with the local anesthetic cardiotoxicity enhanced by cardiac ischemia-relating acidosis.

Besides ischemic acidosis, reactive oxygen species [72] and mitochondrial membrane cardiolipin [54] may be also responsible for enhancing local anesthetic cardiotoxicity. Ischemic and reperfused myocardia produce nitric oxide simultaneously with generating superoxide anion, both of which react to form peroxynitrite that pathologically contributes to the myocardial ischemia-reperfusion injury by peroxidizing membrane lipids [73]. The peroxidation of membrane lipids is accompanied by a change in fluidity of liposomal and biological membranes. Cardiolipin constitutes a significant portion of total mitochondrial phospholipids in mammalian cardiomyocytes and plays an important physiological role for hearts. Since hydrophobic local anesthetics readily reach mitochondrial membranes even when applied extracellularly, they can interact with membrane cardiolipin.

Tsuchiya et al. [74] treated biomimetic model membranes of varying lipid compositions with peroxynitrite and local anesthetics separately or in combination. They found that peroxynitrite reacts with the membranes to decrease the membrane fluidity with the potency being cardiolipin- > SAPC- > DPPC-containing membranes. Biomimetic membranes treated with 0.1–10 μM peroxynitrite were more rigid by increasing the membrane cardiolipin content from 0 to 30 mol%, suggesting that cardiolipin is a possible target for peroxynitrite. Cardiolipin in cardiomyocyte mitochondrial membranes preferentially reacts with peroxynitrite [75]. While the peroxidizability of membrane lipids is enhanced as a function of the number of double bonds in lipid molecules, cardiolipin in mammalian cells predominantly contains linoleic acid (C18 : 2) as a side-chain fatty acid [76]. Linoleic acid constitutes 80–90% acyl chains of cardiolipin and tetralinoleoyl cardiolipin is the most common molecular species in cardiomyocyte mitochondrial membranes. Because of its high unsaturation degree, cardiolipin is more susceptible to peroxynitrite compared with other membrane-constituting unsaturated phospholipids. Bupivacaine and lidocaine of each 200 μM were revealed to exert the greater fluidizing effects on biomimetic membranes containing 10 mol% cardiolipin by pretreating the membranes with 0.1 and 1 μM peroxynitrite [74], which is attributable to the membrane rigidity enhanced by peroxynitrite. The drug and membrane interaction is essentially influenced by the inherent fluidity of membranes as bupivacaine and ropivacaine are more effective in fluidizing the membranes that contain a certain amount of membrane-rigidifying cholesterol [77]. Local anesthetics have the property to exert greater membrane-fluidizing effects on the relatively rigid (less fluid) membranes than those on the relatively fluid (less rigid) ones. Peroxynitrite preferentially decreases the fluidity of cardiolipin-containing biomembranes and the resulting membranes are susceptible to the interaction with local anesthetics, which may be partly associated with the local anesthetic cardiotoxicity enhanced by myocardial ischemia.

One may interpret that the membrane effects of bupivacaine and lidocaine lead to the protection against myocardial ischemic insults, not the cardiotoxicity. The cardioprotective effects of local anesthetics were recently revealed to be mediated by their antioxidant and antiapoptotic activities [78, 79]. Although membrane-fluidizing bupivacaine and lidocaine can counteract the membrane rigidification by peroxynitrite, their membrane interactivities are not correlated to such activities [44, 79]. Membrane lipids are completely peroxidized in a very short time by peroxynitrite, resulting in the structural and functional changes of membrane-constituting cardiolipin [80]. The interaction of local anesthetics with peroxynitrite-treated membranes seems to relate to their cardiotoxic effects, not cardioprotective ones. The membrane interactivity of lidocaine was enhanced when mitochondria-mimetic membranes containing cardiolipin were pretreated with ischemic peroxynitrite, but reduced when nerve cell-mimetic membranes not containing cardiolipin were treated with inflammatory peroxynitrite [46], suggesting that the presence or absence of cardiolipin determines whether the membrane interaction of local anesthetics is increased or decreased.

Myocardial ischemia decreases the content of cardiolipin in mitochondria. The 20–25% depletion was indicated for cardiolipin in rabbit heart subsarcolemmal mitochondria [81]. The effects of local anesthetics on membrane fluidity and permeability are influenced by the composition of cardiolipin in membranes [22, 23]. The responsibility of the membrane interaction for local anesthetic cardiotoxicity may be influenced to some degree by varying cardiolipin membrane content.

8. Discrimination between Stereoisomers

8.1. Local Anesthetic Stereoisomers. More than 50% of currently used drugs are composed of chiral compounds, about 90% of which have been clinically administered as a racemate (racemic mixture) consisting of an equimolar mixture of enantiomers [82]. The chirality of drug molecules generally arises due to the presence of an asymmetric carbon. Enantiomers are a pair of stereoisomers that are mirror images of each other and not superimposable, called chiral.

Drug enantiomers are discriminable in qualitative and quantitative pharmacology. Typically, one enantiomer is more active or more toxic than its enantiomeric counterpart, antipode. Stereoselectivity (selectivity to one stereoisomer) is linked to the clinical advantage of using a single enantiomer over its antipode and racemate, which increases the beneficial effect and decreases the adverse effect. Since the clinical use in the 1960s, bupivacaine had been widely marketed as a racemic mixture of bupivacaine (*rac*-bupivacaine) that consists of equimolar enantiomers: *S*(−)-bupivacaine of the levorotatory configuration and *R*(+)-bupivacaine of the dextrorotatory configuration (Figure 5). In the 1990s, however, an urgent problem of its cardiotoxic effects led to the first development of an *S*(−)-enantiomeric local anesthetic, less toxic ropivacaine [83]. This trend was followed by the introduction of levobupivacaine into clinical practice as a pure *S*(−)-enantiomer of bupivacaine [84].

Vladimirov et al. [85] indicated the inhibition ratio of rat neuronal channels to be 1 : 1.3–3 for *S*(−)-bupivacaine and *R*(+)-bupivacaine. Lyons et al. [86] also reported that the relative analgesic effect of *S*(−)-bupivacaine to *rac*-bupivacaine was 0.87 for epidural pain relief in labor. Lim et al. [87] found the stereoselectivity that the analgesic effect of *rac*-bupivacaine is greater than *S*(−)-bupivacaine for patients in labor, while Vladimirov et al. [85] showed that the in vivo nerve block by bupivacaine was less enantioselective (selective to one enantiomer) at clinically used concentrations.

Compared with the analgesic potency, local anesthetics show a greater difference in cardiotoxicity between stereoisomers [51]. Graf et al. [88] found that an *R*(+)-enantiomer prolongs the atrioventricular conduction time

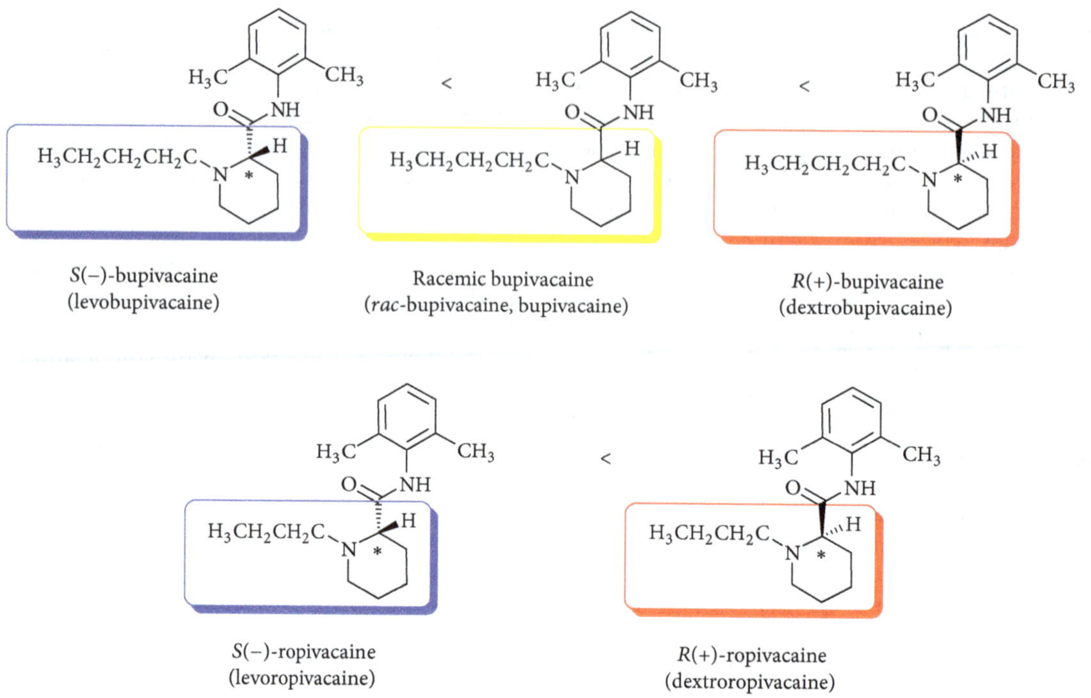

FIGURE 5: Local anesthetic stereoisomers and their relative cardiotoxicity.

more significantly than a racemate and an $S(-)$-enantiomer in isolated guinea pig hearts perfused with 0.5–10 μM bupivacaine stereoisomers. The relative atrioventricular time was 1.54 for $R(+)$-bupivacaine and 1.30 for *rac*-bupivacaine versus 1.00 for $S(-)$-bupivacaine in the perfusion of each 10 μM. Groban et al. [24] carried out the incremental escalating infusions of local anesthetics on open-chest dogs to the point of cardiovascular collapse. Consequently, they found that the mortality is lidocaine, ropivacaine, $S(-)$-bupivacaine, and *rac*-bupivacaine in the increasing order and that the comparative cardiotoxicity is 1.7 for *rac*-bupivacaine versus 1.0 for $S(-)$-bupivacaine. Morrison et al. [89] determined the electrocardiographic cardiotoxic effects of bupivacaine stereoisomers on swine injected with increasing anesthetic doses and showed that the relative median lethal dose was 1.87 for $S(-)$-bupivacaine versus 1.00 for *rac*-bupivacaine.

The major mode of action of local anesthetics is referred to as the block of sodium, potassium, and calcium channels in the nervous and cardiovascular system. Valenzuela et al. [90] found that bupivacaine blocks the relevant sodium channels so enantioselectively that $R(+)$-enantiomer is 1.2–1.7 times more potent than $S(-)$-enantiomer in isolated guinea pig ventricular myocytes. Valenzuela et al. [91] also reported that the relative potency to block cloned human cardiac potassium channels was 1.6 for $R(+)$-bupivacaine versus 1.0 for $S(-)$-bupivacaine. Pharmacological studies have been exclusively focusing on the interactions of local anesthetics with proteinous ion channels, receptors, and enzymes. This is mainly due to the stereostructure-specific actions on functional proteins that can be understood by the enantioselective affinity of drugs for proteins [83]. However, the protein-interacting theory does not fully explain the pharmacodynamic difference between bupivacaine stereoisomers, requiring an alternative or additional explanation for the discriminable effects of local anesthetic stereoisomers.

8.2. Enantioselective Membrane Interactivity. Tsuchiya and Mizogami [20] reported that local anesthetic stereoisomers increased the fluidity of nerve cell-mimetic membranes with the potency being $S(-)$-enantiomer < racemate < $R(+)$-enantiomer and also the fluidity of cardiomyocyte-mimetic membranes with the potency being $S(-)$-ropivacaine < $S(-)$-bupivacaine < $R(+)$-bupivacaine. However, these stereoisomers were not discriminated in interactivity with the membranes devoid of cholesterol. When 40 mol% and more cholesterol were contained in membranes, the membrane interactivity was $S(-)$-bupivacaine < *rac*-bupivacaine < $R(+)$-bupivacaine and $S(-)$-ropivacaine < $R(+)$-ropivacaine, which agreed with the rank order of their cardiotoxicity [77]. Mizogami et al. [92] also reported that bupivacaine stereostructure-specifically interacted with biomimetic membranes containing cholesterol to show the relative potency consistent with the clinical features of bupivacaine stereoisomers. Membrane cholesterol is essential to the enantiomeric discrimination of local anesthetics.

The membrane lipid-interacting theory is still controversial as to whether local anesthetics actually act on biomembranes at cardiotoxically relevant concentrations. At 5–200 μM covering the free plasma concentrations for bupivacaine stereoisomers to cause cardiovascular collapse [24], Tsuchiya and Mizogami [93] proved that bupivacaine stereoisomers are able to modify the fluidity of cardiomyocyte-mimetic membranes even at low micromolar concentrations with the potency being $S(-)$-bupivacaine < *rac*-bupivacaine < $R(+)$-bupivacaine. While the bupivacaine-induced changes in DPH fluorescence polarization are considered relevant to the clinical effects [23], the difference between stereoisomers varied depending on their tested concentrations [93], which may account for the inconsistent results of previous studies. The comparative effects of $R(+)$-bupivacaine, *rac*-bupivacaine, and $S(-)$-bupivacaine to produce arrhythmia and cardiovascular collapse differed in experimental and clinical studies [24, 51, 89]. An analgesic effect of *rac*-bupivacaine was greater than that of $S(-)$-bupivacaine in humans [87], whereas bupivacaine was much less enantioselective in the in vivo rat nerve block at clinically used concentrations [85]. When comparing the blocking effects on human nerves, $S(-)$-bupivacaine showed an almost similar potency to *rac*-bupivacaine [84]. These inconsistencies are attributable to the concentration-dependent enantiomeric discrimination that the difference in membrane interactivity between $R(+)$-bupivacaine and $S(-)$-bupivacaine steeply increases at concentrations lower than 50 μM [93].

8.3. Chirality of Lipid Membranes. Because drug enantiomers absolutely differ in spatial configuration, they should behave differently when interacting with chiral systems, while not being in achiral environments such as an aqueous solution. In fact, enantiomeric compounds of each other show the different interaction with other compounds that are also enantiomers. Almost all of substances in the body are composed of enantiomeric biocompounds, therefore chiral drugs could interact enantioselectively with such chiral macromolecular targets. The conventional protein-interacting theory emphasizes the importance of proteinous acting sites because proteins are entirely made up of L-amino acids, not D-amino acids. Drug enantiomers form the different spatial relationship in the asymmetric environments of functional proteins that are composed of only L-amino acids. However, the action of enantiomeric local anesthetics on ion channels is not necessarily consistent with the stereoselectivity that an $R(+)$-enantiomer is more potent than an $S(-)$-enantiomer. Previous comparisons showed that $S(-)$-bupivacaine blocked ion channels with the potency equal to or greater than *rac*-bupivacaine [94, 95].

Considering that amphiphilic drugs pharmacodynamically and pharmacokinetically interact with lipid bilayers, it is reasonable to presume that membrane lipids could play a significant role in the in vivo discriminative recognition of such drug molecules. Local anesthetics penetrate into membrane lipid bilayers, align between phospholipid acyl chains, and occupy the space to perturb the phospholipid acyl chain alignment. If local anesthetics stereostructure-specifically interact with chiral components in lipid bilayers, they would modify membrane fluidity with the potency being different between stereoisomers. Tsuchiya and Mizogami [96] hypothesized that drugs interact enantioselectively with chiral lipid membranes to induce membrane fluidity, order, and permeability changes that were discriminable between drug enantiomers. The enantioselective lipid environments to discriminate stereoisomers may be provided by phospholipids and/or cholesterol with the chirality.

The enantiomeric discrimination arises from the direct interaction with chiral centers. Based on the hypothesis that a chiral carbon in their glycerol backbone may allow phospholipids to behave as a chiral component in membranes, phospholipids were speculated to interact preferentially with molecules having the same chirality and exhibit the selectivity to one enantiomer over its counterpart [97]. However, any membrane phospholipids were not found to produce the discrimination of local anesthetic $S(-)$-enantiomers from their antipodes [77]. Compared with phospholipids, cholesterol has much more chiral carbons. It is very likely that cholesterol enhances the chirality of lipid bilayers and its absolute configuration modulates the membrane stereoselectivity [98].

In comparisons of the membrane interactivity between bupivacaine stereoisomers [20, 77, 93], the used probe DPH partitions into the center of lipid bilayers [92], the membrane component cholesterol is located in lipid bilayers with its backbone embedded in the hydrocarbon core [99], and bupivacaine is preferentially localized in the hydrophobic membrane core [19]. Different polarization changes are attributed to the enantioselective interaction of bupivacaine, not to the differential affinity of bupivacaine enantiomers for specific membrane regions. The opposite configurations are considered to allow drug enantiomers to be discriminated by their interaction with another chiral molecule in biomembranes. Membrane cholesterol contributes to such an enantioselective interaction by increasing the chirality of lipid bilayers. The stereostructure and membrane interactivity relationship supports the clinical use of $S(-)$-enantiomers to decrease the adverse effects of local anesthetics on the cardiovascular system.

9. Interaction Preference for Membrane Microdomain Lipid Rafts

In the late 1990s, the fluid mosaic model of Singer and Nicholson for biomembranes was evolved to a more sophisticated concept, especially concerning the membrane lipid composition and molecular organization. It has become clear that biomembranes are not the simple bilayer structure with uniformly distributed lipids but organized into phase-separated microdomains, called lipid rafts, with specific lipid components and molecular dynamics that differ from the surrounding liquid crystalline phase and bulk membranes [100]. In lipid rafts, cholesterol and sphingolipids are packed in a highly ordered structure (liquid ordered) distinct from the rest of membranes (liquid disordered). There is accumulating evidence to indicate that lipid rafts are the target of various drugs including general anesthetic agents [101]. However, the interaction of local anesthetics with membrane microdomain lipid rafts is unclear.

Ion channels, β-adrenergic receptors, and signaling proteins were discovered to be localized to membrane microdomains within the cardiovascular system [102, 103]. Drugs and chemicals were also revealed to initiate and facilitate their effects by interacting with membrane microdomain lipid rafts [104, 105]. As one of possible pharmacological mechanisms, it is of much interest to know whether local anesthetics more intensively or selectively interact with the lipid rafts surrounding ion channels compared with overall lipid bilayers. Kamata et al. [106] recently reported that lidocaine disrupted the raft structures in human erythrocyte membranes. They also reported that lidocaine reversibly prevented the raft formation in human erythrocyte membranes, suggesting the involvement of raft-related signal transduction in the mode of local anesthetic action [107].

In order to verify the hypothesis that local anesthetics could interact preferentially with lipid rafts over nonraft membranes, Tsuchiya et al. [108] compared the effects of 50–200 μM local anesthetics on raft model membranes, cardiolipin-containing biomimetic membranes, and cardiomyocyte mitochondria-mimetic membranes. Local anesthetics interacted with nonraft membranes to increase the membrane fluidity with the potency being *R*(+)-bupivacaine > *rac*-bupivacaine > *S*(−)-bupivacaine > ropivacaine > lidocaine > prilocaine, which is consistent with the rank order of cardiotoxic potency. These local anesthetics also acted on raft-like liquid-ordered membranes, but any raft model membranes showed neither drug structure dependence nor stereoselectivity in membrane interaction, leading to the conclusion that the mechanistic relevance of membrane microdomain lipid rafts to local anesthetics is questionable at least in their effects on raft model membranes. Bandeiras et al. [109] also reported that lidocaine interacted with raft model membranes, although its interactivity was weaker compared with nonraft membranes.

10. Anesthetic and Phytochemical Membrane Interaction

10.1. Drug Interaction with Phytochemicals. While the concomitant use of medicines with medicinal plants or herbs has been increasing in popularity, it potentially causes the beneficial or adverse drug interaction with plant components. Unlike the drug-drug interaction, however, the interaction between drugs and phytochemicals (bioactive chemical substances in plants) has not been extensively investigated despite the possibility of more frequent occurrence than expected [110]. Various drugs appear to show the antagonistic, additive, and synergistic interactions with phytochemicals [111].

10.2. Capsaicin. Topical or systemic lidocaine therapy is expected to provide a novel management of neuropathic pain symptoms together with enhancing the utility by combining with capsaicin [112]. Capsaicin, 8-methyl-*N*-vanillyl-6-nonenamide, is a pungent component of plants belonging to the genus *Capsicum* such as chili pepper. On the initial application, this phytochemical shows an excitatory effect to produce burning pain and hyperalgesia, whereas with the repeated or prolonged application it shows an inhibitory effect on the receptive terminals of nociceptors. Capsaicin activates a transient receptor potential vanilloid (TRPV1) receptor, which belongs to a family of TRP channels, to exert an analgesic or algesic effect depending on its concentrations [113]. Capsaicin-activating TRPV1 receptor is a nonselective cation channel that plays an important role to modulate the nociceptive and pain transmission in the peripheral and central nervous system [114, 115]. Besides the use as a food additive in spicy cuisines, capsaicin is currently used for the therapy to treat painful conditions such as diabetic neuropathy and rheumatoid arthritis.

Binshtok et al. [116] suggested that capsaicin could transport a sodium channel blocker QX-314 to nociceptors through the activation of TRPV1 channels and produce the nociceptive-selective analgesia. In their whole-cell voltage-clamp recordings from rat dorsal root ganglion neurons, externally applied QX-314 showed no effects on the sodium channel activity of small sensory neurons when it was applied alone. By applying together with capsaicin, however, QX-314 blocked sodium channels to induce a long-lasting reduction of pain sensitivity. Ries et al. [117] found that a TRPV1 receptor agonist capsaicin accelerates the onset kinetics of QX-314 in a mouse tail-flick test, whereas a TRPV1 receptor antagonist capsazepine decreases the nerve blocking efficacy of QX-314. Permanently charged cationic QX-314 cannot pass through the lipid bilayers of cell membranes but can gain an access to the cell interior through TRPV1 channels that are opened by capsaicin (Figure 6). Once inside, QX-314 is able to bind to the acting site on sodium channels. Shen et al. [118] reported that the peripheral block of nociceptive afferents by QX-314 combined with capsaicin was effective in reducing neuropathic pain. It was also suggested that capsaicin could be applied in combination with bupivacaine and lidocaine instead of QX-314 [119]. Because the transmembrane access rout for QX-314 occurs only on nociceptors, the combination of QX-314 or local anesthetics with capsaicin is expected to produce the ideal analgesia affecting pain alone or the pain-restricted local anesthesia preserving motor and autonomic responses [120]. Shin et al. [121, 122] found that capsaicin significantly potentiates at 50 μM the rat sciatic nerve block by lidocaine. The cooperative drug interaction with capsaicin also would be useful for increasing and prolonging local anesthetic effects.

Capsaicin acts on lipid bilayers to modify the membrane fluidity as well as local anesthetics and QX-314 [123]. Experimental data show that capsaicin interacts with nerve cell-mimetic membranes to change the membrane fluidity and that the combined use with 50 μM capsaicin additively increases the membrane effects of lidocaine and bupivacaine of clinically relevant concentrations [124]. Capsaicin may influence the effects of local anesthetics by cooperatively enhancing their interactivity with biomembranes.

10.3. Phloretin. Flavonoid phloretin is a polyphenol primarily contained in apples and their products, which has been suggested to possess the antioxidant and cancer-preventive activity [125]. Tsuchiya and Mizogami [124] reported the membrane interaction between phloretin and local anesthetics. They treated biomimetic model membranes with lidocaine, bupivacaine, or phloretin alone and in combination and then determined the membrane fluidity changes by

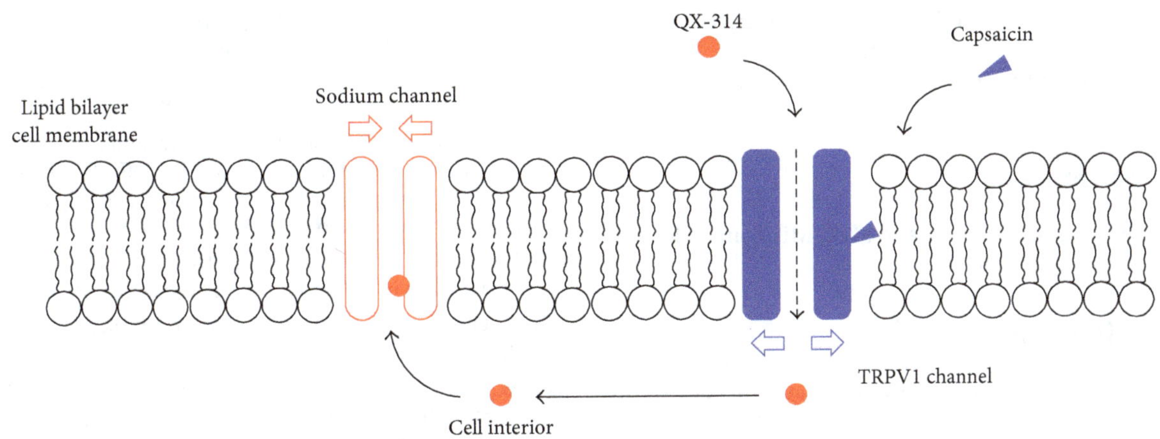

FIGURE 6: Combined use of QX-314 and capsaicin.

measuring DPH fluorescence polarization. Consequently, phloretin was revealed to act on nerve cell-mimetic membranes and decrease the membrane fluidity in contrast to local anesthetics increasing the membrane fluidity. The combined use with 25 μM phloretin antagonistically inhibited the membrane effects of lidocaine and bupivacaine of clinically relevant concentrations. Phloretin was also reported to affect the membrane structure and the local anesthetic permeability of lipid monolayers and bilayers [126, 127].

A phloretin derivative (polymeric mixture of polyesters of phloretin and phosphoric acid) was found to shorten the duration time of infiltration anesthesia of guinea pigs by lidocaine, bupivacaine, and prilocaine and to terminate their local anesthetic effects [128]. Its local anesthetic-inhibitory effect was also proved in the infiltration anesthesia of human teeth [129]. As a clinical utility of the drug and phytochemical interaction, phloretin may be valuable to discontinue local anesthesia as soon as the treatment is completed.

11. Conclusions

Membrane-embedded ion channels, especially sodium channels, have been recognized to be primarily responsible for the pharmacologic and toxic effects of local anesthetics. However, the drug and lipid membrane interaction is not disregardable as the mode of local anesthetic action. While channel proteins have the affinity specific to individual ligand structures, they cannot necessarily interact with all of structurally different drugs. Membrane lipids also play an important role in the differential recognition of drug structures. A substantial number of administered local anesthetic molecules must be transported to the target through the lipid barriers of nerve sheaths and penetrate into or across the lipid bilayers of cell membranes. Amphiphilic local anesthetics hydrophobically and electrostatically interact with lipid bilayers to modify the fluidity of biomembranes with the potency correlating to the anesthetic activity and the cardiac toxicity. Such interactions result in not only the direct influence on membrane functions but also the influence on channel functions by changing the conformation of transmembrane proteins. Membrane components, phospholipids, and cholesterol, rich in molecular species and chirality, allow the membrane interaction of local anesthetics to be structure dependent and stereostructure selective.

The interaction between local anesthetics and membrane lipids would be associated with both the basic mechanisms for anesthetic and cardiotoxic effects and the clinical features such as the activity and toxicity altered by pathophysiological conditions, the cardiotoxicity varying by structural differences and discriminating between stereoisomers, the utility of a lipid emulsion to treat cardiotoxicity, and the combination with phytochemicals. The interaction with only functional proteins cannot explain all of the pharmacological and toxicological characteristics of local anesthetics nor can the interaction with only membrane lipids. Membrane lipid-interacting theory and membrane protein-interacting theory are complimentary to each other, suggesting the modified lipid-protein interaction mechanism for local anesthetics.

Abbreviations

DPH: 1,6-Diphenyl-1,3,5-hexatriene
DPPC: 1,2-Dipalmitoyl-*sn*-glycero-3-phosphocholine
n-AS: *n*-(9-Anthroyloxy)stearic acid ($n = 2, 6, 9$ and 12)
PNA: *N*-Phenyl-1-naphthylamine
POPA: 1-Palmitoyl-2-oleoyl-*sn*-glycero-3-phosphate
POPC: 1-Palmitoyl-2-oleoyl-*sn*-glycero-3-phosphocholine
POPE: 1-Palmitoyl-2-oleoyl-*sn*-glycero-3-phosphoethanolamine
POPG: 1-Palmitoyl-2-oleoyl-*sn*-glycero-3-[phospho-*rac*-(1-glycerol)]
POPI: 1-Palmitoyl-2-oleoyl-*sn*-glycero-3-phospho-(1′-myo-inositol)
POPS: 1-Palmitoyl-2-oleoyl-*sn*-glycero-3-[phospho-L-serine]
QX-314: *N*-Ethyl lidocaine
SM: Sphingomyelin

TMA-DPH: 1-(4-Trimethylammoniumphenyl)-6-phenyl-1,3,5-hexatriene
TRPV1 receptor: Transient receptor potential vanilloid receptor.

Conflict of Interests

The authors (Hironori Tsuchiya and Maki Mizogami) declare there is no conflict of interests.

Acknowledgments

This work was supported by grants-in-aid for Scientific Research 20592381 and 23593005 from Japan Society for the Promotion of Science and a grant from San-Ei Gen Foundation for Food Chemical Research.

References

[1] G. R. Strichartz, V. Sanchez, G. R. Arthur, R. Chafetz, and D. Martin, "Fundamental properties of local anesthetics. II. Measured octanol: buffer partition coefficients and pK_a values of clinically used drugs," *Anesthesia and Analgesia*, vol. 71, no. 2, pp. 158–170, 1990.

[2] A. B. López and M. P. Diago, "Failure of locoregional anesthesia in dental practice. Review of the literature," *Medicina Oral, Patología Oral y Cirugía Bucal*, vol. 11, no. 6, pp. E510–E513, 2006.

[3] D. E. Becker and K. L. Reed, "Essentials of local anesthetic pharmacology," *Anesthesia Progress*, vol. 53, no. 3, pp. 98–109, 2006.

[4] J. H. C. Tan and D. A. Saint, "Interaction of lidocaine with the cardiac sodium channel. Effects of low extracellular pH are consistent with an external blocking site," *Life Sciences*, vol. 67, no. 22, pp. 2759–2766, 2000.

[5] F. Yanagidate and G. R. Strichartz, "Local anesthetics," in *Handbook of Experimental Pharmacology*, vol. 177, pp. 95–127, Springer, Berlin, Germany, 2007.

[6] G. McCleane, "Intravenous lidocaine: an outdated or underutilized treatment for pain?" *Journal of Palliative Medicine*, vol. 10, no. 3, pp. 798–805, 2007.

[7] W. Kopeć, J. Telenius, and H. Khandelia, "Molecular dynamics simulations of the interactions of medicinal plant extracts and drugs with lipid bilayer membranes," *FEBS Journal*, vol. 280, no. 12, pp. 2785–2805, 2013.

[8] J. G. Paiva, P. Paradiso, A. P. Serro, A. Fernandes, and B. Saramago, "Interaction of local and general anaesthetics with liposomal membrane models: a QCM-D and DSC study," *Colloids and Surfaces B*, vol. 95, pp. 65–74, 2012.

[9] C. Högberg and A. P. Lyubartsev, "Effect of local anesthetic lidocaine on electrostatic properties of a lipid bilayer," *Biophysical Journal*, vol. 94, no. 2, pp. 525–531, 2008.

[10] M. Pasenkiewicz-Gierula, T. Róg, J. Grochowski et al., "Effects of a carane derivative local anesthetic on a phospholipid bilayer studied by molecular dynamics simulation," *Biophysical Journal*, vol. 85, no. 2, pp. 1248–1258, 2003.

[11] A. Alberola-Die, J. Martinez-Pinna, J. M. González-Ros, I. Ivorra, and A. Morales, "Multiple inhibitory actions of lidocaine on Torpedo nicotinic acetylcholine receptors transplanted to *Xenopus oocytes*," *Journal of Neurochemistry*, vol. 117, no. 6, pp. 1009–1019, 2011.

[12] K. Hara and T. Sata, "The effects of the local anesthetics lidocaine and procaine on glycine and γ-aminobutyric acid receptors expressed in *Xenopus oocytes*," *Anesthesia and Analgesia*, vol. 104, no. 6, pp. 1434–1439, 2007.

[13] T. W. R. Lee, H. P. Grocott, D. Schwinn, and E. Jacobsohn, "High spinal anesthesia for cardiac surgery: effects on β-adrenergic receptor function, stress response, and hemodynamics," *Anesthesiology*, vol. 98, no. 2, pp. 499–510, 2003.

[14] J. T. Jastak, J. A. Yagiela, and D. Donaldson, *Local Anesthesia of the Oral Cavity*, WB Saunders, Philadelphia, Pa, USA, 1995.

[15] C. Lynch III, "Meyer and Overton revisited," *Anesthesia and Analgesia*, vol. 107, no. 3, pp. 864–867, 2008.

[16] M. Eeman and M. Deleu, "From biological membranes to biomimetic model membranes," *Biotechnology, Agronomy and Society and Environment*, vol. 14, no. 4, pp. 719–736, 2010.

[17] I. Yun, E. Cho, H. Jang et al., "Amphiphilic effects of local anesthetics on rotational mobility in neuronal and model membranes," *Biochimica et Biophysica Acta*, vol. 1564, no. 1, pp. 123–132, 2002.

[18] H. Tsuchiya, M. Mizogami, and K. Takakura, "Reversed-phase liquid chromatographic retention and membrane activity relationships of local anesthetics," *Journal of Chromatography A*, vol. 1073, no. 1-2, pp. 303–308, 2005.

[19] M. Mizogami, H. Tsuchiya, and J. Harada, "Membrane effects of ropivacaine compared with those of bupivacaine and mepivacaine," *Fundamental and Clinical Pharmacology*, vol. 16, no. 4, pp. 325–330, 2002.

[20] H. Tsuchiya and M. Mizogami, "Membrane interactivity of charged local anesthetic derivative and stereoselectivity in membrane interaction of local anesthetic enantiomers," *Local and Regional Anesthesia*, vol. 1, pp. 1–9, 2008.

[21] K. J. McClellan and D. Faulds, "Ropivacaine: an update of its use in regional anaesthesia," *Drugs*, vol. 60, no. 5, pp. 1065–1093, 2000.

[22] H. Önyüksel, V. Sethi, G. L. Weinberg, P. K. Dudeja, and I. Rubinstein, "Bupivacaine, but not lidocaine, disrupts cardiolipin-containing small biomimetic unilamellar liposomes," *Chemico-Biological Interactions*, vol. 169, no. 3, pp. 154–159, 2007.

[23] H. Tsuchiya, T. Ueno, M. Mizogami, and K. Takakura, "Local anesthetics structure-dependently interact with anionic phospholipid membranes to modify the fluidity," *Chemico-Biological Interactions*, vol. 183, no. 1, pp. 19–24, 2010.

[24] L. Groban, D. D. Deal, J. C. Vernon, R. L. James, and J. Butterworth, "Cardiac resuscitation after incremental overdosage with lidocaine, bupivacaine, levobupivacaine, and ropivacaine in anesthetized dogs," *Anesthesia and Analgesia*, vol. 92, no. 1, pp. 37–43, 2001.

[25] L. Groban, D. D. Deal, J. C. Vernon, R. L. James, and J. Butterworth, "Ventricular arrhythmias with or without programmed electrical stimulation after incremental overdosage with lidocaine, bupivacaine, levobupivacaine, and ropivacaine," *Anesthesia and Analgesia*, vol. 91, no. 5, pp. 1103–1111, 2000.

[26] J. Wang and G. Zhang, "Influence of membrane physical state on lysosomal potassium ion permeability," *Cell Biology International*, vol. 29, no. 6, pp. 393–401, 2005.

[27] G. Balogh, I. Horváth, E. Nagy et al., "The hyperfluidization of mammalian cell membranes acts as a signal to initiate the heat shock protein response," *FEBS Journal*, vol. 272, no. 23, pp. 6077–6086, 2005.

[28] S. Schreier, S. V. P. Malheiros, and E. de Paula, "Surface active drugs: self-association and interaction with membranes and surfactants. Physicochemical and biological aspects," *Biochimica et Biophysica Acta*, vol. 1508, no. 1-2, pp. 210–234, 2000.

[29] A. Pohorille, M. A. Wilson, M. H. New, and C. Chipot, "Concentrations of anesthetics across the water-membrane interface; the Meyer-Overton hypothesis revisited," *Toxicology Letters*, vol. 100-101, pp. 421–430, 1998.

[30] A. Sunami, I. W. Glaaser, and H. A. Fozzard, "A critical residue for isoform difference in tetrodotoxin affinity is a molecular determinant of the external access path for local anesthetics in the cardiac sodium channel," *Proceedings of the National Academy of Sciences of the United States of America*, vol. 97, no. 5, pp. 2326–2331, 2000.

[31] T. K. Y. Lim, B. A. MacLeod, C. R. Ries, and S. K. W. Schwarz, "The quaternary lidocaine derivative, QX-314, produces long-lasting local anesthesia in animal models *in vivo*," *Anesthesiology*, vol. 107, no. 2, pp. 305–311, 2007.

[32] G. K. Wang, "Local anesthetics," in *Neural Mechanisms of Anesthesia*, J. F. Antognini, E. E. Carstens, and D. E. Raines, Eds., Humana Press, Totowa, NJ, USA, 2003.

[33] K. A. Slaviero, S. J. Clarke, and L. P. Rivory, "Inflammatory response: an unrecognised source of variability in the pharmacokinetics and pharmacodynamics of cancer chemotherapy," *The Lancet Oncology*, vol. 4, no. 4, pp. 224–232, 2003.

[34] S. Sattari, W. F. Dryden, L. A. Eliot, and F. Jamali, "Despite increased plasma concentration, inflammation reduces potency of calcium channel antagonists due to lower binding to the rat heart," *British Journal of Pharmacology*, vol. 139, no. 5, pp. 945–954, 2003.

[35] E. Claffey, A. Reader, J. Nusstein, M. Beck, and J. Weaver, "Anesthetic efficacy of articaine for inferior alveolar nerve blocks in patients with irreversible pulpitis," *Journal of Endodontics*, vol. 30, no. 8, pp. 568–571, 2004.

[36] N. Srinivasan, M. Kavitha, C. S. Loganathan, and G. Padmini, "Comparison of anesthetic efficacy of 4% articaine and 2% lidocaine for maxillary buccal infiltration in patients with irreversible pulpitis," *Oral Surgery, Oral Medicine, Oral Pathology, Oral Radiology and Endodontology*, vol. 107, no. 1, pp. 133–136, 2009.

[37] I. Potočnik and F. Bajrović, "Failure of inferior alveolar nerve block in endodontics," *Dental Traumatology*, vol. 15, no. 6, pp. 247–251, 1999.

[38] A. Punnia-Moorthy, "Evaluation of pH changes in inflammation of the subcutaneous air pouch lining in the rat, induced by carrageenan, dextran and *Staphylococcus aureus*," *Journal of Oral Pathology*, vol. 16, no. 1, pp. 36–44, 1987.

[39] D. de Backer, "Lactic acidosis," *Minerva Anestesiologica*, vol. 69, no. 4, pp. 281–284, 2003.

[40] H. Tsuchiya, M. Mizogami, T. Ueno, and K. Takakura, "Interaction of local anaesthetics with lipid membranes under inflammatory acidic conditions," *Inflammopharmacology*, vol. 15, no. 4, pp. 164–170, 2007.

[41] T. Ueno, H. Tsuchiya, M. Mizogami, and K. Takakura, "Local anesthetic failure associated with inflammation: verification of the acidosis mechanism and the hypothetic participation of inflammatory peroxynitrite," *Journal of Inflammation Research*, vol. 1, pp. 41–48, 2008.

[42] A. Punnia-Moorthy, "Buffering capacity of normal and inflamed tissues following the injection of local anaesthetic solutions," *British Journal of Anaesthesia*, vol. 61, no. 2, pp. 154–159, 1988.

[43] B. Gunaydin and A. T. Demiryurek, "Interaction of lidocaine with reactive oxygen and nitrogen species," *European Journal of Anaesthesiology*, vol. 18, no. 12, pp. 816–822, 2001.

[44] H. Tsuchiya, T. Ueno, M. Mizogami, and K. Takakura, "Antioxidant activity analysis by liposomal membrane system and application to anesthetics," *Analytical Sciences*, vol. 24, no. 12, pp. 1557–1562, 2008.

[45] T. Ueno, M. Mizogami, K. Takakura, and H. Tsuchiya, "Membrane effect of lidocaine is inhibited by interaction with peroxynitrite," *Journal of Anesthesia*, vol. 22, no. 1, pp. 96–99, 2008.

[46] T. Ueno, M. Mizogami, K. Takakura, and H. Tsuchiya, "Peroxynitrite affects lidocaine by acting on membrane-constituting lipids," *Journal of Anesthesia*, vol. 22, no. 4, pp. 475–478, 2008.

[47] N. M. Flake and M. S. Gold, "Inflammation alters sodium currents and excitability of temporomandibular joint afferents," *Neuroscience Letters*, vol. 384, no. 3, pp. 294–299, 2005.

[48] J. Wang, J. A. Strong, W. Xie, and J. Zhang, "Local inflammation in rat dorsal root ganglion alters excitability and ion currents in small-diameter sensory neurons," *Anesthesiology*, vol. 107, no. 2, pp. 322–332, 2007.

[49] J. M. Dippenaar, "Local anaesthetic toxicity," *Southern African Journal of Anaesthesia and Analgesia*, vol. 13, no. 3, pp. 23–28, 2007.

[50] C. Gevirtz, "Local anesthetic systemic toxicity: prevention and treatment," *Topics in Pain Management*, vol. 27, no. 12, pp. 1–6, 2012.

[51] J. E. Heavner, "Cardiac toxicity of local anesthetics in the intact isolated heart model: a review," *Regional Anesthesia and Pain Medicine*, vol. 27, no. 6, pp. 545–555, 2002.

[52] L. Pardo, T. J. J. Blanck, and E. Recio-Pinto, "The neuronal lipid membrane permeability was markedly increased by bupivacaine and mildly affected by lidocaine and ropivacaine," *European Journal of Pharmacology*, vol. 455, no. 2-3, pp. 81–90, 2002.

[53] P. Friederich, "Basic concepts of ion channel physiology and anaesthetic drug effects," *European Journal of Anaesthesiology*, vol. 20, no. 5, pp. 343–353, 2003.

[54] R. H. Houtkooper and F. M. Vaz, "Cardiolipin, the heart of mitochondrial metabolism," *Cellular and Molecular Life Sciences*, vol. 65, no. 16, pp. 2493–2506, 2008.

[55] K. Felice and H. Schumann, "Intravenous lipid emulsion for local anesthetic toxicity: a review of the literature," *Journal of Medical Toxicology*, vol. 4, no. 3, pp. 184–191, 2008.

[56] J. Muhonen, J. M. Holopainen, and S. K. Wiedmer, "Interactions between local anesthetics and lipid dispersions studied with liposome electrokinetic capillary chromatography," *Journal of Chromatography A*, vol. 1216, no. 15, pp. 3392–3397, 2009.

[57] G. Weinberg, R. Ripper, D. L. Feinstein, and W. Hoffman, "Lipid emulsion infusion rescues dogs from bupivacaine-induced cardiac toxicity," *Regional Anesthesia and Pain Medicine*, vol. 28, no. 3, pp. 198–202, 2003.

[58] R. J. Litz, M. Popp, S. N. Stehr, and T. Koch, "Successful resuscitation of a patient with ropivacaine-induced asystole after axillary plexus block using lipid infusion," *Anaesthesia*, vol. 61, no. 8, pp. 800–801, 2006.

[59] G. Foxall, R. McCahon, J. Lamb, J. G. Hardman, and N. M. Bedforth, "Levobupivacaine-induced seizures and cardiovascular collapse treated with Intralipid," *Anaesthesia*, vol. 62, no. 5, pp. 516–518, 2007.

[60] S. Ciechanowicz and V. Patil, "Lipid emulsion for local anesthetic systemic toxicity," *Anesthesiology Research and Practice*, vol. 2012, Article ID 131784, 11 pages, 2012.

[61] J. A. Warren, R. B. Thoma, A. Georgescu, and S. J. Shah, "Intravenous lipid infusion in the successful resuscitation of local anesthetic-induced cardiovascular collapse after supraclavicular brachial plexus block," *Anesthesia and Analgesia*, vol. 106, no. 5, pp. 1578–1580, 2008.

[62] E. Calenda and S. A. Dinescu, "Failure of lipid emulsion to reverse neurotoxicity after an ultrasound-guided axillary block with ropivacaine and mepivacaine," *Journal of Anesthesia*, vol. 23, no. 3, pp. 472–473, 2009.

[63] E. Bourne, C. Wright, and C. Royse, "A review of local anesthetic cardiotoxicity and treatment with lipid emulsion," *Local and Regional Anesthesia*, vol. 3, no. 1, pp. 11–19, 2010.

[64] J. Mazoit, R. Le Guen, H. Beloeil, and D. Benhamou, "Binding of long-lasting local anesthetics to lipid emulsions," *Anesthesiology*, vol. 110, no. 2, pp. 380–386, 2009.

[65] AAGBI, *Management of Severe Local Anaesthetic Toxicity 2 (2010)*, AAGBI Guidelines, 2010, http://www.aagbi.org/publications/publications-guidelines/M/R.

[66] P. Tsibiribi, C. Bui-Xuan, B. Bui-Xuan et al., "The effects of ropivacaine at clinically relevant doses on myocardial ischemia in pigs," *Journal of Anesthesia*, vol. 20, no. 4, pp. 341–343, 2006.

[67] D. J. Pacini, G. Boachie-Ansah, and K. A. Kane, "Modification by hypoxia, hyperkalaemia and acidosis of the cardiac electrophysiological effects of a range of antiarrhythmic drugs," *British Journal of Pharmacology*, vol. 107, no. 3, pp. 665–670, 1992.

[68] M. Freysz, Q. Timour, L. Bertrix, J. Loufoua-Moundanga, S. Omar, and G. Faucon, "Enhancement by ischemia of the risk of cardiac disorders, especially fibrillation, in regional anesthesia with bupivacaine," *Acta Anaesthesiologica Scandinavica*, vol. 37, no. 4, pp. 350–356, 1993.

[69] R. Ferrari, A. Cargnoni, P. Bernocchi et al., "Metabolic adaptation during a sequence of no-flow and low-flow ischemia: a possible trigger for hibernation," *Circulation*, vol. 94, no. 10, pp. 2587–2596, 1996.

[70] Y. Watanabe, S. Dohi, H. Iida, and T. Ishiyama, "The effects of bupivacaine and ropivacaine on baroreflex sensitivity with or without respiratory acidosis and alkalosis in rats," *Anesthesia and Analgesia*, vol. 84, no. 2, pp. 398–404, 1997.

[71] H. Tsuchiya, M. Mizogami, T. Ueno, and K. Shigemi, "Cardiotoxic local anesthetics increasingly interact with biomimetic membranes under ischemia-like acidic conditions," *Biological and Pharmaceutical Bulletin*, vol. 35, no. 6, pp. 988–992, 2012.

[72] G. Paradies, G. Petrosillo, M. Pistolese, N. Di Venosa, A. Federici, and F. M. Ruggiero, "Decrease in mitochondrial complex I activity in ischemic/reperfused rat heart: involvement of reactive oxygen species and cardiolipin," *Circulation Research*, vol. 94, no. 1, pp. 53–59, 2004.

[73] M. M. Lalu, W. Wang, and R. Schulz, "Peroxynitrite in myocardial ischemia-reperfusion injury," *Heart Failure Reviews*, vol. 7, no. 4, pp. 359–369, 2002.

[74] H. Tsuchiya, M. Mizogami, and K. Shigemi, "Increasing membrane interactions of local anaesthetics as hypothetic mechanism for their cardiotoxicity enhanced by myocardial ischaemia," *Basic and Clinical Pharmacology and Toxicology*, vol. 111, no. 5, pp. 303–308, 2012.

[75] E. J. Lesnefsky and C. L. Hoppel, "Cardiolipin as an oxidative target in cardiac mitochondria in the aged rat," *Biochimica et Biophysica Acta*, vol. 1777, no. 7-8, pp. 1020–1027, 2008.

[76] G. Paradies, G. Petrosillo, V. Paradies, and F. M. Ruggiero, "Role of cardiolipin peroxidation and Ca^{2+} in mitochondrial dysfunction and disease," *Cell Calcium*, vol. 45, no. 6, pp. 643–650, 2009.

[77] H. Tsuchiya, T. Ueno, and M. Mizogami, "Stereostructure-based differences in the interactions of cardiotoxic local anesthetics with cholesterol-containing biomimetic membranes," *Bioorganic and Medicinal Chemistry*, vol. 19, no. 11, pp. 3410–3415, 2011.

[78] D. J. Kaczmarek, C. Herzog, J. Larmann et al., "Lidocaine protects from myocardial damage due to ischemia and reperfusion in mice by its antiapoptotic effects," *Anesthesiology*, vol. 110, no. 5, pp. 1041–1049, 2009.

[79] F. Lenfant, J. Lahet, C. Courderot-Masuyer, M. Freysz, and L. Rochette, "Lidocaine has better antioxidant potential than ropivacaine and bupivacaine: *in vitro* comparison in a model of human erythrocytes submitted to an oxidative stress," *Biomedicine and Pharmacotherapy*, vol. 58, no. 4, pp. 248–254, 2004.

[80] S. Pope, J. M. Land, and S. J. R. Heales, "Oxidative stress and mitochondrial dysfunction in neurodegeneration; cardiolipin a critical target?" *Biochimica et Biophysica Acta*, vol. 1777, no. 7-8, pp. 794–799, 2008.

[81] E. J. Lesnefsky, T. J. Slabe, M. S. K. Stoll, P. E. Minkler, and C. L. Hoppel, "Myocardial ischemia selectively depletes cardiolipin in rabbit heart subsarcolemmal mitochondria," *American Journal of Physiology*, vol. 280, no. 6, pp. H2770–H2778, 2001.

[82] K. M. Rentsch, "The importance of stereoselective determination of drugs in the clinical laboratory," *Journal of Biochemical and Biophysical Methods*, vol. 54, no. 1-3, pp. 1–9, 2002.

[83] C. Nau and G. R. Strichartz, "Drug chirality in anesthesia," *Anesthesiology*, vol. 97, no. 2, pp. 497–502, 2002.

[84] R. H. Foster and A. Markham, "Levobupivacaine: a review of its pharmacology and use as a local anaesthetic," *Drugs*, vol. 59, no. 3, pp. 551–579, 2000.

[85] M. Vladimirov, C. Nau, W. M. Mok, and G. Strichartz, "Potency of bupivacaine stereoisomers tested *in vitro* and *in vivo*: biochemical, electrophysiological, and neurobehavioral studies," *Anesthesiology*, vol. 93, no. 3, pp. 744–755, 2000.

[86] G. Lyons, M. Columb, R. C. Wilson, and R. V. Johnson, "Epidural pain relief in labour: potencies of levobupivacaine and racemic bupivacaine," *British Journal of Anaesthesia*, vol. 81, no. 6, pp. 899–901, 1998, Erratum in: *British Journal of Anaesthesia*, vol. 82, no. 3, p. 488, 1998.

[87] Y. Lim, C. E. Ocampo, and A. T. Sia, "A comparison of duration of analgesia of intrathecal 2.5 mg of bupivacaine, ropivacaine, and levobupivacaine in combined spinal epidural analgesia for patients in labor," *Anesthesia and Analgesia*, vol. 98, no. 1, pp. 235–239, 2004.

[88] B. M. Graf, E. Martin, Z. J. Bosnjak, and D. F. Stowe, "Stereospecific effect of bupivacaine isomers on atrioventricular conduction in the isolated perfused guinea pig heart," *Anesthesiology*, vol. 86, no. 2, pp. 410–419, 1997.

[89] S. G. Morrison, J. J. Dominguez, P. Frascarolo, and S. Reiz, "A comparison of the electrocardiographic cardiotoxic effects of racemic bupivacaine, levobupivacaine, and ropivacaine in anesthetized swine," *Anesthesia and Analgesia*, vol. 90, no. 6, pp. 1308–1314, 2000.

[90] C. Valenzuela, D. J. Snyders, P. B. Bennett, J. Tamargo, and L. M. Hondeghem, "Stereoselective block of cardiac sodium channels by bupivacaine in guinea pig ventricular myocytes," *Circulation*, vol. 92, no. 10, pp. 3014–3024, 1995.

[91] C. Valenzuela, E. Delpón, M. M. Tamkun, J. Tamargo, and D. J. Snyders, "Stereoselective block of a human cardiac potassium channel (Kv1.5) by bupivacaine enantiomers," *Biophysical Journal*, vol. 69, no. 2, pp. 418–427, 1995.

[92] M. Mizogami, H. Tsuchiya, T. Ueno, M. Kashimata, and K. Takakura, "Stereospecific interaction of bupivacaine enantiomers with lipid membranes," *Regional Anesthesia and Pain Medicine*, vol. 33, no. 4, pp. 304–311, 2008.

[93] H. Tsuchiya and M. Mizogami, "R(+)-, Rac-, and S(−)-bupivacaine stereostructure-specifically interact with membrane lipids at cardiotoxically relevant concentrations," *Anesthesia and Analgesia*, vol. 114, no. 2, pp. 310–312, 2012.

[94] T. González, C. Arias, R. Caballero et al., "Effects of levobupivacaine, ropivacaine and bupivacaine on HERG channels: stereoselective bupivacaine block," *British Journal of Pharmacology*, vol. 137, no. 8, pp. 1269–1279, 2002.

[95] P. Friederich, A. Solth, S. Schillemeit, and D. Isbrandt, "Local anaesthetic sensitivities of cloned HERG channels from human heart: comparison with HERG/MiRP1 and HERG/MiRP1T8A," *British Journal of Anaesthesia*, vol. 92, no. 1, pp. 93–101, 2004.

[96] H. Tsuchiya and M. Mizogami, "The membrane interaction of drugs as one of mechanisms for their enantioselective effects," *Medical Hypotheses*, vol. 79, no. 1, pp. 65–67, 2012.

[97] N. Nandi and D. Vollhardt, "Chiral discrimination and recognition in Langmuir monolayers," *Current Opinion in Colloid and Interface Science*, vol. 13, no. 1-2, pp. 40–46, 2008.

[98] S. Lalitha, A. S. Kumar, K. J. Stine, and D. F. Covey, "Chirality in membranes: first evidence that enantioselective interactions between cholesterol and cell membrane lipids can be a determinant of membrane physical properties," *Journal of Supramolecular Chemistry*, vol. 1, no. 2, pp. 53–61, 2001.

[99] A. Kessel, N. Ben-Tal, and S. May, "Interactions of cholesterol with lipid bilayers: the preferred configuration and fluctuations," *Biophysical Journal*, vol. 81, no. 2, pp. 643–658, 2001.

[100] K. Simons and D. Toomre, "Lipid rafts and signal transduction," *Nature Reviews Molecular Cell Biology*, vol. 1, no. 1, pp. 31–39, 2000.

[101] M.-O. Parat, "Could endothelial caveolae be the target of general anaesthetics?" *British Journal of Anaesthesia*, vol. 96, no. 5, pp. 547–550, 2006.

[102] K. M. S. O'Connell, J. R. Martens, and M. M. Tamkun, "Localization of ion channels to lipid raft domains within the cardiovascular system," *Trends in Cardiovascular Medicine*, vol. 14, no. 2, pp. 37–42, 2004.

[103] Y. Xiang, V. O. Rybin, S. F. Steinberg, and B. Kobilka, "Caveolar localization dictates physiologic signaling of β_2-adrenoceptors in neonatal cardiac myocytes," *The Journal of Biological Chemistry*, vol. 277, no. 37, pp. 34280–34286, 2002.

[104] Y. Fujimura, H. Tachibana, and K. Yamada, "Lipid raft-associated catechin suppresses the FcεRI expression by inhibiting phosphorylation of the extracellular signal-regulated kinase1/2," *FEBS Letters*, vol. 556, no. 1-3, pp. 204–210, 2004.

[105] A. Ausuili, A. Torrecillas, F. J. Aranda et al., "Edelfosine is incorporated into rafts and alters their organization," *Journal of Physical Chemistry B*, vol. 112, no. 37, pp. 11643–11654, 2008.

[106] K. Kamata, S. Manno, M. Ozaki, and Y. Takakuwa, "Functional evidence for presence of lipid rafts in erythrocyte membranes: Gsα in rafts is essential for signal transduction," *American Journal of Hematology*, vol. 83, no. 5, pp. 371–375, 2008.

[107] K. Kamata, S. Manno, Y. Takakuwa, and M. Ozaki, "Reversible effect of lidocaine on raft formation," *International Congress Series*, vol. 1283, pp. 281–282, 2005.

[108] H. Tsuchiya, T. Ueno, M. Mizogami, and K. Takakura, "Do local anesthetics interact preferentially with membrane lipid rafts? Comparative interactivities with raft-like membranes," *Journal of Anesthesia*, vol. 24, no. 4, pp. 639–642, 2010.

[109] C. Bandeiras, A. P. Serro, K. Luzyanin, A. Fernandes, and B. Saramago, "Anesthetics interacting with lipid rafts," *European Journal of Pharmaceutical Sciences*, vol. 48, no. 1-2, pp. 153–165, 2013.

[110] C. Ioannides, "Drug-phytochemical interactions," *Inflammopharmacology*, vol. 11, no. 1, pp. 7–42, 2003.

[111] S. Zhou, Z. Zhou, C. Li et al., "Identification of drugs that interact with herbs in drug development," *Drug Discovery Today*, vol. 12, no. 15-16, pp. 664–673, 2007.

[112] Y. Vorobeychik, V. Gordin, J. Mao, and L. Chen, "Combination therapy for neuropathic pain: a review of current evidence," *CNS Drugs*, vol. 25, no. 12, pp. 1023–1034, 2011.

[113] D. Špicarová and J. Paleček, "The role of spinal cord vanilloid (TRPV1) receptors in pain modulation," *Physiological Research*, vol. 57, supplement 3, pp. S69–S77, 2008.

[114] M. J. Caterina, M. A. Schumacher, M. Tominaga, T. A. Rosen, J. D. Levine, and D. Julius, "The capsaicin receptor: a heat-activated ion channel in the pain pathway," *Nature*, vol. 389, no. 6653, pp. 816–824, 1997.

[115] K. Venkatachalam and C. Montell, "TRP channels," *Annual Review of Biochemistry*, vol. 76, pp. 387–417, 2007.

[116] A. M. Binshtok, B. P. Bean, and C. J. Woolf, "Inhibition of nociceptors by TRPV1-mediated entry of impermeant sodium channel blockers," *Nature*, vol. 449, no. 7162, pp. 607–610, 2007.

[117] C. R. Ries, R. Pillai, C. C. Chung, J. T. Wang, B. A. MacLeod, and S. K. Schwarz, "QX-314 produces long-lasting local anesthesia modulated by transient receptor potential vanilloid receptors in mice," *Anesthesiology*, vol. 111, no. 1, pp. 122–126, 2009.

[118] J. Shen, L. E. Fox, and J. Cheng, "Differential effects of peripheral versus central coadministration of QX-314 and capsaicin on neuropathic pain in rats," *Anesthesiology*, vol. 117, no. 2, pp. 365–380, 2012.

[119] P. Gerner, A. M. Binshtok, C. Wang et al., "Capsaicin combined with local anesthetics preferentially prolongs sensory/nociceptive block in rat sciatic nerve," *Anesthesiology*, vol. 109, no. 5, pp. 872–878, 2008.

[120] E. W. McCleskey, "Neuroscience: a local route to pain relief," *Nature*, vol. 449, no. 7162, pp. 545–546, 2007.

[121] H. Shin, H. J. Park, S. A. Raymond, and G. R. Strichartz, "Potentiation by capsaicin of lidocaine's tonic impulse block in isolated rat sciatic nerve," *Neuroscience Letters*, vol. 174, no. 1, pp. 14–16, 1994.

[122] H. Shin, H. J. Park, and S. A. Raymond, "Potentiation by capsaicin of lidocaine's phasic impulse block in isolated rat sciatic nerve," *Pharmacological Research*, vol. 30, no. 1, pp. 73–79, 1994.

[123] H. Tsuchiya, "Biphasic membrane effects of capsaicin, an active component in *Capsicum* species," *Journal of Ethnopharmacology*, vol. 75, no. 2-3, pp. 295–299, 2001, Erratum in: *Journal of Ethnopharmacology*, vol. 76, no. 3, p. 313, 2001.

[124] H. Tsuchiya and M. Mizogami, "Plant components exhibit pharmacological activities and drug interactions by acting on lipid membranes," *Pharmacognosy Communications*, vol. 2, no. 4, pp. 58–71, 2012.

[125] K. Yang, C. Tsai, Y. Wang et al., "Apple polyphenol phloretin potentiates the anticancer actions of paclitaxel through induction of apoptosis in human Hep G2 cells," *Molecular Carcinogenesis*, vol. 48, no. 5, pp. 420–431, 2009.

[126] R. Cseh and R. Benz, "Interaction of phloretin with lipid monolayers: relationship between structural changes and dipole potential change," *Biophysical Journal*, vol. 77, no. 3, pp. 1477–1488, 1999.

[127] B. G. Auner and C. Valenta, "Influence of phloretin on the skin permeation of lidocaine from semisolid preparations," *European Journal of Pharmaceutics and Biopharmaceutics*, vol. 57, no. 2, pp. 307–312, 2004.

[128] G. Åberg and G. Sydnes, "An inhibitory effect of polyphloretin phosphate (PPP) on local anaesthesia," *Acta Anaesthesiologica Scandinavica*, vol. 19, no. 5, pp. 377–383, 1975.

[129] A. Nordenram and K. Danielsson, "The effect of polyphloretin phosphate (PPP) on oral infiltration anaesthesia. An experimental investigation," *Swedish Dental Journal*, vol. 12, no. 6, pp. 217–220, 1988.

4

Recent Advances in Epidural Analgesia

Maria Bauer,[1] John E. George III,[2] John Seif,[2] and Ehab Farag[1,2]

[1] *Department of Outcomes Research, Cleveland Clinic, Cleveland, OH 44195, USA*
[2] *Anesthesiology Institute, Cleveland Clinic, Cleveland, OH 44195, USA*

Correspondence should be addressed to Ehab Farag, farage@ccf.org

Academic Editor: Andrea Trescot

Neuraxial anesthesia is a term that denotes all forms of central blocks, involving the spinal, epidural, and caudal spaces. Epidural anesthesia is a versatile technique widely used in anesthetic practice. Its potential to decrease postoperative morbidity and mortality has been demonstrated by numerous studies. To maximize its perioperative benefits while minimizing potential adverse outcomes, the knowledge of factors affecting successful block placement is essential. This paper will provide an overview of the pertinent anatomical, pharmacological, immunological, and technical aspects of epidural anesthesia in both adult and pediatric populations and will discuss the recent advances, the related rare but potentially devastating complications, and the current recommendations for the use of anticoagulants in the setting of neuraxial block placement.

1. Introduction

Neuraxial anesthesia is the term for central blocks involving the spinal, epidural, and caudal spaces. While it is now an invaluable adjunct and even occasionally an alternative to general anesthesia, its use is not a new phenomenon. Physicians such as Corning published studies documenting success with neuraxial blocks as early as 1885 [1]. Even more ambitious physician-scientists such as Bier became knowledgeable about spinal anesthesia, in particular, through self-investigation [2]. It unfortunately was also through this type of dedication that he became all too familiar with postdural puncture headaches. Despite its early use, though, much of the gains we have with neuraxial blocks did not occur until the early 1900's. Limitations in this particular area of anesthesia were limited to lack of drug diversity and a lack of adequate equipment. Prior to 1904, the only drug available for neuraxial use was cocaine, and development of epidural technology was still a ways off. With a larger drug base and equipment advancements came an expansion of the role of neuraxial anesthesia in anesthesia practice.

Excluding the obvious fact that surgical conditions primarily dictate the type of anesthesia performed, most operations below the neck can be performed under neuraxial anesthesia. Various studies have shown a decrease in postoperative morbidity and even mortality when used either with general anesthesia or alone. Neuraxial blocks have even been shown to reduce the incidence of venous thrombosis and pulmonary embolism while also minimizing transfusion requirements and respiratory compromise following thoracic and upper abdominal surgery. A decreased stress response has also been noted which may have positive cardiac benefits such as reduced perioperative and postoperative ischemia. Despite these proposed advantages of neuraxial blocks, adverse reactions and complications can occur. These can range from self-limited back soreness to permanent neurologic deficits and even death. Because an expansive review of neuraxial blocks is beyond the scope of this review, we have chosen to focus our discussion to epidural and caudal anesthesia. In doing so, we will review pertinent epidural knowledge, and present cutting edge advances specific to epidural and caudal anesthesia.

2. Anatomy for Epidural Placement

The anatomy for the placement of an epidural goes beyond the epidural space itself. It is for this reason that this section will not only cover anatomy of this space, but also important surrounding anatomy.

The epidural space extends from the base of the skull to the sacral hiatus. Its lateral boundaries are the vertebral pedicles, while the anterior and posterior boundaries are the dura mater and ligamentum flavum, respectively. The contents of the space include fat, lymphatics, and veins with nerve roots that cross it. Determinants of epidural fat include age and body habitus with obese patients having the greatest amount of epidural fat [2]. The amount of epidural fat within the space is just one of the factors that determine volume necessary for adequate anesthesia or analgesia.

Veins within the epidural space form a plexus called Batson's venous plexus. These veins connect with the iliac and azygos veins and are significant because of a lack of valves commonly found in veins. It is the lack of these valves in conjunction with a compressed inferior vena cava from a gravid uterus, which results in the venous engorgement of epidural veins found in parturients.

Traditional thought on epidural anatomy was that it is one continuous space. A more recent thought is the concept of it being a potential space with septations or crevices formed by layering of epidural contents (fat). The anatomic layering and texture of epidural contents create inconsistent paths that ultimately make flow through it less uniform [3]. The idea of these septations or crevices forming variable paths for the flow of a solution is the rationale given for unilateral or partial epidural blockade [4].

Vertebral spinous processes help define the midline. In the cervical and lumbar areas they are horizontal, while in the thoracic vertebrae (specifically T4 through T9) they are caudally angulated. The space between these caudally angulated spinous processes are often difficult to access leading some to favor a paramedian approach to thoracic epidural placement as opposed to the traditional midline approach. While the surgical site dictates the level of the epidural placement, the safest location is one whereby inadvertent spinal cord damage can be avoided. In adults, the spinal cord typically ends at the lower border of the L1 vertebra while in children it is at the level of the lower border of L3. By the age of 8 years, one can safely target the same lumbar levels for safe epidural placement as in the adult, while under the age of 7 years, a caudal approach to the epidural space is safest. One generally accepted landmark for assessing lumbar level for epidural placement is the superior aspect of the iliac crest. A horizontal line drawn between the superior borders of either iliac crest corresponds to the L4 vertebral body or the L4-5 interspace. For thoracic epidural placement, the inferior border of the scapula is the usual site of the T7 vertebral body/spinous process, and is typically used to approximate thoracic level of epidural placement for thoracic or intraabdominal surgical procedures. The approximate distance from the skin to the epidural space in 80% of individuals is 4–6 cm with the caveat that thin and obese patients may vary outside of this range [5].

3. Choices for Epidural Infusions

Local anesthetics are the mainstay of therapy for obtaining analgesia or anesthesia with an epidural. Understanding the pharmacology of local anesthetics is therefore paramount. Specifically, factors such as surgical location and duration, desire to have a sensory and/or motor block, or the expected potency and duration of a specific local anesthetic agent should be considered prior to placing an epidural block. The choice of which local anesthetic agent to use can be categorized based on desired length of action. Regardless of the class of local anesthetic, these drugs can be divided into ones that are short, intermediate, or long acting. The shortest-acting local anesthetic agent is chloroprocaine. Its short length provides ample anesthesia for short surgical procedures, and its quick elimination obviates the need for prolonged recovery room discharges.

Lidocaine has traditionally been the agent of choice for slightly longer surgical procedures that require an intermediate-acting local anesthetic. In place of lidocaine, some centers have also adopted the use of mepivacaine for its longer length of action with a similar onset profile. The intermediate length of action of either agent can be prolonged by the addition of epinephrine. Of note is the potential for an increased incidence of hypotension due to venous pooling from the beta effects of epinephrine containing solutions. This phenomenon seems to be especially true of patients receiving lumbar epidural analgesia.

Longer-acting local anesthetics used for epidural blockade typically consist of either bupivacaine or ropivacaine in varying concentrations. Greater concentrations of either will produce a greater motor block in addition to the sensory block that is typically desired. Ropivacaine, an analog of mepivacaine, has a lesser intense and shorter duration of motor block in addition to a lower toxicity profile than an equipotent dose of bupivacaine [6]. The cardiac toxicity profile of bupivacaine is the highest among all the choices of local anesthetics. It is due to a high degree of protein binding and a greater blocking effect on cardiac sodium channels.

Multiple attempts have been made to find various additives to improve the onset and duration of an epidural block. Alkalinization with sodium bicarbonate has proven effective in a dose of 1 mEq/10 mL local anesthetic for chloroprocaine, lidocaine, or mepivacaine. A lower concentration of sodium bicarbonate (0.1 mEq/10 mL of local anesthetic) is necessary for bupivacaine and ropivacaine due to the potential of precipitation with higher concentrations. The addition of epinephrine to a local anesthetic increases the duration of action by decreasing the vascular absorption. While this phenomenon has been shown to be true with the short- and intermediate-acting local anesthetic agents, it appears to be less effective with longer-acting agents. With the low doses typically used in the epidural space, the overall cardiovascular response seems to be vasodilation (causing a decrease in mean arterial pressure), in addition to an increase in heart rate and contractility. These effects ultimately result in maintenance of cardiac output. Phenylephrine has also been used to prolong the effects of neuraxial local anesthetics. In contrast to the use of epinephrine in the epidural space, it causes an increase in peripheral vascular resistance without the added benefits of an increase in chronotropy or contractility. The resulting drop in cardiac output is the reason most anesthesiologists avoid phenylephrine in the epidural space.

Opioids remain the analgesic adjuvant of choice for augmenting the effects of local anesthetics in the epidural space. Epidural administration of fentanyl intraoperatively has been shown to significantly reduce volatile agent requirements by more than twofold in some instances [7]. Despite the benefits of neuraxial opioids, side effects do occur. Some of the more common side effects are pruritus (specifically in the mid-facial area), nausea, and urinary retention. Hypotension can also occur which is attributed to the reduction of sympathetic outflow via opioid receptors in the sympathetic ganglia.

Another class of analgesic adjuvants includes alpha-adrenergic agonists. Clonidine is the main drug used in this class due to its production as a preservative-free preparation. The effects of epidurally administered clonidine are seen as early as 20 minutes after injection, with peak effects occurring in 1 hour. The analgesic potency has been described as being comparable to epidurally administered morphine [8]. Adding clonidine to opioids in the epidural space has an additive effect, which results in a lower dose of narcotic necessary for optimal pain control. This as a consequence diminishes the incidence of respiratory depression that potentially occurs with neuraxial opioids. Clonidine is lipophilic, and as a result is quickly redistributed systemically despite neuraxial injection. It therefore has both central and peripheral effects. At lower doses, the central effects cause sympatholysis leading to hypotension, while the peripheral effects at higher doses cause vasoconstriction. Clonidine administered in the low thoracic or lumbar region typically produces blood pressure effects similar to that seen with intravenous administration [9]. When given in the mid or upper thoracic regions, epidurally administered clonidine causes an even greater decrease in blood pressure [10]. This more substantial drop in blood pressure is attributed to blocking thoracic dermatomes that contribute to sympathetic fibers innervating the heart. In addition to the hypotensive potential of clonidine, bradycardia, and nausea with or without vomiting are also potential side effects. The cause of bradycardia is twofold. Clonidine has vagomimetic effects in addition to inhibiting norepinephrine release. Additional side effects such as sedation and dry mouth are possible, but seem to be dose related. Even more esoteric compounds such as neostigmine, ketamine, ketorolac, midazolam, and dexamethasone are being studied with hopes to develop additional tools to supplement or even replace the neuraxial analgesia and anesthesia of local anesthetics. While this discussion focuses on epidural use of these agents, their clinical use may have far greater application. Current studies are not only investigating these agents in the acute pain setting, but are also for use in various chronic pain disorders.

4. The Effect of Anesthetic Technique on Immune Function

Surgery is associated with a wide range of metabolic, endocrine, hematological, and inflammatory/immunological responses, known collectively as surgical stress response. Surgical stress response has been identified as a major factor accounting for perioperative immune suppression [11]. The extent to which this adaptive response can be modified appears to be dependent on the anesthetic and analgesic technique used, and with regards to postoperative outcomes, has been extensively studied [12, 13]. There is evidence that regional anesthesia, particularly epidural blockade, attenuates or inhibits surgical stress by blocking afferent neural stimuli from reaching the central nervous system, as well as by blocking the efferent activation of the sympathetic nervous system [14, 15]. The nervous system accounts for the main common pathway mediating the surgical stress response [16]. Immune response is subject to neuroendocrine regulation and elicits neuroendocrine changes [17], augmenting or blunting the neuroendocrine response. It therefore affects postoperative immune function, and ultimately long-term outcomes [18, 19].

5. Perioperative Immunosuppression and the Impact of Anesthetic Technique on Postoperative Outcomes

Impaired perioperative immunity is related to the neuroendocrine stress response. Evidence suggests that the factors that are associated with immunosuppression during surgery are surgical stress response, general anesthesia, and opioid analgesia.

Surgical trauma in itself induces the release of catecholamines, adrenocorticotropic hormone, and cortisol, depresses cell-mediated immune responses including natural killer cell and cytotoxic T-cell function [13, 19–21], and promotes tumor vascularization [22, 23]. Additionally, risk factors, such as pain [24], blood transfusion [25], hypothermia [26], and hyperglycemia [27], further impair immunity. Pain activates the HPA axis, and may induce accelerated lymphocyte apoptosis [28]. Hypothermia impairs neutrophil oxidative killing by causing thermoregulatory vasoconstriction and thus decreasing oxygen supply [29]. Perioperative hyperglycemia impairs phagocytic activity and oxidative burst, as there is less NADPH available due to the activation of the NADPH consuming polyol pathway [30–32]. Earlier studies suggested that cell-mediated immune function [33, 34] is reduced by allogenic blood transfusion. Transfusion has more recently been suggested to facilitate host T_h2 cells to produce immunosuppressive IL-4 and IL-10; however, the exact mechanism of causality is yet unclear [25].

General anesthesia is also considered to be immunosuppressive, either by directly affecting immune mechanisms, or by activating the hypothalamic-pituitary-adrenal (HPA) axis and the sympathetic nervous system [12, 29]. Volatile anesthetics, by mechanisms that are only partially elucidated, impair NK cell, T cell, dendritic cell, neutrophil, and macrophage functions. Furthermore, opioid analgesics were found to inhibit both cellular and humoral immune function in humans [35, 36]. Melamed and colleagues showed that ketamine, thiopental, and halothane, but not propofol, had inhibitory effects on NK cell activity and increased metastatic burden in rats [37].

Opioids suppress the innate and adaptive immune responses [38, 39]. While neural and neuroendocrine responses are also involved [40], the presence of opioid-related receptors on the surface of immune cells increases the likelihood of a direct immune-modulating effect [41]. De

Waal and colleagues found different opioids to have differing immunosuppressive effects [42]. Synthetic opioids, however, do not appear to attenuate immune response [43, 44].

These immunosuppressive factors occur simultaneously during surgery and in the immediate postoperative period. The perioperative period is therefore a decisive period during which interventions that promote host defense may especially benefit the patient [11]. This may be of particular interest in patients undergoing tumor resection. While surgery is essential to reduce tumor burden, and among various treatment options, it is considered to be the most effective treatment for solid tumors; a rapid spread and growth of malignant tissue is often observed after tumor resection [45]. Cancer surgery, even with the best technique, is usually associated with dissemination of malignant cells through the lymphatics and the systemic circulation, and, at the time of surgery, many patients have already established micrometastases [46]. The clinical manifestation of this minimal residual disease is a function of both the host immune competence (particularly NK cell function) and the tumor's proliferative and angiogenic abilities [22, 23, 45, 47]. Regional anesthesia reduces the amount of intraoperative general anesthetics required, has opioid sparing effects, and markedly attenuates the neuroendocrine stress response to surgery as well as preserving NK cell function and T_h1 cell activity better than general anesthesia [48]. It is hypothesized that regional anesthesia and analgesia help preserve control of tumor progression. Modification to anesthetic management might thus reduce the risk of recurrence [18].

6. Imaging Techniques during Epidural Catheterization

Identifying the epidural space and correct needle positioning is often challenging for the novice anesthesiologist. Epidural catheter placement is thought to be among the most difficult techniques to acquire [49], with a success rate of as low as 60% at the first attempt [50], and an overall success rate of nearly 90% [51]. Factors contributing to the success or failure of catheter placement can be surgery related, as the type of surgery determines the specific region of the vertebral column for block placement [52]; patient dependent, such as body habitus, presence or absence of identifiable anatomical landmarks, or spinal anatomy; or operator dependent, such as the degree of personal experience, patient positioning, needle size, or the use of conventional "blind" versus imaging-guided techniques [53]. Previous reports suggest that the conventional "loss of resistance" technique used in the thoracic and lumbar region may have a false-positive success rate of as high as 30%, and, although generally considered reliable for epidural anesthesia, when used as a sole tool, this clinical sign may not offer the same potential to accurately identify the epidural space, as when complemented with an imaging tool [54, 55]. Visualization of the interlaminar space, accurate estimation of the depth to the epidural space, and optimal needle insertion angle are known to facilitate epidural block placement [50, 56, 57]. With the rapidly evolving imaging technology, there has been an increasing interest in the use of various imaging tools, to improve success rates of neuraxial blocks. Several studies have shown the usefulness of both ultrasound guided and fluoroscopically guided catheter insertion techniques [49, 58, 59].

6.1. Ultrasound Guided Epidural Catheter Placement. Ultrasound is a radiation-free imaging tool that is now widely used in clinical practice. The first successful sonographic measurement of the epidural space dates back to the 1980s, when Cork and colleagues [60], and Currie [61] were able to localize and estimate the distance from the skin to the epidural space. More recently, Bonazzi and de Gracia identified the ligamentum flavum in the lumbar vertebral region [62]. Technical improvement in sonographic visualization, such as the ability to digitally depict anatomical structures at high resolution, has much increased the clinical feasibility of ultrasound in epidural catheter insertion and visualization [57, 58]. The increasing popularity of this technique over the past three decades has been attributed to a more accurate estimation of epidural space depth, a more optimal determination of the needle insertion point, and insertion angle particularly in cases of difficult anatomy (such as obesity, especially during obstetric anesthesia, or scoliosis), or the presence of implanted hardware [63], and reduced failure rate [56]. While the use of ultrasound offers a greater likelihood of successful catheter placement in the obese patient, morbid obesity may pose technical difficulties to the visualization of the vertebral anatomy and the epidural space.

Besides the obvious benefits of this radiation-free technique compared to the conventional "blind" method, there are disadvantages of ultrasound use in the setting of epidural block placement. Technically, it can be difficult to simultaneously stabilize and advance the Tuohy needle, and maintain the acoustic window, holding the ultrasound probe in the optimal position. Also, it can be difficult to maintain continuous visualization of the Tuohy needle tip during advancement. The use of ultrasound in adults is helpful for anatomical identification, but there is limited published evidence available for the same degree of usefulness of real time needle insertion, compared to the pediatric population. A recent study by Belavy and colleagues, evaluating the feasibility of real-time 4D ultrasound for epidural catheter placement in cadavers, found that 4D ultrasound potentially improves operator orientation of the vertebral column at the cost of needle visibility and resolution [64–67]. Slight discrepancy between the sonographically and clinically measured epidural space depth should be anticipated, likely due to factors such as tissue deformation during needle passage, deviation from the midline, and deviation from the 90 degree insertion angle that has been found to most precisely correlate with the sonographically measured skin-epidural space distance. When compared to the fluoroscopic visualization, ultrasound guidance does not offer the advantage of placing the epidural catheter exactly at the desired vertebral level; also, the depth of the inserted needle may not always be adequately assessed.

6.2. Fluoroscopically Guided Epidural Catheter Placement. The usefulness of fluoroscopic guidance in epidural block placement in various regions of the vertebral column has been established [49, 55, 61]. Previous studies have shown that more than 50% of lumbar epidurals, in the absence of appropriate imaging tools, were actually performed at a level other than the one predicted [68]. A study by Renfrew and colleagues found that caudal blocks without the use of fluoroscopy resulted in a 52% incidence of erroneous needle placement [69], likely due to the subfascial compartment that provides low resistance to injection. Fluoroscopic guidance offers the advantages of precise needle angulation and localization of the catheter at the targeted vertebral level even in the presence of difficult or unreliable surface anatomy, as well as accurate identification of the epidural space, or the assessment of injectate dispersal, with the use of contrast dye to confirm the epidural placement. These factors may also obviate complications [59]. Fluoroscopy therefore improves the success rate of epidural block and provides a reliable delivery of therapeutic substances into the epidural space; however, both the patient and the operator are exposed to radiation. Furthermore, this method may only be safe in patients without contraindication to the use of contrast dye or radiation itself.

While the use of imaging tools for epidural catheter placement is gaining increasing popularity for their potential to increase success rate and reduce complications, the potential risks and benefits of these methods should be thoroughly assessed, and the choice of imaging technique should be determined on an individual basis. It should be remembered that the use of ultrasound guidance does not eliminate the need for using the conventional "loss of resistance" technique, and it is as important as when using the blind insertion technique.

7. Considerations in the Pediatric Population

With the development of advanced skills with ultrasound, guided techniques has attracted an increased interest in its use for neuraxial blocks. The benefits of identifying anatomy and directly visualizing needles and catheters, as found with peripheral blocks, can be of great value for improved success and confirmation of neuraxial blocks. Because of the large variation of each patient's body habitus due to age, it can be difficult to predict the puncture depth to reach either the epidural or intrathecal spaces [70].

In pediatric population, checking the anatomy with the ultrasound before and during performing the procedure gains and assures a lot of success. Visualization is clearer than in the adult population due to less ossification of the vertebral column and easiness to predict the epidural and/or the intrathecal spaces. Loss-of-resistance technique to identify the epidural space can be very challenging in neonates due to presence of less fibrous tissue limiting the tactile feedback [71].

Visibility of the spread of fluid is a promising technique during injection through the needle and catheter, which could confirm the position. Using an epidural electrical stimulation test is another method but the clinical value of electrical stimulation in caudal needle placement has not been extensively studied [72].

7.1. Caudal Needle and Catheter Placement under Ultrasound. Caudal anesthesia is one of the most popular regional blocks in the pediatric population to provide perioperative analgesia. Placement of a single shot caudal block or a lumbar/thoracic epidural catheter achieved through the caudal epidural space is an advanced skill. This technique becomes even more complex when considering variation in patient age, weight, and varying levels of bone ossification. Ultrasound guidance for this procedure is helpful in identifying the underlying anatomic structures. The ones most commonly of interest include the sacral hiatus, sacral cornua, coccyx, and sacrococcygeal ligament. While probe orientation can be done using either a transverse or longitudinal view of the midline, it is typically best to orient and assess landmarks prior to performing the procedure (Figures 1, 2, 3, 4, and 5).

When introducing a catheter into the caudal space to reach the lumbar or thoracic spine, a technique similar to the above is used for cannula placement. The catheter can then be directly visualized during advancement with the ultrasound at each level of the spine above the sacrum (Figures 2(a), 2(b), and 3).

As is the case during the assessment, either the longitudinal or transverse axes can be used to visualize the underlying structures and catheter position.

Confirmation of catheter placement can be performed through visualization of local anesthetic spread as well as through direct visualization of the catheter within the epidural space. Catheter tip visibility may be improved with the injection of a bubble-based fluid or local anesthetic spread and a swoosh test (using a stethoscope to listen to fluid movement).

7.2. Tunneling of Caudal Epidural Catheter. Bacterial colonization is regarded as a causative factor for infectious complications of caudal catheters in children [73]. In addition to the routine measures of wearing personal protective equipment (hats, masks, and gloves), prepping the area with an alcohol-based solution, and maintaining a sterile field, another option is to tunnel the catheter after placement. A small subcutaneous placement of the proximal portion of the catheter not only decreases the length of tubing potentially exposed to contamination, but it also helps in gaining a more secure catheter placement. Both of these features become especially advantageous in prolonged epidural catheter use.

8. Complications of Epidural Anesthesia

Epidural anesthesia and analgesia are generally considered to be safe with regards to adverse post procedural events, as their complications, resulting in permanent deficits, are rare. Besides their indications and obvious benefits, knowledge of adverse outcomes should also comprise an essential part of clinical decision making.

Complications of central neuraxial blockade, much depending on the experience in patient management, as well

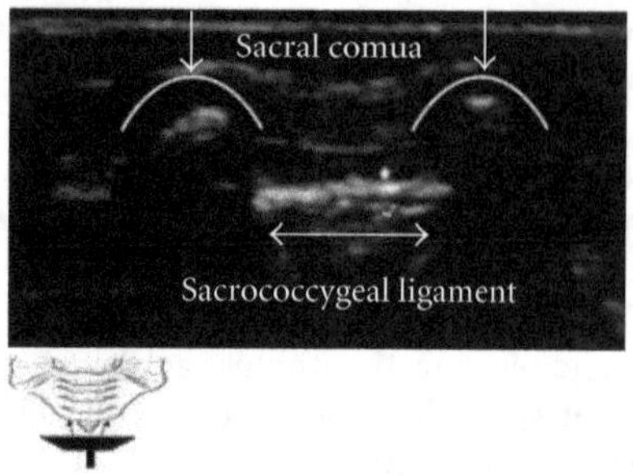

Figure 1: Placing the probe transverse plane at the coccyx, the sacral cornua (represented in white arrows heading down) are viewed laterally as humps. Sacral hiatus is located between an upper hyperechoic line, representing the sacrococcygeal membrane or ligament and an inferior hyperechoic line representing the dorsum of the pelvic surface of the sacrum (bidirectional sided arrow).

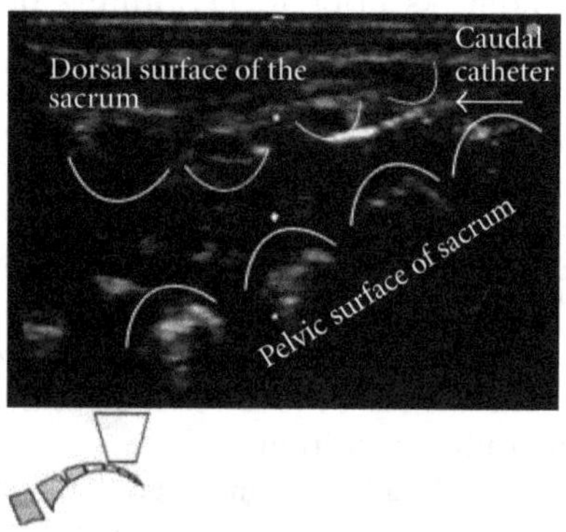

(a)

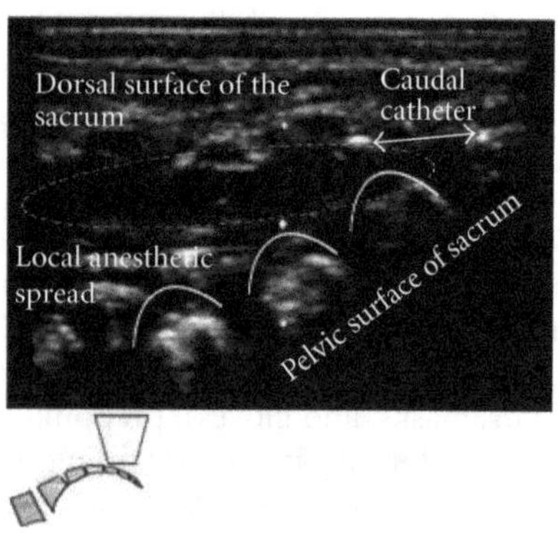

(b)

Figure 2: (a) Placing the probe longitudinally between the sacral cornua will capture the dorsal surface of the sacrum, the dorsal aspect of the pelvic surface of the sacrum, and the sacrococcygeal ligament. Angiocatheter penetrated the sacrococcygeal ligament and lies in the epidural space. (b) Local Anesthetic spread through Caudal Angiocatheter in caudal epidural space.

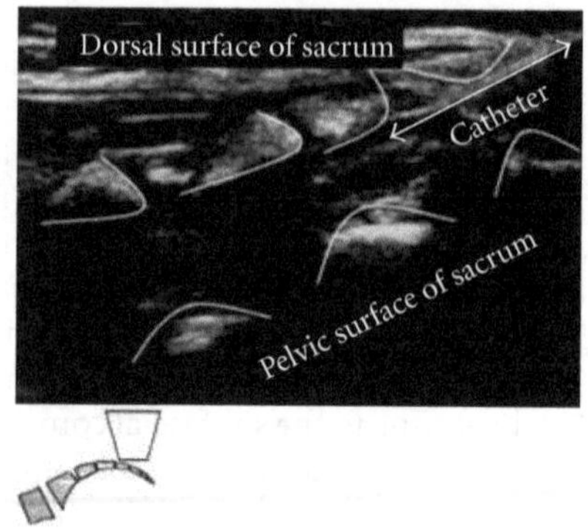

Figure 3: Caudal epidural catheter passing through Angiocatheter in the epidural space.

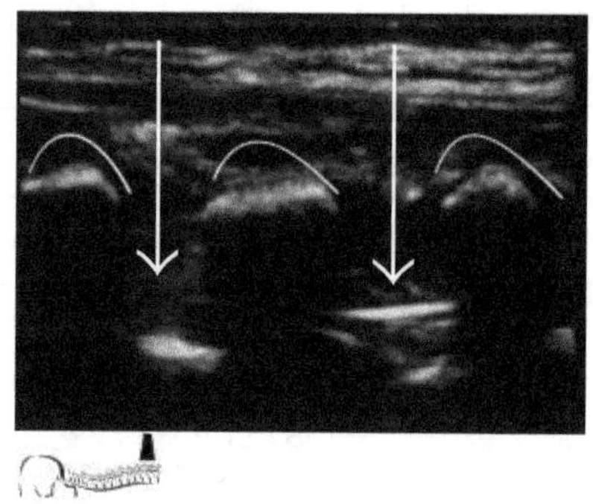

Figure 4: Longitudinal view at the thoracic spine level, viewing the advancement of the caudal epidural catheter. Curved lines show spinous processes. Arrows show epidural catheter in between spinous processes.

as materials, equipment, and the presence of risk factors, have been reported to occur at various frequencies [74, 75]. An epidemiologic study conducted in Sweden over a period of 10 years revealed an increasing trend (1 in 10,000 neuraxial anesthetics) of severe complications after central neuraxial blockade [74]. Relatively recent literature suggests that most of these occur with the perioperative use of epidural block [74, 76]. The incidence of major complications (permanent harm including death) of epidural and combined spinal-epidural anesthesia were at least twice as high as those of spinal and caudal blocks, as reported by Cook and colleagues. This study also found that the incidence of epidural catheter-related serious morbidity and mortality was higher when blocks were placed in the perioperative setting, as opposed to catheter placement in obstetric and pediatric populations, when inserted for chronic pain management, or when placed by non-anesthetists [77]. While prognosis is infrequently reported, retrospective reviews report full recovery in 61–75% of patients, epidural hematoma accounting for two-thirds of residual neurological deficits [77, 78]. Serious complications, if not recognized and treated at an early stage, may thus result in permanent loss of function [74, 79]. With regards to the timing of catheter placement, there is still substantial controversy: while many anesthesia providers believe that epidural catheters should be placed in awake or mildly sedated patients capable of providing feedback [80], Horlocker's retrospective review found no evidence of an increased risk for neural injury in anesthetized patients receiving epidural anesthetic [81]. Thoracic epidural placement, however, should never be attempted on an anesthetized patient. Having increasingly become

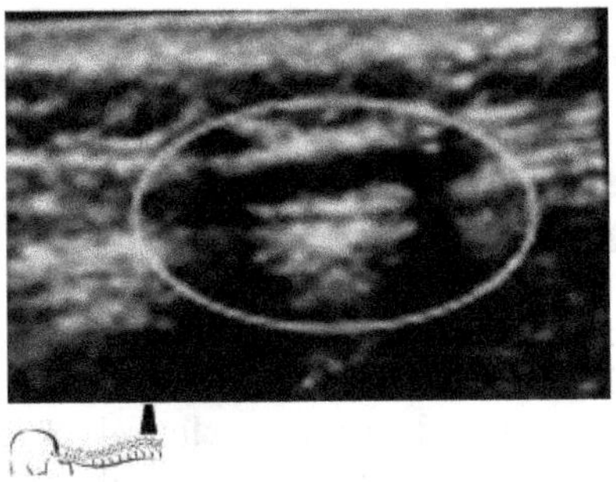

FIGURE 5: Longitudinal view at the lumbar spine. Visualization of the local anesthetic spread confirmed the position.

the focus of attention, and as a result of both meticulous adherence to sterile, atraumatic catheter insertion technique and management, as well as careful risk-benefit assessment, major complications of epidural anesthesia are now rare, particularly those not involving infection or bleeding, and many resolving within 6 months [74]. The estimation of the incidence of all adverse outcomes, however, is often inaccurate.

Complications may occur early if related to traumatic catheter insertion, or later in the operative-postoperative course if caused by catheter-related spinal space-occupying lesions such as epidural hematoma or abscess formation, and are infrequent among the general population. Although its incidence is lower than when associated with spinal anesthesia [80], transient neurological injury has been found to account for the majority of short-term epidural catheter related complications (1 in 6,700) in a meta-analysis by Ruppen and colleagues, followed by deep epidural infections (1 in 145,000), epidural hematoma (1 in 150,000–168,000), and persistent neurological injury (1 in 257,000) in women receiving epidural catheter for childbirth [82, 83]. Spinal epidural hematoma, however, has been recently suggested to occur in a rate as high as 1 in 3,600 in female patients undergoing knee arthroplasty [74, 84, 85]. These findings were consistent with those previously reported in the ASA Closed Claims Project database analysis by Lee et al; however, limitations of that study design and database do not allow risk quantification specific to regional anesthetic techniques or populations [86].

Adverse events may result from direct mechanical injury or adverse physiological responses. Neurological complications resulting from accidental penetration of the dura are similar to those that occur with spinal anesthesia. Inadvertent dural puncture and postdural puncture headache, direct neural injury, total spinal anesthesia, and subdural block have been commonly reported. The incidence of inadvertent dural puncture ranges between 0.19–0.5% of epidural catheter placements. Postdural puncture headache (PDPH), described as a positional, bilateral frontal-occipital, nonthrobbing pain, may develop in as much as 75% of patients [87–89]. PDPH is thought to develop as a result of persistent transdural leakage of cerebrospinal fluid (CSF) at a rate that is faster than that of CSF production. The subsequently decreasing CSF volume and pressure causes traction on the meninges and intracranial vessels, which refer pain to the frontal-occipital region, often extending to the neck and shoulders, more pronounced in the upright position. Available measures of prevention besides conservative measures are immediate intrathecal catheter placement, prophylactic epidural blood patch, epidural or intrathecal administration of saline, and epidural administration of morphine [90]. Direct neural injury has a reported incidence of 0.006% [82], and has been associated with paresthesias during needle placement and pain on injection [80]. Total spinal anesthesia may occur if the solution used for epidural anesthesia is inadvertently administered into the intrathecal space in large volumes. Symptoms are of a rapidly arising subarachnoid block, potentially resulting in cardiovascular collapse and apnea requiring prompt resuscitation. Provided that immediate, skilled resuscitative efforts are made, complete recovery should be expected [91]. While clinically not always distinguishable from epidural blocks, the incidence of clinically recognized subdural block was found to be 0.024% in a prospective study [92]. A subdural block may present as high sensory block, often with sparing of motor and sympathetic fibers, is slow in onset, and the blockade is disproportionately extensive for the volume of anesthetic injected. Clinical signs and symptoms may be mistaken for accidental intrathecal injection, migration of epidural catheter, or an asymmetrical, patchy or inadequate epidural block. Subdural placement is thought to occur independently of the operator's expertise. Although there are no established risk factors, recent lumbar puncture and rotation of the needle may predispose to subdural injection [93].

Hemorrhagic complications are serious adverse outcomes that may arise from neuraxial anesthesia. Epidural hematoma is a rare, but potentially devastating, complication that requires emergency decompression in case of clinical deterioration. It is rarely attributed to an arterial source, and can develop spontaneously [94, 95]. While paralysis may occur even after hematoma evacuation, it is still not precisely understood why several of the spinal epidural hematomas associated with concurrent anticoagulant use involving less blood than the volume injected when performing a therapeutic blood patch [85]. Clinically significant bleeding is more likely with congenital or acquired coagulation abnormalities, thrombocytopenia, vascular anomalies or anatomical abnormalities, advanced age and female gender, repetitive attempts at catheter insertion, and traumatic block placement [74, 96–98]. The risk is reported to increase 15-fold when there is a concomitant use of anticoagulants, and appropriate precautions are not taken [85]. Appropriate timing of anticoagulant administration is important in decreasing the risk of bleeding [99]. The commonest presenting symptoms of spinal epidural hematoma are new back pain, radicular pain, and progressive lower extremity weakness. Symptoms rarely present immediately after surgery, but may develop while the catheter is still in place. These symptoms can occur 15 hours to 3 days after catheter insertion [78, 98]. The diagnostic investigation of choice is MRI. A delay in diagnostic imaging may lead to devastating outcomes, and is a common error, as manifesting neurological symptoms and back pain may be attributed to the use of epidural infusion and a prolonged effect of local anesthetic, and to musculoskeletal origin [78, 100]. Cauda equina syndrome due to hematoma formation, a rare complication with a reported incidence of 2.7/100,000 epidural blocks, was found to result in permanent deficit in more than two-third of the cases [74]. Classic manifestation is low back pain, altered proprioception and decreased sensation to pinprick and temperature in the lumbar and sacral nerve distribution, voiding and defecation disturbances, and progressive loss of muscle strength. Outcomes are primarily function of interval to hematoma evacuation and the severity of the neurological deficit, and are favorable if decompression is performed within 8 hours of the development of symptoms [98].

Epidural catheter related infections are rare complications both in adult and in pediatric patients. A retrospective database analysis by Sethna et al. found an expected incidence ranging between 3–13/10,000 catheters in children [101]. Epidural abscess and meningitis has been reported to occur in 1 : 1000 and 1 : 50,000 catheter placements, respectively [74]. Although epidural catheters are placed under aseptic conditions, needle or catheter contamination does occur even during aseptic puncture and sterile handling of devices [102]. Of patient risk factors, skin colonization at the puncture site and bacterial migration along the catheter is proposed to be the most likely route of infection; however, immunosuppression [74, 103], diabetes mellitus [104], chronic renal failure, steroid administration, cancer, herpes zoster, rheumatoid arthritis [105], systemic or local sepsis, and prolonged infusion duration are also identifiable risk factors. The rate of skin colonization at puncture sites is reported to be higher in children than in adults, with an overall incidence as high as 35% [101]. The incidence of infection increases after three days [106]. The classic presentation signs and symptoms are severe midline back pain, fever, and leukocytosis, with or without neurological symptoms (worsening lower limb weakness and paraplegia, incontinence, irradiating pain, nuchal rigidity, and headache). Symptoms commonly appear after removal of the epidural catheter [78]. Neurological deficits have been found to be persistent in more than 50% of patients developing epidural abscess [105]. Barrier precautions, skin disinfection [107], as well as the use of closed epidural system, and patient-controlled epidural analgesia [101] have been suggested as ways to decrease the incidence of epidural catheter-associated infections. Frequent syringe changes, on the other hand, may be associated with a higher rate of epidural infections [108]. Frequently implicated infecting organisms are Methicillin-resistant Staphylococcus aureus (MRSA), Staphylococcus aureus, and Coagulase-negative Staphylococcus [101, 109]. Outcomes are favorable when diagnosed and treated promptly. Adhesive arachnoiditis, presenting in various forms, is a sterile inflammatory response to accidental subarachnoid injection of local anesthetics, preservatives, detergents, or antiseptics [110–112], and has also resulted from traumatic puncture or epidural abscess. Medical literature suggests an extremely low incidence [113, 114].

Complications of epidural anesthesia are rare events that may result in detrimental sequelae. Strict adherence to prophylactic measures and treatment without delay is essential to further lower the incidence of adverse outcomes.

9. Epidural Anesthesia and Thromboprophylaxis

Some controversy exists with regards to reduced coagulation and neuraxial anesthesia and challenges are emerging as new agents are introduced into clinical practice. Spinal epidural hematoma, although still considered to be a rare complication occurring at a previously reported rate of less than 1 in 150,000 epidural and less than 1 in 220,000 spinal anesthetics in patients with normal coagulation status, is now suggested to occur in a rate as high as 1 in 3,000 in some patient populations [84, 85]. Patients receiving antithrombotic or antiplatelet therapies are more at risk for this potentially dramatic adverse event, in particular after invasive procedures [98]. In the United States, the estimated incidence of spinal epidural hematoma with concurrent administration of antithrombotic drugs (low molecular weight heparins) is 1 : 40,800 for spinal anesthesia, 1 : 6,600 for single-shot epidural anesthesia, and 1 : 3,100 for continuous epidural anesthesia [85]. Risk factors for epidural bleeding were established as coagulation disorders, antithrombotic or fibrinolytic therapy, or the use of any agents interfering with coagulation, female gender, age, difficult vertebral or spinal cord anatomy, difficult or traumatic catheter insertion, and lack of guidelines [96, 98, 115, 116]. Catheter removal carries nearly the same risk as insertion [98]. Appropriate time intervals between the administration of anticoagulants, neuraxial block placement, and catheter removal are crucial in the prevention of hematoma formation [117, 118].

The American Society of Regional Anesthesia and Pain Medicine (ASRA), and more recently, the European Society of Anaesthesiology (ESA) published their consensus statements on neuraxial anesthesia and the use of antithrombotic and thrombolytic agents [99, 119]. While providing guidelines in clinical decision making, and having the aim of minimizing hemorrhagic complications, these recommendations do not guarantee a specific outcome, and allow of variations based on the judgment of the anesthesiologist. The guidelines of the American Society of Regional Anesthesia and Pain Medicine and the European Society of Anaesthesiology are based on previously published national recommendations, hematology, pharmacology, and risk factors for surgical bleeding, and incorporate updated information since the time of their publication.

With regards to epidural catheter placement, the ASRA recommends that patients receiving thrombolytic therapy be queried and their medical records reviewed for a recent history of lumbar puncture or neuraxial analgesia. Neuraxial anesthesia should be avoided, or, if received concurrently with the fibrinolytic/thrombolytic therapy, close neurological monitoring should be continued along with the administration of neuraxial solutions that minimize sensory and motor block. There is no definitive recommendation for epidural catheter removal in patients receiving fibrinolytic and thrombolytic therapy. Thrombolytics, if scheduled, should be avoided for 10 days after puncture of noncompressible vessels [99].

Patients receiving unfractionated heparin (UFH) thrice a day, if recommended by recent thromboprophylaxis guidelines, may be at an increased risk of surgical-related bleeding. The ASRA recommends that the patient's—potentially simultaneous—anticoagulant and antiplatelet medication be daily reviewed. There is no contraindication to epidural blockade in patients receiving subcutaneous UFH prophylaxis at daily doses of 2 × 5000 U. The risk of bleeding may be increased in debilitated patients receiving prolonged therapy, and may be decreased by delaying the heparin injection until after neuraxial block placement. The safety of central neural block in patients receiving subcutaneous UFH in a dosing regimen of more than 10,000 U daily has not been established, and an increased risk of a spinal epidural hematoma has also not been elucidated. Patients receiving heparin for greater than 4 days should be assessed for heparin-induced thrombocytopenia (HIT). In patients with known coagulopathies, combining neuraxial techniques with intraoperative heparinization should be avoided however, this technique is acceptable in patients with no other coagulation disorders, if

(1) heparin administration is delayed for 1 hour after puncture,
(2) epidural catheters are removed 2 to 4 hours after the last heparin dose and the patient's coagulation status is assessed. the next heparin dose may be administered 1 hour after catheter removal,
(3) patient is closely monitored for early signs of neurologic dysfunction while receiving neuraxial solutions that minimize sensory and motor block postoperatively.

Per the ASRA guidelines, in contrast with the ESA recommendations that suggest considering postponement of the procedure, difficult or traumatic block placement should not necessarily prompt postponing surgery; however, the potential benefits should be carefully weighed against all potentially detrimental outcomes in each individual. With regards to the full anticoagulation of patients undergoing cardiac surgery, the ASRA finds insufficient evidence available to determine an increased risk of neuraxial hematoma. Close postoperative monitoring of neurologic function, as well as administration of neuraxial solutions that minimize sensory and motor block to facilitate detection of signs and symptoms of cord compression, is however suggested [99, 119].

Patients on low molecular weight heparin (LMWH) anticoagulation have not been found to be at an increased risk of bleeding in high-risk groups, contrasting with patients receiving UFH-thromboprophylaxis. Also, compared to UFH, LMWH-therapy has been associated with a significant decrease in the risk of HIT, as demonstrated by Warkentin and colleagues [120]; nonetheless, LMWHs are contraindicated in such condition due to the high level of cross-reactivity. To avoid an elevated risk of bleeding complications, an interval of 10 to 12 hours between preoperative LMWH administration at prophylactic doses and needle placement or catheter removal is recommended. Administration of LMWH the night before surgery does not thus interfere with epidural block placement on the day of surgery. In patients on therapeutic doses of LMWH, catheter placement should be delayed for a minimum of 24 hours after the last dose. Patients undergoing general surgery and receiving LMWH 2 hours prior to surgery are not ideal candidates for a neuraxial blockade, and are thus recommended against neuraxial techniques. Patients receiving postoperative LMWH thromboprophylaxis may safely be administered both single-dose and continuous catheter techniques. With regards to management, timing of the first postoperative dose, dosing schedule, and total daily dose are authoritative. Concerning the management of patients receiving LMWH, the ASRA recommends against the routine monitoring of anti-Xa level and concurrent administration of medication affecting hemostasis, regardless of LMWH dosing regimen [99, 119].

The management of patients receiving perioperative oral anticoagulants is still controversial. In the United States, much like in Europe, therapeutic oral anticoagulation is considered as a contraindication to central neuraxial blockade. As opposed to Europe, however, perioperative thromboprophylaxis is still possible in the United States. According to the recommendation of the American Society of Regional Anesthesia and Pain Medicine, warfarin therapy must be stopped ideally 4-5 days before the scheduled procedure, and the INR checked before neuraxial block placement. In patients receiving an initial preoperative dose of warfarin, INR should be measured before needle puncture if the administration of the first dose exceeded 24 hours, or if a second dose of such anticoagulant has been administered. In patients at risk for an enhanced response to oral anticoagulants, a reduced dose of drug should be administered. In patients receiving low-dose warfarin during epidural analgesia, INR should be monitored daily. Epidural catheters should be removed when the INR is less than 1.5. If the INR is greater than 1.5 but less than 3, indwelling epidural catheters should be done with caution. The ASRA recommends against concurrent use of agents, such as UFH, LMWH, or platelet aggregation inhibitors, that influence other components of the clotting system, as these, without affecting the INR, may increase the risk of bleeding. Medical records should be reviewed for such agents. Neurologic testing of sensory and motor function should be performed routinely during epidural analgesia for patients on oral anticoagulants, and should be continued for at least 24 hours after catheter removal, until the INR returns to the desired prophylactic range. In patients with INR greater than 3, the American Society of Regional Anesthesia and Pain Medicine recommends that the warfarin be held or reduced, without making a definitive recommendation regarding the management to facilitate catheter removal in these patients [99, 119].

Platelet aggregation inhibitors, such as acetylsalicylic acid, thienopyridines (clopidogrel, ticlopidine, and prasugrel), glycoprotein (GP) IIb/IIIa antagonists (eptifibatide, tirofiban, and abciximab), the novel ADP P2Y12 receptor antagonist ticagrelor, and the selective phosphodiesterase IIIA inhibitor cilostazol, have diverse effects on platelet function. No wholly accepted test exists to guide antiplatelet therapy. It is therefore critical to perform a careful pre-operative risk assessment to identify factors that might potentially contribute to bleeding. Although administration of nonsteroidal anti-inflammatory drugs (including aspirin) does not appear to significantly increase the incidence of hematoma formation, concurrent administration of LMWH, UFH, or oral anticoagulants resulted in a higher rate of complications in both surgical and medical patients, their use along with NSAIDs, including aspirin, is therefore not recommended. Cyclooxygenase-2 inhibitors have minimal inhibitory effect on platelet aggregation, and should be considered in patients requiring anti-inflammatory therapy in the presence of anticoagulation. The actual incidence of spinal epidural hematoma related to thienopyridines and GP IIb/IIIa inhibitors is not known. Management should be based on labeling precautions and the experience of professionals involved in the clinical care of the patient. However, as it has been suggested by recent guidelines, ticlopidine and clopidogrel therapy should be discontinued 14 and 7days prior to neuraxial block, respectively. If needle puncture is indicated between 5 and 7 days of discontinuation of clopidogrel, normalization of platelet function should be documented. GP IIb/IIIa antagonists exert a dose-dependent effect on platelet aggregation. After the last administered dose, the time to normal aggregation is 4 to 8 hours for eptifibatide and tirofiban, and 24 to 48 hours for abciximab. Neuraxial blockade should be avoided until normal platelet function is achieved. Should a patient, despite the contraindication, be administered GP IIb/IIIa inhibitors within 4 weeks of surgery, careful neurological monitoring should be performed [99, 119].

Both the ASRA and the ESA guidelines recommend against the mandatory discontinuation of herbal agents (most commonly: garlic, Echinacea, Gingko biloba, ginseng, aloe vera, and ephedra of dwarf palm), neither should neuraxial techniques be avoided, as there is insufficient evidence that these, by themselves, significantly increase the risk for spinal hematoma formation. There is insufficient evidence to conclude that thrombin inhibitors, such as lepirudin, desirudin, bivalirudin, or argatroban, are safer to use in patients receiving spinal or epidural anesthesia; performance of these techniques in the presence of these agents is thus not recommended. Until sufficient evidence is available, neuraxial techniques in patients receiving fondaparinux should only be performed if single needle pass, atraumatic block placement, and avoidance of indwelling catheters are feasible, or a different method of prophylaxis should be considered [99, 119].

10. Summary

Epidural and caudal anesthesia is a versatile neuraxial anesthetic technique with an expanding area of indication. It can be used in the perioperative setting as the sole anesthetic, or in combination with general or spinal anesthesia. Its potential to decrease postoperative complication rate by its beneficial physiological effects has been clearly demonstrated in several studies. The absolute contraindications to its use have traditionally been well defined. Despite its rare, but potentially devastating complications, neuraxial anesthesia is considered to be safe. Performing such procedures in the presence of anticoagulants is however controversial. With patients presenting with medical conditions that predispose to clinically significant bleeding and an increased number of patients taking various anticoagulants, there is greater concern for an increased incidence of epidural hematomas. The key to maximizing the advantages while minimizing the disadvantages of epidural and caudal anesthesia is to become familiar with the anatomical, physiological, pharmacological, and technical aspects of block placement. The review and advances discussed here allow both adult and pediatric populations a form of care that is often considered indispensable.

Conflict of Interests

The authors declare no conflict of interest.

References

[1] J. Corning, "Spinal anesthesia and local medications of the cord," *New York Journal of Medicine*, vol. 42, pp. 483–485, 1885.

[2] D. Brown, "Spinal, epidural, and caudal anesthesia," in *Miller's Anesthesia*, R. D. Miller, Ed., pp. 1653–1683, Elsevier, Philadelphia, Pa, USA, 6th edition, 2005.

[3] Q. H. Hogan, "Lumbar epidural anatomy. A new look by cryomicrotome section," *Anesthesiology*, vol. 75, no. 5, pp. 767–775, 1991.

[4] Q. Hogan, "Distribution of solution in the epidural space: examination by cryomicrotome section," *Regional Anesthesia and Pain Medicine*, vol. 27, no. 2, pp. 150–156, 2002.

[5] B Deschner, M. Allen, and O. de Leon, "Epidural blockade," in *Textbook of Regional Anesthesia and Acute Pain Management*, A. Hadzic, Ed., pp. 237–269, McGraw–Hill, New York, NY, USA, 1st edition, 2006.

[6] J. H. McClure, "Ropivacaine," *British Journal of Anaesthesia*, vol. 76, no. 2, pp. 300–307, 1996.

[7] I. Harukuni, H. Yamaguchi, S. Sato, and H. Naito, "The comparison of epidural fentanyl, epidural lidocaine, and intravenous fentanyl in patients undergoing gastrectomy," *Anesthesia and Analgesia*, vol. 81, no. 6, pp. 1169–1174, 1995.

[8] A. Tamsen and T. Gordh, "Epidural clonidine produces analgesia," *The Lancet*, vol. 2, no. 8396, pp. 231–232, 1984.

[9] M. De Kock, B. Crochet, C. Morimont, and J. L. Scholtes, "Intravenous or epidural clonidine for intra- and postoperative analgesia," *Anesthesiology*, vol. 79, no. 3, pp. 525–531, 1993.

[10] M. De Kock, "Site of hemodynamic effects of alpha sub 2 -adrenergic agonists," *Anesthesiology*, vol. 75, pp. 715–716, 1991.

[11] B. Biki, E. Mascha, D. C. Moriarty, J. M. Fitzpatrick, D. I. Sessler, and D. J. Buggy, "Anesthetic technique for radical prostatectomy surgery affects cancer recurrence: a retrospective analysis," *Anesthesiology*, vol. 109, no. 2, pp. 180–187, 2008.

[12] J. P. Desborough, "The stress response to trauma and surgery," *British Journal of Anaesthesia*, vol. 85, no. 1, pp. 109–117, 2000.

[13] S. Ben-Eliyahu, G. G. Page, R. Yirmiya, and G. Shakhar, "Evidence that stress and surgical interventions promote tumor development by suppressing natural killer cell activity," *International Journal of Cancer*, vol. 80, no. 6, pp. 880–888, 1999.

[14] S. C. O'Riain, D. J. Buggy, M. J. Kerin, R. W. G. Watson, and D. C. Moriarty, "Inhibition of the stress response to breast cancer surgery by regional anesthesia and analgesia does not affect vascular endothelial growth factor and prostaglandin E2," *Anesthesia and Analgesia*, vol. 100, no. 1, pp. 244–249, 2005.

[15] H. Kehlet, "Modification of responses to surgery by neural blockade: clinical implications," in *Neural Blockade in Clinical Anesthesia and Management of Pain*, M. Cousins and P. Bridenbaugh, Eds., pp. 129–178, J. B. Lippincott, Philadelphia, Pa, USA, 1998.

[16] H. Kehlet, "Surgical stress: the role of pain and analgesia," *British Journal of Anaesthesia*, vol. 63, no. 2, pp. 189–195, 1989.

[17] H. O. Besedovsky, A. E. Del Rey, and E. Sorkin, "Immune-neuroendocrine interactions," *Journal of Immunology*, vol. 135, no. 2, pp. 750–754, 1985.

[18] D. I. Sessler, "Long-term consequences of anesthetic management," *Anesthesiology*, vol. 111, no. 1, pp. 1–4, 2009.

[19] S. Ben-Eliyahu, G. Shakhar, G. G. Page, V. Stefanski, and K. Shakhar, "Suppression of NK cell activity and of resistance to metastasis by stress: a role for adrenal catecholamines and β-adrenoceptors," *NeuroImmunoModulation*, vol. 8, no. 3, pp. 154–164, 2000.

[20] K. Buttenschoen, K. Fathimani, and D. C. Buttenschoen, "Effect of major abdominal surgery on the host immune response to infection," *Current Opinion in Infectious Diseases*, vol. 23, no. 3, pp. 259–267, 2010.

[21] D. J. Buggy and G. Smith, "Epidural anaesthesia and analgesia: better outcome after major surgery?" *British Medical Journal*, vol. 319, no. 7209, pp. 530–531, 1999.

[22] M. S. O'Reilly, T. Boehm, Y. Shing et al., "Endostatin: an endogenous inhibitor of angiogenesis and tumor growth," *Cell*, vol. 88, no. 2, pp. 277–285, 1997.

[23] M. S. O'Reilly, L. Holmgren, Y. Shing et al., "Angiostatin: a novel angiogenesis inhibitor that mediates the suppression of metastases by a Lewis lung carcinoma," *Cell*, vol. 79, no. 2, pp. 315–328, 1994.

[24] M. Yokoyama, Y. Itano, S. Mizobuchi et al., "The effects of epidural block on the distribution of lymphocyte subsets and natural-killer cell activity in patients with and without pain," *Anesthesia and Analgesia*, vol. 92, no. 2, pp. 463–469, 2001.

[25] S. A. Kirkley, "Proposed mechanisms of transfusion-induced immunomodulation," *Clinical and Diagnostic Laboratory Immunology*, vol. 6, no. 5, pp. 652–657, 1999.

[26] L. Reynolds, J. Beckmann, and A. Kurz, "Perioperative complications of hypothermia," *Best Practice and Research*, vol. 22, no. 4, pp. 645–657, 2008.

[27] M. Turina, D. E. Fry, and H. C. Polk, "Acute hyperglycemia and the innate immune system: clinical, cellular, and molecular aspects," *Critical Care Medicine*, vol. 33, no. 7, pp. 1624–1633, 2005.

[28] G. Delogu, S. Moretti, G. Famularo et al., "Mitochondrial perturbations and oxidant stress in lymphocytes from patients undergoing surgery and general anesthesia," *Archives of Surgery*, vol. 136, no. 10, pp. 1190–1196, 2001.

[29] G. P. Chrousos, F. Epstein, J. Flier, S. Reichlin, and S. Pavlou, "The hypothalamic-pituitary-adrenal axis and immune-mediated inflammation," *New England Journal of Medicine*, vol. 332, no. 20, pp. 1351–1362, 1995.

[30] A. J. Rassias, A. L. Givan, C. A. S. Marrin, K. Whalen, J. Pahl, and M. P. Yeager, "Insulin increases neutrophil count and phagocytic capacity after cardiac surgery," *Anesthesia and Analgesia*, vol. 94, no. 5, pp. 1113–1119, 2002.

[31] C. P. Nielson and D. A. Hindson, "Inhibition of polymorphonuclear leukocyte respiratory burst by elevated glucose concentrations in vitro," *Diabetes*, vol. 38, no. 8, pp. 1031–1035, 1989.

[32] A. J. Rassias, C. A. S. Marrin, J. Arruda, P. K. Whalen, M. Beach, and M. P. Yeager, "Insulin infusion improves neutrophil function in diabetic cardiac surgery patients," *Anesthesia and Analgesia*, vol. 88, no. 5, pp. 1011–1016, 1999.

[33] I. Beck, J. S. Scott, M. Pepper, and E. H. Speck, "The effect of neonatal exchange and later blood transfusion on lymphocyte cultures," *American Journal of Reproductive Immunology*, vol. 1, no. 5, pp. 224–225, 1981.

[34] P. I. Tartter, B. Steinberg, D. M. Barron, and G. Martinelli, "Transfusion history, T cell subsets and natural killer cytotoxicity in patients with colorectal cancer," *Vox Sanguinis*, vol. 56, no. 2, pp. 80–84, 1989.

[35] K. Yuki, N. S. Astrof, C. Bracken, G. S. Sulpicio, and M. Shimaoka, "Sevoflurane binds and allosterically blocks integrin lymphocyte function-associated antigen-1," *Anesthesiology*, vol. 113, no. 3, pp. 600–609, 2010.

[36] P. Sacerdote, M. Bianchi, L. Gaspani et al., "The effects of tramadol and morphine on immune responses and pain after surgery in cancer patients," *Anesthesia and Analgesia*, vol. 90, no. 6, pp. 1411–1414, 2000.

[37] R. Melamed, S. Bar-Yosef, G. Shakhar, K. Shakhar, and S. Ben-Eliyahu, "Suppression of natural killer cell activity and promotion of tumor metastasis by ketamine, thiopental, and halothane, but not by propofol: mediating mechanisms and prophylactic measures," *Anesthesia and Analgesia*, vol. 97, no. 5, pp. 1331–1339, 2003.

[38] J. M. Risdahl, K. V. Khanna, P. K. Peterson, and T. W. Molitor, "Opiates and infection," *Journal of Neuroimmunology*, vol. 83, no. 1-2, pp. 4–18, 1998.

[39] S. Roy and H. H. Loh, "Effects of opioids on the immune system," *Neurochemical Research*, vol. 21, no. 11, pp. 1375–1386, 1996.

[40] T. Hori, T. Katafuchi, S. Take, Y. Kaizuka, T. Ichijo, and N. Shimizu, "The hypothalamo-sympathetic nervous system modulates peripheral cellular immunity," *Neurobiology*, vol. 3, no. 3-4, pp. 309–317, 1995.

[41] M. H. Makman, "Morphine receptors in immunocytes and neurons," *Advances in Neuroimmunology*, vol. 4, no. 2, pp. 69–82, 1994.

[42] E. J. De Waal, J. W. Van Der Laan, and H. Van Loveren, "Effects of prolonged exposure to morphine and methadone on in vivo parameters of immune function in rats," *Toxicology*, vol. 129, no. 2-3, pp. 201–210, 1998.

[43] K. Jaeger, D. Scheinichen, J. Heine et al., "Remifentanil, fentanyl, and alfentanil have no influence on the respiratory burst of human neutrophils in vitro," *Acta Anaesthesiologica Scandinavica*, vol. 42, no. 9, pp. 1110–1113, 1998.

[44] B. Larsen, G. Hoff, W. Wilhelm, H. Buchinger, G. A. Wanner, and M. Bauer, "Effect of intravenous anesthetics on spontaneous and endotoxin- stimulated cytokine response in cultured human whole blood," *Anesthesiology*, vol. 89, no. 5, pp. 1218–1227, 1998.

[45] P. Buinauskas, G. McDonald, and W. Cole, "Role of operative stress on the resistance of the experimental animal to inoculated cancer cells," *Annals of Surgery*, vol. 148, pp. 642–648, 1958.

[46] M. G. Denis, C. Lipart, J. Leborgne et al., "Detection of disseminated tumor cells in peripheral blood of colorectal cancer patients," *International Journal of Cancer*, vol. 74, no. 5, pp. 540–544, 1997.

[47] G. Shakhar and S. Ben-Eliyahu, "Potential prophylactic measures against postoperative immunosuppression: could they reduce recurrence rates in oncological patients?" *Annals of Surgical Oncology*, vol. 10, no. 8, pp. 972–992, 2003.

[48] W. A. Koltun, M. M. Bloomer, A. F. Tilberg et al., "Awake epidural anesthesia is associated with improved natural killer cell cytotoxicity and a reduced stress response," *American Journal of Surgery*, vol. 171, no. 1, pp. 68–72, 1996.

[49] T. Nagaro, T. Yorozuya, M. Kamei, N. Kii, T. Arai, and S. Abe, "Fluoroscopically guided epidural block in the thoracic and lumbar regions," *Regional Anesthesia and Pain Medicine*, vol. 31, no. 5, pp. 409–416, 2006.

[50] P. Marhofer, M. Greher, and S. Kapral, "Ultrasound guidance in regional anaesthesia," *British Journal of Anaesthesia*, vol. 94, no. 1, pp. 7–17, 2005.

[51] P. H. Pan, T. D. Bogard, and M. D. Owen, "Incidence and characteristics of failures in obstetric neuraxial analgesia and anesthesia: a retrospective analysis of 19,259 deliveries," *International Journal of Obstetric Anesthesia*, vol. 13, no. 4, pp. 227–233, 2004.

[52] P. Lirk, H. Messner, M. Deibl et al., "Accuracy in estimating the correct intervertebral space level during lumbar, thoracic and cervical epidural anaesthesia," *Acta Anaesthesiologica Scandinavica*, vol. 48, no. 3, pp. 347–349, 2004.

[53] H. Willschke, P. Marhofer, A. Bosenberg et al., "Epidural catheter placement in children: comparing a novel approach using ultrasound guidance and a standard loss-of-resistance technique," *British Journal of Anaesthesia*, vol. 97, no. 2, pp. 200–207, 2006.

[54] A. H. White, R. Derby, and G. Wynne, "Epidural injections for the diagnosis and treatment of low-back pain," *Spine*, vol. 5, no. 1, pp. 78–86, 1980.

[55] A. H. White, "Injection techniques for the diagnosis and treatment of low back pain," *Orthopedic Clinics of North America*, vol. 14, no. 3, pp. 553–567, 1983.

[56] C. P. C. Chen, S. F. T. Tang, T. C. Hsu et al., "Ultrasound guidance in caudal epidural needle placement," *Anesthesiology*, vol. 101, no. 1, pp. 181–184, 2004.

[57] T. Grau, R. W. Leipold, R. Conradi, E. Martin, and J. Motsch, "Ultrasound imaging facilitates localization of the epidural space during combined spinal and epidural anesthesia," *Regional Anesthesia and Pain Medicine*, vol. 26, no. 1, pp. 64–67, 2001.

[58] T. Grau, R. W. Leipold, R. Conradi, E. Martin, and J. Motsch, "Efficacy of ultrasound imaging in obstetric epidural anesthesia," *Journal of Clinical Anesthesia*, vol. 14, no. 3, pp. 169–175, 2002.

[59] B. A. Johnson, K. P. Schellhas, and S. R. Pollei, "Epidurography and therapeutic epidural injections: technical considerations and experience with 5334 cases," *American Journal of Neuroradiology*, vol. 20, no. 4, pp. 697–705, 1999.

[60] R. C. Cork, J. J. Kryc, and R. W. Vaughan, "Ultrasonic localization of the lumbar epidural space," *Anesthesiology*, vol. 52, no. 6, pp. 513–516, 1980.

[61] J. M. Currie, "Measurement of the depth to the extradural space using ultrasound," *British Journal of Anaesthesia*, vol. 56, no. 4, pp. 345–347, 1984.

[62] M. Bonazzi and L. B. de Gracia, "Individuazione ecoguidata dello spazio epidurale lombare," *Minerva Anesthesiol*, vol. 61, pp. 201–205, 1995.

[63] D. H. Wallace, J. M. Currie, L. C. Gilstrap, and R. Santos, "Indirect sonographic guidance for epidural anesthesia in obese pregnant patients," *Regional Anesthesia*, vol. 17, no. 4, pp. 233–236, 1992.

[64] H.-J. Rapp, A. Folger, and T. Grau, "Ultrasound-guided epidural catheter insertion in children," *Anesthesia and Analgesia*, vol. 101, no. 2, pp. 333–339, 2005.

[65] D. Belavy, M. J. Ruitenberg, and R. B. Brijball, "Feasibility study of real-time three-/four-dimensional ultrasound for epidural catheter insertion," *British Journal of Anaesthesia*, vol. 107, no. 3, pp. 438–445, 2011.

[66] M. K. Karmakar, X. Li, A. M.-H. Ho, W. H. Kwok, and P. T. Chui, "Real-time ultrasound-guided paramedian epidural access: evaluation of a novel in-plane technique," *British Journal of Anaesthesia*, vol. 102, no. 6, pp. 845–854, 2009.

[67] H. Yamagami, Y. Yuda, M. Shiotani, K. Ooseto, Y. Naganuma, and H. Karasawa, "The administration of continuous epidural block under proneposition with fluoroscopic guidance," *Japanese Journal of Anesthesiology*, vol. 38, no. 2, pp. 229–235, 1989.

[68] B. Fredman, M. B. Nun, E. Zohar et al., "Epidural steroids for treating "failed back surgery syndrome": is fluoroscopy really necessary?" *Anesthesia and Analgesia*, vol. 88, no. 2, pp. 367–372, 1999.

[69] D. L. Renfrew, T. E. Moore, M. H. Kathol, G. Y. El-Khoury, J. H. Lemke, and C. W. Walker, "Correct placement of epidural steroid injections: fluoroscopic guidance and contrast administration," *American Journal of Neuroradiology*, vol. 12, no. 5, pp. 1003–1007, 1991.

[70] O. J. Arthurs, M. Murray, M. Zubier, J. Tooley, and W. Kelsall, "Ultrasonographic determination of neonatal spinal canal depth," *Archives of Disease in Childhood*, vol. 93, no. 6, pp. f451–f454, 2008.

[71] J. G. McCormack and S. Malherbe, "Applications of ultrasound in paediatric anaesthesia," *Current Anaesthesia and Critical Care*, vol. 19, no. 5-6, pp. 302–308, 2008.

[72] B. C. H. Tsui, P. Tarkkila, S. Gupta, and R. Kearney, "Confirmation of caudal needle placement using nerve stimulation," *Anesthesiology*, vol. 91, no. 2, pp. 374–378, 1999.

[73] W. Fujinaka, N. Hinomoto, S. Saeki, A. Yoshida, and S. Uemura, "Decreased risk of catheter infection in infants and children using subcutaneous tunneling for continuous caudal anesthesia," *Acta Medica Okayama*, vol. 55, no. 5, pp. 283–287, 2001.

[74] V. Moen, N. Dahlgren, and L. Irestedt, "Severe neurological complications after central neuraxial blockades in Sweden 1990–1999," *Anesthesiology*, vol. 101, no. 4, pp. 950–959, 2004.

[75] N. Dahlgren and K. Tornebrandt, "Neurological complications after anaesthesia. A follow-up of 18,000 spinal and epidural anaesthetics performed over three years," *Acta Anaesthesiologica Scandinavica*, vol. 39, no. 7, pp. 872–880, 1995.

[76] U. Aromaa, M. Lahdensuu, and D. A. Cozanitis, "Severe complications associated with epidural and spinal anaesthesias in Finland 1987–1993. A study based on patient insurance

claims," *Acta Anaesthesiologica Scandinavica*, vol. 41, no. 4, pp. 445–452, 1997.

[77] T. M. Cook, D. Counsell, and J. A. W. Wildsmith, "Major complications of central neuraxial block: report on the Third National Audit Project of the Royal College of Anaesthetists," *British Journal of Anaesthesia*, vol. 102, no. 2, pp. 179–190, 2009.

[78] I. W. Christie and S. McCabe, "Major complications of epidural analgesia after surgery: results of a six-year survey," *Anaesthesia*, vol. 62, no. 4, pp. 335–341, 2007.

[79] A. A. N. M. Royakkers, H. Willigers, A. J. Van der Ven, J. Wilmink, M. Durieux, and M. Van Kleef, "Catheter-related epidural abscesses—Don't wait for neurological deficits," *Acta Anaesthesiologica Scandinavica*, vol. 46, no. 5, pp. 611–615, 2002.

[80] Y. Auroy, P. Narchi, A. Messiah, L. Litt, B. Rouvier, and K. Samii, "Serious complications related to regional anesthesia: results of a prospective survey in France," *Anesthesiology*, vol. 87, no. 3, pp. 479–486, 1997.

[81] T. T. Horlocker, M. D. Abel, J. M. Messick, and D. R. Schroeder, "Small risk of serious neurologic complications related to lumbar epidural catheter placement in anesthetized patients," *Anesthesia and Analgesia*, vol. 96, no. 6, pp. 1547–1552, 2003.

[82] W. Ruppen, S. Derry, H. McQuay, and R. A. Moore, "Incidence of epidural hematoma, infection, and neurologic injury in obstetric patients with epidural analgesia/anesthesia," *Anesthesiology*, vol. 105, no. 2, pp. 394–399, 2006.

[83] C. L. Wu, R. W. Hurley, G. F. Anderson, R. Herbert, A. J. Rowlingson, and L. A. Fleisher, "Effect of postoperative epidural analgesia on morbidity and mortality following surgery in medicare patients," *Regional Anesthesia and Pain Medicine*, vol. 29, no. 6, pp. 525–533, 2004.

[84] A. Tyagi and A. Bhattacharya, "Central neuraxial blocks and anticoagulation: a review of current trends," *European Journal of Anaesthesiology*, vol. 19, no. 5, pp. 317–329, 2002.

[85] D. R. Schroeder, "Statistics: detecting a rare adverse drug reaction using spontaneous reports," *Regional Anesthesia and Pain Medicine*, vol. 23, no. 6, pp. 183–189, 1998.

[86] L. A. Lee, K. L. Posner, K. B. Domino, R. A. Caplan, and F. W. Cheney, "Injuries associated with regional anesthesia in the 1980s and 1990s: a closed claims analysis," *Anesthesiology*, vol. 101, no. 1, pp. 143–152, 2004.

[87] C. M. Gleeson and F. Reynolds, "Accidental dural puncture rates in UK obstetric practice," *International Journal of Obstetric Anesthesia*, vol. 7, no. 4, pp. 242–246, 1998.

[88] B. Darvish, A. Gupta, S. Alahuhta et al., "Management of accidental dural puncture and post-dural puncture headache after labour: a Nordic survey," *Acta Anaesthesiologica Scandinavica*, vol. 55, no. 1, pp. 46–53, 2011.

[89] M. Van de Velde, R. Schepers, N. Berends, E. Vandermeersch, and F. De Buck, "Ten years of experience with accidental dural puncture and post-dural puncture headache in a tertiary obstetric anaesthesia department," *International Journal of Obstetric Anesthesia*, vol. 17, no. 4, pp. 329–335, 2008.

[90] C. C. Apfel, A. Saxena, O. S. Cakmakkaya, R. Gaiser, E. George, and O. Radke, "Prevention of postdural puncture headache after accidental dural puncture: a quantitative systematic review," *British Journal of Anaesthesia*, vol. 105, no. 3, pp. 255–263, 2010.

[91] K. Hara and T. Sata, "Unintentional total spinal anesthesia during cervical epidural block with ropivacaine," *Japanese Journal of Anesthesiology*, vol. 55, no. 9, pp. 1168–1169, 2006.

[92] J. G. Jenkins, "Some immediate serious complications of obstetric epidural analgesia and anaesthesia: a prospective study of 145 550 epidurals," *International Journal of Obstetric Anesthesia*, vol. 14, no. 1, pp. 37–42, 2005.

[93] D. Agarwal, M. Mohta, A. Tyagi, and A. K. Sethi, "Subdural block and the anaesthetist," *Anaesthesia and Intensive Care*, vol. 38, no. 1, pp. 20–25, 2010.

[94] S. M. Hussenbocus, M. J. Wilby, C. Cain, and D. Hall, "Spontaneous spinal epidural hematoma: a case report and literature review," *Journal of Emergency Medicine*. In press.

[95] T. T. Horlocker, "What's a nice patient like you doing with a complication like this? Diagnosis, prognosis and prevention of spinal hematoma," *Canadian Journal of Anesthesia*, vol. 51, no. 6, pp. 527–534, 2004.

[96] H. Wulf, "Epidural anaesthesia and spinal haematoma," *Canadian Journal of Anaesthesia*, vol. 43, no. 12, pp. 1260–1271, 1996.

[97] H. Renck, "Neurological complications of central nerve blocks," *Acta Anaesthesiologica Scandinavica*, vol. 39, no. 7, pp. 859–868, 1995.

[98] E. Vandermeulen, H. van Aken, and J. Vermylen, "Anticoagulants and spinal-epidural anaesthesia," *Anesthesia & Analgesia*, vol. 79, pp. 1165–1177, 1994.

[99] T. T. Horlocker, D. J. Wedel, J. C. Rowlingson et al., "Regional Anesthesia in the patient receiving antithrombotic or thrombolytic therapy; American Society of Regional Anesthesia and Pain Medicine evidence-based guidelines (Third Edition)," *Regional Anesthesia and Pain Medicine*, vol. 35, no. 1, pp. 64–101, 2010.

[100] F. W. Cheney, K. B. Domino, R. A. Caplan, and K. L. Posner, "Nerve injury associated with anesthesia: a closed claims analysis," *Anesthesiology*, vol. 90, no. 4, pp. 1062–1069, 1999.

[101] N. F. Sethna, D. Clendenin, U. Athiraman, J. Solodiuk, D. P. Rodriguez, and D. Zurakowski, "Incidence of epidural catheter-associated infections after continuous epidural analgesia in children," *Anesthesiology*, vol. 113, no. 1, pp. 224–232, 2010.

[102] C. Raedler, C. Lass-Flörl, F. Pühringer, C. Kolbitsch, W. Lingnau, and A. Benzer, "Bacterial contamination of needles used for spinal and epidural anaesthesia," *British Journal of Anaesthesia*, vol. 83, no. 4, pp. 657–658, 1999.

[103] L. P. Wang, J. Hauerberg, and J. F. Schmidt, "Incidence of spinal epidural abscess after epidural analgesia: a national 1-year survey," *Anesthesiology*, vol. 91, no. 6, pp. 1928–1936, 1999.

[104] A. S. Baker, R. G. Ojemann, M. N. Swartz, and E. P. Richardson, "Spinal epidural abscess," *New England Journal of Medicine*, vol. 293, no. 10, pp. 463–468, 1975.

[105] W. D. Ngan Kee, M. R. Jones, P. Thomas, and R. J. Worth, "Extradural abscess complicating extradural anaesthesia for Caesarean section," *British Journal of Anaesthesia*, vol. 69, no. 6, pp. 647–652, 1992.

[106] S. Grewal, G. Hocking, and J. A. W. Wildsmith, "Epidural abscesses," *British Journal of Anaesthesia*, vol. 96, no. 3, pp. 292–302, 2006.

[107] I. Haraga, S. Shono, S. Abe, and K. Higa, "Aseptic precautions in epidural catheterization for surgery," *Japanese Journal of Anesthesiology*, vol. 59, no. 5, pp. 585–588, 2010.

[108] D. B. Scott and B. M. Hibbard, "Serious non-fatal complications associated with extradural block in obstetric practice," *British Journal of Anaesthesia*, vol. 64, no. 5, pp. 537–541, 1990.

[109] H. B. Yuan, Z. Zuo, K. W. Yu, W. M. Lin, H. C. Lee, and K. H. Chan, "Bacterial colonization of epidural catheters

used for short-term postoperative analgesia: microbiological examination and risk factor analysis," *Anesthesiology*, vol. 108, no. 1, pp. 130–137, 2008.

[110] K. Drasner, M. L. Rigler, D. I. Sessler, and M. L. Stoller, "Cauda equina syndrome following intended epidural anesthesia," *Anesthesiology*, vol. 77, no. 3, pp. 582–585, 1992.

[111] A. Sghirlanzoni, R. Marazzi, D. Pareyson, A. Olivieri, and M. Bracchi, "Epidural anaesthesia and spinal arachnoiditis," *Anaesthesia*, vol. 44, no. 4, pp. 317–321, 1989.

[112] J. A. Aldrete, "Neurologic deficits and arachnoiditis following neuroaxial anesthesia," *Acta Anaesthesiologica Scandinavica*, vol. 47, no. 1, pp. 3–12, 2003.

[113] I. Rice, M. Y. K. Wee, and K. Thomson, "Obstetric epidurals and chronic adhesive arachnoiditis," *British Journal of Anaesthesia*, vol. 92, no. 1, pp. 109–120, 2004.

[114] D. M. Long, "Chronic adhesive spinal arachnoiditis: pathogenesis, prognosis, and treatment," *Neurosurgery Quarterly*, vol. 2, no. 4, pp. 296–319, 1992.

[115] D. K. Wysowski, L. Talarico, J. Bacsanyi, P. Botstein, P. Chaikin, and J. Lim, "Spinal and epidural hematoma and low-molecular-weight heparin," *New England Journal of Medicine*, vol. 338, no. 24, pp. 1774–1775, 1998.

[116] W. H. Geerts, D. Bergqvist, G. F. Pineo et al., "Prevention of venous thromboembolism: American College of Chest Physicians evidence-based clinical practice guidelines (8th edition)," *Chest*, vol. 133, no. 6, pp. 381S–453S, 2008.

[117] M. Stafford-Smith, "Impaired haemostasis and regional anaesthesia," *Canadian Journal of Anaesthesia*, vol. 43, no. 5, pp. R129–R141, 1996.

[118] E. Vandermeulen, F. Singelyn, M. Vercauteren, J. F. Brichant, B. E. Ickx, and P. Gautier, "Belgian guidelines concerning central neural blockade in patients with drug-induced alteration of coagulation: an update," *Acta Anaesthesiologica Belgica*, vol. 56, no. 2, pp. 139–146, 2005.

[119] W. Gogarten, E. Vandermeulen, H. Van Aken, S. Kozek, J. V. Llau, and C. M. Samama, "Regional anaesthesia and antithrombotic agents: Recommendations of the European Society of Anaesthesiology," *European Journal of Anaesthesiology*, vol. 27, no. 12, pp. 999–1015, 2010.

[120] T. E. Warkentin, M. N. Levine, J. Hirsh et al., "Heparin-induced thrombocytopenia in patients treated with low-molecular- weight heparin or unfractionated heparin," *New England Journal of Medicine*, vol. 332, no. 20, pp. 1330–1335, 1995.

5

A Triple-Masked, Randomized Controlled Trial Comparing Ultrasound-Guided Brachial Plexus and Distal Peripheral Nerve Block Anesthesia for Outpatient Hand Surgery

Nicholas C. K. Lam,[1] Matthew Charles,[1] Deana Mercer,[2] Codruta Soneru,[1] Jennifer Dillow,[1] Francisco Jaime,[1] Timothy R. Petersen,[1,3] and Edward R. Mariano[4,5]

[1] *Department of Anesthesiology & Critical Care Medicine, University of New Mexico, Albuquerque, NM 87131, USA*
[2] *Department of Orthopaedics & Rehabilitation, University of New Mexico, Albuquerque, NM 87131, USA*
[3] *Department of Anthropology, University of New Mexico, Albuquerque, NM 87131, USA*
[4] *Department of Anesthesiology, Perioperative and Pain Medicine, Stanford University School of Medicine, Stanford, CA, USA*
[5] *Anesthesiology and Perioperative Care Service, Veterans Affairs Palo Alto Health Care System, 3801 Miranda Avenue (112A), Palo Alto, CA 94304, USA*

Correspondence should be addressed to Edward R. Mariano; emariano@stanford.edu

Academic Editor: Chih Shung Wong

Background. For hand surgery, brachial plexus blocks provide effective anesthesia but produce undesirable numbness. We hypothesized that distal peripheral nerve blocks will better preserve motor function while providing effective anesthesia. *Methods.* Adult subjects who were scheduled for elective ambulatory hand surgery under regional anesthesia and sedation were recruited and randomly assigned to receive ultrasound-guided supraclavicular brachial plexus block or distal block of the ulnar and median nerves. Each subject received 15 mL of 1.5% mepivacaine at the assigned location with 15 mL of normal saline injected in the alternate block location. The primary outcome (change in baseline grip strength measured by a hydraulic dynamometer) was tested before the block and prior to discharge. Subject satisfaction data were collected the day after surgery. *Results.* Fourteen subjects were enrolled. Median (interquartile range [IQR]) strength loss in the distal group was 21.4% (14.3, 47.8%), while all subjects in the supraclavicular group lost 100% of their preoperative strength, $P = 0.001$. Subjects in the distal group reported greater satisfaction with their block procedures on the day after surgery, $P = 0.012$. *Conclusion.* Distal nerve blocks better preserve motor function without negatively affecting quality of anesthesia, leading to increased patient satisfaction, when compared to brachial plexus block.

1. Introduction

Ultrasound-guided regional anesthesia is commonly performed for patients undergoing hand surgery [1]. However, the inability to use the affected limb due to motor block has been shown to reduce patient satisfaction [2, 3]. To address this issue, alternative regional anesthesia techniques have been suggested [4, 5]; for wrist and hand surgery, one approach involves short-acting brachial plexus block combined with long-acting distal peripheral nerve blocks [6, 7]. Unfortunately, this approach does not avoid the necessary period of immobility caused by a proximal brachial plexus block and may not improve patient satisfaction [8].

For outpatient hand surgery, distal peripheral nerve blocks alone should preserve motor function and may provide effective anesthesia [9, 10], thereby leading to greater patient satisfaction with the regional anesthetic technique and the surgical experience. However, the degree of motor sparing with this technique has not been established yet. We designed this randomized, triple-masked, clinical trial to test the primary hypothesis that ultrasound-guided distal peripheral nerve blocks in the forearm will preserve motor function to a greater extent than ultrasound-guided supraclavicular blocks while holding total local anesthetic dose constant.

2. Materials and Methods

The Human Research Review Committee at the University of New Mexico Health Sciences Center (Albuquerque, NM) approved this study, and the protocol was registered prospectively with ClinicalTrials.gov (NCT01927289). All subjects provided written informed consent.

Eligible subjects were 18 years or older, ASA I to III, and scheduled for elective ambulatory hand surgery with an expected surgical time of less than 15 minutes under regional anesthesia and intravenous sedation. Exclusion criteria were surgery outside the median and ulnar nerve distributions, bilateral surgery, body mass index of more than 45 kg/m^2, neck or clavicle deformities, infection at the planned injection site, existing neurologic disease, chronic pain diagnosis, opioid use greater than two weeks in the last six months, insulin dependent diabetes mellitus or diabetes with end-organ damage, allergy to local anesthetics, coagulopathy, previous surgery on the operative limb, and inability to comprehend study-related procedures.

2.1. Randomization. Randomization for group allocation was performed using a computer-generated random sequence (http://www.random.org/) to produce a series of sealed envelopes containing allocation instructions. One envelope was selected for each subject after consent was obtained and the unopened allocation envelope was immediately delivered to the anesthesiologist responsible for preparing study drugs. This anesthesiologist was not involved in any subsequent study procedures. Each subject was randomly assigned to one of two groups: distal (distal peripheral nerve blocks) or proximal (supraclavicular block). Regardless of group assignment, all subjects received the same volume and concentration of local anesthetic to keep dose constant, 15 mL of 1.5% mepivacaine at the assigned injection site with 15 mL of normal saline injected in the alternate location. The order of procedures was the same for all subjects: distal peripheral nerve injections of masked study solution first followed by proximal supraclavicular injection of masked study solution.

2.2. Masking. After informed consent was obtained, a 20 mL syringe containing 15 mL of 1.5% mepivacaine and a 20 mL syringe containing 15 mL of normal saline were filled and labeled as to block site according to the allocation. This preparation was performed by an anesthesiology provider not involved in block administration, care of the subject, or assessment. The subject, regional anesthesiologist performing the block, assessor, all health care providers, and the data analyst were masked to the allocation.

2.3. Patient and Procedural Preparation. All subjects were given celecoxib 400 mg orally before surgery unless contraindicated. All block procedures were performed preoperatively in a holding room by a single regional anesthesiologist trained in both proximal brachial plexus and distal peripheral nerve blocks under ultrasound guidance. Subjects' motor function was assessed by testing their hand grip strength using a hydraulic hand dynamometer (JAMAR©, Lafayette Instrument Company, Lafayette, IL). Three baseline measurements were recorded on both the ipsilateral and contralateral sides. Before nerve blockade, all subjects received intravenous access, supplemental oxygen, and standard monitoring which included noninvasive blood pressure, electrocardiogram, and pulse oximetry. Sedation and anxiolysis were achieved with intravenously administered midazolam in 1 to 2 mg increments and fentanyl in 25 mcg increments as needed for subject comfort.

2.4. Distal Peripheral Nerve Blocks

2.4.1. Ulnar Nerve. The subject was placed supine with the ipsilateral arm abducted and externally rotated with the palm facing up. The palmar and medial side of the ipsilateral forearm was disinfected using chlorhexidine gluconate (ChloraPrep; CareFusion, San Diego, CA). A 28 mm high-frequency ultrasound probe (L28, S-Nerve, Fujifilm SonoSite Inc., Bothell, WA) covered with a sterile dressing was placed at the mid-forearm level to identify the flexor digitorum superficialis muscles and flexor digitorum profundus muscles where the median nerve is located [11]. A long axis slide was used to trace the median nerve distally to 5 cm from the proximal wrist crease [10]. A short axis slide was then performed medially to locate the ulnar artery and the ulnar nerve adjacent to it [12]. Upon location of these structures, 1.5 mL of 0.5% lidocaine with 5 mcg/mL epinephrine was injected subcutaneously at the medial border of the ultrasound probe. This was the point of needle insertion for both ulnar and median nerve block [10]. A 22 gauge 80 mm insulated echogenic needle (SonoPlex Stim Cannula; Pajunk Medizintechnologie, Germany) was inserted through the skin at the medial border of the probe and advanced in plane from medial to lateral toward the ulnar nerve. Five mL of masked study solution was injected around the ulnar nerve, and circumferential spread was confirmed by ultrasound.

2.4.2. Median Nerve. Following ulnar nerve injection, a short axis slide laterally allowed for the visualization of the median nerve at the same level as the injection point for the ulnar nerve. The same needle was then redirected further laterally towards the median nerve using an in-plane approach. Five mL of masked study solution was injected around the median nerve (Figure 1). Redirection of the needle at the discretion of the regional anesthesiologist was allowed to achieve circumferential spread [10]. At the end of the ulnar and median nerve block procedures, 5 mL of masked study solution was used to raise a wheal on the volar side of the wrist at the level of the palmar crease.

2.5. Supraclavicular Block. Supraclavicular brachial plexus block was performed with the subject supine with the head of the bed slightly elevated. The anticipated block site in the ipsilateral supraclavicular fossa was prepared using the same antiseptic precautions as the distal group, and the same ultrasound equipment was used. With the ultrasound transducer

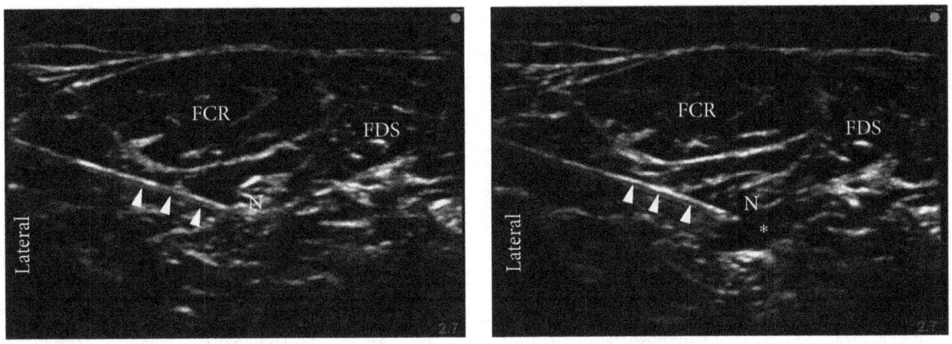

(a) (b)

FIGURE 1: Short-axis sonograms of ultrasound-guided median nerve block at two time points: preinjection (a) and postinjection (b); arrows identify the needle; N = nerve; FCR = flexor carpi radialis muscle; FDS = flexor digitorum superficialis muscle; $*$ = injectate solution.

placed in the supraclavicular fossa in a coronal-oblique plane posterior to the clavicle, the brachial plexus was identified in proximity to the subclavian artery above the first rib [13]. The first rib and pleura were identified in all subjects. After subcutaneous infiltration of 3 mL of a premixed commercially available 0.5% lidocaine with 5 mcg/mL epinephrine at the planned insertion site lateral to the ultrasound transducer, the same type of needle used in the distal group was inserted and advanced in plane toward the brachial plexus [13]. The needle tip was positioned under US guidance lateral to the subclavian artery and cephalad to the first rib (i.e., "corner pocket") adjacent to the hypoechoic neural structures of the brachial plexus [13, 14]. After negative aspiration, 15 mL of the masked study solution was injected incrementally to ensure circumferential spread; 5 mL was injected in the corner pocket with the remaining 10 mL distributed evenly within the neural compartment to produce circumferential spread around the plexus.

The procedural time (seconds) for each block was recorded. This duration was defined for the individual block procedure as the interval from the ultrasound transducer's first contact with the subject to the time the block needle exited the skin. Total procedural time was defined as the interval from first ultrasound transducer contact for the first distal block to completion of the supraclavicular block with removal of the last block needle.

2.6. Block Assessment. After completion of all block procedures, sensory and motor blockade were evaluated every five minutes for 30 minutes. Data collection was performed by an independent observer who was masked to each subject's group allocation. The extent of sensory blockade was tested in the median nerve and ulnar nerve distribution of the hand using ice on the palmar surface of the index finger and the little finger, respectively: 0 = no perception, 1 = decreased sensation, or 2 = normal sensation. Successful blockade was defined as complete sensory blockade (i.e., sensory block score = 0) in both peripheral nerve distributions within 30 minutes of completing the supraclavicular block.

2.7. Perioperative Care. If complete sensory blockade was not achieved within 30 minutes, the affected subject was excluded from the study and categorized as a block failure. The subject was offered a supplementary nerve block, if there was sufficient time prior to surgery, or general anesthesia to achieve surgical anesthesia. A single upper arm pneumatic tourniquet was used for all subjects. Intravenous sedation using midazolam and/or propofol were provided intraoperatively as per routine clinical practice and titrated to the comfort of the subject, while maintaining verbal contact. Short-acting opioids were given intraoperatively only if the subject complained of pain. No other anesthetics or analgesics, such as dexmedetomidine, ketamine, ketorolac, or intravenous acetaminophen, were given intraoperatively. Any subject who required moderate or deep sedation, general anesthesia, or supplementary blocks was noted. After surgery, 5 mL of 0.25% bupivacaine incisional infiltration was performed by the surgeon in all subjects as per routine clinical practice. Postoperatively, all subjects were prescribed intravenous and oral opioids as needed for breakthrough pain in the postanesthesia care unit (PACU). In the PACU, three hand grip strength measurements were recorded for all subjects using the same dynamometer on both the ipsilateral and contralateral sides. Subjects were discharged from PACU to home with prescriptions for oral ibuprofen 400 mg and two tablets of hydrocodone 5 mg with acetaminophen 325 mg to be taken every four hours as needed for pain. Subjects were advised to consume both analgesics when they first felt the hand numbness resolving.

2.8. Outcomes. The primary outcome of this study was postoperative change in hand grip strength in the operative limb as a percent reduction of preoperative baseline strength. Secondary outcomes on the day of surgery included procedural time, block success/failure, onset time, block duration, sedative and analgesic requirements, and surgery duration. Each surgeon was interviewed by an assessor blinded to the allocation of the subject at the end of surgery to assess his/her satisfaction using a seven-point Likert scale: "On a scale of 1 to 7 with 1 being *not at all*, 4 being *neutral*, and 7 being *completely satisfied*, how satisfied were you with the surgical conditions provided for this subject?"

On postoperative day one, subjects were interviewed by an assessor blinded to group allocation regarding their

Table 1: Demographic and surgical observations.

	Distal group ($n = 7$)	Proximal group ($n = 7$)	P value
Age, years	54.0 (5.1)	53.7 (5.6)	0.92
Sex, n (m/f)	3/4	3/4	0.99
Height, cm	163.0 (9.1)	164.7 (11.8)	0.77
Weight, kg	86.5 (16.2)	87.6 (17.1)	0.90
Surgery duration, min	12.1 (2.6)	15.7 (4.5)	0.09
Tourniquet duration, min	8.0 (2.2)	10.0 (3.4)	0.21
Surgeon's satisfaction, 1–7	7 (7, 7)	7 (7, 7)	0.39

Continuous data are presented as mean (SD) when normally distributed or median (interquartile range) when not normally distributed; count data are presented as number of subjects as appropriate.

satisfaction with the block via telephone. Subject satisfaction was assessed with a standardized question scored on a seven-point Likert scale: "Thinking about your nerve blocks, how satisfied were you with them: where 1 is *not at all*, 4 is *neutral*, and 7 is *completely satisfied*?" The interview also included inquiries on the time that the subjects first felt the return of sensation and the time they first felt full recovery of strength. Subjects were asked about the occurrence of any adverse events or potential block-related complications, including paresthesias, motor deficits, persistent pain, and bruising. If complications occurred, they were followed up as per routine clinical practice and noted for the study.

2.9. Sample Size Estimate. Based on a pilot study performed at the authors' institution (unpublished data), we assumed that the distal block group will experience a 10% decrease in hand grip strength from baseline compared to a 90% decrease in the supraclavicular block group. Assuming a similar effect size, 80% power, and $\alpha = 0.05$ using a two-sample test of proportions, we estimated that seven subjects per group would be required.

2.10. Statistical Analysis. Normality of data distribution was determined using the Shapiro-Wilk test. Continuous data with normal distribution were presented as mean (standard deviation [SD]) and analyzed with Student's t-test; continuous data with nonnormal distribution were presented as median (interquartile range [IQR]) and analyzed using the Mann-Whitney U test. Categorical data were analyzed with the Chi square test or Fisher's exact test ($n < 5$ in any field). Correlation between change in hand grip strength and patient satisfaction was assessed with two nonparametric measures of association: Spearman's rho and Kendall's tau. For the primary outcome, $P < 0.05$ was considered statistically significant. The results from secondary outcome analyses should be interpreted as suggestive and not conclusive.

3. Results

Thirty-one patients were assessed for eligibility and offered enrollment in this study. Five eligible patients refused to participate, and 12 were excluded based on study criteria (e.g., bilateral surgery, previous surgery on the operative limb, and diabetes with nerve or end organ damage), leaving 14 subjects who were enrolled and successfully completed study procedures (Figure 2).

Demographic and surgical data are presented in Table 1; no statistically significant differences in these variables were noted between study groups. All subjects received preoperative celecoxib except for one subject in the proximal group with sulfur allergy. There were no failed blocks in either group, and no subjects required breakthrough analgesia or experienced postoperative nausea or vomiting in the PACU.

3.1. Primary Outcome. Median (IQR) strength loss in the surgical limb for the distal group was 21.4% (14.3%, 47.8%), while all subjects in the proximal group lost 100% (100%, 100%) of their preoperative strength, $P = 0.001$.

3.2. Secondary Outcomes. Block procedures in the proximal group required less time [mean (SD)] than in the distal group: 226.8 (38.5) versus 408.8 (82.3) seconds, respectively ($P < 0.0001$; 95% CI for difference 131.0–232.9 seconds). Subjects in the distal group reported higher satisfaction scores [median (interquartile range)] with their block procedures than those in the proximal group on the day after surgery: 7 (7, 7) versus 6 (6, 6), respectively ($P = 0.012$). Subject satisfaction correlated inversely with operative limb strength loss based on Spearman's rho −0.62 ($P = 0.016$) and Kendall's tau is −0.55 ($P = 0.025$). Subject-reported mean (SD) time to return of sensation in the distal group was 261 (91.6) minutes, while that in the proximal group was 358 (53.5) minutes ($P = 0.03$, 95% CI for the difference: 40.1–96.4 minutes). There were no differences in other secondary outcomes (Table 2).

One subject exhibited symptoms of persistent paresthesia in the proximal group, but this had resolved by the second postoperative day. There were no protocol violations or other adverse events.

4. Discussion

Both ultrasound-guided distal peripheral nerve blocks and proximal brachial plexus blocks can be used as the primary anesthetic for outpatient hand surgery, but distal peripheral nerve blocks are superior at preserving motor function of the operative limb and may lead to modest improvements in patient satisfaction.

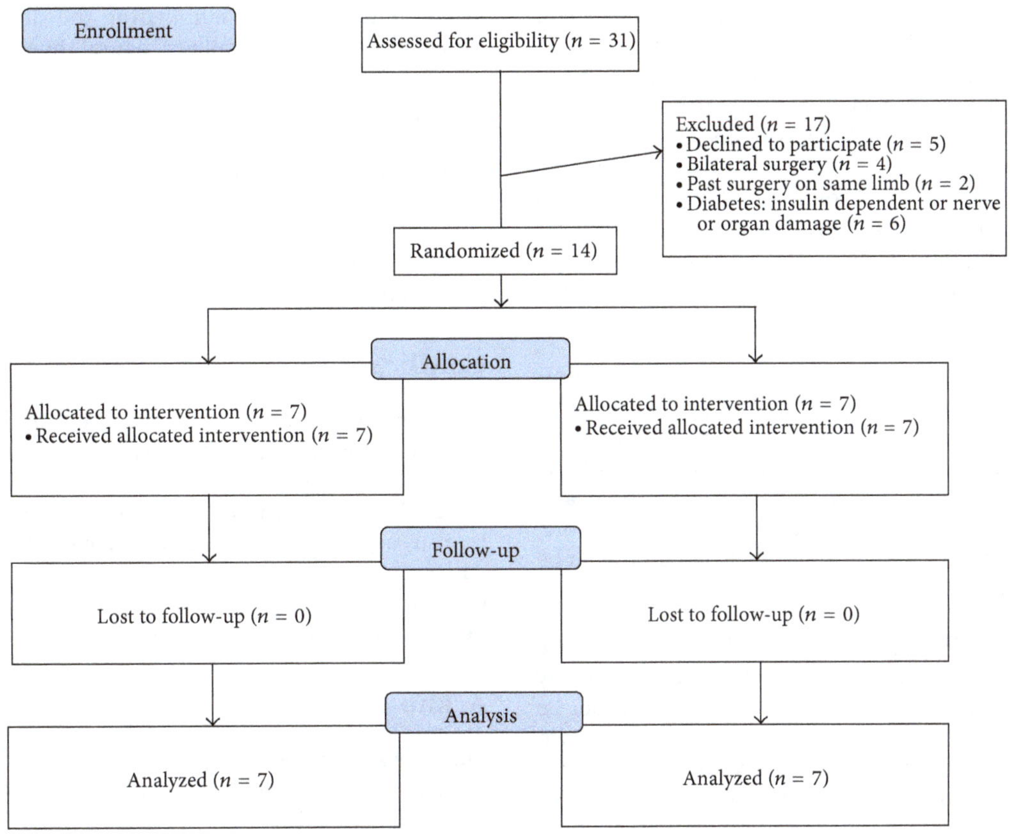

FIGURE 2: CONSORT study flow diagram.

TABLE 2: Secondary outcomes observations.

	Distal group ($n = 7$)	Proximal group ($n = 7$)	P value
Anesthetic onset time, min	5 (5, 15)	10 (10, 20)	0.12
Bruising, n	3	2	0.99
Paresthesia, n	0	1	0.99
Total anesthesia preparation time (both blocks + onset time), min	16.1 (14.8, 26.0)	21.8 (18.5, 28.8)	0.20
Assigned block procedural time + onset time, min	12.1 (11.0, 22.2)	14.8 (13.5, 22.8)	0.31

Data are presented as median (interquartile range) or number of subjects, as appropriate.

Unlike the present study, Fredrickson and colleagues did not find a difference in subject satisfaction when the combination of short-acting brachial plexus block and distal nerve blocks was compared to long-acting brachial plexus block; however, the median satisfaction score on a 0–10 scale (with 10 = "very satisfied overall") was 10 in each group [8]. Since all subjects in the Fredrickson study experienced complete upper extremity motor block, albeit of different duration, and would have expected this type of block postoperatively, we speculate that these pain scores reflect managed expectations. Perhaps, if presented with the alternative of avoiding motor block, these satisfaction results may have been different. We designed the present study based on this assumption, given the published feasibility of distal peripheral nerve blocks as an anesthetic technique for minor hand surgery [15–17], and subjects in our distal group did experience less motor block and subsequently rated their satisfaction higher than the proximal group. The present study is the first to rigorously compare the anesthetic quality of the distal peripheral nerve block technique to an established standard (brachial plexus blockade).

4.1. Importance of Preserving Motor Function. The use of distal peripheral nerve blocks as a primary anesthetic technique for trigger finger or carpal tunnel release, with preservation of motor function, may allow patients to move the affected digit(s) or hand when instructed to do so during surgery. While local anesthetic infiltration alone [18] and intravenous regional anesthesia (IVRA or Bier block) [19] are also acceptable techniques for minor hand surgery, surgeons at our institution prefer distal peripheral nerve blocks to avoid local anesthetic-induced distortion of the surgical field. Distal peripheral nerve blocks have been associated with shorter surgical time when compared to IVRA for carpal tunnel release [9]. One potential patient safety advantage of distal peripheral nerve blocks is avoiding the upper limb immobility and lack of protective reflexes resulting from brachial plexus blockade especially for outpatients. Studies on ambulatory brachial plexus catheter patients with lower local anesthetic concentrations have not been able to eliminate self-reported numbness [20, 21]. Avoiding motor block through the use of distal peripheral nerve blocks alone eliminates the need for a sling (and its associated cost) and may allow patients to better protect the operative limb from inadvertent injury [22].

4.2. System Considerations. The procedural time for supraclavicular block is shorter than that for distal peripheral nerve blocks by three minutes on average, consistent with previous-published procedural times [9]. However, the total anesthesia preparation time combining block performance time and time for anesthetic onset is similar between groups; therefore, this minor procedural time difference does not appear to be clinically relevant.

4.3. Local Anesthetic Dosing. The total local anesthetic dosage in the present study was held constant between groups so any difference in postoperative hand grip strength could not be attributed to a difference in dose. A previous study has shown that the minimum effective volume (MEV) of 1.5% *lidocaine* for ultrasound-guided supraclavicular block when injecting in the corner pocket and superior compartment is 30 mL [23]. Compared to our study, the study by Tran and colleagues enrolled a sample of patients undergoing a more diverse set of surgical procedures (hand, wrist, forearm, and elbow) versus strictly minor hand surgery and used lidocaine instead of mepivacaine [23]. A more recent study of ultrasound-guided supraclavicular blocks using 1.5% mepivacaine, although the technique slightly differs from the one used in the present study, has shown that the MEV90 (estimated for 90% of patients) is 15 mL—the same volume used in the present study [24]. No subjects in the proximal group had failed blocks or required analgesics in the recovery room; therefore, we conclude that the observed difference in patient satisfaction is not likely related to a difference in anesthetic efficacy.

4.4. Study Limitations. Only surgeries of brief duration (<15 minutes expected surgical time) were included in our study in order to minimize tourniquet pain which would not be covered by the distal forearm blocks. Regarding the primary outcome of hand grip strength, we recognize that performance is dependent on subject effort; if a subject is tired or distracted, he or she may not perform as well on a trial even though the same innate muscle strength is present. We attempted to minimize this variability by taking three measurements at each assessment and by blinding the assessor and providers. The results of the present study may only apply to practices employing similar regional anesthetic and surgical techniques and equipment; in particular, this study did not involve the use of nerve stimulation, so we do not know how this nerve localization modality may have influenced outcomes. Finally, the use of a second sham block in all subjects for the purposes of masking is not a part of usual clinical practice; eliminating the sham block can be expected to reduce overall procedural time.

5. Conclusions

In summary, this study suggests that ultrasound-guided distal peripheral nerve blocks can be an effective alternative to brachial plexus blockade as the primary anesthetic for outpatient hand surgery and offers the potential advantage of preserved motor function.

Conflict of Interests

Dr. Mariano has received unrestricted funding paid to his institution for developing educational programs from I-Flow/Kimberly-Clark (Lake Forest, CA, USA) and B Braun (Bethlehem, PA, USA). These companies had absolutely no input into any aspect of the present study conceptualization, design, and implementation; data collection, analysis, and interpretation; or paper preparation. None of the other authors has any personal financial interests to disclose.

Acknowledgment

This work is supported by Department of Anesthesiology & Critical Care Medicine, University of New Mexico, Albuquerque, NM, USA.

References

[1] M. Roy, M.-J. Nadeau, D. Côté et al., "Comparison of a single- or double-injection technique for ultrasound-guided supraclavicular block: a prospective, randomized, blinded controlled study," *Regional Anesthesia and Pain Medicine*, vol. 37, no. 1, pp. 55–59, 2012.

[2] M. J. Fredrickson and D. J. Price, "Analgesic effectiveness of ropivacaine 0.2% vs 0.4% via an ultrasound-guided C5-6 root/superior trunk perineural ambulatory catheter," *British Journal of Anaesthesia*, vol. 103, no. 3, pp. 434–439, 2009.

[3] M. J. Fredrickson, K. R. Smith, and A. C. Wong, "Importance of volume and concentration for ropivacaine interscalene block in preventing recovery room pain and minimizing motor block after shoulder surgery," *Anesthesiology*, vol. 112, no. 6, pp. 1374–1381, 2010.

[4] P. Marhofer, W. Harrop-Griffiths, S. C. Kettner, and L. Kirchmair, "Fifteen years of ultrasound guidance in regional anaesthesia: Part 1," *British Journal of Anaesthesia*, vol. 104, no. 5, pp. 538–546, 2010.

[5] P. Marhofer, W. Harrop-Griffiths, H. Willschke, and L. Kirchmair, "Fifteen years of ultrasound guidance in regional anaesthesia: Part 2—recent developments in block techniques," *British Journal of Anaesthesia*, vol. 104, no. 6, pp. 673–683, 2010.

[6] M. J. Fredrickson, F. S. H. Ting, S. Chinchanwala, and M. R. Boland, "Concomitant infraclavicular plus distal median, radial, and ulnar nerve blockade accelerates upper extremity anaesthesia and improves block consistency compared with infraclavicular block alone," *British Journal of Anaesthesia*, vol. 107, no. 2, pp. 236–242, 2011.

[7] B. E. Smith, J. F. Challands, M. Suchak, and D. Siggins, "Regional anaesthesia for surgery of the forearm and hand. A technique of

combined supraclavicular and discrete blocks," *Anaesthesia*, vol. 44, no. 9, pp. 747–749, 1989.

[8] M. J. Fredrickson, P. J. Wolstencroft, S. Chinchanwala, and M. R. Boland, "Does motor block related to long-acting brachial plexus block cause patient dissatisfaction after minor wrist and hand surgery? A randomized observer-blinded trial," *British Journal of Anesthesia*, vol. 109, pp. 809–815, 2012.

[9] E. R. Mariano, M. K. Lehr, V. J. Loland, and M. L. Bishop, "Choice of loco-regional anesthetic technique affects operating room efficiency for carpal tunnel release," *Journal of Anesthesia*, vol. 27, pp. 611–614, 2013.

[10] P. Macaire, F. Singelyn, P. Narchi, and X. Paqueron, "Ultrasound- or nerve stimulation-guided wrist blocks for carpal tunnel release: a randomized prospective comparative study," *Regional Anesthesia and Pain Medicine*, vol. 33, no. 4, pp. 363–368, 2008.

[11] C. J. L. McCartney, D. Xu, C. Constantinescu, S. Abbas, and V. W. S. Chan, "Ultrasound examination of peripheral nerves in the forearm," *Regional Anesthesia and Pain Medicine*, vol. 32, no. 5, pp. 434–439, 2007.

[12] A. Kathirgamanathan, J. French, G. L. Foxall, J. G. Hardman, and N. M. Bedforth, "Delineation of distal ulnar nerve anatomy using ultrasound in volunteers to identify an optimum approach for neural blockade," *European Journal of Anaesthesiology*, vol. 26, no. 1, pp. 43–46, 2009.

[13] L. G. Soares, R. Brull, J. Lai, and V. W. Chan, "Eight ball, corner pocket: the optimal needle position for ultrasound-guided supraclavicular block," *Regional Anesthesia and Pain Medicine*, vol. 32, no. 1, pp. 94–95, 2007.

[14] S. Kapral, P. Krafft, K. Eibenberger, R. Fitzgerald, M. Gosch, and C. Weinstabl, "Ultrasound-guided supraclavicular approach for regional anesthesia of the brachial plexus," *Anesthesia and Analgesia*, vol. 78, no. 3, pp. 507–513, 1994.

[15] J. A. Dilger and R. E. Wells Jr., "The use of peripheral nerve blocks at the elbow for carpal tunnel release," *Journal of Clinical Anesthesia*, vol. 17, no. 8, pp. 621–623, 2005.

[16] P. Macaire, O. Choquet, D. Jochum, V. Travers, and X. Capdevila, "Nerve blocks at the wrist for carpal tunnel release revisited: The use of sensory-nerve and motor-nerve stimulation techniques," *Regional Anesthesia and Pain Medicine*, vol. 30, no. 6, pp. 536–540, 2005.

[17] L. Delaunay and J. E. Chelly, "Blocks at the wrist provide effective anesthesia for carpal tunnel release," *Canadian Journal of Anesthesia*, vol. 48, no. 7, pp. 656–660, 2001.

[18] M. M. Tomaino, D. Ulizio, and M. T. Vogt, "Carpal tunnel release under intravenous regional or local infiltration anaesthesia," *Journal of Hand Surgery*, vol. 26, no. 1, pp. 67–68, 2001.

[19] S. Brill, W. Middleton, G. Brill, and A. Fisher, "Bier's block; 100 years old and still going strong!," *Acta Anaesthesiologica Scandinavica*, vol. 48, no. 1, pp. 117–122, 2004.

[20] B. M. Ilfeld, L. T. Le, J. Ramjohn et al., "The effects of local anesthetic concentration and dose on continuous infraclavicular nerve blocks: A multicenter, randomized, observer-masked, controlled study," *Anesthesia and Analgesia*, vol. 108, no. 1, pp. 345–350, 2009.

[21] L. T. Le, V. J. Loland, E. R. Mariano et al., "Effects of local anesthetic concentration and dose on continuous interscalene nerve blocks: a dual-center, randomized, observer-masked, controlled Study," *Regional Anesthesia and Pain Medicine*, vol. 33, no. 6, pp. 518–525, 2008.

[22] A. Saporito, E. Sturini, J. Petri, A. Borgeat, and J. A. Aguirre, "Case report: unusual complication during outpatient continuous regional popliteal analgesia," *Canadian Journal of Anesthesia*, vol. 59, pp. 958–962, 2012.

[23] D. Q. H. Tran, S. Dugani, J. A. Correa, A. Dyachenko, N. Alsenosy, and R. J. Finlayson, "Minimum effective volume of lidocaine for ultrasound-guided supraclavicular block," *Regional Anesthesia and Pain Medicine*, vol. 36, no. 5, pp. 466–469, 2011.

[24] J. G. Song, D. G. Jeon, B. J. Kang, and K. K. Park, "Minimum effective volume of mepivacaine for ultrasound-guided supraclavicular block," *Korean Journal of Anesthesiology*, vol. 65, pp. 37–41, 2013.

6

Spinal Cord Stimulation: The Clinical Application of New Technology

Dominic Hegarty[1, 2]

[1] *Department of Anaesthesia and Intensive Care, Cork University Hospital, Cork, Ireland*
[2] *Department of Pharmacology and Therapeutics, University College Cork, Clinical Sciences Building, Cork, Ireland*

Correspondence should be addressed to Dominic Hegarty, dominichegarty@hotmail.com

Academic Editor: Andrea Trescot

The use of neuromodulation for pain relief is among the fastest-growing areas of medicine, involving many diverse specialties and impacting on hundreds of thousands of patients with numerous disorders worldwide. As the evidence of efficacy improves, the interest in spinal cord stimulation (SCS) will increase because it is minimally invasive, safe, and a reversible treatment modality with limited side effect profile. While the mechanism of action evades complete understanding, the technological improvements have been considerable and current neuromodulation developments have been coupled with the rapid growth of the neuromodulation device industry resulting in the development of the next-generation neuromodulation systems. The development, the newest technicaliti and the future for the clinical application of spinal cord stimulation (SCS) are reviewed here.

1. Introduction

Neuromodulation is among the fastest-growing areas of medicine, involving many diverse specialties and impacting on hundreds of thousands of patients with numerous disorders worldwide [1]. Historically, electricity, either in the form of the torpedo fish or man-made electrotherapy, has been used to try and cure various ailments [2]. For example, in the middle of the 18th century "electroanalgesia" became advocated for the treatment of angina pectoris, gout, headaches, pleuritic pain, and sciatica. However, by the 20th century the enthusiasm for the medical use of electricity became associated with "quackery" [3] and was banned from clinical practice. In 1965 Melzack and Wall presented the "Gate Theory" [4], which postulated that stimulation of nonpainful stimuli can inhibit painful afference, thereby offering the opportunity to align basic research with the clinical application of electricity which has resulted in the development of neuromodulation techniques as we know them today [5–7]. While the mechanism of action evades complete understanding, the technological improvements have been considerable and current neuromodulation developments have been coupled with the rapid growth of the neuromodulation device industry resulting in the development of the next-generation neuromodulation systems. The development, the newest technicalities, and the future for the clinical application of spinal cord stimulation (SCS) are reviewed here.

2. Principles of Neuromodulation

Essentially there are two components of a fully implanted SCS system: the electrodes (or lead) and an implantable pulse generator (IPG). In SCS the placement of epidural electrodes is generally targeted at the dorsal column of the spinal cord; however, in patients with segmental pain (single dermatome), stimulation is focused at the corresponding dorsal root. This is where the ascending tracts pass without decussation to the gracile and cuneate nuclei of the medulla oblongata. These tracts are composed of a wide range of fiber diameters which are the central processes of the primary afferent neurons located in the spinal ganglia. As the tracts ascend, they receive accession from the dorsal roots, resulting in a somatotopic organization [6]. The recruitment of fibers is correlated directly with the diameter of the fiber and inversely with the distance between the electrode contacts and the fibers [6]. Hence the thickness of the cerebrospinal fluid layers [8], the individual anatomy, and the electrodes each influence the recruitment of the dorsal column [8–11] and dorsal root fibers [12].

In addition the large diameter fibers of the dorsal root and dorsal column have different orientation with respect to the spinal anatomy and hence in a different position in the electrical field evoked by the stimulation pulses. Furthermore, the distance between the electrode and the thickness of the dorsal cerebral spinal fluid (dCSF) layer influences the sensitivity of the fibers to the stimulation. Computer modeling predicted that a "bipolar" or a narrow guarded cathode programming sequence selectively stimulates dorsal cord fibers when the dCSF is small. In contrast, dorsal root stimulation is favored the most in "monopolar" stimulation when dCSF is wide [8–10]. In pain patients with segmental pain, stimulation can be focused on dorsal root fibers of the corresponding dermatome, whereas in patients with complex pain a multitude of dorsal column fibers related to multiple dermatomes should be stimulated. The results of these computer-based model studies led to the development of electrode arrays with similar geometric properties [13].

Once an electrode/lead is suitability positioned, the most common way to increase the intensity of the stimulation is to increase the amplitude (i.e., the current, the voltage provided); increasing the pulse rate beyond physiological limits (approximately 300 pulse per second) is not traditionally seen as providing therapeutic benefit as neural transmission may become blocked. Similarly the pulse width was traditionally set at 200 μs in order to provide adequate amplitude while conserving the energy of the battery. With modern technological advancements, these concepts are now facing an interesting challenge and may influence the future of some aspects of SCS.

3. New Electrode Contact and Lead Design

Remarkable technological advances have been achieved in terms of electrode contact/lead design. Firstly, the new multicontact arrays available in traditional and five-column paddle leads (St. Jude Medical, Inc, USA) have resulted in the ability to provide improved programmable capability and possible treatment outcome. Mathematical modeling has highlighted the potential benefits of tight-electrode spacing in electrode contact design whereby gaps in stimulation are avoided (Boston Scientific Neuromodulation, Valencia, Calif, USA). Indeed, to obtain large paraesthesia coverage, all active contacts (anodes and cathodes at one or more arrays) should be closely spaced.

In the beginning SCS stimulation involved only a single channel, which meant that the stimulator had only one cathodal voltage output and one anodal voltage output, each one being connected to one or more lead contacts. Only recently multichannel systems have been produced (Boston Scientific Neuromodulation, Valencia, Calif, USA). In these systems any active lead contact is driven independently with a preprogrammed current pulse. The only condition is that the sum of all cathodal and anodal currents is zero and that all pulses are synchronized. The number of settings increases exponentially from 50 combinations with four electrode contacts to tens of millions when 16 electrode contacts are available [14]. Intuitively one would be forgiven for assuming that with the newer multicontact or the multichannel systems [15] significant clinical improvements would follow, but these technical advantages have not necessarily improved treatment in all indications [16]. In fact, despite the large number of contacts available, the actual number of active contacts will generally be small (bipole, tripole, or quadruple).

Secondly, the improved "steerability" of the leads combined with a variety of stylets to guide the positioning of the electrodes has resulted in a preference for the less invasive percutaneous insertion of the leads into the epidural space via a Touhy needle. The design of the Epiducer lead delivery system (St. Jude Medical, Inc, USA) is proposed to allow the advancement of a paddle lead without the use of a laminectomy.

Importantly, the improved flexibility of the leads has not compromised the lead fracture rate; this has fallen from 6% in earlier studies [17] to 3% [18]. Lead migration usually occurs in the first 12 months of implantation and varies between 8% [19] and 27% [20]. Migration may be related to the anchoring technique and not the actual lead design. The industry is striving to identify a solution to migration through the development of consistent and verifiable anchoring technology. Another development based on computer modeling is transverse tripolar stimulation, allowing the mediolateral steering of the electric field to correct for an inaccurate lead position [21]. Transverse tripolar steering principle led to even more complex configurations like the development of a 5-column paddle lead (Penta, St. Jude Medical).

A third technical challenge that remains is the lack of compatibility of the leads with magnetic resonance imaging (MRI) and radiofrequency diathermy which can be a significant limitation for some patients. Metallic implants (including nonferrous) are prone to heating when exposed to MRI or diathermy. In vitro comparisons showed that temperature changes near SCS electrodes were higher than those found with other metallic implants, reaching up to $4.88^{\circ}C/s^{-1}$ [22]. While the safe use of MRI in patients with SCS leads in place has been reported [23], so too has nonreversible damage and death [20, 24]. Most manufacturers are addressing the issue, and safer leads are expected.

4. IPG Advancements

Originally regarded as just a battery, the IPG has now evolved to become an engineer's paradise. Long gone are the nickel-cadmium systems which are replaced by lithium-based batteries thereby prolonging the lifespan of the device. With the advent of complex stimulation settings involving the activation of an increasing number of contacts the premature exhaustion of the battery is avoided by using automatic nocturnal, time-cycled, or manual interruption of stimulation. The industry has developed a variety of new generation of compact rechargeable IPGs to meet the new requirements of SCS; thereby, energy consumption becomes less of a problem.

As previously mentioned the recruitment of dorsal horn fibers is correlated inversely with the distance between the electrode contact and the fiber [6]. Hence the thickness of the cerebrospinal fluid layers [8] the recruitment of the dorsal column [8–11] and dorsal root fibers [12]. Therefore as electrode/leads placement varies and stimulation intensity can vary depending on the position of the patient (e.g., supine or standing) to such an extent that patients cannot use the IPG without manually changing the program in order to avoid painful overstimulation.

The RestoreSensor (Medtronic Inc, USA) is the first implantable neurostimulator for spinal cord stimulation (SCS) that automatically adapts stimulation settings in response to position changes and provides objective patient activity data. The adaptive SCS is based on acceleration sensor that enables chronic motion sensing in battery-powered applications. It is robust to shock and represents the first practical, packaged, three-axis accelerometer suitable for chronic physiological measurements. The sensor's performance is also desirable for more general micropower applications like package tracking, vibration, and tilt detection.

Initial results from the Testing RestoreSensor Usability and Satisfaction (TRUST) survey [25] in 30 patients, mainly suffering from predominant leg pain due to failed back surgery syndrome or complex regional pain syndrome type I, followed up over a 10-week period are very promising. 80% of patients reported more effective pain relief. Use of the patient programmer became less difficult, and less necessary, with adaptive stimulation. Adaptive stimulation had a positive effect on sleep quality in all patients, which may have led to a perception of greater sleep quantity. In total, 58% of patients reported the ability to perform more activities with the therapy (e.g., standing, walking, sleeping, and staying in a particular position longer). Overall patient satisfaction was 97% at the end of the 10-week follow-up period [25].

5. Modification of the Pulse Width

In SCS, the pulse amplitude is usually the focus of stimulation control as it is intuitively understood by clinician and patient alike [26–29]. With advances in SCS technology, particularly rechargeable IPG implantable devices, pulse width (PW) programming ranges of now match that of older radiofrequency systems (with programmability up to 1000 μs). Traditionally PW was only changed when other parameter adjustments fail to achieve therapeutic goals. In neurostimulation the pulse amplitude and width relate directly to the depolarization of the cell membrane and are therefore critical parameters for determining the locus of excited tissue [30]. The value of PW programming was investigated in 19 subjects who had a fully implanted SCS in place for over 3 months to treat chronic intractable low back and/or leg pain. It was shown that the baseline median PW parameter was 295 μs (range 242–326 μs) with a median amplitude of 2.5 mA (1.3–3.3 mA). Following independent modification of the PW, the median PW of all patients' programs increased to 400 μs, approximately 48% higher (P = 0.01) and showed a significant increase in the paraesthesia-pain overlap (56%, P = 0.04). It was estimated that 10/19 patients appeared to have greater paraesthesia coverage, 7/19 patients selected the new PW programs, and 8/19 patients appeared to display a "caudal shift" of paraesthesia coverage with increased PW [31].

Mathematical modelling suggests that the mechanism behind such paraesthesia steering is due to the different selectivity of PW for larger and smaller fibers. The model considered incorporated realistic fiber size, density, and distributions in the dorsal columns, based upon human anatomic data. With a greater relative density of smaller fibers located more medial in the dorsal columns, an increase in PW will recruit smaller fibers more readily and thus result in greater midline axon recruitment. Clinically, this appeared to manifest as a caudal shift in paraesthesia. In summary variable PW programming in SCS appears to have clinical value, demonstrated by some patients improving their paraesthesia-pain overlap, as well as the ability to increase and even "steer" paraesthesia coverage [31].

6. High-Frequency Stimulation

Although SCS is a recommended treatment for patients with failed back surgery syndrome (FBSS) [32], if paraesthesia over the lumbar dermatomes cannot be obtained, then axial low back pain is very difficult to treat and clinical results are poor [33]. Ongoing multicentred European prospective trials [34] using dual octapolar, percutaneous leads placed sequentially near anatomic midline and connected to a rechargeable IPG capable of delivering waveforms with frequencies up to 10 kHz. (Nevro, Menlo Park, Calif) have shown that of 34 cases with full implantation the average back pain VAS decreased by 77% (8.9 cm baseline to 2.0 cm at 6 months, $P < .001$) and leg pain VAS decreased by 82% at 6-month follow-up. (5.5 cm baseline to 0.7 cm at 6 months, $P < .001$). In addition the average Oswestry Disability Index score decreased by 36% (from 58 to 37, $P < .001$). This approach is novel for several reasons: (a) the use of high-frequency stimulation provides sustained analgesia in a previously difficult patient cohort without paraesthesia—thus adequate axial low back pain relief is achieved without the overwhelming leg sensation one would have expected by increasing the frequency using a traditional IPG; (b) anatomical placement of the leads is possible and intraoperative paraesthesia mapping is avoided; (c) it has decreased programming requirements; (d) continued use of the system independent of position including night-time use is possible. To date, no adverse effect of such high-frequency stimulation has been reported however, the clinical outcome in the longer term is awaited. Pre-clinical studies in goats who received 10 days of continuous stimulation at amplitudes up to the sensory/motor threshold showed no difference in the behaviour or spinal cord neural histology between the therapy and control groups. Why such stimulation has this remarkable effect still remains to be understood and may influence our approach to this co-cohort heretofore unsatisfactorily managed with conventional SCS technology.

7. New Clinical Applications

There are several established indications for SCS such as neuropathic back and leg pain, complex regional pain syndrome, spinal cord injury, and ischemic pain (vascular and angina pectoris). While it is beyond the remit of this paper to discuss each clinical indication, there is a growing database of clinical-based evidence to support the use of SCS. The economic evaluation in these areas is limited but the initial costs of SCS is generally both more effective and less costly then conventional management over a period of 3–5 years [33]. Unfortunately SCS is regarded as a last-resort option by many healthcare providers, and the real economic benefits may lie in the earlier introduction of the technique.

The recognition of new treatment modalities and the new application of SCS techniques will redefine our understanding of the pathophysiological concepts involved in different medical conditions. For example, painful bladder syndrome/interstitial cystitis and diffuse chronic abdominal/pelvic pain may be considered as neuropathic pain thereby offering the potential for exciting development. The evidence that cervical SCS increases cerebral blood flow (CBF) may lead to a role in cerebral ischemia. The modification of the autonomic system, particularly its sympathetic component by SCS, suggests that body functions under significant autonomic control could be subjected to modulation. It is suggested that in the future bronchospasm, gastrointestinal motility, and possibily metabolic disorders could become the focus of neuromodulation [35].

8. Conclusion

Modern medicine requires that any treatment modality is based on rational knowledge and well-documented theories; however, some conditions, particularly those involving chronic pain, often remain imprecise. SCS may be one of the few examples of a treatment that has significantly contributed to a change in attitudes and providing satisfactory relief to patients who in the past would have been left untreated.

Spinal cord stimulation has significant implications for the healthcare system offering a safe reversible treatment modality with a limited side effect profile. To ensure the deliverance of a high-standard quality of care spinal cord stimulation should be provided in small well-resourced centres able to address the aftercare needs of this patient cohort. Cost-effectiveness and efficacy are fundamental if SCS is to be accepted as the therapy of choice by the public, physicians, and the healthcare decision makers. Earlier introduction of the technique may prove to be critical. Research into the mechanism of pain, the diseases, and the action of SCS requires randomized control trials (RCTs). The inability (a) to blind patients (owning to the paraesthesia), (b) to select a comparative therapy (medical, surgical, rehabilitation), and/or (c) to address the ethical implications to participate in a trial are specific issues in the design of such a RCT.

As the evidence of efficacy improves and the number of indications increases, the interest in the neuromodulation and SCS will undoubtedly increase. SCS is minimally invasive, safe, and reversible treatment modality with limited side effect profile. It is only through the combined efforts of the biomedical industry, basic science researchers, and frontline healthcare providers will the technological advancements already made in this area continue to make significant clinical impact on the patients of tomorrow.

References

[1] E. S. Krames, P. H. Peckham, A. R. Rezai, and F. Aboelsaad, "What is neuromodulation?" in *Neuromodulation*, Krames et al., Ed., pp. 3–8, Elsevier, 2009.

[2] D. Kellaway, "The william osler medical essay; the part played by electric fish in the early history of bioelectricity and electrotherapy," *Bulletin of the History of Medicine*, vol. 20, pp. 112–137, 1946.

[3] R. M. Macklis, "Magnetic healing, quackery, and the debate about the health effects of electromagnetic fields," *Annals of Internal Medicine*, vol. 118, no. 5, pp. 376–383, 1993.

[4] R. Melzack and P. D. Wall, "Pain mechanisms: a new theory," *Science*, vol. 150, no. 3699, pp. 971–979, 1965.

[5] U. Rossi, "The history of electrical stimulation of the nervous system for the control of pain," in *Electric Stimulation and the Relief of Pain*, B. A. Simpson, Ed., pp. 5–16, Elsevier, London, UK, 2003.

[6] A. Foletti, A. Durrer, and E. Buchser, "Neurostimulation technology for the treatment of chronic pain: a focus on spinal cord stimulation," *Expert Review of Medical Devices*, vol. 4, no. 2, pp. 201–214, 2007.

[7] C. N. Shealy, J. T. Mortimer, and J. B. Reswick, "Electrical inhibition of pain by stimulation of the dorsal columns: preliminary clinical report," *Anesthesia and Analgesia*, vol. 46, no. 4, pp. 489–491, 1967.

[8] J. Holsheimer and J. J. Struijk, "How do geometric factors influence epidural spinal cord stimulation? A quantitative analysis by computer modeling," *Stereotactic and Functional Neurosurgery*, vol. 56, no. 4, pp. 234–249, 1991.

[9] J. Holsheimer and W. A. Wesselink, "Optimum electrode geometry for spinal cord stimulation: the narrow bipole and tripole," *Medical and Biological Engineering and Computing*, vol. 35, no. 5, pp. 493–497, 1997.

[10] J. Holsheimer, J. J. Struijk, and N. R. Tas, "Effects of electrode geometry and combination on nerve fibre selectivity in spinal cord stimulation," *Medical and Biological Engineering and Computing*, vol. 33, no. 5, pp. 676–682, 1995.

[11] N. J. M. Rijkhoff, J. Holsheimer, F. M. J. Debruyne, and H. Wijkstra, "Modelling selective activation of small myelinated nerve fibres using a monopolar point electrode," *Medical and Biological Engineering and Computing*, vol. 33, no. 6, pp. 762–768, 1995.

[12] J. J. Struijk, J. Holsheimer, and H. B.K. Boom, "Excitation of dorsal root fibers in spinal cord stimulation: a theoretical study," *IEEE Transactions on Biomedical Engineering*, vol. 40, no. 7, pp. 632–639, 1993.

[13] L. Manola, J. Holsheimer, P. H. Veltink, K. Bradley, and D. Peterson, "Theoretical investigation into longitudinal cathodal

field steering in spinal cord stimulation," *Neuromodulation*, vol. 10, no. 2, pp. 120–132, 2007.

[14] B. A. Simpson, "Spinal cord stimulation," *Pain Reviews*, vol. 1, pp. 199–230, 1994.

[15] R. B. North, M. G. Ewend, M. T. Lawton, and S. Piantadosi, "Spinal cord stimulation of chronic, intractable pain: superiority of 'multi-channel' devices," *Pain*, vol. 44, no. 2, pp. 119–130, 1991.

[16] R. B. North, D. H. Kidd, J. Olin, J. N. Sieracki, and L. Petrucci, "Spinal cord stimulation for axial low back pain: a prospective controlled trial comparing 16-contact insulated electrodes with 4-contact percutaneous electrodes," *Neuromodulation*, vol. 9, no. 1, pp. 56–67, 2006.

[17] R. Davis and E. Gray, "Technical factors important to dorsal column stimulation," *Applied Neurophysiology*, vol. 44, no. 1-3, pp. 160–170, 1981.

[18] G. H. Spincemaille, H. M. Klomp, E. W. Steyerberg, H. Van Urk, and J. D.F. Habbema, "Technical data and complications of spinal cord stimulation: data from a randomized trial on critical limb ischemia," *Stereotactic and Functional Neurosurgery*, vol. 74, no. 2, pp. 63–72, 2000.

[19] M. S. May, C. Banks, and S. J. Thomson, "A retrospective, long-term, third-party follow-up of patients considered for spinal cord stimulation," *Neuromodulation*, vol. 5, no. 3, pp. 137–144, 2002.

[20] M. J. L. De Jongste, D. Nagelkerke, C. M. Hooyschuur et al., "Stimulation characteristics, complications, and efficacy of spinal cord stimulation systems in patients with refractory angina: a prospective feasibility study," *Pacing and Clinical Electrophysiology*, vol. 17, no. 11 I, pp. 1751–1760, 1994.

[21] J. C. Oakley, F. Espinosa, H. Bothe et al., "Transverse tripolar spinal cord stimulation: results of an international multicenter study," *Neuromodulation*, vol. 9, no. 3, pp. 192–203, 2006.

[22] P. S. Ruggera, D. M. Witters, G. von Maltzahn, and H. I. Bassen, "In vitro assessment of tissue heating near metallic medical implants by exposure to pulsed radio frequency diathermy," *Physics in Medicine and Biology*, vol. 48, no. 17, pp. 2919–2928, 2003.

[23] R. V. Sha, H. K. Smith, J. Chung, A. Hegazi, and G. B. Racz, "Cervical spinal cord neoplasm in a patient with an implanted cervical spinal cord stimulator: the controversial role of magnetic resonance imaging," *Pain Physician*, vol. 7, no. 2, pp. 273–278, 2004.

[24] J. M. Henderson, J. Thach, M. Phillips, K. Baker, F. G. Shellock, and A. R. Rezai, "Permanent neurological deficit related to magnetic resonance imaging in a patient with implanted deep brain stimulation electrodes for Parkinson's disease: case report," *Neurosurgery*, vol. 57, no. 5, p. E1063, 2005.

[25] J. W. Kallewaard, J. Koy, P. Rigoard, D. Abejon, and K. Gatzinksy, "Adaptive spinal cord stimulation: results from the testing restore sensor usability and satisfaction (TRUST) survey," *INS London*, 2011.

[26] M. Tulgar, G. Barolat, and B. Ketcik, "Analysis of parameters for epidural spinal cord stimulation," *Stereotactic and Functional Neurosurgery*, vol. 61, no. 3, pp. 129–139, 1993.

[27] J. D. Law and L. V. Miller, "Importance and documentation of an epidural stimulating position," *Applied Neurophysiology*, vol. 45, no. 4-5, pp. 461–464, 1982.

[28] R. Segal, B. R. Stacey, T. E. Rudy, S. Baser, and J. Markham, "Spinal cord stimulation revisited," *Neurological Research*, vol. 20, no. 5, pp. 391–396, 1998.

[29] J. P. van Buyten, "The performance and safety of an implantable spinal cord stimulation system in patients with chronic pain: a 5-year study," *Neuromodulation*, vol. 6, no. 2, pp. 79–87, 2003.

[30] J. T. Mortimer, "Motor prostheses," in *Handbook of Physiology—The Nervous System III*, V. Brooks, Ed., pp. 155–187, American Physiological Society, Bethesda, Md, USA, 1981.

[31] T. L. Yearwood, B. Hershey, K. Bradley, and D. Lee, "Pulse width programming in spinal cord stimulation: a clinical study," *Pain Physician*, vol. 13, no. 4, pp. 321–335, 2010.

[32] K. Kumar, R. S. Taylor, L. Jacques et al., "Spinal cord stimulation versus conventional medical management for neuropathic pain: a multicentre randomised controlled trial in patients with failed back surgery syndrome," *Pain*, vol. 132, no. 1-2, pp. 179–188, 2007.

[33] J. C. Oakley, "Spinal cord stimulation in axial low back pain: solving the dilemma," *Pain Medicine*, vol. 7, no. 1, pp. S58–S63, 2006.

[34] I. Smet, J. P. van Buyten, and A. Al-Kaisy, "Successful treatment of low back pain with a novel neuromodulation device," in *Proceedings of the 14th North American Neuromodulation Society Annual Meeting*, Las Vegas, Nev, USA, 2010.

[35] E. Buchser and S. Thompson, "The future of spinal cord stimulation and related "neuroaugmentative" procedures," in *Electrical Stimulation and the Relief of Pain*, B. A. Simpson, Ed., pp. 251–267, Elsevier, London, UK, 2003.

7

Real-Time Ultrasound-Guided Spinal Anaesthesia

P. H. Conroy,[1] C. Luyet,[2] C. J. McCartney,[3] and P. G. McHardy[3]

[1] *Department of Anaesthesia, Adelaide and Meath National Children's Hospital, Tallaght, Dublin, Ireland*
[2] *Universitätsklinik für Anästhesiologie und Schmerztherapie, Inselspital, Bern University Hospital, 3010 Bern, Switzerland*
[3] *Department of Anesthesia, Sunnybrook Health Sciences Centre, Room M3-200, 2075 Bayview Avenue, Toronto, ON, Canada M4N 3M5*

Correspondence should be addressed to P. G. McHardy; paul.mchardy@sunnybrook.ca

Academic Editor: Jean Jacques Lehot

Identification of the subarachnoid space has traditionally been achieved by either a blind landmark-guided approach or using prepuncture ultrasound assistance. To assess the feasibility of performing spinal anaesthesia under real-time ultrasound guidance in routine clinical practice we conducted a single center prospective observational study among patients undergoing lower limb orthopaedic surgery. A spinal needle was inserted unassisted within the ultrasound transducer imaging plane using a paramedian approach (i.e., the operator held the transducer in one hand and the spinal needle in the other). The primary outcome measure was the success rate of CSF acquisition under real-time ultrasound guidance with CSF being located in 97 out of 100 consecutive patients within median three needle passes (IQR 1–6). CSF was not acquired in three patients. Subsequent attempts combining landmark palpation and pre-puncture ultrasound scanning resulted in successful spinal anaesthesia in two of these patients with the third patient requiring general anaesthesia. Median time from spinal needle insertion until intrathecal injection completion was 1.2 minutes (IQR 0.83–4.1) demonstrating the feasibility of this technique in routine clinical practice.

1. Introduction

Since the first description of spinal anaesthesia in humans by Bier in 1898 [1] the identification of the subarachnoid space has traditionally been achieved by an anatomical landmark guided approach. While surface anatomical landmarks are useful, they are nevertheless surrogate markers. They may be difficult to palpate in obese patients as well as those with edema. Landmark-based approaches do not take into account all anatomical variations or abnormalities, and frequently lead to incorrect identification of a given lumbar interspace [2]. Accurate identification of the subarachnoid space is paramount as multiple attempts at needle placement may cause patient discomfort, higher incidence of spinal hematoma [3], postdural puncture headache [4, 5], and trauma to neural structures [6–8]. Having alternative approaches may help improve success and mitigate the limitations of the current techniques.

Neuraxial sonography allows the operator to preview spinal anatomy, identify midline, and determine the interspace for needle insertion. Even if the preliminary scout scan has already been shown to be helpful [9], a real-time ultrasound guided approach may further improve on the limitations of the ultrasound-assisted pre-puncture techniques. In particular this technique avoids the potential for error in the process of having to "remember" the degree of cephalad to caudad and lateral to medial angulation required after pre-puncture skin marking. To date we can find only one case report [10] and one report of a series of 10 patients [11] where the technique of real time ultrasound guided spinal anaesthesia has been employed. The aim of this single center prospective observational study was to investigate the feasibility of performing a systematic method for real-time ultrasound guided paramedian access to the subarachnoid space with the spinal needle inserted in the plane (in-plane) of the ultrasound beam by a single operator.

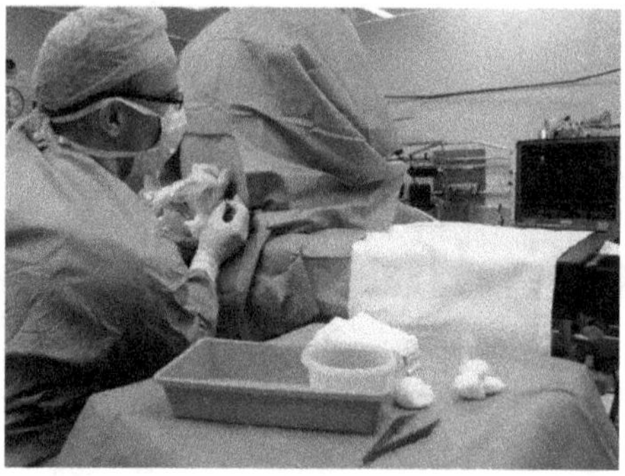

FIGURE 1: Typical positioning of the operator, ultrasound transducer and the patient during, real-time ultrasound-guided spinal anaesthesia.

2. Methods

After ethical approval (Toronto Academic Health Sciences Network), registration at Clinicaltrials.gov (NCT01326988), and obtaining informed consent we recruited 100 patients scheduled to undergo spinal anaesthesia for elective lower limb surgery between May and September 2011. Other inclusion criteria were age 18 to 90 years, ASA I–III, and ability to provide written informed consent. Standard exclusion criteria for spinal anaesthesia included coagulopathy, INR ≥ 1.5, platelet count $<75 \times 10^9$/L, local infection at the site of injection, indeterminate neurologic disease, or allergy to local anaesthetics. Routine monitoring (ECG, heart rate, noninvasive arterial pressure, and arterial oxygen saturation) was established and intravenous sedation with midazolam (1-2 mg) was given. Any peripheral nerve block procedures appropriate to the patients' surgical procedure were performed prior to spinal anaesthesia (e.g., continuous femoral nerve block for knee replacement surgery). Spinal anaesthesia was administered either by a staff anaesthetist or one of 2 regional anaesthesia fellows, each with experience of more than 30 neuraxial ultrasound-assisted procedures.

The block procedure was performed with the patient, at the operator's discretion, in the sitting or lateral position. Full aseptic technique with gloves, gown, mask, and sterile transducer cable sheath were employed. A standard curvilinear 2–5 MHz transducer attached to an ultrasound device (either a Sonosite M Turbo, Bothell, Washington, or a Phillips HD11Xe, Bothell, Washington) was applied to the patient's back, lateral to the midline (paramedian sagittal scan) in the preferred hand of the operator. The spinal needle was held in the opposite hand and the ultrasound screen positioned in the line of sight of the operator (see Figure 1). The US image was optimized by setting an appropriate scanning depth (6–10 cm), selecting a transducer frequency, and adjusting the gain to obtain the best possible image.

The sacrum was identified first and then the probe was moved cephalad in the paramedian axis with a 10–15 degree tilt toward the midline. The lumbar lamina were identified and a target space between L2-3 and L5-S1 was chosen. The probe was positioned with its midline point directly above the selected space. The transducer was then rotated 45 degrees towards midline, into an oblique, paramedian sagittal view (Figure 1). This maneuver affords a view of the spinous process of the upper vertebral body and the lamina of the lower vertebral body simultaneously. The angle between these two structures represents the paramedian window into the spinal canal. Selecting this approach reduces the risk of the facet joints obstructing the needle path as frequently occurs during a paramedian needle insertion within a transverse scanning plane.

With this view it is possible to visualize the lamina, the intervertebral space, and the posterior longitudinal ligament-vertebral body complex (seen as a white line deep in the intervertebral space). Unlike previous descriptions of real-time techniques, this maneuver provides an ergonomic advantage for simultaneous needle handling specifically because more room is created between the needle entry point and the bed surface. It also allows for a needle approach that more closely approximates the traditional paramedian technique as well as all the other advantages that a paramedian approach has been shown to afford when using neuraxial ultrasound [12]. As a final maneuver the probe is moved towards the patient's midline (craniomedial) in the same axis already established. The entry point of the needle would otherwise be too lateral when using a curvilinear probe. The final position of the probe and the image of the spine it provides can be seen in Figure 2.

Ultrasound gel was placed on the back directly under the transducer. Any ultrasound gel near the selected skin puncture site was carefully removed using sterile gauze prior to needle insertion. As a further precaution the point of needle entry through the skin was physically outside the footprint area of the transducer. Lidocaine 1%, (2-3 mL) was used for skin infiltration prior to the procedure. A standard spinal needle (90 mm long) was chosen at the discretion of the operator which provided the optimum balance of characteristics needed for ultrasound visibility and ability to steer in the tissues while at the same time considering the risk of postdural puncture headache. The needle was inserted in plane from the caudal end of the ultrasound transducer with its tip directed towards the interlaminar space. The angle of needle insertion, that is, the trajectory for needle insertion, was then optimized while the spinal needle was still in the erector spinae muscle (Figure 3).

The needle was gradually advanced to the interlaminar space, under real-time in-plane US guidance, until the tip was judged to have broken through the ligamentum flavum/dura complex—frequently a distinct "give" could usually be felt at this point. Depending on the quality of the image and the size of the interlaminar space, the needle tip was occasionally lost from view if it entered the acoustic shadow formed by the spinous process. At this point the operator would feel the needle enter the ligamentum flavum and entry into the thecal space was typically achieved in less than one centimeter. With dosages varying according to the planned surgery plain 0.5% bupivacaine (5–15 mg) with fentanyl (5–15 μg) was injected over 15–20 s and the patient was then returned to, or left

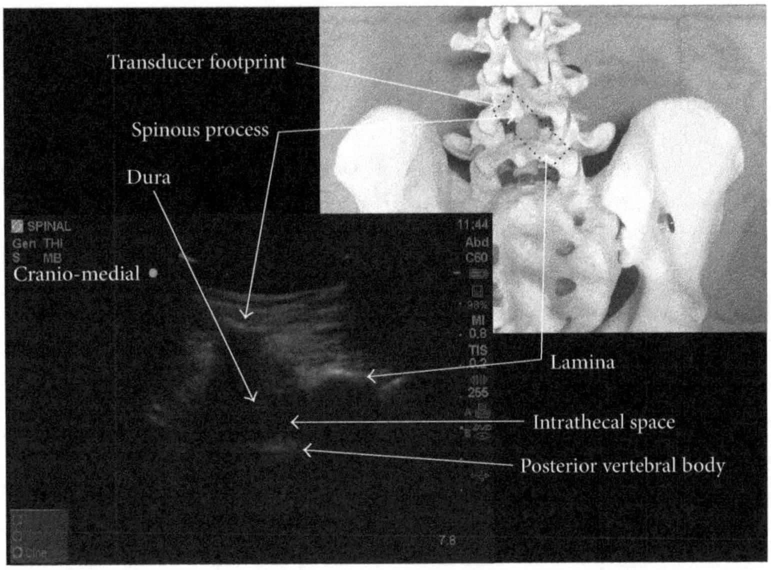

FIGURE 2: Spine model showing the paramedian oblique transducer orientation (rotated by 45 degrees) used during real-time scanning with a typical ultrasound image.

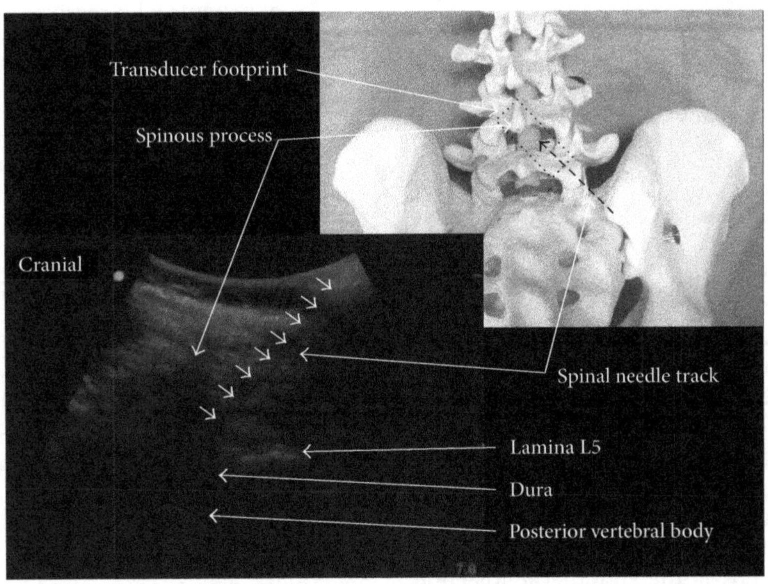

FIGURE 3: Ultrasound image showing the paramedian spinal needle insertion path compared with a schematic overlay of the transducer orientation on a spinal model.

in, the lateral position with the surgical side uppermost. The patient was determined to be ready for surgery at the discretion of the attending anesthetist.

Propofol (1-2 mg·kg^{-1}·hr^{-1}) was used for intraoperative sedation, and oxygen (4 L/min) administered via a facemask. The spinal anaesthetic was deemed to have failed if the procedure was converted to general anaesthesia within the first two hours after intrathecal injection. Postoperative care in the ward was entirely at the discretion of the orthopedic surgeons except for the analgesic management which was managed by the acute pain team.

The primary outcome measure was the success rate of CSF acquisition by real-time ultrasound guidance. Secondary outcome measures included the number of needle passes it took to access the subarachnoid space. Every ventral advancement of the needle was considered as a "needle pass" even if no further skin puncture was performed. Needle passes were limited to a maximum of 6 per skin puncture. Skin punctures were limited to a maximum of 3 per patient. The number of different spinal levels attempted, procedure time from first needle insertion to completion of the intrathecal injection and the number of separate skin punctures were recorded.

Scores were also recorded relating to the following aspects of the procedure

(1) Preprocedure clinical scoring for potential predictors of difficulty in the event of a blind landmark based approach [13, 14].

(2) Summary difficulty score according to the anesthetist's subjective opinion: Easy/Normal = 0, Difficult = 1.

(3) Bony landmark palpability: 0 = easily palpable; 1 = poorly palpable; 2 = impalpable.

(4) Presence of spinal curvature abnormality: None = 0; Yes = 1.

In the event that the permitted number of needling attempts was reached without acquiring CSF then the real-time US technique was defined as a failure. In such cases the spinal block was performed using either a traditional landmark based approach and/or pre-puncture ultrasound assistance at the discretion of the attending anaesthetist. Complications were recorded including those directly related to the technique (e.g., vascular puncture), inadequacies of the block that required rescue spinal injection of local anaesthetic, or conversion to general anaesthesia within 2 hours of the initial spinal anaesthetic injection. All study data were recorded by the operator after performing the procedure and patients were followed up by telephone at 6 weeks postoperatively.

2.1. Statistics. A convenience sample of 100 consecutive patients was planned in order to represent the typical patient population presenting for elective spinal anaesthesia. Descriptive statistics were calculated for all variables of interest. Normally distributed data are presented as mean and standard deviation—non-normally distributed data are presented as median (interquartile range [range]). Normality was tested using the Shapiro-Wilk test. Correlation between Preprocedure clinical scoring for predictors of difficulty in the event of a blind landmark based approach and measurements made during the puncture such as total number of needle advancements, total number of skin punctures, and the time to completion of the intrathecal injection were calculated using Spearmans rank correlation coefficient for non-normally distributed data or the Pearson Product Moment correlation coefficient for normally distributed data. All calculations were carried out using Sigma Plot 12 for Windows (Systat Software Inc. GmbH, Germany).

3. Results

100 patients were completed and patient characteristics are detailed in Table 1. Using real-time ultrasound guidance CSF was acquired in 97% of cases within the predefined limits set in the study protocol. There was failure to acquire CSF by real-time guidance in 3 patients. Subsequent attempts using a combination of the traditional landmark palpation method and pre-puncture ultrasound scanning resulted in successful spinal anaesthesia in 2 of these patients. The third patient received elective general anaesthesia following multiple failed attempts to acquire CSF using a combination of all the approaches described above by 2 different operators.

Table 1: Patient characteristics.

		Surgery performed (n)	
Total Patients (n)	100		
Gender (n)	M: 37, F: 63	Total knee arthroplasty	61
Age (yrs)	66 ± 11 Range 39–86	Total hip arthroplasty (THA)	24
Height (m)	1.7 ± 0.1 Range 1.7–1.9	Revision THA	3
Weight (kg)	83.5 ± 18.1 Range 45–146	Other knee surgery	4
BMI (kg·m^{-2})	30.4 ± 5.9 Range 17.6–52.1	Other lower limb surgery	9

Values expressed as number n (= % patients) or mean ± SD.

5% of patients who received intrathecal local anaesthetic injection were subsequently converted to general anaesthesia intraoperatively—2 patients had poor CSF flow during injection, 1 had no block despite 2 easy injections of LA into free-flowing CSF, 1 patient became very restless while sedated 50 minutes into a total knee arthroplasty, and 1 patient had inadequate block height for surgery with insufficient time to perform a repeat block.

The median number of needle passes required to acquire a satisfactory flow of CSF for spinal anaesthetic injection was 3 (IQR 1–6 [range 1–18]). The median number of skin punctures was 1 (IQR 1-2 [range 1–3]). 65% patients required only one skin puncture for CSF acquisition with 12% patients needing the maximum allowed three skin punctures to successfully complete the injection. The number of median spinal levels punctured was 1 [IQR 1-2]). 30% patients required only a single needle pass with CSF being obtained in 80% cases within 6 needle passes. An average of 1.46 spinal interspaces was punctured.

The median time required for sterile preparation of the ultrasound equipment and initial pre-puncture scanning was 3.9 mins (IQR 2.7–5.2 [range 1.4–15.3]). The median time required from spinal needle insertion until completion of the intrathecal injection was 1.2 mins (IQR 0.8–4.1 [range 0.2–15]). Total procedure time (excluding patient positioning and local anaesthetic preparation) was 8 minutes (IQR 4.4–10.2 [range 2.9–19.7]). Patients were in the seated position in 95% of cases (lateral position in 5 cases)—one of the 3 patients where real-time US guidance failed to locate CSF was in the lateral position. CSF was acquired using real-time needle guidance through a 22 G Quincke spinal needle in 86% of cases and a 25 G Whitacre needle in the remainder (all needles used were 90 mm in length). All patients were followed up by telephone interview at 6 weeks post procedure for procedure-related complications with a telephone response rate of 67%. An orthostatic post dural

TABLE 2: Predicted difficulty of spinal anaesthesia.

Anaesthetists subjective prediction of Difficulty	Easy	64
	Difficult	36
Palpability of bony landmarks	Easily palpable	53
	Poorly palpable	35
	Impalpable	12
Predicted spinal anaesthesia difficulty scoring (after Atallah)	Easy (grade 0–3)	63
	Easy (grade ≥4)	37

Data are presented as n (= %). Atallah's spinal anaesthesia difficulty score comprises nine difficulty grades. Grade 4 is the difficulty grade at or above which difficulty is expected. Grades are calculated based on the sum of specific scores assigned for BMI, age, bony landmark palpability, radiological characteristics, and spinal deformity [13].

puncture headache was reported by one patient on whom a 22 G Quincke needle was used.

Data relating to the preintervention predicted difficulty of performing spinal anaesthesia are presented in Table 2. There was no significant correlation between the total number of skin punctures, time to acquire CSF, or the total number of needle advancements and either the patients BMI, the anaesthetist's subjective Preprocedure prediction of difficulty or the palpability of bony landmarks. There was, however, a significant correlation observed between the presence of a spinal curve abnormality and both the number of skin punctures required (correlation coefficient 0.251; $P = 0.0124$) as well as the total number of needle advancements required (correlation coefficient 0.307, $P = 0.002$). Overall 63% of patients recruited were predicted to be difficult according to the previously validated pre-procedural difficulty scoring system by Atallah et al. [13].

4. Discussion

This study demonstrates that real-time ultrasound guided spinal anaesthesia is a clinically feasible procedure among this unselected population of patients undergoing lower limb orthopaedic surgery. This a patient group among whom the greatest outcome benefits are to be gained from neuraxial block [15]. A success rate of 97% in CSF acquisition using real-time US guidance appears to be broadly similar to that achieved in other studies of the adult orthopaedic patient population using traditional landmark [16] or ultrasound guided pre-puncture [9] approaches for spinal anaesthesia. Administration of spinal anaesthesia under real time ultrasound guidance failed in 3 patients within the predefined limits specified in the real-time study protocol. 2 of these patients eventually had successful spinal anesthesia using a combination of traditional landmark palpation and ultrasound pre-puncture scanning outside of the real-time study protocol (i.e., according to routine clinical practice in our institution with no predefined limitations on the number of needle insertions/skin puncture attempts). As this was a non-comparative trial a definitive conclusion cannot be drawn from this data as to the relative merits of the real-time guidance method versus landmark only or ultrasound prepuncture techniques.

Acquisition of CSF in and of itself does not necessarily reflect the number of needle passes or skin punctures required to achieve this endpoint and thus may not reflect the actual procedural difficulty encountered—assessment of the usefulness of this technique according to these clinically relevant outcomes requires a prospective randomised trial comparing these 3 different methods for the administration of spinal anaesthesia.

Use of real-time ultrasound guidance for combined spinal-epidural insertion as part of a randomised controlled trial in a younger obstetrics population has previously found that real-time guidance significantly reduces the number of needle passes required when compared to a traditional landmark based approach [17]. Our success rate for correct identification of the subarachnoid space on the first skin puncture (65%) is similar with others previously reported (64% [14], 61.5% [18], and 61.9–68.3% [19]). Minimising the number of skin punctures is important due to the risks associated with multiple attempts at needle placement as described earlier (i.e., a higher incidence of spinal hematoma, postdural puncture headache, and trauma to neural structures) [3–8].

Patients were in the sitting position in 95% cases (5% were in the lateral position) which is typical of our pre-existing institutional practice. Performing real-time US guided spinal anaesthesia in the prone position as reported by Lee et al. [11] can be difficult for patients to tolerate and introduces other practical issues. In this study, choice of patient positioning was left to individual operator discretion who found both the lateral and sitting positions to be ergonomically feasible.

Total procedure time was 8 ± 4.68 minutes (average ± SD). Typical procedure times reported for a landmark based approach range from 4.4 ± 3.2 mins [19] to 4.8 ± 4.4 mins [16]. Real-time US guided spinal anaesthesia takes longer because extra time is required to identify a satisfactory acoustic window coupled with the need to maintain needle-probe alignment. The time spent for sterile preparation of the probe and initial "scout" scanning prior to insertion of the needle (average 4.4 min ± 2.6 min) appears longer than that reported for ultrasound assisted neuraxial techniques by Carney and Hunt (2.7 min (±0.6 min)) [20]. However the mean time taken for real-time scanning of the spinal needle approach until completion of the intrathecal injection was an average of 3 min (±3.5)—in effect this was the duration of combined real-time scanning and "needling".

4.1. Failure Rate. Failure of spinal anaesthesia has been defined as the need to convert to general anaesthesia or to repeat the intrathecal injection following the initial block—this occurred in 5% of patients in this study. There are widely varying reports of the failure rate of spinal anaesthesia in the literature ranging from <1% to 17% [21]. Contemporary reports of spinal anaesthesia failure rate continue to be in the range of 11.6% [16].

Our technique had a 97% success rate of CSF acquisition in this study. The only other real-time ultrasound guided neuraxial procedures in which this outcome was reported were in two studies of combined spinal-epidural anaesthesia which had failure rates of 22% (4/18 patients [22]) and 14% (2/14 patients [23]), respectively. However given the different nature of the techniques and different reasons for failure (as detailed in a recent review by Cook [24]) direct comparison is not possible.

4.2. Difficult Spinal Insertion. The ease of palpation of spinal bony landmarks (classified as easy, poorly, or totally impalpable spinous processes) has been shown to be the most significant independent predictor of difficulty with spinal anaesthesia administration in two previous studies [13, 14].

Atallah et al. have previously developed a difficulty scoring system for predicting difficult spinal anaesthesia where patients are given a score ranging from 0 to 4 for each of the variables age, BMI, surface landmark palpability, spinal bony deformity, and radiological characteristics [13]. A score ≥4 is predictive of difficulty even if the radiological score is omitted. By this yardstick 63% of our patients were predicted to be difficult. However on the other hand the average BMI of this sample of patients was not very different to that of average North American adults in the 40–79 year old age range. The mean BMI of adults in this age range in Canada for the period 2007–2009 was 27.7 kg/m^2 while that of Americans was 29.1 kg/m^2 [25]. In other words our patients were not always "difficult" and further data are needed for difficult patients in which traditional landmark or even pre-puncture scanning may prove to be inferior to real time ultrasound guidance.

Conversely using our guidance technique only 7% of spinal insertions in this study were found to be "difficult" according to separate difficulty criteria proposed by Weed et al. (i.e., ≥10 needle passes associated with spinal needling time of >400 seconds or cases where CSF failed to be obtained) [26]. In contrast Weed et al. found 28% of their patients to be difficult by these criteria when using a landmark based approach. This apparent reduction in predicted difficulty when using our technique could be due to the improved visualisation and guidance of the needle path offered by real-time scanning as opposed to a pre-scan or landmark technique.

4.3. Spinal Needle Size. An audit of spinal anesthesia practice was conducted 1 year prior to this study at our institution. Data collected relating to the size of spinal needles used at that stage indicates 25 G Whitaker needles were used in 81% of our patients (a 22 G Quincke was used in the remainder). This is markedly different from the pattern in our study where we used 22 G needles in 96% patients. This change was motivated by the fact that 22 G needles are stiffer and more echogenic than finer 25 G needles thereby making them easier to visualise and to steer within the ultrasound beam towards the target. This consideration however can be obviated by using a longer introducer needle with cornerstone ultrasound reflectors or indeed by using a 22 G needle as an introducer and then stopping short of the dura before inserting a 25 G needle through the lumen as suggested by Medd et al. [27]. However despite our predominant use of 22 G needles only one patient reported postdural puncture headache during follow-up giving an estimated incidence of 1%.

4.4. Study Limitations. Our study is a single centre descriptive observational study of real-time US guided spinal anaesthesia and not a comparative randomised controlled trial. We cannot, therefore, make any direct comparisons between this approach versus a pre-puncture ultrasound or landmark only technique. To this end we are currently planning a randomised controlled trial comparing these techniques directly paying particular attention to that subset of patients with a high Preprocedure difficulty score according to Atallah et al.

It was not practicable to blind the study and the individual operators self-reported the study outcomes directly following performance of the procedure. This introduces the possibility of observer bias [26].

5. Conclusion

In summary we have demonstrated that real-time ultrasound-guided spinal anaesthesia is a clinically feasible procedure. Performance of the technique assessed across a broad range of measures appears similar to the traditional landmark based technique as well as pre-puncture ultrasound assisted approaches.

Conflict of Interests

No external funding and no conflict of interests declared apart from Dr. Cedric Luyet who has received consultancy fees from Pajunk Inc. related to research about novel catheters in regional anaesthesia—however there is no relation to this study/paper.

Acknowledgment

The authors wish to thank Patrick Twohig for provision of his audit data on spinal anaesthesia (conducted in 2010 at the Holland Orthopaedic and Arthritic Centre prior to this study) and also for helping with data entry for this study. This work was supported by departmental resources only.

References

[1] A. Bier, "Versuche über cocainisirung des rückenmarkes," *Deutsch Zeitschrift für Chirurgie*, vol. 51, no. 3, pp. 352–358, 1899.

[2] C. R. Broadbent, W. B. Maxwell, R. Ferrie, D. J. Wilson, M. Gawne-Cain, and R. Russell, "Ability of anaesthetists to identify a marked lumbar interspace," *Anaesthesia*, vol. 55, no. 11, pp. 1122–1126, 2000.

[3] H. Wulf, "Epidural anaesthesia and spinal haematoma," *Canadian Journal of Anaesthesia*, vol. 43, no. 12, pp. 1260–1271, 1996.

[4] H. Flaatten, J. Felthaus, R. Larsen, S. Bernhardsen, and H. Klausen, "Postural post-dural puncture headache after spinal and epidural anaesthesia. A randomised, double-blind study,"

Acta Anaesthesiologica Scandinavica, vol. 42, no. 7, pp. 759–764, 1998.

[5] D. A. Harrison and B. T. Langham, "Spinal anaesthesia for urological surgery. A survey of failure rate, postdural puncture headache and patient satisfaction," *Anaesthesia*, vol. 47, no. 10, pp. 902–903, 1992.

[6] Y. Auroy, P. Narchi, A. Messiah, L. Litt, B. Rouvier, and K. Samii, "Serious complications related to regional anesthesia: Results of a prospective survey in France," *Anesthesiology*, vol. 87, no. 3, pp. 479–486, 1997.

[7] R. Puolakka, J. Haasio, M. T. Pitkänen, M. Kallio, and P. H. Rosenberg, "Technical aspects and postoperative sequelae of spinal and epidural anesthesia: a prospective study of 3,230 orthopedic patients," *Regional Anesthesia and Pain Medicine*, vol. 25, no. 5, pp. 488–497, 2000.

[8] T. T. Horlocker, D. G. McGregor, D. K. Matsushige, D. R. Schroeder, and J. A. Besse, "A retrospective review of 4767 consecutive spinal anesthetics: central nervous system complications," *Anesthesia and Analgesia*, vol. 84, no. 3, pp. 578–584, 1997.

[9] K. J. Chin, A. Perlas, V. Chan, D. Brown-Shreves, A. Koshkin, and V. Vaishnav, "Ultrasound imaging facilitates spinal anesthesia in adults with difficult surface anatomic landmarks," *Anesthesiology*, vol. 115, no. 1, pp. 94–101, 2011.

[10] K. J. Chin, V. W. S. Chan, R. Ramlogan, and A. Perlas, "Real-time ultrasound-guided spinal anesthesia in patients with a challenging spinal anatomy: two case reports," *Acta Anaesthesiologica Scandinavica*, vol. 54, no. 2, pp. 252–255, 2010.

[11] P. J. Lee, R. Tang, A. Sawka, C. Krebs, and H. Vaghadia, "Real-time ultrasound-guided spinal anesthesia using taylor's approach," *Anesthesia and Analgesia*, vol. 112, no. 5, pp. 1236–1238, 2011.

[12] T. Grau, R. U. W. Leipold, J. Horter, R. Conradi, E. O. Martin, and J. Motsch, "Paramedian access to the epidural space: the optimum window for ultrasound imaging," *Journal of Clinical Anesthesia*, vol. 13, no. 3, pp. 213–217, 2001.

[13] M. M. Atallah, A. D. Demian, and A. A. Shorrab, "Development of a difficulty score for spinal anaesthesia," *British Journal of Anaesthesia*, vol. 92, no. 3, pp. 354–360, 2004.

[14] J. Sprung, D. L. Bourke, J. Grass et al., "Predicting the difficult neuraxial block: a prospective study," *Anesthesia and Analgesia*, vol. 89, no. 2, pp. 384–389, 1999.

[15] A. Rodgers, N. Walker, S. Schug et al., "Reduction of postoperative mortality and morbidity with epidural or spinal anaesthesia: results from overview of randomised trials," *British Medical Journal*, vol. 321, no. 7275, pp. 1493–1497, 2000.

[16] J. Weed, K. Finkel, M. L. Beach, C. B. Granger, J. D. Gallagher, and B. D. Sites, "Spinal anesthesia for orthopedic surgery: a detailed video assessment of quality," *Regional Anesthesia and Pain Medicine*, vol. 36, pp. 51–55, 2011.

[17] T. Grau, R. W. Leipold, S. Fatehi, E. Martin, and J. Motsch, "Real-time ultrasonic observation of combined spinal-epidural anaesthesia," *European Journal of Anaesthesiology*, vol. 21, no. 1, pp. 25–31, 2004.

[18] G. R. De Oliveira Filho, H. P. Gomes, M. H. Z. Da Fonseca, J. C. Hoffman, S. G. Pederneiras, and J. H. S. Garcia, "Predictors of successful neuraxial block: a prospective study," *European Journal of Anaesthesiology*, vol. 19, no. 6, pp. 447–451, 2002.

[19] M. J. Tessler, K. Kardash, R. M. Wahba, S. J. Kleiman, S. T. Trihas, and M. Rossignol, "The performance of spinal anesthesia is marginally more difficult in the elderly," *Regional Anesthesia and Pain Medicine*, vol. 24, no. 2, pp. 126–130, 1999.

[20] A. Carney and V. Hunt, "The use of neuraxial scanning can facilitate spinal anaesthesia for lower limb joint arthroplasty," in *Proceedings of the 15th Annual Scientific congress of the British Society of Orthopaedic Anaesthetists*, vol. 66, pp. 407–408, Nottingham, UK, Novemeber 2010.

[21] P. D. W. Fettes, J. R. Jansson, and J. A. W. Wildsmith, "Failed spinal anaesthesia: mechanisms, management, and prevention," *British Journal of Anaesthesia*, vol. 102, no. 6, pp. 739–748, 2009.

[22] D. Tran, A. A. Kamani, E. Al-Attas, V. A. Lessoway, S. Massey, and R. N. Rohling, "Single-operator real-time ultrasound-guidance to aim and insert a lumbar epidural needle," *Canadian Journal of Anesthesia*, vol. 57, no. 4, pp. 313–321, 2010.

[23] M. K. Karmakar, X. Li, A. M. H. Ho, W. H. Kwok, and P. T. Chui, "Real-time ultrasound-guided paramedian epidural access: evaluation of a novel in-plane technique," *British Journal of Anaesthesia*, vol. 102, no. 6, pp. 845–854, 2009.

[24] T. M. Cook, "Combined spinal-epidural techniques," *Anaesthesia*, vol. 55, no. 1, pp. 42–64, 2000.

[25] Body Composition of Canadian Adults 2007 to 2009. Canadian Health Measures Survey, 2007 to 2009. National Health and Nutrition Examination Survey, 2007-2008.

[26] J. T. Weed, A. H. Taenzer, K. J. Finkel, and B. D. Sites, "Evaluation of pre-procedure ultrasound examination as a screening tool for difficult spinal anaesthesia," *Anaesthesia*, vol. 66, pp. 925–930, 2011.

[27] C. Medd, R. Chandrashekar, and G. Simon, "Needle-through-Quincke needle technique for establishing spinal anaesthesia in the obese patient," *Anaesthesia*, vol. 66, no. 5, pp. 400–401, 2011.

8

Measurements of Epidural Space Depth using Preexisting CT Scans Correlate with Loss of Resistance Depth during Thoracic Epidural Catheter Placement

Nathaniel H. Greene,[1] Benjamin G. Cobb,[1] Ken F. Linnau,[2] and Christopher D. Kent[1]

[1]*Department of Anesthesiology and Pain Medicine, University of Washington School of Medicine, Seattle, WA 98195, USA*
[2]*Department of Radiology, University of Washington School of Medicine, Seattle, WA 98195, USA*

Correspondence should be addressed to Nathaniel H. Greene; nathanielgreene@me.com

Academic Editor: Enrico Camporesi

Background. Thoracic epidural catheters provide the best quality postoperative pain relief for major abdominal and thoracic surgical procedures, but placement is one of the most challenging procedures in the repertoire of an anesthesiologist. Most patients presenting for a procedure that would benefit from a thoracic epidural catheter have already had high resolution imaging that may be useful to assist placement of a catheter. *Methods.* This retrospective study used data from 168 patients to examine the association and predictive power of epidural-skin distance (ESD) on computed tomography (CT) to determine loss of resistance depth acquired during epidural placement. Additionally, the ability of anesthesiologists to measure this distance was compared to a radiologist, who specializes in spine imaging. *Results.* There was a strong association between CT measurement and loss of resistance depth ($P < 0.0001$); the presence of morbid obesity (BMI > 35) changed this relationship ($P = 0.007$). The ability of anesthesiologists to make CT measurements was similar to a gold standard radiologist (all individual ICCs > 0.9). *Conclusions.* Overall, this study supports the examination of a recent CT scan to aid in the placement of a thoracic epidural catheter. Making use of these scans may lead to faster epidural placements, fewer accidental dural punctures, and better epidural blockade.

1. Introduction

Local anesthetics and opioid medications administered by thoracic epidural catheters provide the best quality postoperative pain relief for major abdominal and thoracic surgical procedures [1]. The process of placing a catheter into the epidural space between the thoracic vertebrae can be challenging due to variations in thoracic spinal anatomy and narrow intervertebral spaces. One of the consequent risks is excessively deep placement of the needle with the potential complication of dural puncture headache and, rarely, needle induced injury to the spinal cord, making thoracic epidural placement a riskier procedure than a lumbar epidural.

Anesthesiologists increasingly use ultrasound imaging to guide the placement of needles into the body for the purpose of doing medical procedures. The bony vertebral column largely precludes the use of bedside sonography for steep angle neuraxial procedures owing to the lack of ultrasound transmission in bone. These challenges are magnified in the patients in whom neuraxial procedures are most difficult (those with morbid obesity or spinal abnormalities). While most anesthesiologists have a general idea at what depth they should expect to encounter the epidural space, there can be a wide range of variability between individuals [2]. The depth from the skin to the epidural space is influenced by both patient factors including body mass index [3] and procedural factors such as the needle angle required to enter the epidural space between the posterior elements of the vertebrae [4]. For any individual patient it would be helpful to know the specific depth to the epidural space prior to epidural needle placement.

With increased utilization of computed tomography (CT) for not only diagnostic purposes but also preoperative planning, most patients undergoing epidural catheter placement

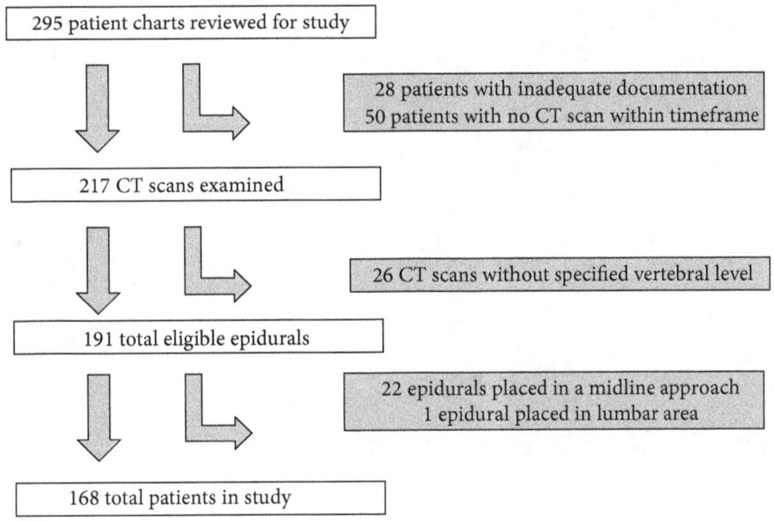

FIGURE 1: Patient selection procedure.

for pain control after major thoracic and abdominal surgeries will have recent abdominal and thoracic imaging available for review preoperatively.

The goal of this study was to compare measurements taken by anesthesiologists from CT imaging to the depth of loss of resistance as recorded during epidural placement. The secondary goal of this study was to compare the ability of anesthesiologists to measure this distance on a CT scan to a radiologist.

2. Materials and Methods

2.1. Patient Selection. After local IRB approval, we conducted a retrospective cohort study using electronic medical records to identify eligible patients. Individual patient records were assessed for documentation of placement of a thoracic epidural catheter between March and August of 2011 at the University of Washington Medical Center. Patients were excluded if a CT scan of the respective spinal level was not available either 6 months prior to or during hospitalization following epidural catheter placement. If a patient had more than one appropriate imaging study, the scan closest in time to the epidural placement date was used. Given the high proportion of thoracic epidurals placed in the paramedian approach, we excluded thoracic epidurals placed in a midline approach from this analysis. We initially examined 295 patient records and included 168 records in our study (Figure 1).

2.2. Measuring Imaging Distances. All images were viewed using the institutional online PACS (Centricity Enterprise Web; GE Healthcare, Waukesha, WI) tool with measurements being made within the program. After identification of the image that optimized the view of both pedicles of the upper vertebra of the interspace accessed when placing the epidural catheter (e.g., T7 vertebra if a T7-T8 epidural catheter was placed), a line was drawn between midline at the skin and the most posterior part of the spinal canal (Figure 2). This epidural-skin distance (ESD) was measured in the axial plane (Figure 2) and was recorded from the value automatically generated by the PACS software when drawing the connecting line. Measurements for all 168 epidurals made by the lead author of the study were used for analysis.

2.3. Assessing Anesthesiologists' Radiologic Abilities. In order to ensure an anesthesiologist would be able to reliably measure the distance from the skin to the epidural space, the imaging measurements made by three different anesthesiologists (Nathaniel H. Greene, Christopher D. Kent, and Benjamin G. Cobb) were compared with a radiologist who specializes in imaging of the spine (Ken F. Linnau). A random sample of 50 patients of the 168 in the study was selected for review by all authors. Each author independently made their own measurements of the epidural-skin distance. Agreement between the measurements made by anesthesiologists and the gold standard radiologist was assessed by calculating exact concordance, concordance within 5 and 10 mm, root mean squared error (RMSE), and intraclass correlation coefficient (ICC) for each anesthesiologist.

2.4. Clinical Prediction Rules. Based on simple trigonometric principles, we hypothesized that the ESD should be linearly related to the needle path when placing an epidural in a paramedian approach. The linear transformation required could theoretically be estimated using the angles of approach in the axial plane and sagittal plane (Figure 2). Thus, fitting a linear regression model using ordinary least squares would seem to best approximate the true relationship between the ESD and loss of resistance (LOR) depth. The best fit line would yield an equation with a slope and an intercept. Given that trigonometric principles demonstrate that our CT measurement should be directly proportional to the loss of resistance depth, there is likely some degree of tissue compression which would make us predict *a priori* that there will be a positive intercept value to account for this

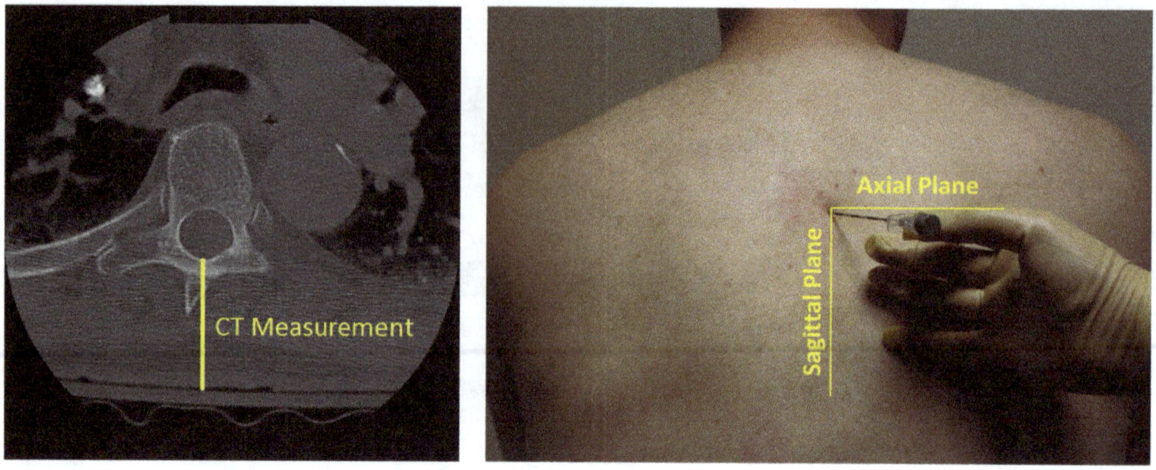

(a) (b)

Figure 2: (a) Axial computed tomography (CT) image of thorax with demonstrated measurement technique; (b) demonstration of appropriate planes with epidural needle placed on back.

fact. It is likely that tissue compression would be higher in morbidly obese patients, as a greater proportion of the CT measurement is compressible adipose tissue. Because some of our patients were morbidly obese (BMI > 35), we included a variable in our model that reflected the presence of morbid obesity. Multivariable linear regression assuming robust standard errors was used with LOR depth as the dependent variable and ESD and presence of morbid obesity as an independent variable to test for association. As we hypothesized this CT measurement would be most useful to identify patients with abnormally shallow and abnormally deep epidural spaces, receiver operating curves (ROC) were generated for two outcomes, LOR depth less than or equal to 4 cm and LOR depth greater than or equal to 8 cm. All statistical analyses were done using Stata Intercooled 12 (StataCorp; College Station, TX).

3. Results

3.1. Patient Characteristics. There were a total of 166 patients analyzed (Table 1). They had an average age of 57 years and ranged from 20 to 90 years old. The average BMI was 28, with wide range represented from 15.5 to 53.9. Approximately 13% of the sample had a BMI of greater than 35. The population was 51% male and all portions of the thoracic spine were represented with epidurals being most commonly placed at the T8-T9 interspace (28%).

3.2. Assessing Anesthesiologists' Radiologic Abilities. There was significant agreement between all three anesthesiologists' and the radiologist's measurements with expected variance as evidenced by the lack of agreement when the measurements were the same (Table 2). Additionally, the root mean squared error was consistently low, with the maximum error of 3.7, approximately 8% of the mean measurement of 47 mm. All anesthesiologists' measurements also exhibited a very high intraclass correlation (>0.9) with the radiologist's measurement (gold standard).

Table 1: Patient characteristics of sample ($N = 166$).

Continuous variable	Mean (SD)	Range
Age	56.8 (15.1)	20–90
BMI	28.1 (7.0)	15.5–53.9
CT epidural skin distance (mm)	46.7 (11.7)	27–86
Loss of resistance depth (cm)	6.1 (1.1)	3.5–8*
Categorical variable	Number	%
Male (%)	85	51
BMI > 35 (%)	21	13
Epidural level (%)		
T3	2	1.2
T4	9	5.4
T5	16	9.6
T6	24	14.5
T7	27	16.3
T8	46	27.7
T9	23	13.9
T10	12	7.2
T11	4	2.4
T12	3	1.9

*LOR depth > 8 classified as 8 (see text).

3.3. Clinical Prediction Rule. There appears to be a linear relationship between loss of resistance depth and epidural-skin distance (Figure 3). This relationship appears to be slightly different in the presence of obesity. Linear regression suggests a strong relationship between ESD and LOR for paramedian epidurals. Obesity was also significantly associated with loss of resistance depth after adjusting for the CT measurement.

TABLE 2: Analysis result.

	Anesthesiologists' measurements versus radiologist's measurement		
	Anesthesiologist 1	Anesthesiologist 2	Anesthesiologist 3
Measurements within 1 cm	98%	98%	100%
Measurements within 0.5 cm	98%	96%	86%
Measurements were the same	22%	34%	18%
Root mean squared error	2.5	2.3	3.7
Intraclass correlation coefficient	0.98	0.99	0.97

TABLE 3: Regression analysis.

	Multivariable regression analysis		
	Coefficient	95% Cl	*P* value
CT epidural skin distance (mm)	0.053	[0.050, 0.075]	<0.0001
BMI > 35	−0.59	[−1.01, −0.16]	0.007
Constant	3.30	[2.71, 3.88]	<0.0001

The intercept in the model was significantly above zero as well (Table 3). The area under the curve (AUC) of the ROC generated using ESD to predict a LOR greater than or equal to 8 cm was 0.7876 while the AUC of the ROC generated using ESD to predict a LOR less than or equal to 4 cm was 0.8009 (Figure 4).

4. Discussion

We found a strong relationship between the distance from the skin to the epidural space as measured on CT imaging and the clinically recorded depth of loss of resistance. The linear model appeared to be different for morbidly obese patients. The ESD measurement appeared to perform reasonably well in identifying very deep loss of resistance depths, potentially requiring the use of a nonstandard Tuohy needle, and very shallow depths, possibly alerting a clinician to prevent an inadvertent dural puncture. The anesthesiologists' measurements of this distance were very similar to the radiologist's measurements, indicating anesthesiologists may not need the assistance of a radiologist to measure the distance between the skin and the epidural space.

One limitation of our analysis is that it is retrospective in nature. There was no way to verify the loss of resistance depth each practitioner reported as the true loss of resistance. In our experience, clinicians may not always be completely accurate with the values reported, as documentation of placement of the epidural can be somewhat removed in time from the time of the procedure. Also, our analysis relies on the accurate identification of the vertebral interspace at which the epidural catheter was placed. It has been shown [5, 6] that clinicians are commonly one or two interspaces away from the targeted space. The relative precision of the CT ESD and LOR depth measurements are also dissimilar. The radiological software we used gave us precision down to the millimeter while the

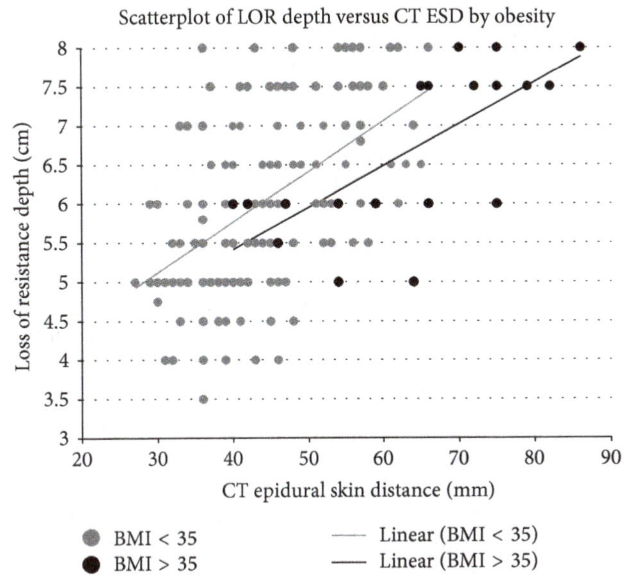

FIGURE 3: Scatterplot of loss of resistance (LOR) depth versus epidural-skin distance (ESD) separated by the presence of morbid obesity. Best fit linear lines projected on data.

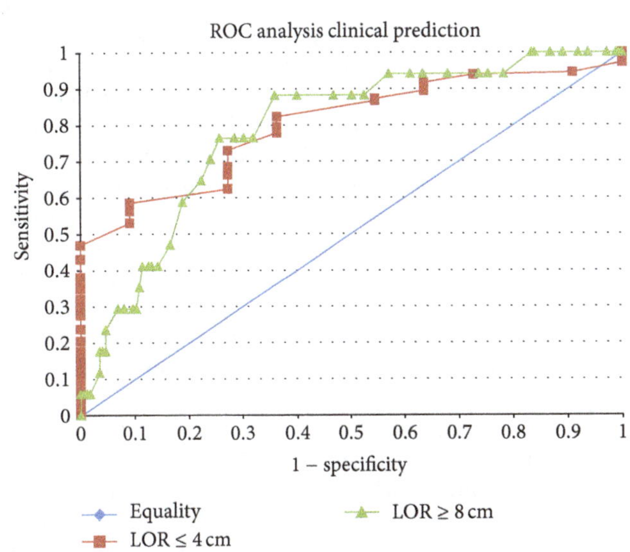

FIGURE 4: Receiver operating curve (ROC) of using epidural-skin distance (ESD) as measured by computed tomography (CT) to predict shallow or deep loss of resistance depths.

finest degree of precision routinely reported within loss of resistance measurements is down to 0.5 cm. When placing a thoracic epidural, it is also possible for a clinician to start at one interspace and traverse up to one or two interspaces if a steep angle is used thus obtaining a much deeper LOR than would have been produced by a more perpendicular approach. We also could not verify that the putative epidural catheter was in the true epidural space. Of the 168 epidurals examined, there were over 20 different anesthesiologists who actually performed the catheter placement. Based on our clinical experience with these anesthesiologists, there were several different techniques utilized which likely resulted in varying angles of approach which is the most likely explanation why there was still such variation in LOR depths for a given CT measurement distance.

Despite these limitations, this study shows the potential impact that careful review of already available CT scans can provide. Our findings are in agreement with two other published studies that have found good correlation between CT scan measurements to loss of resistance depth [4, 7]. The information derived from these previous studies is somewhat limited in its clinical utility. Both studies examine only one or two interspaces whereas epidurals can be placed at almost any thoracic level as required by the location of the surgical incision. In both of these previous studies, the description of how the measurements were made was not specific enough to indicate how an anesthesiologist might reproduce and use measurement information taken from a CT scan. This study helps support that the examination of a CT scan can be applicable at various interspaces in the thoracic spine. Additionally, the measurements can easily be made by anesthesiologist without the assistance of a radiologist. The anesthesiologists in this study have had no additional formal training in radiology outside of what was learned in medical school and anesthesiology residency.

This study also adds benefit in interpreting the CT measurements differently for obese patients. As can be seen in the scatterplot and best fit lines, although morbidly obese patients tended to have deeper LOR depths and higher ESD measurements, the relationship is different. As can be inferred from the linear regression model, the coefficient is negative suggesting shallower LOR depths than a normal weight patient with a similar CT measurement. This makes sense scientifically, as one would expect the tissue measured in a morbidly obese patient would be more compressible and an adjustment would need to be made. The true degree of compression seen in the CT image may also depend on the interspace as CTs are taken in the supine position and the kyphosis of the spine dictates differential pressures on the tissue posterior to the spine potentially causing differential compression.

Given the large number of patients examined in this study, the results do seem generalizable despite a relative lack of precision of our model. *A priori*, we predicted a pure linear transformation based on an angle in the sagittal plane of 30° and an angle in the axial plane of 15° which would estimate a ratio of 1.2. This line can be drawn on the scatterplot and approximate some of the data, but our ordinary least squares regression suggests that this is not the best fit model. The true model describing the relationship between CT ESD and LOR depth probably does have an intercept that accounts for tissue compression and a coefficient that is based on the angles of approach, but we cannot expect that a study of 168 epidurals in different patients would have the same angles of approach making the coefficient the aggregate "average" of coefficients calculated by the various angles used to place an epidural.

The value of having a sense of distance to the epidural space prior to starting a procedure could be particularly helpful. For example, if the predicted depth by imaging was never less than the actual loss of resistance depth then overly tentative epidural placements with false loss of resistance at shallow depths could be avoided. Closer examination of the scatterplot almost seems to reveal such a relationship in both populations, although this population is different. In our sample, 8% of patients had observed loss of resistance depths of 8 cm or greater suggesting that a longer nonstandard needle may have been useful. On the other end of the spectrum and perhaps more importantly, epidural-skin distance on imaging appears to also be useful in predicting abnormally shallow loss of resistance depths, which could help prevent dural punctures and thus nerve injury with potential for permanent damage.

5. Conclusions

In summary, our results suggest that making a simple measurement on a CT scan of a patient prior to placing an epidural catheter can be helpful in determining loss of resistance depth. This measurement can be adequately made by an anesthesiologist without the assistance of a radiologist. Further prospective data are needed to determine how precise this prediction could be and future studies should consider addressing obese populations separately.

Conflict of Interests

The authors declare that there is no conflict of interests regarding the publication of this paper.

Acknowledgment

The authors are indebted to Bala Nair, Ph.D., for assistance with extracting data from their local electronic medical record.

References

[1] B. M. Block, S. S. Liu, A. J. Rowlingson, A. R. Cowan, J. A. Cowan Jr., and C. L. Wu, "Efficacy of postoperative epidural analgesia: a meta-analysis," *Journal of the American Medical Association*, vol. 290, no. 18, pp. 2455–2463, 2003.

[2] K. P. Chen, Y. Y. Poon, and C. H. Wong, "The depth to the epidural space," *Anaesthesiologica Sinica*, vol. 27, no. 4, pp. 353–356, 1989.

[3] C. M. Brummett, B. S. Williams, R. W. Hurley, and M. A. Erdek, "A prospective, observational study of the relationship between body mass index and depth of the epidural space during lumbar

transforaminal epidural steroid injection," *Regional Anesthesia and Pain Medicine*, vol. 34, no. 2, pp. 100–105, 2009.

[4] M. C. Kao, S. K. Tsai, W. K. Chang et al., "Prediction of the distance from skin to epidural space for low-thoracic catheter insertion by computed tomography," *British Journal of Anaesthesia*, vol. 92, no. 2, pp. 271–273, 2004.

[5] D. A. Teoh, K. L. Santosham, C. C. Lydell, D. F. Smith, and M. T. Beriault, "Surface anatomy as a guide to vertebral level for thoracic epidural placement," *Anesthesia and Analgesia*, vol. 108, no. 5, pp. 1705–1707, 2009.

[6] C. Arzola, S. Avramescu, U. Tharmaratnam, K. J. Chin, and M. Balki, "Identification of cervicothoracic intervertebral spaces by surface landmarks and ultrasound," *Canadian Journal of Anesthesia*, vol. 58, no. 12, pp. 1069–1074, 2011.

[7] J. Carnie, J. Boden, and F. G. Smith, "Prediction by computerised tomography of distance from skin to epidural space during thoracic epidural insertion," *Anaesthesia*, vol. 57, no. 7, pp. 701–704, 2002.

9

New Delivery Systems for Local Anaesthetics

Edward A. Shipton

Department of Anaesthesia, University of Otago, Christchurch 8042, New Zealand

Correspondence should be addressed to Edward A. Shipton, shiptonea@xtra.co.nz

Academic Editor: James B. Eisenkraft

Part 2 of this paper deals with the techniques for drug delivery of topical and injectable local anaesthetics. The various routes of local anaesthetic delivery (epidural, peripheral, wound catheters, intra-nasal, intra-vesical, intra-articular, intra-osseous) are explored. To enhance transdermal local anaesthetic permeation, additional methods to the use of an eutectic mixture of local anaesthetics and the use of controlled heat can be used. These methods include iontophoresis, electroporation, sonophoresis, and magnetophoresis. The potential clinical uses of topical local anaesthetics are elucidated. Iontophoresis, the active transportation of a drug into the skin using a constant low-voltage direct current is discussed. It is desirable to prolong local anaesthetic blockade by extending its sensory component only. The optimal release and safety of the encapsulated local anaesthetic agents still need to be determined. The use of different delivery systems should provide the clinician with both an extended range and choice in the degree of prolongation of action of each agent.

1. Introduction

A drug delivery system should have minimal tissue reaction, a reliable drug release profile, and well-defined degradation rate for biodegradable carrier until all nontoxic products are excreted [1]. For local anaesthetics (LAs), the development of new effective delivery systems intends to suitably modulate the release rate of these drugs, extend their anaesthetic effect, and enhance their localisation; this reduces problems of systemic toxicity. Part 2 of this paper deals with the innovations pertaining to formulations, and techniques for drug delivery of topical and injectable local anaesthetics.

2. Routes of Local Anaesthetic Delivery

2.1. Epidural. Patient controlled epidural analgesia (PCEA) allows patients to self-administer drug doses according to their analgesic needs. This route relies on a staff-programmed pump and skilled and qualified members of the hospital staff for administration. Both local anaesthetics and opioids are agents for epidural analgesia. The use of epidural local anaesthetics is associated with a higher incidence of hypotension, motor block, and urinary retention, compared with use of opioids [2]. However, in a recent meta-analysis, only a continuous infusion of epidural local anaesthetics was superior to intravenous opioids in improving pain control and reducing adverse effects [3].

2.2. Peripheral. Patient-controlled regional analgesia (PCRA) encompasses a variety of techniques that provide effective postoperative pain relief without systemic exposure to opioids. Using PCRA, patients initiate the delivery of small doses of local anaesthetics (ropivacaine, bupivacaine) via an indwelling catheter that can be placed in different regions of the body depending upon the type of surgery. In some cases, a combination of local anaesthetic and opioid is administered. Infusions are controlled either by a staff-programmed electronic pump (Figure 1) or by a disposable elastomeric pump [3]. An elastomeric pump is a device that has a distensible bulb inside a protective bulb with a built-in filling port, delivery tube, and an antibacterial filter. Antibacterial filters are recommended with blocks involving a nerve plexus (and in neuraxial blocks). Analgesia can be delivered directly into a surgical incision (incisional PCRA), the intra-articular tissue (IA PCRA), or the perineural site (perineural PCRA) (Figure 2) [2].

2.3. Wound Catheters. The insertion of wound catheters allows for continuous infusions of local anaesthetics into the surgical wound at the end of the procedure (Figure 3).

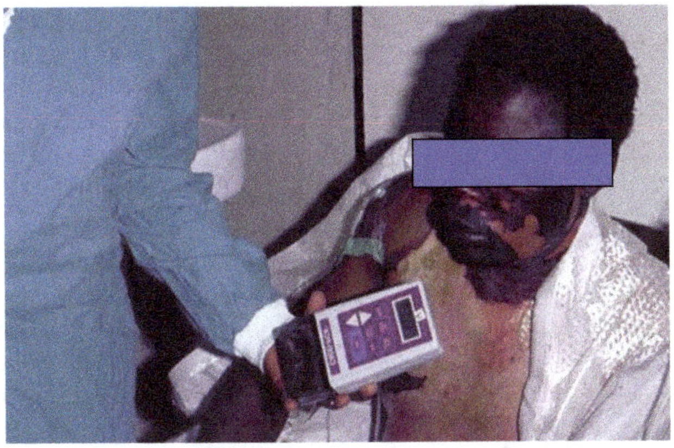

Figure 1: Pharmacia Deltec CADD Ambulatory Infusion Pump.

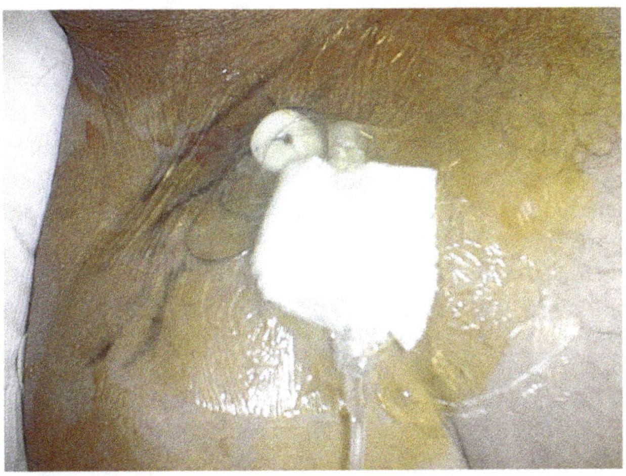

Figure 2: Patient-controlled perineural analgesia via infraclavicular brachial plexus catheter.

Continuous wound catheters can confer several benefits, including improved analgesia, reduced opioid use and adverse effects, increased patient satisfaction, and reduced hospital stay [4].

The use of continuous wound catheters consistently reduces the need for opioids (both rescue and total dose). Patients have consistently rated postoperative nausea and vomiting (PONV) as a primary concern after surgery [5, 6]. The reduced need for opioids (though an infrequently measured result in Randomised Controlled Trials) might contribute to increased patient satisfaction [4]. Reduced length of hospital stay has been associated with continuous wound catheters, especially in the cardiothoracic and orthopaedic surgery subgroups [4]. Meta-analysis suggested the potential saving of one day of hospital stay [4]. Incidences of technical failure and local anaesthetic toxicity from wound catheters are low. Several reports have raised potential concern about wound infections from the presence of a catheter [7]. However, reported wound infection rates were found to be similar between active (0.7%) and control groups (1.2%) [4].

2.4. Intranasal Route. The nasal mucosa acts as an anatomical obstacle hard to get over, except for compounds with low molecular weight or highly lipophilic compounds. For the manipulation of nasal fractures, lignocaine and cocaine have been used in topical local anaesthesia in the form of a spray, paste, or on cotton wool and pledgets; this appears to be a safe and effective alternative to general anaesthesia. A systematic review has found no significant differences between local anaesthesia and general anaesthesia as regards pain, cosmesis or nasal patency after nasal fracture manipulation performed under topical local anaesthesia [8]. A recent Cochrane review showed that nasopharyngeal topical local anaesthetic or vasoconstrictor preparations prior to the use of a fibre-optic nasal endoscope did not demonstrate any advantages in using a topical treatment prior to endoscopy [9]. In contrast, the very lipophilic opioids, such as fentanyl are rapidly absorbed via intranasal administration (with a bioavailability close to 90% for fentanyl) and are used for the treatment of breakthrough pain [10].

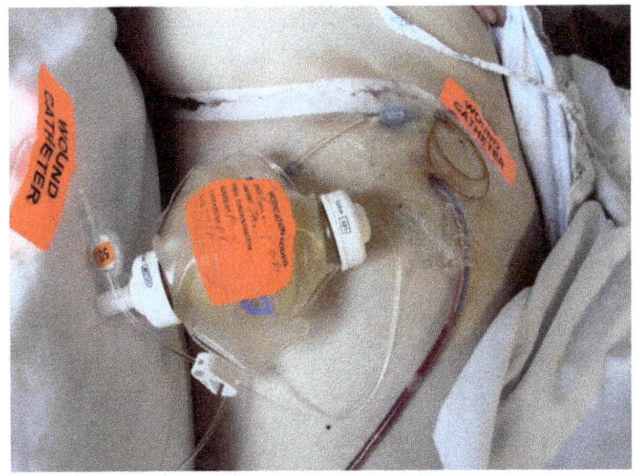

Figure 3: Elastomeric pump for a wound catheter.

2.5. Intravesical (Bladder) Route. The transport of local anaesthetics through the urothelium into deeper layers of the bladder has been significantly enhanced by electromotive drug administration (Figure 4) [11]. It is a cost-effective way to deliver lignocaine with greatly improved penetration rate into the bladder wall [12]. Vehicles such as electromotive drug administration, new in situ delivery systems, and bioadhesive liposomes make it possible to extend intravesical therapy and drug administration to many bladder diseases [11].

2.6. Intra-Articular (IA) Route. For microspheres destined for intra-articular delivery, the following properties have been identified as important, namely, size (within the range of 4-5 μm in diameter), resistance to in vivo degradation, minimal leakage of drug, and biocompatibility [13]. Prolonging the intra-articular drug residence time of LAs may be met by formulating microspheres that have been rationally designed to optimise uptake by the synovium [13]. However, the causes of 23 cases of postarthroscopic glenohumeral chondrolysis were recently analysed. Several common factors were found, but no single mechanism was shown. Multiple

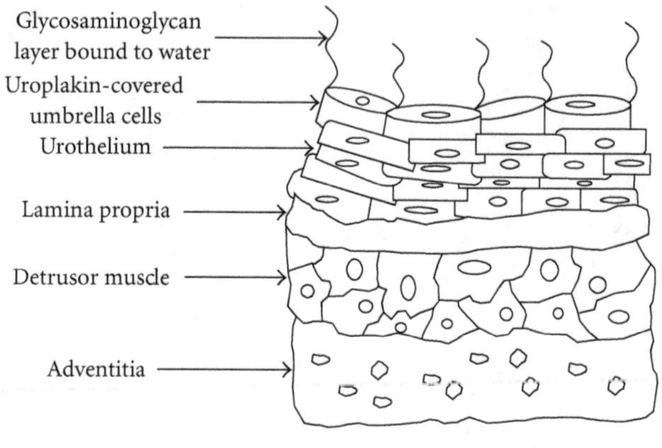

FIGURE 4: The structure of the urinary bladder wall and urothelium.

factors seemed to be implicated. The use of intra-articular local anaesthetics is probably not advisable until the role of local anaesthetics in this regard has been clarified, as chondrolysis has been the subject of many lawsuits [14].

2.7. Intra-Osseous Route. Computer-controlled local anaesthetic delivery devices (C-CLAD) and systems for intraosseous injection are important additions to the dental anaesthesia armamentarium [15]. C-CLAD using slow infusion rates can significantly reduce the discomfort of local anaesthetic infusions, especially in palatal tissues; C-CLAD facilitates palatal approaches to pulpal nerve block. It should find special use in cosmetic dentistry, periodontal therapy, and paediatric dentistry [15].

3. Transdermal Route of Local Anaesthetic Drug Delivery

Transdermal drug delivery is one of the most patient-compliant routes of drug administration. However, the stratum corneum, the outer most layer of the skin resists the penetration of drugs across the skin (Figure 5). Hydrophilic, ionised, and macromolecular substances are poorly permeable across the skin [16]. To enhance drug permeation in a passive manner, transdermal drugs should be lipophilic and should ideally have a molecular weight less than 500 Daltons [17]. Alternatively, energy-dependent active measures can be used to enhance drug delivery across the skin. These include physical permeabilisation of skin or by driving the drug molecule across the skin. In addition to the use of an eutectic mixture of local anaesthetics, and the use of controlled heat, other methods such as iontophoresis, electroporation, sonophoresis, and magnetophoresis can be used [16].

3.1. Magnetophoresis. Magnetophoresis is a method of enhancement of drug permeation across the biological barriers by the application of a magnetic field (Figure 6). The predominant mechanism responsible for magnetically mediated drug permeation enhancement is known as "magnetokinesis" [17]. The octanol/water partition coefficient of drugs increases when exposed to the magnetic field [17]. Magnetophoretic patch systems deliver drugs at a higher rate than nonmagnetic patch systems. In the rat model, the dermal bioavailability (Area Under the Curve 0–6 hours) from the magnetophoretic patch system was significantly higher compared to a non-magnetic control patch [17].

3.2. Sonophoresis/Phonophoresis. The use of ultrasound for the delivery of drugs to, or through, the skin is commonly known as sonophoresis or phonophoresis (Figure 7). The frequency of the ultrasound wave corresponds to the number of times that the transducer tip is displaced per second of application time. High-frequency sonophoresis includes frequencies in the range of 0.7–16 MHz (most commonly 1–3 MHz) [18]. Low-frequency sonophoresis includes frequencies in the range of 20–100 kHz and allows transdermal delivery of both hydrophilic and high-molecular mass permeants at therapeutic levels [19].

The main contributor responsible for skin permeability enhancement by sonophoresis is acoustic cavitation. This causes the formation of acoustic microjets on the surface of the skin in a nonuniform manner [19]. When surfactant is included in the treatment of skin with low-frequency sonophoresis, a strong synergistic enhancement in skin permeability occurs, allowing delivery of hydrophilic permeants. Additionally, low-frequency sonophoresis-mediated transdermal delivery can be used to deliver macromolecules, including liposomes and nanoparticles [19]. This technology is currently approved for use by the Federal Drug Administration (FDA) for local anaesthetics. In volunteers, a transducer has been used to administer an anaesthetic drug transdermally. When 0.5 MHz ultrasound in phonophoresis used for conduction anaesthesia with lignocaine hydrochloride, it was found to be more effective than the 1 MHz widely used in clinical situations (Figure 7) [20].

3.3. Microporation Technologies. Skin microporation may be considered a minimally invasive technology that can be broadly divided into microneedle technology, thermal microporation, and laser ablation [21]. To improve the rate and extent of transdermal lignocaine across porcine ear skin, the application of novel laser microporation technology (Painless Laser Epidermal System) has been used to create well-defined conduits in the skin [22].

3.4. Electroporation. Electroporation is the application of short high voltage pulses that result in formation of transient aqueous pathways for diffusion of molecules across the skin [16]. In case of electroporation, the electrical pulses are applied only for fraction of a second; the interval between subsequent pulses allows the skin to depolarise [16]. Therefore, polarisation of skin does not interfere with the current flow or drug diffusion. In the porcine epidermis, the transport of lignocaine hydrochloride in case of low voltage electropulsation was found to be 8-fold more than the control [16]. The amount of lignocaine hydrochloride present in the epidermis was found to be 2-fold higher as well.

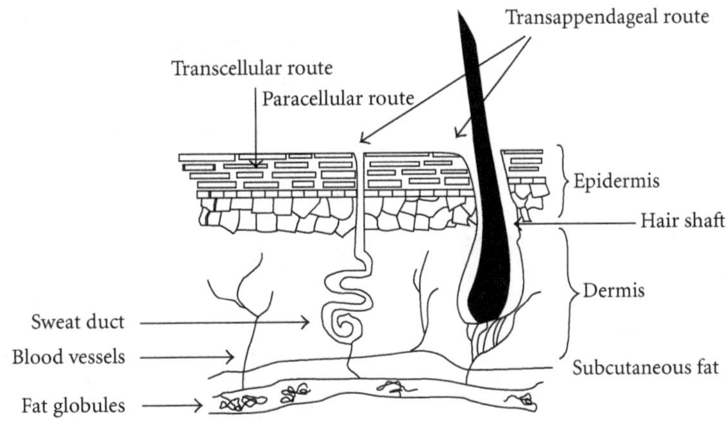

Figure 5: Transdermal routes of absorption of local anaesthetics.

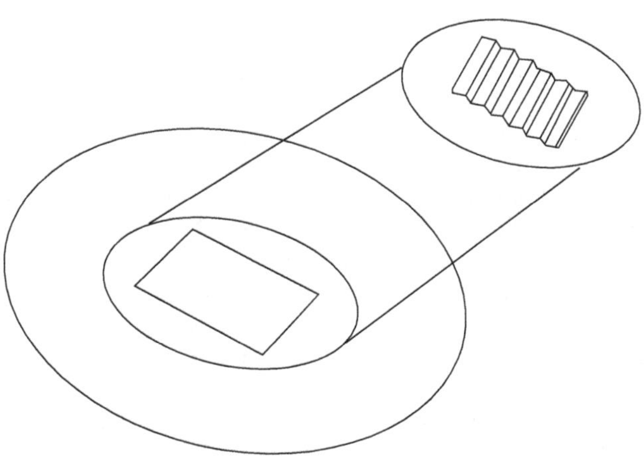

Figure 6: Magnetophoresis.

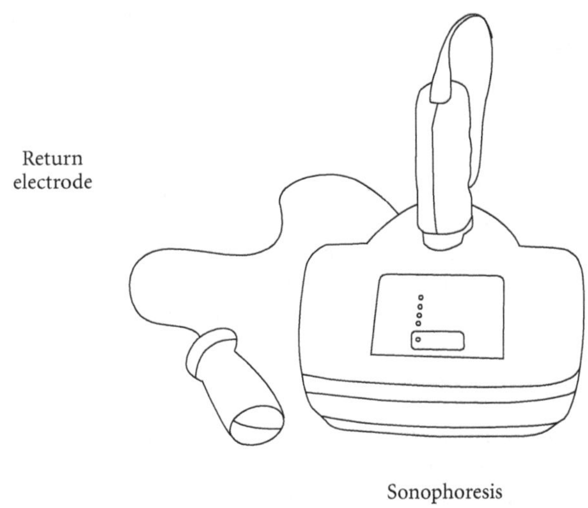

Figure 7: Sonophoresis—an ultrasonic skin permeation device.

Electrokinesis (electrophoresis and or electro-osmosis) and permeabilisation of membranes are responsible for enhanced transdermal drug transport by low voltage electroporation. The total duration of electrical current application during 20 minutes of low voltage electroporation is only one minute. Low voltage electroporation enhances drug permeation relatively more efficiently than constant direct current iontophoresis [16].

3.5. Eutectic Patches. A new topical local anaesthetic eutectic patch consisting of a mixture of lignocaine 70 mg and tetracaine 70 mg (Synera in the United States, Rapydan in Europe) has been developed [23]. This patch has an integrated heating element intended to enhance the flux of the tetracaine and lignocaine leading to more rapid and effective delivery of the local anaesthetics to the target area. The patch starts heating once removed from the pouch and exposed to atmospheric oxygen; it may increase skin temperature by up to 5°C [23].

To study the use of lignocaine/tetracaine-medicated plasters in patients undergoing minor dermatological or vascular access procedures, patients were randomised in a double-blind clinical trial [24]. Patient-reported median pain scores with the use of lignocaine/tetracaine-medicated plasters were found to be significantly lower than those with an identical plaster-containing placebo [24].

3.6. Clinical. With the use of topical local anaesthetics for dermal laceration repair, a meta-analysis reviewed 22 trials with more than 3000 randomised patients; it concluded that topical tetracaine, bupivacaine, and lignocaine had an equivalent or superior analgesic efficacy to the intradermal infiltration of cocaine-containing anaesthetics. The topical preparations proved less expensive and were safer [23, 25]. In another recent meta-analysis of 25 trials with more than 2000 subjects, three topical anaesthetics, (tetracaine, liposome-encapsulated tetracaine, and liposome-encapsulated lignocaine) were found to be equally efficacious [26]. Tetracaine had the added advantage of a longer duration and was reported not to cause methemoglobinemia [27]. Another study has demonstrated that the lignocaine/tetracaine patch provided better local anaesthesia than the control at all application times under 60 minutes [28].

Potential uses of topical anaesthetics include the following: for gaining pain-free vascular access; for skin or punch

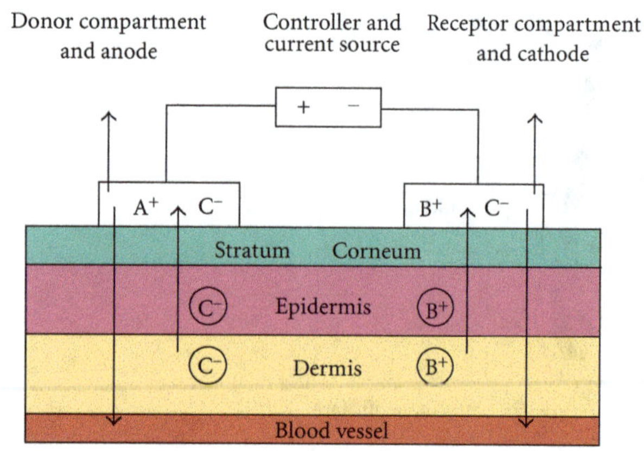

A^+ cationic drug: B^+ biological cations, C^- biological anions

Figure 8: Iontophoresis. Components of an anodal iontophoretic device are a current source; a current control device; anode (donor) reservoir system (with a positively charged drug/ion in solution); cathode reservoir system (on a different skin site). With an electric current, all cations move away from the anode and into the skin, and negatively charged ions move from the body into donor reservoir.

biopsies; for bone marrow aspiration; for treatment of postherpetic neuralgia; for immunisation; for myofascial pain due to trigger points; for nerve entrapment such as carpal tunnel syndrome; for regional block placement; and for dermal procedures requiring laser treatment.

4. Iontophoresis

Iontophoresis involves the active transportation of a drug into the skin using a constant low-voltage direct current. Ions migrate between electrodes of opposite charges, promoting ion transport through the skin (Figure 8) [29]. A direct electrical current facilitates the dermal penetration of positively charged lignocaine molecules when placed under a positive electrode for local anaesthesia. Physicochemical properties, such as good aqueous solubility, and the presence of charged groups that render peptides and proteins "difficult to deliver" by other approaches, are ideal for iontophoresis [30] The amount of drug delivered via iontophoresis is dependent on the current and the duration of delivery. The control afforded by constant current iontophoresis over transport rates means that peptide/protein delivery kinetics could mimic endogenous secretion profiles [30]. Moreover, complex input kinetics can be used to optimise and individualise therapy.

Iontophoresis has been known to cause skin irritation at higher current densities or upon longer application [16, 31, 32]. Moreover, when direct current electric field is applied over longer durations, an electrochemical polarisation occurs in the skin which decreases the magnitude of current flow through the skin [16]. This in turn could affect the amount of drug ions driven across the skin.

Small, portable iontophoresis devices have been developed. Dermal anaesthesia can be achieved fairly rapidly using lignocaine iontophoresis without needles [29]. Adrenaline added to the lignocaine solution enhances the effect and duration of local anaesthesia during iontophoresis; this is due to the local vasoconstriction inhibiting lignocaine absorption into the systemic circulation.

Delivery can be hastened by using ultrasound. In a Randomised Controlled Trial, ultrasound pretreatment plus two-minute low-voltage iontophoresis provided better skin anaesthesia than sham-ultrasound plus two-minute low-voltage iontophoresis, and similar to standard, 10-minute high-voltage iontophoresis [33]. Lignocaine HCl 10%/Adrenaline 0.1% topical iontophoretic patch (LidoSite) is the first FDA-approved prefilled active anaesthetic patch. In volunteers, it was found that 2% lidocaine could be delivered up to 5 mm below the surface of the skin when the drug compound contained adrenaline, and when passive delivery occurred for at least 50 minutes after the active delivery has terminated [34].

5. Future

It is desirable to acquire the ability to prolong local anaesthetic blockade and, if possible, extend only its sensory component. This paper portrayed the innovative techniques for the drug delivery of topical and injectable local anaesthetics. However, the optimal release and safety of the encapsulated LA agents still need to be determined. Using encapsulation to avoid systemic toxicity, the nonconventional local anaesthetics (tetrodotoxin, saxitoxin) show promising efficacy [1]. Recently, lignocaine-coated microneedles have been developed for rapid, safe, and prolonged local analgesic action [35]. These delivery systems should provide the clinician with both an extended range and a choice in the degree of prolongation of action of each agent [36].

Disclosure

No funds were received in support of this work. No benefits in any form have been or will be received from a commercial party related directly or indirectly to the subject of this manuscript. There is no conflict of interests.

References

[1] C. F. Weiniger, M. Golovanevski, M. Sokolsky-Papkov, and A. J. Domb, "Review of prolonged local anesthetic action," *Expert Opinion on Drug Delivery*, vol. 7, no. 6, pp. 737–752, 2010.

[2] E. R. Viscusi, "Patient-controlled drug delivery for acute postoperative pain management: a review of current and emerging technologies," *Regional Anesthesia and Pain Medicine*, vol. 33, no. 2, pp. 146–158, 2008.

[3] A. H. Taenzer and C. Clark, "Efficacy of postoperative epidural analgesia in adolescent scoliosis surgery: a meta-analysis," *Paediatric Anaesthesia*, vol. 20, no. 2, pp. 135–143, 2010.

[4] S. S. Liu, J. M. Richman, R. C. Thirlby, and C. L. Wu, "Efficacy of continuous wound catheters delivering local anesthetic for postoperative analgesia: a quantitative and qualitative systematic review of randomized controlled trials," *Journal of the American College of Surgeons*, vol. 203, no. 6, pp. 914–932, 2006.

[5] T. J. Gan, T. Meyer, C. C. Apfel et al., "Consensus guidelines for managing postoperative nausea and vomiting," *Anesthesia and Analgesia*, vol. 97, no. 1, pp. 62–71, 2003.

[6] C. C. Apfel, K. Korttila, M. Abdalla et al., "A factorial trial of six interventions for the prevention of postoperative nausea and vomiting," *New England Journal of Medicine*, vol. 350, no. 24, pp. 2441–2534, 2004.

[7] S. L. Brown and A. E. Morrison, "Local anesthetic infusion pump systems adverse events reported to the food and drug administration," *Anesthesiology*, vol. 100, no. 5, pp. 1305–1306, 2004.

[8] N. K. Chadha, C. Repanos, and A. J. Carswell, "Local anaesthesia for manipulation of nasal fractures: systematic review," *Journal of Laryngology and Otology*, vol. 123, no. 8, pp. 830–836, 2009.

[9] V. S. Sunkaraneni and S. E. Jones, "Topical anaesthetic or vasoconstrictor preparations for flexible fibre-optic nasal pharyngoscopy and laryngoscopy," *Cochrane Database of Systematic Reviews*, vol. 3, p. CD005606, 2011.

[10] P. Watts and A. Smith, "PecSys: in situ gelling system for optimised nasal drug delivery," *Expert Opinion on Drug Delivery*, vol. 6, no. 5, pp. 543–552, 2009.

[11] A. Giannantoni, S. M. Di Stasi, M. B. Chancellor, E. Costantini, and M. Porena, "New frontiers in intravesical therapies and drug delivery," *European Urology*, vol. 50, no. 6, pp. 1183–1193, 2006.

[12] S. GuhaSarkar and R. Banerjee, "Intravesical drug delivery: challenges, current status, opportunities and novel strategies," *Journal of Controlled Release*, vol. 148, no. 2, pp. 147–159, 2010.

[13] S. H. R. Edwards, "Intra-articular drug delivery: the challenge to extend drug residence time within the joint," *Veterinary Journal*, vol. 190, no. 1, pp. 15–21, 2010.

[14] D. S. Bailie and T. S. Ellenbecker, "Severe chondrolysis after shoulder arthroscopy: a case series," *Journal of Shoulder and Elbow Surgery*, vol. 18, no. 5, pp. 742–747, 2009.

[15] T. M. Clark and J. A. Yagiela, "Advanced techniques and armamentarium for dental local anesthesia," *Dental Clinics of North America*, vol. 54, no. 4, pp. 757–768, 2010.

[16] S. M. Sammeta, S. R. K. Vaka, and S. N. Murthy, "Transdermal drug delivery enhanced by low voltage electropulsation (LVE)," *Pharmaceutical Development and Technology*, vol. 14, no. 2, pp. 159–164, 2009.

[17] S. N. Murthy, S. M. Sammeta, and C. Bowers, "Magnetophoresis for enhancing transdermal drug delivery: mechanistic studies and patch design," *Journal of Controlled Release*, vol. 148, no. 2, pp. 197–203, 2010.

[18] B. E. Polat, D. Hart, R. Langer, and D. Blankschtein, "Ultrasound-mediated transdermal drug delivery: mechanisms, scope, and emerging trends," *Journal of Controlled Release*, vol. 152, no. 3, pp. 330–348, 2011.

[19] B. E. Polat, D. Blankschtein, and R. Langer, "Low-frequency sonophoresis: application to the transdermal delivery of macromolecules and hydrophilic drugs," *Expert Opinion on Drug Delivery*, vol. 7, no. 12, pp. 1415–1432, 2010.

[20] T. Y. Kim, D. I. Jung, Y. I. Kim, J. H. Yang, and S. C. Shin, "Anesthetic effects of lidocaine hydrochloride gel using low frequency ultrasound od 0.5 MHz," *Journal of Pharmacy and Pharmaceutical Sciences*, vol. 10, no. 1, pp. 1–8, 2007.

[21] A. K. Banga, "Microporation applications for enhancing drug delivery," *Expert Opinion on Drug Delivery*, vol. 6, no. 4, pp. 343–354, 2009.

[22] Y. G. Bachhav, S. Summer, A. Heinrich, T. Bragagna, C. Böhler, and Y. N. Kalia, "Effect of controlled laser microporation on drug transport kinetics into and across the skin," *Journal of Controlled Release*, vol. 146, no. 1, pp. 31–36, 2010.

[23] S. Masud, R. D. Wasnich, J. L. Ruckle et al., "Contribution of a heating element to topical anesthesia patch efficacy prior to vascular access: results from two randomized, double-blind studies," *Journal of Pain and Symptom Management*, vol. 40, no. 4, pp. 510–519, 2010.

[24] J. D. Croxtall, "Lidocaine/tetracaine medicated plaster: in minor dermatological and needle puncture procedures," *Drugs*, vol. 70, no. 16, pp. 2113–2120, 2010.

[25] A. Eidelman, J. M. Weiss, I. K. Enu, J. Lau, and D. B. Carr, "Comparative efficacy and costs of various topical anesthetics for repair of dermal lacerations: a systematic review of randomized, controlled trials," *Journal of Clinical Anesthesia*, vol. 17, no. 2, pp. 106–116, 2005.

[26] A. Eidelman, J. M. Weiss, J. Lau, and D. B. Carr, "Topical anesthetics for dermal instrumentation: a systematic review of randomized, controlled trials," *Annals of Emergency Medicine*, vol. 46, no. 4, pp. 343–351, 2005.

[27] M. Brisman, B. M. L. Ljung, Otterbom, L. E. Larsson, and S. E. Andreasson, "Methaemoglobin formation after the use of EMLA cream in term neonates," *Acta Paediatrica*, vol. 87, no. 11, pp. 1191–1194, 1998.

[28] J. Sawyer, S. Febbraro, S. Masud, M. A. Ashburn, and J. C. Campbell, "Heated lidocaine/tetracaine patch (Synera, Rapydan) compared with lidocaine/prilocaine cream (EMLA) for topical anaesthesia before vascular access," *British Journal of Anaesthesia*, vol. 102, no. 2, pp. 210–215, 2009.

[29] R. Wakita, Y. Oono, S. Oogami, S. Hayashi, and M. Umino, "The relation between epinephrine concentration and the anesthetic effect of lidocaine iontophoresis," *Pain Practice*, vol. 9, no. 2, pp. 115–121, 2009.

[30] T. Gratieri, D. Kalaria, and Y. N. Kalia, "Non-invasive iontophoretic delivery of peptides and proteins across the skin," *Expert Opinion on Drug Delivery*, vol. 8, no. 5, pp. 645–663, 2011.

[31] J. Hirvonen, F. Hueber, and R. H. Guy, "Current profile regulates iontophoretic delivery of amino acids across the skin," *Journal of Controlled Release*, vol. 37, no. 3, pp. 239–249, 1995.

[32] M. Kanebako, T. Inagi, and K. Takayama, "Transdermal delivery of indomethacin by iontophoresis," *Biological and Pharmaceutical Bulletin*, vol. 25, no. 6, pp. 779–782, 2002.

[33] E. L. H. Spierings, J. A. Brevard, and N. P. Katz, "Two-minute skin anesthesia through ultrasound pretreatment and iontophoretic delivery of a topical anesthetic: a feasibility study," *Pain Medicine*, vol. 9, no. 1, pp. 55–59, 2008.

[34] D. O. Draper, M. Coglianese, and C. Castel, "Absorption of iontophoresis-driven 2% lidocaine with epinephrine in the tissues at 5 mm below the surface of the skin," *Journal of Athletic Training*, vol. 46, no. 3, pp. 277–281, 2011.

[35] Y. Zhang, K. Brown, K. Siebenaler, A. Determan, D. Dohmeier, and K. Hansen, "Development of lidocaine-coated microneedle product for rapid, safe, and prolonged local analgesic action," *Pharmaceutical Research*. In press.

[36] M. D. Wiles and M. H. Nathanson, "Local anaesthetics and adjuvants—future developments," *Anaesthesia*, vol. 65, supplement 1, pp. 22–37, 2010.

10

The Role of Continuous Peripheral Nerve Blocks

José Aguirre,[1] Alicia Del Moral,[2] Irina Cobo,[2] Alain Borgeat,[1] and Stephan Blumenthal[3]

[1] *Division of Anesthesiology, Balgrist University Hospital, 8008 Zurich, Switzerland*
[2] *Department of Anesthesiology, General University Hospital of Valencia, 46014 Valencia, Spain*
[3] *Department of Anesthesiology, Triemli Hospital, 8063 Zurich, Switzerland*

Correspondence should be addressed to José Aguirre, jose.aguirre@balgrist.ch

Academic Editor: Didier Morau

A continuous peripheral nerve block (cPNB) is provided in the hospital and ambulatory setting. The most common use of CPNBs is in the peri- and postoperative period but different indications have been described like the treatment of chronic pain such as cancer-induced pain, complex regional pain syndrome or phantom limb pain. The documented benefits strongly depend on the analgesia quality and include decreasing baseline/dynamic pain, reducing additional analgesic requirements, decrease of postoperative joint inflammation and inflammatory markers, sleep disturbances and opioid-related side effects, increase of patient satisfaction and ambulation/functioning improvement, an accelerated resumption of passive joint range-of-motion, reducing time until discharge readiness, decrease in blood loss/blood transfusions, potential reduction of the incidence of postsurgical chronic pain and reduction of costs. Evidence deriving from randomized controlled trials suggests that in some situations there are also prolonged benefits of regional anesthesia after catheter removal in addition to the immediate postoperative effects. Unfortunately, there are only few data demonstrating benefits after catheter removal and the evidence of medium- or long-term improvements in health-related quality of life measures is still lacking. This review will give an overview of the advantages and adverse effects of cPNBs.

1. Background

Since its first description in 1946, cPNB has evolved from a case report of a needle inserted through a cork taped to a patient's chest to a wide-spread and validated analgesic technique in the postoperative setting [1]. The earliest reports of cPNB focused on prolonging intraoperative surgical anesthesia and the treatment of intractable hiccups [1–3]. The indication for cPNB has evolved since then, and many indications have been described in the literature: treatment of vasospasm induced by Raynaud disease [4]; induction of sympathectomy and vasodilation for improvement of blood flow after vascular surgery/trauma [5, 6], replantation or limb salvage [7, 8]; treatment of peripheral embolism [9, 10]; analgesia in the setting of trauma [11]; treatment of chronic pain syndrome such as trigeminal neuralgia [12], complex regional pain syndrome [13], terminal cancer pain, [14], and phantom limb pain [15, 16]. Independently of these indications, the majority of publications dealing with cPNB focus on postsurgical pain treatment, where evidence supports the concept that regional anesthesia and analgesia offers superior pain relief to systemic opioid analgesia following major surgery [17]. However, postsurgical pain is the only indication which has been validated using randomized controlled trials (RCTs) [18–22]. Compared with opioid analgesics cPNBs provide superior analgesia with a lower incidence of opioid-induced side effects like nausea, vomiting, pruritus, and sedation [21]. Moreover, in a meta-analysis Rodgers et al. suggested that mortality associated with major surgery was reduced by 30% when central regional anesthesia was used combined or not with general anesthesia [23]. On the other hand, a Cochrane review showed no impact of regional anesthesia compared to general anesthesia on mortality after hip fracture. Only the acute postoperative confusion was reduced after regional anesthesia [24]. However, for continuous peripheral regional anesthesia these findings cannot be extrapolated. Though, continuous peripheral regional anesthesia offers improved functional outcomes after extremity surgery at least for a short term period (up to 6 months) [25–27].

Despite this evidence of value, the hypothesis that regional anesthesia has an overall beneficial and long-lasting

TABLE 1: Incidence of persistent postsurgical pain and associated disability. Based on data from [37, 71–73].

Surgery	Incidence	Severe disability
Amputation	30–85%	5–10%
Thoracotomy	5–67%	10%
Inguinal hernia repair	10–30%	2–4%
Breast surgery	11–65%	5–10%
Coronary artery bypass graft	30–50%	5–10%
Cesarean section	10–18%	4%

effect on patient outcome following surgery still remains difficult to prove and has been challenged, especially in times with reduced resources. For more than 30 years, regional anesthesia has challenged anesthesiologists to determine whether it offers real benefits over other types of anesthesia, such as preserving cognitive function after major surgery compared to general anesthesia, improving long-term joint function and rehabilitation leading to earlier return to work, reducing costs, reducing the need for blood transfusions and increasing patient-reported outcomes such as satisfaction, quality of life, and quality of recovery.

The implications of regional anesthesia after major surgery are multifaceted and not fully elucidated, thus requiring future studies with a focus on evaluating issues like implicating roles of mismanaged pain, environmental factors, stress responses associated with the perioperative period, long-term followups focusing on joint mobilisation and quality of life.

This paper will elucidate the benefits of cPNB over intravenous analgesia and single-shot perineural blocks (sPNB) according to the published literature and show some aspects for possible future directions.

2. The Need for Optimal Postsurgical Analgesia

In western countries, 50–70% of in hospital patients suffer from moderate-to-severe pain after surgery [28], and 40% of ambulatory surgical patients have moderate/severe pain during the first 24–48 h [29]. Orthopedic surgery remains the major indication for peripheral nerve blocks for anesthesia and postoperative analgesia [30]. Orthopedic surgery is one of the most if not the most painful surgery [31, 32]. In fact, after orthopedic surgery significant increases in pain scores may persist for 2 to 3 days [33, 34]. In postoperative evaluations of hip and knee surgeries using questionnaires 28% of patients after total hip arthroplasty [35] and 33% of patients after total knee arthroplasty [36] suffered from chronic pain. The common finding between these patients was the intensity of immediate postoperative pain. Intense persistent postsurgical pain has indeed been described as a risk factor for the development of chronic pain [37, 38]. Therefore, an improvement in postsurgical pain therapy could be an important factor to reduce pain chronification and its adverse effects on health system costs [39] (Table 1).

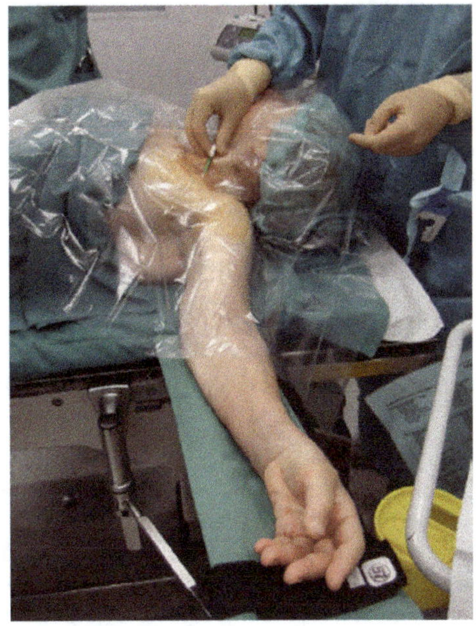

FIGURE 1: Sterile precautions for regional anesthesia.

3. cPNB Insertion Techniques

3.1. Skin Preparation and Patient Draping. Sterility is of utmost importance for the performance of cPNB independently of the technique performed (neurostimulation or ultrasound). The American Society of Regional Anesthesia and Pain Medicine (ASRA) recommends antiseptic hand washing, sterile gloves, surgical mask and hats, and the use of alcohol-based chlorhexidine antiseptic solutions [40]. Further sterile protection of the ultrasound probe is essential [41]. The catheter dressing after insertion has to be sterile and transparent to avoid and recognize catheter infection (Figures 1 and 2).

3.2. Needle Choice. Short bevel needles are widely accepted as standard practice in regional anesthesia. The literature is not conclusive to support the notion that nerve injury is minimized using short bevel needles [42–44]. The use of ultrasound for catheter placement is increasing and apart from thin-walled needles also Tuohy needles remain popular with this technique. However, despite the use of ultrasound, the risk of intraepineurial local anesthetic injections may be quite common as described by Liu et al. in a large prospective study on ultrasound-guided interscalene and supraclavicular blockade for shoulder surgery [45] and different case reports [46, 47]. For fascia iliaca blocks a blunt needle (pencil point or Tuohy) offers a better recognition of a "pop" as tactile feedback when the different fascias are pierced [48].

3.3. Nerve Stimulation. Before introduction of portable nerve stimulators in 1962 [49], PNB were performed using induced paresthesia ("no paresthesia and no analgesia"), [50] fascial "pop," [51] or even with fluoroscopic guidance [52]. Despite the fact that there has never been a repeated comparison of nerve stimulation and paresthesia which has

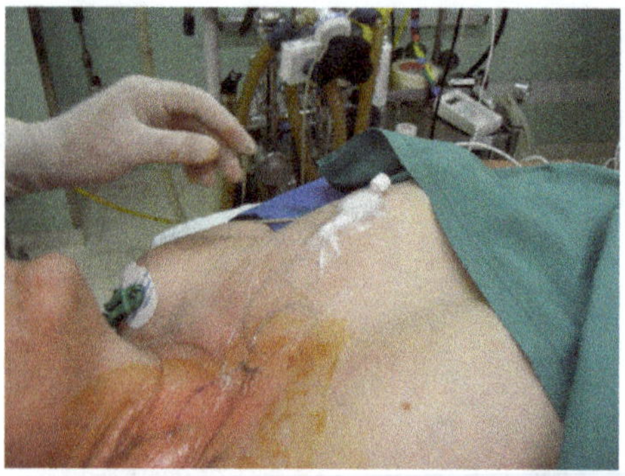

Figure 2: Sterile catheter dressing after catheter tunneling.

been for a long time the most wide-spread technique and is still used, nerve stimulation has been considered the gold standard at least until the introduction of ultrasound in 1989 [53]. Using electrical current to place an insulated needle close to a peripheral nerve to inject local anesthetic or place a perineural catheter is the basic principle of nerve stimulation [54]. Without doubt, if properly used nerve stimulation offers a high success rate for sPNB and for cPNB [55–62]. The most important rules to achieve competitive success rates for sPNB are

(i) use a proper technique with logical (adaptable to all patients, independent of body height and weight) and reproducible landmarks [56–59];

(ii) accept only responses with previously described high success rate (e.g., distal responses of the posterior cord for infraclavicular block; inversion for popliteal block) [56, 57, 63];

(iii) inject only at following nerve stimulator setting (with still weak motor response visible): amplitude width: 0.1 ms, frequency: 2 Hz, and impulse: 0.3–0.4 mA;

(iv) use the correct block for the planned surgery (e.g., not an interscalene block for elbow surgery [64] but an infraclavicular block) (Table 2).

Often comparative studies which described unacceptable low success rate for nerve stimulation are based on violation of at least one of the above-mentioned principles [64–67]. Although unclear data exists showing a consistent relationship between stimulating current and proximity to the nerve [68–70], the above-mentioned nerve stimulator setting is associated with high success and low complication rates [56].

For catheter placement, it is of prime importance that the needle is guided tangentially to the nerve to avoid nerve injury and to guarantee a catheter placement parallel to the nerve (Figure 3). In this case, a 3-orifice catheter will facilitate a spread of the local anesthetic along the nerve compared with an end-orifice catheter. To avoid early catheter displacement, the insertion should be performed before injection of local anesthetic [74]. To our mind, for catheter placement the cannula over the needle technique [26] threading the perineural catheter 3-4 cm past the tip of

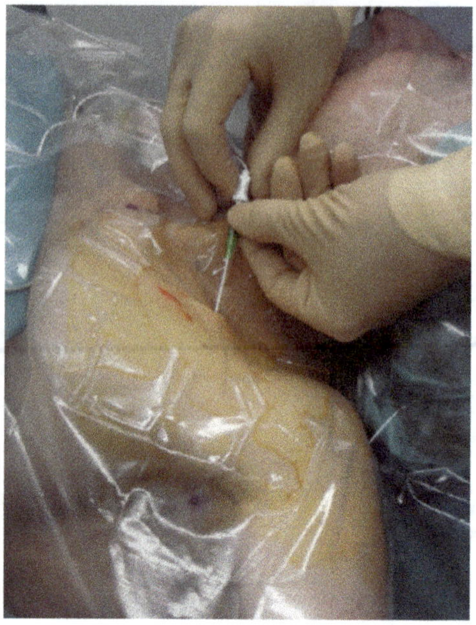

Figure 3: Cannula over the needle technique.

the cannula with subsequent subcutaneous tunneling for 4-5 cm to avoid displacement after insertion is the technique of choice (Figures 3, 4, 5 and 6). The optimal distance to advance a perineural catheter past the needle tip remains unknown according to the literature, but data suggests that increasing the insertion distance >5 cm is correlated with an increased risk of catheter coiling [75]. As there is no data suggesting insertion lengths >5 cm, the maximal insertion depth should be considered 5 cm [75, 76].

An further option is the use of stimulating catheters: with an insulated needle electrical current is used to locate the target nerve, followed by the insertion of a perineural catheter that conducts current to its tip [77]. Although there is evidence supporting some advantages in certain anatomic locations (popliteal fossa, femoral, and interscalene region) [78–80], the clinical relevance considering the significantly increased material costs remains unclear [81–83].

3.4. Ultrasound. The introduction of ultrasound for regional anesthesia has been an important development. First it was considered a supplement to nerve stimulation, now it is recognized as a "stand-alone" technique [84]. Unfortunately, a nonending dispute between nerve stimulation and ultrasound has distracted the focus of interest from clinically important questions [85, 86]. Almost all comparative studies violate in a way or another at least one of the crucial points for correct nerve stimulation mentioned above and have been subject to criticism [87–89]. The recent review by Abrahams et al. [90] dealing with this topic emphasized the superiority of ultrasound according to the present "evidence" and was severely disputed in web publications of letters to the editor [91]. There are also some publications comparing ultrasound-guided catheter insertion versus nerve stimulation catheter insertion [92–95]. Actually, some of these studies report at least similar analgesia between

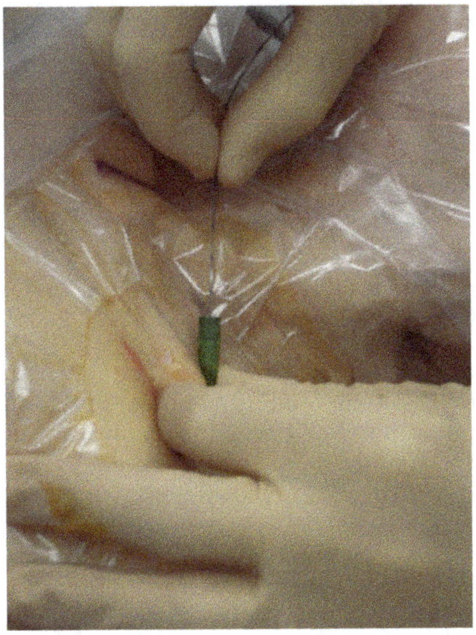

Figure 4: Catheter insertion through the cannula. Catheter is advanced up to 5 cm over the cannula tip.

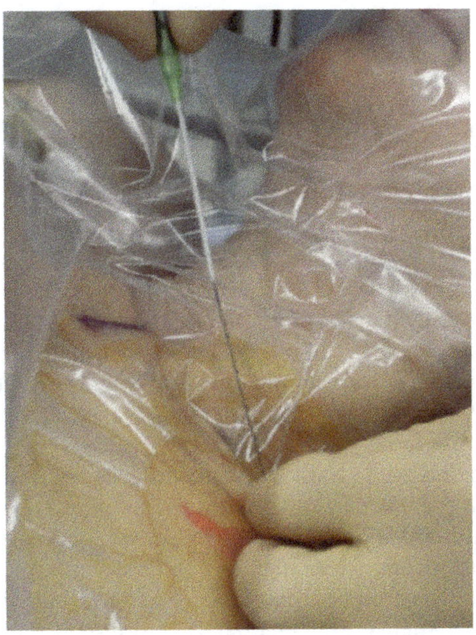

Figure 5: Cannula removal leaving the catheter in place.

both techniques [96–98]. Regrettably, in most of these publications the inappropriate use of neurostimulation lead to intolerable low success rates (<80%). Moreover, surrogate outcome like needle passes through the skin, needle time under the skin, patient satisfaction, local anesthetic volume, and other parameters of doubtful clinical importance have been introduced to compare these techniques. The comparison of ultrasound with stimulating catheters shows a similar picture: ultrasound is at least as effective with improvement of insertion-related discomfort and insertion time [93, 99]. The limited length and the main focus of this

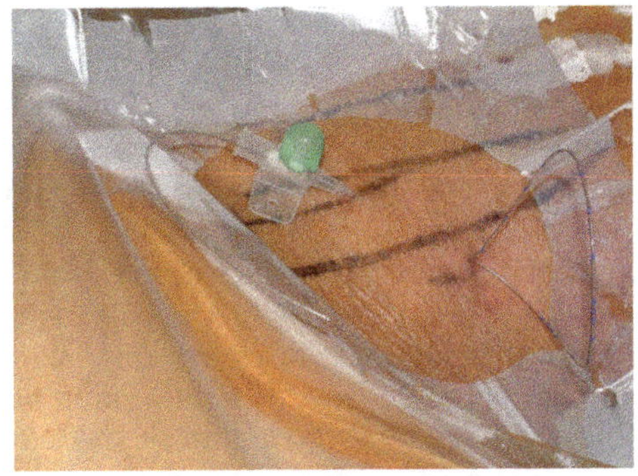

Figure 6: Catheter tunneling.

Table 2: Suggested catheter insertions for different surgical procedures. First choice is the first mentioned. The used literature for interscalene [58, 103, 104], cervical paravertebral [105–109], infraclavicular [59, 110–113], supraclavicular [114–116], axillary block [117–119], psoas compartment [120, 121], fascia iliaca [122–124], femoral [125–127], obturator [128, 129], popliteal sciatic [56, 57], and proximal sciatic [130–133].

Surgery	Catheter insertion location
Shoulder/proximal humerus	Interscalene; cervical paravertebral
Distal humerus, elbow, forearm, and hand	Infraclavicular; supraclavicular; axillary block
Hip	Psoas compartment; fascia iliaca; femoral
Thigh/knee	Femoral; fascia iliaca; obturator; proximal sciatic
Calf/ankle/foot	Sciatic (popliteal; proximal); add femoral nerve block for major ankle surgery [26]

review preclude a further indepth discussion of this topic. Indeed, there are randomized controlled trials suggesting that stimulating catheters for popliteal blocks [100], and the combination of ultrasound and nerve stimulation for catheter insertion improve analgesia [101]. Both techniques have to be considered equal if properly used with the respective advantages and disadvantages. This statement is in accordance with the most recent recommendation of the ASRA [102].

Data from controlled trials involving ultrasound-guided sPNB is not automatically applicable to ultrasound-guided cPNB. However, many reports confirm the feasibility of ultrasound-guided catheter-insertion with a great success rate [134, 135] also if there are few RCTs available [19, 136–138]. The description of the different techniques for ultrasound-guided catheter insertion (needle out-of-plane with nerve in short-axis approach and needle in-plane with nerve in short-axis or long-axis approaches) are well described in a recent editorial [139].

The combination of nerve stimulation (insulated needle or stimulating catheter) and ultrasound guidance for catheter placement is controversially discussed in the literature, and often the difficulties are major compared to the single use of either technique [101, 140–142].

In certain situations ultrasound might be, at least theoretically, superior to nerve stimulation for example when sensory nerves are the target [143], after limb amputations [144] if there is no phantom sensation to guide nerve stimulation [145], when vascular puncture is an absolute contraindication like in anticoagulated patients [146], or when an electrically induced muscle response is impossible [147] or not desired [148]. However, ultrasound needle and catheter tip visualization are often difficult specially in deep structures. In these cases, nerve stimulation might prove beneficial [149].

4. Local Anesthetics, Infusion Rates, and Delivery Strategies

4.1. Local Anesthetics & Adjuncts. The most commonly used local anesthetics for cPNB are bupivacaine and ropivacaine, and both seem to provide adequate analgesia without major toxicity. However, ropivacaine is known to be more "motor sparing" [55] and less cardiotoxic compared to bupivacaine [150]. However, cases of toxicity involving both bupivacaine and ropivacaine are almost exclusively related to a single large injection of local anesthetic. At the concentrations of 0.15% for bupivacaine and 0.2% for ropivacaine, they seem to provide similar analgesia with little difference in hand strength preservation [151, 152]. Recently, for interscalene cPNB after open rotator cuff repair ropivacaine 0.3% was compared to 0.2% showing a decrease in morphine consumption, a better sleep quality, and no impairment in hand strength [55].

To prolong the effect of local anesthetics, the addition of different drugs to local anesthetics has been suggested for sPNB and cPNB like opioids [165, 166], epinephrine [167], and clonidine [168], but their safety or clinical benefits like reduction of local anesthetic use for cPNB remain unclear [169, 170].

4.2. Infusion Rates and Delivery Strategies. Preliminary evidence does not suggest a rigid local anesthetic delivery system for all cPNB. According to the literature, total local anesthetic dose and not its concentration or its delivery rate mainly influences clinical effects, although this issue is currently disputed in the literature [55, 162, 171–176]. At the moment, insufficient information is available to base recommendations on the optimal basal rate, bolus volume, and lockout period for the different variables that may affect these values (catheter location, catheter type, surgical procedure, etc.). As a rule, we can state that basal infusion of local anesthetic reduces breakthrough pain and improves sleep quality [33, 173, 177]. The addition of patient-controlled bolus doses further improves analgesia allowing a reduction of the basal rate and further allowing a reduction of opioids and their related side effects [33]. However, the comparison of basal-bolus and basal-only techniques related to pain scores and patient satisfaction is controversially disputed in the literature [33, 34, 177].

Reducing the basal rate might reduce the risk of toxicity and the reduction of motor and sensory block could prevent the risk for patient falls [178].

Until prospectively collected data are available, possible dose recommendations based on randomized controlled studies and clinical experience are given in Table 3. Although the maximum recommended hourly total dose of all local anesthetics during perineural infusion is still unknown [179], a wide safety margin has been reported in numerous clinical trials [180, 181].

For the outpatient setting, many types of pumps are on the market: reusable and disposable, nonelectronic and electronic, basal-only and basal-bolus capable [22, 182]. Nonelectronic disposable infusion pumps are divided in elastomeric, positive-pressure (spring-powered and gas-pressure-powered), and negative-pressure (vacuum) pumps [183]. The model chosen has to be adapted to the needs of the patient and meet with the costs. In clinical trials comparing electronic-programmable pumps with elastomeric pumps, elastomeric pumps have been shown to offer similar postoperative analgesia for fewer technical problems and lower costs [184]. In clinical practice, they were easy to use and accurate in function [185].

5. Why cPNB Instead of sPNB?

5.1. Pain Therapy. Different case reports suggest beneficial effects of cPNB for different indications [12, 186, 187], but published RCTs include only postoperative patients and address mainly pain relief, which is considered to be the main indication for cPNB [21].

Although single-injection nerve blocks (sPNB) also provide excellent analgesia, cPNB increases the flexibility of both duration and density of local anesthetic effect depending on the chosen dose. SPNB offers a good pain therapy for up to 24 hours but for this duration a dense motor block and important sensory loss must be taken into account. In situations like trauma surgery, where compartment syndrome might be masked by these dense and long-lasting blocks, these properties are not wished by the surgeon. However, there is not enough evidence to support the thesis that patient-controlled analgesia with opioids or regional analgesia delay the diagnosis of compartment syndrome provided patients are adequately monitored [188, 189]. Continuous peripheral nerve blocks offer the possibility to adapt to the different needs by lowering the volume or the concentration of the local anesthetic [153, 190]. This flexibility reduces the need for a large initial bolus reducing the risk of systemic toxicity. Moreover, the reduction of dense motor and sensory blocks reduces the risk of falls and positioning injury [178, 191, 192]. An increase of local anesthetic concentration can also improve patient outcome. Borgeat et al. increased the ropivacaine concentration for interscalene blocks from 0.2 to 0.3% after rotator cuff repair and described a significant reduction of morphine consumption and a better sleep quality for the first postoperative night without increasing the intensity of motor block or side effects [55].

Table 3: Recommended doses of different local anesthetics for different catheter locations and their administration regimen according to clinical practice of the authors (CP), own publications or based on selected randomized controlled trials. Ropi: ropivacaine; Bupi: bupivacaine; B: basal rate (ml/h); Bo: bolus (ml); L: lockout (min). The used literature for Interscalene [55, 58, 153–157], infraclavicular [33, 59], axillary, [7] femoral [158–160], Fascia iliaca [161], subgluteal sciatic [162], and popliteal sciatic [51, 52, 78, 163, 164].

Catheter location	Local anesthetic	Infusion rate
Interscalene	(i) Ropi 0.2% (ii) Ropi 0.3% (iii) Bupi 0.125% (sufentanil 0.1 μg/ml and clonidine 1 μg/ml)	(i) CP: B: 4–6; Bo: 4–6; L: 20–30 (ii) CP: B: 3–5; Bo: 3-4; L: 20–30 (ii) CP: B: 5; Bo: 2.5; L: 30
Infraclavicular	(i) Ropi 0.2%	(i) CP: B: 4–6; Bo:4–6; L: 20–60
Axillary	(i) Bupi 0.25%	(i) B: 10 / B: 0; Bo: 10; L: 60
Femoral (i) Hip surgery (ii) Knee surgery	(i) Hip (a) Ropi 0.2% (b) Bupi 0.125% (+sufentanil 0.1 μg/ml and clonidine 1 μg/ml) (ii) Knee (a) Ropi 0.2% (b) Bupi 0.125% (clonidine 1 μg/ml)	(i) Hip (a) B: 6; Bo: 4; L: 30 (b) B: 10 / B: 0; Bo: 10; L: 60 / B: 0; Bo 5; L: 30 (ii) Knee (a) CP: B: 3–6; Bo: 2–4; L: 20–30 min (b) B: 5; Bo: 2.5; L: 30
Fascia iliaca (knee surgery)	(i) Ropi 0.2%	(i) B: 5; Bo: 5; L: 60 / B: 0; Bo: 10; L: 60
Subgluteal sciatic	(i) Ropi 0.2%	(i) B: 5; Bo: 5; L: 60
Popliteal sciatic	(i) Ropi 0.2% (ii) Levobupi 0.125%	(i) CP: B:4–6; Bo: 4–6; L: 20 (ii) B: 5; Bo: 3; L:15

5.2. Upper Extremity. Most of cPNB benefits are mainly dependent on successfully improving pain control, reducing opioid consumption and its related side effects and increasing patient satisfaction [21]. Like for shoulder and elbow surgery, potent analgesia is achieved and maintained with cPNB due to their complete innervation by nerves affected by the perineural infusion [55, 58, 59].

For shoulder and upper arm surgery, the interscalene nerve block (ISNB) has become a standard procedure in specialized centers [193]. This technique has been evaluated in different RCTs using either neurostimulator or ultrasound and as has been shown to be superior to settings using subcutaneous/oral opioids or even opioid-based patient controlled analgesia (PCA) [27, 34, 58, 138, 153–155, 194–200]. The superiority of continuous interscalene block (cISNB) towards single-shot interscalene block (sISNB) was demonstrated for moderate painful and extremely painful surgery in different studies [153–155, 196, 200, 201].

The benefits for elbow surgery using continuous infraclavicular perineural block is well validated [202], but good analgesia needs a high dose of local anesthetic leading to insensate extremities [175]. However, for surgical procedures distal to the elbow, brachial plexus infusions seem to provide less impressive analgesia [202]. Moreover, benefits of axillary [203] and supraclavicular [204, 205] continuous infusions demonstrated by RCTs are still lacking.

5.3. Lower Extremity. Femoral or posterior lumbar plexus infusions are well validated for hip [158, 187, 206, 207] and knee surgery in RCTs [208–210] but might result in dangerous quadriceps femoris and hip adductor weakness if high doses of local anesthetic are administered to optimize analgesia [178]. Moreover, contrary to the brachial plexus, in the lower extremity a single perineural infusion will not cover all surgical sites as these are innervated by multiple nerves. Therefore, a single perineural infusion might not provide optimal analgesia without the concurrent use of additional analgesics [171, 211]. A valid method to achieve optimal analgesia is the supplementation of a continuous perineural infusion with a separate single-injection peripheral nerve block as is often done for knee arthroplasty (continuous femoral nerve block complemented by a sciatic block) [212]. Inserting a second catheter for continuous perineural infusion has been suggested [26, 206, 213], but limited available data are conflicting and not useful to establish a clear clinical practice [26, 214]. Moreover, the recent review by Paul et al. [215] has brought new light into the clinical standard for pain management after total knee arthroplasty. Only two RCTs [211, 216] compared single-shot femoral nerve block to continuous infusion of local anesthetic according to his inclusion criteria. The additional use of single-shot sciatic nerve block was also investigated. According to the chosen methodology he suggested that at the moment, there is not enough evidence to support the use of neither a single-shot sciatic nerve block nor a continuous perineural femoral nerve block in addition to a single-injection femoral nerve block [217]. Despite the emotional reactions to this review [218] fearing that the use of cPNB will be questioned by surgeons according to the missing evidence, further studies should address this question to establish the correct approach for this surgery [212].

Also if lumbar epidural provides generally equivalent analgesia to femoral perineural infusion for both, hip and knee arthroplasty cPNB offers a more favorable side effect profile avoiding the risk of epidural hematoma during anticoagulant administration [25, 207]. Therefore, cPNB has to be considered the method of choice if regional anesthesia is indicated for the lower extremity.

For foot and ankle surgery, the use of cPNB has clearly demonstrated its superiority to other analgesia regimens. It has been shown to decrease hospital costs and length of stay [219]. Several studies have shown that regional anesthesia for foot surgery is safe and does lead to reduced perioperative opioid requirements [56, 57, 220]. Patients have reported improved sleep, reduced pain scores, and faster recovery times [162, 190, 221–223]. Patient satisfaction scores improved after regional anesthesia compared with general anesthetic with following systemic analgesia [224–226]. Recently, Blumenthal et al. described, that an additional femoral nerve catheter with ropivacaine 0.2% to a continuous popliteal catheter with ropivacaine 0.2% both for 48 hours for major ankle surgery reduces pain during motion compared to popliteal catheter alone. This effect was still present after 6 months suggesting that short-duration regional anesthesia has a late impact on residual pain after major ankle surgery [26].

6. Functional Outcome

6.1. Short-Term Use of cPNB. The effects of the short-term use of cPNB on functional outcome after orthopedic surgery are still controversially discussed. Ilfeld et al. reported in a retrospective study that in the 3 days after a total shoulder arthroplasty, a continuous interscalene block using ropivacaine 0.2% was associated with increased range of shoulder motion due to the complete analgesia provided [227]. These results were supplemented by a following prospective study analyzing the effects of ambulatory continuous interscalene nerve block after shoulder arthroplasty [27]. Authors concluded that an ambulatory continuous interscalene nerve block considerably decreased the time until readiness for discharge (defined as achievement of a previously established range of motion and good pain control) after shoulder arthroplasty. This result was achieved primarily by providing potent analgesia permitting greater passive shoulder movement and by the avoidance of intravenous opioids. However, recently Hofmann-Kiefer et al. compared a continuous interscalene infusion of local anesthetic with an opioid-based PCA regimen. They reported that continuous interscalene block improved analgesia without improving postoperative function during early rehabilitation of the shoulder joint. [198]. For knee surgery, De Ruyter et al. reported that a continuous femoral nerve block provided satisfactory analgesia, improved rehabilitation, and reduced hospital length of stay compared with opiates [228]. Contrary, Raimer et al. described better analgesia with continuous psoas and sciatic blocks or epidural catheters compared to opioid PCA regarding pain levels, analgesic requirements, and patient satisfaction. However, there was no difference in functional outcome between the 3 groups [229].

6.2. Benefits after Catheter Removal. Despite the overwhelming evidence highlighting cPNB benefits during local anesthetic infusion, there exist few data demonstrating benefits after catheter removal. These data include improved analgesia a few days after removal [61, 186, 216] and after 6 months [26], faster resumption of unassisted standing [186], and improved passive knee flexion leading to earlier discharge from rehabilitation centers [25, 230]. The often cited increase in health-related quality of life has been shown only in 1 study [231] but could not be reproduced in many other more recent studies [232–236].

These results are in accordance with the review by Liu and Wu analyzing the effect of analgesic technique on postoperative patient-reported outcomes [20]. Authors found that regional anesthesia offered better postoperative analgesia control with reduction of opioid-related side effects, but there were insufficient and inconsistent data to support subsequent improvement in quality of life, quality of recovery, satisfaction, and length of hospital stay.

Therefore, more studies focusing on the medium- or long-term improvements in health-related quality-of-life measures are needed [234, 237].

6.3. Impact on Postoperative Cognitive Dysfunction. Postoperative cognitive dysfunction (POCD) is an important issue in an aging society. Postoperative cognitive dysfunction is a poorly defined condition as numerous studies use different definitions and neuropsychological tests to detect potentially altered short- or longer-term memory, motor control or information processing following anesthesia. There is evidence that altered intraoperative physiology may influence POCD and longer-term outcomes. A meta-analysis of 21 studies on POCD and postoperative delirium (POD) found no effect of anaesthesia type on the odds ratio of developing POD (0.88, 95% CI 0.51–1.51) [238]. However, it has been suggested that avoidance of general anesthesia and of central acting analgesics in the elderly leads to reduced postoperative long-term cognitive dysfunction [163]. The most recent study suggesting that anesthesia regimen has no impact on cognitive dysfunction had severe protocol inaccuracies, as the regional anesthesia group (spinal anesthesia) was premedicated with a benzodiazepine, another benzodiazepine was added prior to spinal anesthesia, a bispectral index <60 was achieved with propofol or with gas during surgery, and pain therapy was performed with oral oxycodone and subsequent morphine PCA [164]. Further well-designed studies are needed to assess the impact of continuous regional anesthesia for surgery and postoperative pain treatment on the incidence of POCD.

7. Ambulatory and Home Therapy

Apart from the classical postoperative setting, cPNB has been successfully introduced in the ambulatory surgery setting for both adults [134, 191] and pediatric patients [239].

Continuous peripheral nerve blocks offer the opportunity to deliver effective pain therapy at home and are considered to be a valid alternative to opioid-based analgesia and its related side effects [240]. However, a proper patient selection is essential for safe cPNB at home, as not all patients are willing to accept the extra responsibility of the catheter and pump system [191, 240].

Additionally, patients with known hepatic or renal insufficiency are excluded from ambulatory cPNB to avoid possible local anesthetic toxicity [241]. Obese patients and those with heart or lung disease who cannot compensate for mild hypercarbia and/or hypoxia are excluded from interscalene and cervical paravertebral infusions, which are known to affect the phrenic nerve and ipsilateral diaphragm function [155].

8. Economical Outcome

The advantages of sPNB over general anesthesia related to cost-effectiveness in the operation theatre have been recently described by Gonano et al. for shoulder arthroscopy [242]. Authors could show that ultrasound-guided interscalene blocks lead to an improvement of anesthesia-related workflow and to a reduction of postanesthesia care unit (PACU) time compared to general anesthesia. The positive effects of regional anesthesia on the anesthesia-related costs are well known: reduction of postoperative nausea and vomiting, reduced length of stay, successful same day discharge, reduction of unplanned admission or readmission, reduction of multiple-day hospitalizations to single days, earlier discharge, reduction or even elimination of PACU length of stay leading to reduced postoperative nursing interventions, faster discharge times, and reduction of operating room time without increase in turnover time [211, 243–245]. Fredrickson and Stewart compared recently continuous interscalene nerve block for rotator cuff repair to combined single injection interscalene block with additional postoperative intermittent intra-articular local anaesthetic infiltration and to intermittent intra-articular only local anaesthetic infiltration. Authors concluded that continuous interscalene nerve block following rotator cuff repair in a multiprovider setting was associated with reduced total opioid/tramadol and antiemetic consumption, without a significant increase in the monetary costs [246].

Unfortunately, there are no studies comparing sPNB and cPNB regarding cost-effectiveness. However, the duration of hospitalization [247] or even the need for hospitalization [248] can be reduced by the use of cPNB reducing inpatient treatment costs.

9. Benefits of cPNBs

The impact of cPNBs on analgesia has been described in many RCTs and has been elucidated above [21]. The related dramatic decrease in required supplemental opioids, opioid-related side effects, and sleep disturbances, while simultaneously increasing patient satisfaction are further benefits [190]. Moreover, a decreased time to adequate ambulation with additional optimization of daily activities after ambulatory cPNB compared with intravenous opioids has been described [34]. For continuous regional anesthesia following shoulder and knee arthroplasty, an accelerated improvement of passive joint range of motion potentially leading to shorter hospitalization has been described [25, 27, 216, 230].

Ambulatory shoulder arthroplasty and 23-hour-stay knee and hip arthroplasty using ambulatory continuous interscalene, femoral, and psoas compartment nerve blocks, respectively have been reported [247, 249, 250].

However, although postknee arthroplasty inflammation is reduced after a continuous femoral nerve block [186]. the cPNB could not produce major improvements in long-term outcomes such as decreased chronic pain and improved health-related quality of life [20, 235, 251]. Studies focusing on long-term outcomes are lacking to evaluate the effects of cPNB after 6 and 12 months on costs, functional outcome and socioeconomic aspects.

10. Adverse Effects

Two prospective investigations involving more than 2.100 patients suggest that the incidence of cPNB-related complications is very low and comparable to sPNB techniques [58, 252]. However, different catheter insertion techniques, different anatomic locations, variations in equipment and different infusion regimens make comparisons difficult. In fact, several prospective studies report an incidence of secondary block (during infusion) failure of 1% [253], 20% [197], and 50% [254]. Therefore, all reported complications in this chapter cannot be translated to the different clinical practices.

10.1. Minor Complications. These complications are frequently seen in clinical practice and include catheter obstruction, catheter dislodgement, fluid leakage, disconnection from the pump system, infusion pump malfunction, and skin irritation or allergic reactions to the sterile catheter dressing [202, 252, 253, 255, 256].

10.2. cPNB-Specific Complications. These seldom but possible complications include inaccurate catheter tip placement resulting too far from the target nerve and therefore lacking successful analgesia, [74] or in an undesirable position like intravascular [257], intrapleural [258], intraneural [259], epidural [260] or even intrathecal. [261–263]. However, whether catheter migration is possible after correct placement remains unclear [264, 265].

10.3. Infections. Most studies reporting infection in relation with cPNB derive from hospitalized patients even if data for large outpatient series are increasing. Although the reported rates of inflammation (3%-4%) [86, 252, 253] and catheter bacterial colonization (6%–57%) are apparently high [266, 267], the incidence of catheter infection for inpatients ranges from 0% to 3.2% [252, 266, 268], and for outpatient rates are below 1% [191, 269].

Risk factors for infection in the setting of cPNB include lack of or inappropriate antibiotic prophylaxis, and axillary or femoral catheter location [269]. However, other studies have reported the interscalene location as the most problematic for infection [253, 268]. Further risk factors are admission to an intensive care unit, male sex [252], and increased infusion duration [252]. Though, some case reports demonstrate that prolonged catheter use for more than 30 days is possible without increased rate of infection [15]. There is limited evidence proving that subcutaneous catheter tunneling [270] may decrease the risk of bacterial colonization and infection.

Although life-threatening catheter-related infections and sepsis have been reported in the literature [271, 272], no published case of permanent injury due to cPNB-related infection is reported in the literature [269].

Sterility precautions while filling the infusion pumps are of utmost importance. In a recent case report of a severe, deep cellulitis, evolving to mediastinitis was attributed to contaminated infusate from a pump which was manipulated in nonsterile conditions [272]. Therefore, anesthetists should act upon the recommendations of the American Society of Regional Anesthesia and Pain Medicine (ASRA) using sterile precautions such as antiseptic hand washing, sterile gloves, surgical masks and hats, and using alcohol-based chlorhexidine antiseptic solutions to avoid such complications [40].

10.4. Neurologic Complications. Although neurologic injury associated with cPNB is usually transient ranging from 0.3% to 2.0% [33], it remains the most feared concern performing regional anesthesia. Injury may occur during catheter placement or even in the postoperative period. For regional anesthesia in general the incidence of transient adverse neurologic symptoms associated with cPNB is 0% to 1.4% for interscalene [253, 273], 0.4% to 0.5% for femoral [252, 274], and 0% to 1.0% for sciatic catheters [266, 274]. Neuburger et al. described a 0.2% incidence of neurologic deficits lasting more than 6 weeks in nearly 3.500 catheters from multiple anatomic locations [253]. However, it remains unknown whether the deficits resolved spontaneously after the 6-week study period. Other prospective investigations report that the overwhelming majority of neurologic symptoms still present at 4 to 6 weeks resolve spontaneously within 3 months of surgery [252, 273].

There are also cases of long-term or permanent nerve injury in patients after perineural infusion [275]. In five large, prospective series with patient followups at least three months after, 3 cases of unresolved adverse neurologic events were found [58, 252, 266, 273, 274]. The combination of these results including 4.148 patients suggests that the risk of neurologic injury lasting longer than 9 months associated with cPNB is 0.07%. The role of the continuous infusion for the evolution of these complications remains unclear.

Only few reports of nerve injury in patients sent home with cPNB are described in the current literature. However, pressure injury due to insensate extremity has been implicated as a likely cause [10]. Therefore, particular precautions must be taken when casts or splints are placed on patients with insensate extremities.

A further important neurologic concern associated with in- and out-patient cPNB is the risk of falls. Williams et al. reported recently 1.7% of outpatients treated with continuous femoral nerve block fell due to insensate lower extremity despite adequate instructions how to behave at home [192]. Ilfeld et al. pooled data from 3 previously published, randomized, triple-masked, and placebo-controlled studies of cPNB involving the femoral nerve after knee and hip arthroplasty and demonstrated a causal relationship between cPNB and the risk of falling after these surgical interventions [178].

This complication elucidates the potential benefit in providing low-concentration blocks that preserve more motor function and proprioception. Moreover, the desire to offer complete analgesia should be balanced against the risk of falling. Therefore, the recently published study dealing with multimodal analgesic approaches including regional anesthesia can offer a solution to achieve excellent analgesia while preserving motor function [276].

10.5. Local Anesthetic Toxicity. Most investigators report basal hourly infusion rates of 5 to 10 mL/h using dilute solutions of either ropivacaine or bupivacaine [33, 34]. Despite these low rates of infusion, local anesthetic toxicity is reported as a possible complication of cPNB [277]. Systemic local anesthetic toxicity is a serious but rare complication using cPNB [278, 279]. Although, continuous infusion is unlikely to result in sudden onset of toxicity, patients treated with a pump with bolus capability are at risk if intravascular migration should occur. A further rare complication is myonecrosis after repeated large boluses of bupivacaine [280]. Also if there is in vitro and animal evidence for local anesthetic-caused neurotoxicity [281, 282], there seems to be little evidence that the risk of nerve injury from prolonged local anesthetic exposure might be increased in patients suffering diabetes or preexisting neuropathies [283, 284].

11. Future Directions

Local anesthetics act on the voltage-gated sodium channels [285]. The $Na_{v1.7}$is the main channel for pain transmission in the peripheral nerves [286, 287]. Selective blocking of this channel for the postoperative period could be of special interest for ambulant cPNB avoiding the risk of falls. A high selective $Na_{v1.7}$ local anesthetic would increase the ambulant use of cPNB with probably a remarkable impact in health costs.

Liposomes as reservoirs for drugs are biocompatible due to their biodegradability and low toxicity [288]. They can reduce the exposure of sensitive tissues like nerves to potentially toxic drugs like high concentrations of local anesthetics. Their administration is independent of technical skills required for catheter placement as a variety of routes are possible (topical, intramuscular, nasal, subcutaneous, oral, pulmonary, and intravenous) [289]. Even though not yet approved for peripheral nerve blocks, liposomal formulations of various local anesthetics offer an increase in clinical efficacy compared with the plain drugs [290]. Actual limitations of encapsulated local anesthetics are myotoxicity, neurotoxicity, tachyphylaxis, viscosity, and motor block [291]. Clinical studies describe a prolonged analgesia after infiltration and epidural application [292, 293]. Once the potential adverse effects like a prolonged motor block and toxicity are eliminated, these promising clinical results might be transferred to peripheral regional anesthesia.

12. Conclusions

The Literature provides a plethora of information involving cPNB, but some aspects of perineural infusion remain controversial: the optimal catheter insertion modality, the optimal technique for each indication, the infusates offering the best safety, standardized local anesthetic delivery regimens, and optimization of continuous ambulatory infusion to reduce possible risks (as falling). The optimal analgesic technique for many surgical procedures has to be further elucidated, and cPNB must be compared with possible new analgesic techniques/regimens [231].

The new application areas for local anesthetic such as anti-inflammatory effects/anticancer effects [294, 295] have to be further investigated, and cPNB must be included in clinical trials addressing these topics.

The socioeconomical aspect of anesthesia remains an important issue, and the role of cPNB for in hospital and at home use and their effects in the healing process and the readmission of the patients at work after surgery must be clarified.

Prospective research addressing the above-mentioned issues can maximize the potential benefits and minimize the potential risks of cPNBs.

Conflict of Interests

The authors declare that they have no conflicts of interests.

References

[1] F. P. Ansbro, "A method of continuous brachial plexus block," *The American Journal of Surgery*, vol. 71, no. 6, pp. 716–722, 1946.

[2] J. A. DeKrey, C. F. Schroeder, and D. R. Buechel, "Continuous brachial plexus block," *Anesthesiology*, vol. 30, no. 3, p. 332, 1969.

[3] S. J. Sarnoff and L. C. Sarnoff, "Prolonged peripheral nerve block by means of indwelling plastic catheter; treatment of hiccup; note on the electrical localization of peripheral nerve," *Anesthesiology*, vol. 12, no. 3, pp. 270–275, 1951.

[4] R. A. Greengrass, N. G. Feinglass, P. M. Murray, and S. D. Trigg, "Continuous regional anesthesia before surgical peripheral sympathectomy in a patient with severe digital necrosis associated with Raynaud's phenomenon and scleroderma," *Regional Anesthesia and Pain Medicine*, vol. 28, no. 4, pp. 354–358, 2003.

[5] R. Franz, J. Hartman, and M. Wright, "Comparison of anesthesia technique on outcomes of endovascular repair of abdominal aortic aneurysms: a five-year review of monitored anesthesia care with local anesthesia vs. general or regional anesthesia," *Journal of Cardiovascular Surgery*, vol. 52, no. 4, pp. 567–577, 2011.

[6] E. B. Malinzak and T. J. Gan, "Regional anesthesia for vascular access surgery," *Anesthesia and analgesia*, vol. 109, no. 3, pp. 976–980, 2009.

[7] J. P. Mezzatesta, D. A. Scott, S. A. Schweitzer, and D. E. Selander, "Continuous axillary brachial plexus block for postoperative pain relief intermittent bolus versus continuous infusion," *Regional Anesthesia*, vol. 22, no. 4, pp. 357–362, 1997.

[8] N. Vadivelu, M. Gesquire, S. Mitra et al., "Safety of local anesthesia combined with monitored intravenous sedation for American Society of Anesthesiologists 3 and 4 patients undergoing lower limb-preservation procedures," *Journal of Foot and Ankle Surgery*, vol. 49, no. 2, pp. 152–154, 2010.

[9] S. M. Smith and V. L. Rees, "The use of prolonged continuous spinal anesthesia to relieve vasospasm and pain in peripheral embolism," *Anesthesiology*, vol. 9, pp. 229–238, 1948.

[10] L. N. Cheeley, "Treatment of peripheral embolism by continuous sciatic nerve block," *Current Researches in Anesthesia & Analgesia*, vol. 31, no. 3, pp. 211–212, 1952.

[11] J. J. Wu, L. Lollo, and A. Grabinsky, "Regional anesthesia in trauma medicine," *Anesthesiology Research and Practice*, vol. 2011, Article ID 713281, 7 pages, 2011.

[12] M. Umino, H. Kohase, S. Ideguchi, and N. Sakurai, "Long-term pain control in trigeminal neuralgia with local anesthetics using an indwelling catheter in the mandibular nerve," *Clinical Journal of Pain*, vol. 18, no. 3, pp. 196–199, 2002.

[13] J. Kato, D. Gokan, K. Ueda, M. Shimizu, T. Suzuki, and S. Ogawa, "Successful pain management of primary and independent spread sites in a child with CRPS type I using regional nerve blocks," *Pain Medicine*, vol. 12, no. 1, p. 174, 2011.

[14] K. C. P. Vissers, K. Besse, M. Wagemans et al., "23. Pain in patients with cancer," *Pain Practice*, vol. 11, no. 5, pp. 453–475, 2011.

[15] B. Borghi, M. D'Addabbo, P. F. White et al., "The use of prolonged peripheral neural blockade after lower extremity amputation: the effect on symptoms associated with phantom limb syndrome," *Anesthesia and Analgesia*, vol. 111, no. 5, pp. 1308–1315, 2010.

[16] S. Preißler, C. Dietrich, W. Meissner et al., "Brachial plexus block in phantom limb pain: a case report," *Pain Medicine*, vol. 12, no. 11, pp. 1649–1654, 2011.

[17] L. Le-Wendling and F. K. Enneking, "Continuous peripheral nerve blockade for postoperative analgesia," *Current Opinion in Anaesthesiology*, vol. 21, no. 5, pp. 602–609, 2008.

[18] S. S. Liu, J. Ngeow, and R. S. John, "Evidence basis for ultrasound-guided block characteristics: onset, quality, and duration," *Regional anesthesia and pain medicine*, vol. 35, no. 2, pp. S26–S35, 2010.

[19] S. S. Liu, J. E. Ngeow, and J. T. YaDeau, "Ultrasound-guided regional anesthesia and analgesia: a qualitative systematic review," *Regional Anesthesia and Pain Medicine*, vol. 34, no. 1, pp. 47–59, 2009.

[20] S. S. Liu and C. L. Wu, "The effect of analgesic technique on postoperative patient-reported outcomes including analgesia: a systematic review," *Anesthesia and Analgesia*, vol. 105, no. 3, pp. 789–808, 2007.

[21] J. M. Richman, S. S. Liu, G. Courpas et al., "Does continuous peripheral nerve block provide superior pain control to opioids? A meta-analysis," *Anesthesia and Analgesia*, vol. 102, no. 1, pp. 248–257, 2006.

[22] B. M. Ilfeld, "Continuous peripheral nerve blocks: a review of the published evidence," *Anesthesia & Analgesia*, vol. 113, pp. 904–925, 2011.

[23] A. Rodgers, N. Walker, S. Schug et al., "Reduction of postoperative mortality and morbidity with epidural or spinal anaesthesia: results from overview of randomised trials,"

British Medical Journal, vol. 321, no. 7275, pp. 1493–1497, 2000.

[24] M. J. Parker, H. H. Handoll, and R. Griffiths, "Anaesthesia for hip fracture surgery in adults," *Cochrane Database of Systematic Reviews*, no. 4, Article ID CD000521, 2004.

[25] X. Capdevila, Y. Barthelet, P. Biboulet, Y. Ryckwaert, J. Rubenovitch, and F. D'Athis, "Effects of perioperative analgesic technique on the surgical outcome and duration of rehabilitation after major knee surgery," *Anesthesiology*, vol. 91, no. 1, pp. 8–15, 1999.

[26] S. Blumenthal, A. Borgeat, C. Neudrfer, R. Bertolini, N. Espinosa, and J. Aguirre, "Additional femoral catheter in combination with popliteal catheter for analgesia after major ankle surgery," *British Journal of Anaesthesia*, vol. 106, no. 3, pp. 387–393, 2011.

[27] B. M. Ilfeld, K. Vandenborne, P. W. Duncan et al., "Ambulatory continuous interscalene nerve blocks decrease the time to discharge readiness after total shoulder arthroplasty: a randomized, triple-masked, placebo-controlled study," *Anesthesiology*, vol. 105, no. 5, pp. 999–1007, 2006.

[28] I. Power, "Recent advances in postoperative pain therapy," *British Journal of Anaesthesia*, vol. 95, no. 1, pp. 43–51, 2005.

[29] J. L. Apfelbaum, C. Chen, S. S. Mehta, and T. J. Gan, "Postoperative pain experience: results from a national survey suggest postoperative pain continues to be undermanaged," *Anesthesia and Analgesia*, vol. 97, no. 2, pp. 534–540, 2003.

[30] T. T. Horlocker, "Pain management in total joint arthroplasty: a historical review," *Orthopedics*, vol. 33, no. 9, pp. 14–19, 2010.

[31] H. Y. V. Ip, A. Abrishami, P. W. H. Peng, J. Wong, and F. Chung, "Predictors of postoperative pain and analgesic consumption: a qualitative systematic review," *Anesthesiology*, vol. 111, no. 3, pp. 657–677, 2009.

[32] M. P. Ekstein and A. A. Weinbroum, "Immediate postoperative pain in orthopedic patients is more intense and requires more analgesia than in post-laparotomy patients," *Pain Medicine*, vol. 12, no. 2, pp. 308–313, 2011.

[33] B. M. Ilfeld, T. E. Morey, and F. K. Enneking, "Infraclavicular perineural local anesthetic infusion: a comparison of three dosing regimens for postoperative analgesia," *Anesthesiology*, vol. 100, no. 2, pp. 395–402, 2004.

[34] X. Capdevila, C. Dadure, S. Bringuier et al., "Effect of patient-controlled perineural analgesia on rehabilitation and pain after ambulatory orthopedic surgery: a multicenter randomized trial," *Anesthesiology*, vol. 105, no. 3, pp. 566–573, 2006.

[35] L. Nikolajsen, B. Brandsborg, U. Lucht, T. S. Jensen, and H. Kehlet, "Chronic pain following total hip arthroplasty: a nationwide questionnaire study," *Acta Anaesthesiologica Scandinavica*, vol. 50, no. 4, pp. 495–500, 2006.

[36] P. A. E. Puolakka, M. G. F. Rorarius, M. Roviola, T. J. S. Puolakka, K. Nordhausen, and L. Lindgren, "Persistent pain following knee arthroplasty," *European Journal of Anaesthesiology*, vol. 27, no. 5, pp. 455–460, 2010.

[37] H. Kehlet, T. S. Jensen, and C. J. Woolf, "Persistent postsurgical pain: risk factors and prevention," *Lancet*, vol. 367, no. 9522, pp. 1618–1625, 2006.

[38] F. M. Perkins and H. Kehlet, "Chronic pain as an outcome of surgery: a review of predictive factors," *Anesthesiology*, vol. 93, no. 4, pp. 1123–1133, 2000.

[39] M. N. Raftery, P. Ryan, C. Normand, A. W. Murphy, D. De La Harpe, and B. E. McGuire, "The economic cost of chronic noncancer pain in Ireland: results from the PRIME study, part 2," *Journal of Pain*, vol. 13, no. 2, pp. 139–145, 2012.

[40] J. R. Hebl, "The importance and implications of aseptic techniques during regional anesthesia," *Regional Anesthesia and Pain Medicine*, vol. 31, no. 4, pp. 311–323, 2006.

[41] C. Aveline, H. Le Hetet, A. Le Roux et al., "Perineural ultrasound-guided catheter bacterial colonization: a prospective evaluation in 747 cases," *Regional Anesthesia and Pain Medicine*, vol. 36, no. 6, pp. 579–584, 2011.

[42] D. Selander, K. G. Dhuner, and G. Lundborg, "Peripheral nerve injury due to injection needles used for regional anesthesia. An experimental study of the acute effects of needle point trauma," *Acta Anaesthesiologica Scandinavica*, vol. 21, no. 3, pp. 182–188, 1977.

[43] A. S. C. Rice and S. B. McMahon, "Peripheral nerve injury caused by injection needles used in regional anaesthesia: influence of bevel configuration, studied in a rat model," *British Journal of Anaesthesia*, vol. 69, no. 5, pp. 433–438, 1992.

[44] X. Sala-Blanch, T. Ribalta, E. Rivas et al., "Structural injury to the human sciatic nerve after intraneural needle insertion," *Regional Anesthesia and Pain Medicine*, vol. 34, no. 3, pp. 201–205, 2009.

[45] S. S. Liu, M. A. Gordon, P. M. Shaw, S. Wilfred, T. Shetty, and J. T. YaDeau, "A prospective clinical registry of ultrasound-guided regional anesthesia for ambulatory shoulder surgery," *Anesthesia and Analgesia*, vol. 111, no. 3, pp. 617–623, 2010.

[46] J. M. Cohen and A. T. Gray, "Functional deficits after intraneural injection during interscalene block," *Regional Anesthesia and Pain Medicine*, vol. 35, no. 4, pp. 397–399, 2010.

[47] J. Dooley, M. Fingerman, S. Melton, and S. M. Klein, "Contralateral local anesthetic spread from an outpatient interscalene catheter," *Canadian Journal of Anesthesia*, vol. 57, no. 10, pp. 936–939, 2010.

[48] D. Morau, S. Lopez, P. Biboulet, N. Bernard, J. Amar, and X. Capdevila, "Comparison of continuous 3-in-1 and fascia iliaca compartment blocks for postoperative analgesia: feasibility, catheter migration, distribution of sensory block, and analgesic efficacy," *Regional Anesthesia and Pain Medicine*, vol. 28, no. 4, pp. 309–314, 2003.

[49] G. M. Greenblatt and J. S. Denson, "Needle nerve stimulatorlocator: nerve blocks with a new instrument for locating nerves," *Anesthesia and analgesia*, vol. 41, pp. 599–602, 1962.

[50] D. Kulenkampff, "Anesthesia of the brachial plexus," *Zentralblatt für Chirurgie*, vol. 28, pp. 1337–1350, 1911.

[51] D. Selander, "Catheter technique in axillary plexus block. Presentation of a new method," *Acta Anaesthesiologica Scandinavica*, vol. 21, no. 4, pp. 324–329, 1977.

[52] W. A. Tan and D. G. Spigos, "Sciatic nerve block under fluoroscopic guidance," *CardioVascular and Interventional Radiology*, vol. 9, no. 1, pp. 59–60, 1986.

[53] P. L. Ting and V. Sivagnanaratnam, "Ultrasonographic study of the spread of local anaesthetic during axillary brachial plexus block," *British Journal of Anaesthesia*, vol. 63, no. 3, pp. 326–329, 1989.

[54] J. De Andrés, J. M. Alonso-Iñigo, X. Sala-Blanch, and M. A. Reina, "Nerve stimulation in regional anaesthesia: theory and practice," *Best Practice and Research: Clinical Anaesthesiology*, vol. 19, no. 2, pp. 153–174, 2005.

[55] A. Borgeat, J. Aguirre, M. Marquardt, J. Mrdjen, and S. Blumenthal, "Continuous interscalene analgesia with ropivacaine 0.2% versus ropivacaine 0.3% after open rotator cuff repair: the effects on postoperative analgesia and motor function," *Anesthesia and Analgesia*, vol. 111, no. 6, pp. 1543–1547, 2010.

[56] A. Borgeat, S. Blumenthal, D. Karovic, A. Delbos, and P. Vienne, "Clinical evaluation of a modified postetior anatomical approach to performing the popliteal block," *Regional Anesthesia and Pain Medicine*, vol. 29, no. 3, pp. 290–296, 2004.

[57] A. Borgeat, S. Blumenthal, M. Lambert, P. Theodorou, and P. Vienne, "The feasibility and complications of the continuous popliteal nerve block: a 1001-case survey," *Anesthesia and Analgesia*, vol. 103, no. 1, pp. 229–233, 2006.

[58] A. Borgeat, A. Dullenkopf, G. Ekatodramis, and L. Nagy, "Evaluation of the lateral modified approach for continuous interscalene block after shoulder surgery," *Anesthesiology*, vol. 99, no. 2, pp. 436–442, 2003.

[59] A. Borgeat, G. Ekatodramis, and C. Dumont, "An evaluation of the infraclavicular block via a modified approach of the Raj technique," *Anesthesia and Analgesia*, vol. 93, no. 2, pp. 436–441, 2001.

[60] S. A. Grant, K. C. Nielsen, R. A. Greengrass, S. M. Steele, and S. M. Klein, "Continuous peripheral nerve block for ambulatory surgery," *Regional Anesthesia and Pain Medicine*, vol. 26, no. 3, pp. 209–214, 2001.

[61] B. A. Williams, M. L. Kentor, M. T. Vogt et al., "Reduction of verbal pain scores after anterior cruciate ligament reconstruction with 2-day continuous femoral nerve block: a randomized clinical trial," *Anesthesiology*, vol. 104, no. 2, pp. 315–327, 2006.

[62] W. B. Silverstein, M. U. Saiyed, and A. R. Brown, "Interscalene block with a nerve stimulator: a deltoid motor response is a satisfactory endpoint for successful block," *Regional Anesthesia and Pain Medicine*, vol. 25, no. 4, pp. 356–359, 2000.

[63] H. Lecamwasam, J. Mayfield, L. Rosow, Y. Chang, C. Carter, and C. Rosow, "Stimulation of the posterior cord predicts successful infraclavicular block," *Anesthesia and Analgesia*, vol. 102, no. 5, pp. 1564–1568, 2006.

[64] S. Kapral, M. Greher, G. Huber et al., "Ultrasonographic guidance improves the success rate of interscalene brachial plexus blockade," *Regional Anesthesia and Pain Medicine*, vol. 33, no. 3, pp. 253–258, 2008.

[65] V. W. S. Chan, A. Perlas, C. J. L. McCartney, R. Brull, D. Xu, and S. Abbas, "Ultrasounds guidance improves success rate of axillary brachial plexus block," *Canadian Journal of Anesthesia*, vol. 54, no. 3, pp. 176–182, 2007.

[66] A. Perlas, R. Brull, V. W. S. Chan, C. J. L. McCartney, A. Nuica, and S. Abbas, "Ultrasound guidance improves the success of sciatic nerve block at the popliteal fossa," *Regional Anesthesia and Pain Medicine*, vol. 33, no. 3, pp. 259–265, 2008.

[67] P. Marhofer, K. Schrögendorfer, H. Koinig, S. Kapral, C. Weinstabl, and N. Mayer, "Ultrasonographic guidance improves sensory block and onset time of three-in-one blocks," *Anesthesia and Analgesia*, vol. 85, no. 4, pp. 854–857, 1997.

[68] M. Rigaud, P. Filip, P. Lirk, A. Fuchs, G. Gemes, and Q. Hogan, "Guidance of block needle insertion by electrical nerve stimulation: a pilot study of the resulting distribution of injected solution in dogs," *Anesthesiology*, vol. 109, no. 3, pp. 473–478, 2008.

[69] W. F. Urmey and J. Stanton, "Inability to consistently elicit a motor response following sensory paresthesia during interscalene block administration," *Anesthesiology*, vol. 96, no. 3, pp. 552–554, 2002.

[70] C. A. Bollini, W. F. Urmey, L. Vascello, and F. Cacheiro, "Relationship between evoked motor response and sensory paresthesia in interscalene brachial plexus block," *Regional Anesthesia and Pain Medicine*, vol. 28, no. 5, pp. 384–388, 2003.

[71] J. P. Kainu, J. Sarvela, E. Tiippana, E. Halmesmäki, and K. T. Korttila, "Persistent pain after caesarean section and vaginal birth: a cohort study," *International Journal of Obstetric Anesthesia*, vol. 19, no. 1, pp. 4–9, 2010.

[72] A. S. Poobalan, J. Bruce, P. M. King, W. A. Chambers, Z. H. Krukowski, and W. C. S. Smith, "Chronic pain and quality of life following open inguinal hernia repair," *British Journal of Surgery*, vol. 88, no. 8, pp. 1122–1126, 2001.

[73] W. A. Macrae, "Chronic post-surgical pain: 10 years on," *British Journal of Anaesthesia*, vol. 101, no. 1, pp. 77–86, 2008.

[74] F. V. Salinas, "Location, location, location: continuous peripheral nerve blocks and stimulating catheters," *Regional Anesthesia and Pain Medicine*, vol. 28, no. 2, pp. 79–82, 2003.

[75] X. Capdevila, P. Biboulet, D. Morau et al., "Continuous three-in-one block for postoperative pain after lower limb orthopedic surgery: where do the catheters go?" *Anesthesia and Analgesia*, vol. 94, no. 4, pp. 1001–1006, 2002.

[76] K. Enneking, "Close counts," *Regional Anesthesia and Pain Medicine*, vol. 32, no. 4, pp. 280–281, 2007.

[77] A. M. Morin, P. Kranke, H. Wulf, R. Stienstra, and L. H. J. Eberhart, "The effect of stimulating versus nonstimulating catheter techniques for continuous regional anesthesia: a semiquantitative systematic review," *Regional Anesthesia and Pain Medicine*, vol. 35, no. 2, pp. 194–199, 2010.

[78] A. Casati, G. Fanelli, G. Danelli et al., "Stimulating or conventional perineural catheters after hallux valgus repair: a double-blind, pharmaco-economic evaluation," *Acta Anaesthesiologica Scandinavica*, vol. 50, no. 10, pp. 1284–1289, 2006.

[79] F. V. Salinas, J. M. Neal, L. A. Sueda, D. J. Kopacz, and S. S. Liu, "Prospective comparison of continuous femoral nerve block with nonstimulating catheter placement versus stimulating catheter-guided perineural placement in volunteers," *Regional Anesthesia and Pain Medicine*, vol. 29, no. 3, pp. 212–220, 2004.

[80] M. F. Stevens, R. Werdehausen, E. Golla et al., "Does interscalene catheter placement with stimulating catheters improve postoperative pain or functional outcome after shoulder surgery? A prospective, randomized and double-blinded trial," *Anesthesia and Analgesia*, vol. 104, no. 2, pp. 442–447, 2007.

[81] D. Q. H. Tran, L. Muñoz, G. Russo, and R. J. Finlayson, "Ultrasonography and stimulating perineural catheters for nerve blocks: a review of the evidence," *Canadian Journal of Anesthesia*, vol. 55, no. 7, pp. 447–457, 2008.

[82] M. J. Barrington, D. J. Olive, C. A. McCutcheon et al., "Stimulating catheters for continuous femoral nerve blockade after total knee arthroplasty: a randomized, controlled, double-blinded trial," *Anesthesia and Analgesia*, vol. 106, no. 4, pp. 1316–1321, 2008.

[83] S. M. Hayek, R. M. Ritchey, D. Sessler et al., "Continuous femoral nerve analgesia after unilateral total knee arthroplasty: stimulating versus nonstimulating catheters," *Anesthesia and Analgesia*, vol. 103, no. 6, pp. 1565–1570, 2006.

[84] B. D. Sites, J. M. Neal, and V. Chan, "Editorial: Ultrasound in regional anesthesia: where should the "focus" be set?" *Regional Anesthesia and Pain Medicine*, vol. 34, no. 6, pp. 531–533, 2009.

[85] B. A. Williams, S. L. Orebaugh, B. Ben-David, and P. E. Bigeleisen, "Electrical stimulation: an important force behind the growth of regional anesthesia," *Canadian Journal of Anesthesia*, vol. 54, no. 7, pp. 585–586, 2007.

[86] A. Borgeat and X. Capdevila, "Neurostimulation/ultrasonography: the Trojan War will not take place," *Anesthesiology*, vol. 106, no. 5, pp. 896–898, 2007.

[87] S. Mannion and X. Capdevila, "Ultrasound guidance and success rates of axillary brachial plexus block - II," *Canadian Journal of Anesthesia*, vol. 54, no. 7, p. 584, 2007.

[88] J. Aguirre, S. Blumenthal, and A. Borgeat, "Ultrasound guidance and sucess rates of axillary brachial plexus block - I," *Canadian Journal of Anesthesia*, vol. 54, no. 7, p. 583, 2007.

[89] M. J. Fredrickson, A. Borgeat, J. Aguirre, and A. P. Boezaart, "Ultrasound-guided interscalene block should be compared with the accepted standard for the neurostimulation technique," *Regional Anesthesia and Pain Medicine*, vol. 34, no. 2, p. 180, 2009.

[90] M. S. Abrahams, M. F. Aziz, R. F. Fu, and J. L. Horn, "Ultrasound guidance compared with electrical neurostimulation for peripheral nerve block: a systematic review and meta-analysis of randomized controlled trials," *British Journal of Anaesthesia*, vol. 102, no. 3, pp. 408–417, 2009.

[91] J. Aguirre, "A questionable review will not change facts about neurostimulation compared to ultrasound technique," BJA, 2009, http://bja.oxfordjournals.org/content/102/3/408/reply.

[92] T. F. Bendtsen, T. D. Nielsen, C. V. Rohde, K. Kibak, and F. Linde, "Ultrasound guidance improves a continuous popliteal sciatic nerve block when compared with nerve stimulation," *Regional Anesthesia and Pain Medicine*, vol. 36, no. 2, pp. 181–184, 2011.

[93] E. R. Mariano, G. S. Cheng, L. P. Choy et al., "Electrical stimulation versus ultrasound guidance for popliteal-sciatic perineural catheter insertion a randomized controlled trial," *Regional Anesthesia and Pain Medicine*, vol. 34, no. 5, pp. 480–485, 2009.

[94] E. R. Mariano, V. J. Loland, N. S. Sandhu et al., "Ultrasound guidance versus electrical stimulation for femoral perineural catheter insertion," *Journal of Ultrasound in Medicine*, vol. 28, no. 11, pp. 1453–1460, 2009.

[95] E. R. Mariano, V. J. Loland, R. H. Bellars et al., "Ultrasound guidance versus electrical stimulation for infraclavicular brachial plexus perineural catheter insertion," *Journal of Ultrasound in Medicine*, vol. 28, no. 9, pp. 1211–1218, 2009.

[96] M. J. Fredrickson and T. K. Danesh-Clough, "Ambulatory continuous femoral analgesia for major knee surgery: a randomised study of ultrasound-guided femoral catheter placement," *Anaesthesia and Intensive Care*, vol. 37, no. 5, pp. 758–766, 2009.

[97] M. J. Fredrickson, C. M. Ball, and A. J. Dalgleish, "A prospective randomized comparison of ultrasound guidance versus neurostimulation for interscalene catheter placement," *Regional Anesthesia and Pain Medicine*, vol. 34, no. 6, pp. 590–594, 2009.

[98] M. J. Fredrickson, C. M. Ball, A. J. Dalgleish, A. W. Stewart, and T. G. Short, "A prospective randomized comparison of ultrasound and neurostimulation as needle end points for interscalene catheter placement," *Anesthesia and Analgesia*, vol. 108, no. 5, pp. 1695–1700, 2009.

[99] S. Dhir and S. Ganapathy, "Comparative evaluation of ultrasound-guided continuous infraclavicular brachial plexus block with stimulating catheter and traditional technique: a prospective-randomized trial," *Acta Anaesthesiologica Scandinavica*, vol. 52, no. 8, pp. 1158–1166, 2008.

[100] E. R. Mariano, V. J. Loland, N. S. Sandhu et al., "Comparative efficacy of ultrasound-guided and stimulating popliteal-sciatic perineural catheters for postoperative analgesia," *Canadian Journal of Anesthesia*, vol. 57, no. 10, pp. 919–926, 2010.

[101] C. Aveline, A. Le Roux, H. Le Hetet, P. Vautier, F. Cognet, and F. Bonnet, "Postoperative efficacies of femoral nerve catheters sited using ultrasound combined with neurostimulation compared with neurostimulation alone for total knee arthroplasty," *European Journal of Anaesthesiology*, vol. 27, no. 11, pp. 978–984, 2010.

[102] J. M. Neal, R. Brull, V. W. Chan et al., "The ASRA evidence-based medicine assessment of ultrasound-guided regional anesthesia and pain medicine: executive summary," *Regional anesthesia and pain medicine*, vol. 35, no. 2, pp. S1–S9, 2010.

[103] V. W. S. Chan, "Applying ultrasound imaging to interscalene brachial plexus block," *Regional Anesthesia and Pain Medicine*, vol. 28, no. 4, pp. 340–343, 2003.

[104] A. P. Winnie, S. Ramamurthy, Z. Durrani, and R. Radonjic, "Interscalene cervical plexus block: a single injection technic," *Anesthesia and Analgesia*, vol. 54, no. 3, pp. 370–375, 1975.

[105] A. P. Boezaart, R. Koorn, and R. W. Rosenquist, "Paravertebral approach to the brachial plexus: an anatomic improvement in technique," *Regional Anesthesia and Pain Medicine*, vol. 28, no. 3, pp. 241–244, 2003.

[106] A. P. Boezaart, J. F. De Beer, and M. L. Nell, "Early experience with continuous cervical paravertebral block using a stimulating catheter," *Regional Anesthesia and Pain Medicine*, vol. 28, no. 5, pp. 406–413, 2003.

[107] I. Sandefo, G. Iohom, A. Van Elstraete, T. Lebrun, and B. Polin, "Clinical efficacy of the brachial plexus block via the posterior approach," *Regional Anesthesia and Pain Medicine*, vol. 30, no. 3, pp. 238–242, 2005.

[108] J. G. Antonakakis, B. D. Sites, and J. Shiffrin, "Ultrasound-guided posterior approach for the placement of a continuous interscalene catheter," *Regional Anesthesia and Pain Medicine*, vol. 34, no. 1, pp. 64–68, 2009.

[109] E. R. Mariano, V. J. Loland, and B. M. Ilfeld, "Interscalene perineural catheter placement using an ultrasound-guided posterior approach," *Regional Anesthesia and Pain Medicine*, vol. 34, no. 1, pp. 60–63, 2009.

[110] C. H. Salazar and W. Espinosa, "Infraclavicular brachial plexus block: variation in approach and results in 360 cases," *Regional Anesthesia and Pain Medicine*, vol. 24, no. 5, pp. 411–416, 1999.

[111] J. L. Wilson, D. L. Brown, G. Y. Wong, R. L. Ehman, and D. R. Cahill, "Infraclavicular brachial plexus block: parasagittal anatomy important to the coracoid technique," *Anesthesia and Analgesia*, vol. 87, no. 4, pp. 870–873, 1998.

[112] Z. J. Koscielniak-Nielsen, H. Rasmussen, L. Hesselbjerg, Y. Gũrkan, and B. Belhage, "Clinical evaluation of the lateral sagittal infraclavicular block developed by MRI studies," *Regional Anesthesia and Pain Medicine*, vol. 30, no. 4, pp. 329–334, 2005.

[113] H. C. Rettig, M. J. M. Gielen, E. Boersma, J. Klein, and G. J. Groen, "Vertical infraclavicular block of the brachial plexus: effects on hemidiaphragmatic movement and ventilatory function," *Regional Anesthesia and Pain Medicine*, vol. 30, no. 6, pp. 529–535, 2005.

[114] A. P. Winnie and V. J. Collins, "The subclavian perivascular technique of brachial plexus anesthesia," *Anesthesiology*, vol. 25, pp. 353–363, 1964.

[115] D. L. Brown, D. R. Cahill, and L. D. Bridenbaugh, "Supraclavicular nerve block: anatomic analysis of a method to prevent pneumothorax," *Anesthesia and Analgesia*, vol. 76, no. 3, pp. 530–534, 1993.

[116] V. W. S. Chan, A. Perlas, R. Rawson, and O. Odukoya, "Ultrasound-guided supraclavicular brachial plexus block," *Anesthesia and Analgesia*, vol. 97, no. 5, pp. 1514–1517, 2003.
[117] H. Bouaziz, P. Narchi, F. J. Mercier et al., "Comparison between conventional axillary block and a new approach at the midhumeral level," *Anesthesia and Analgesia*, vol. 84, no. 5, pp. 1058–1062, 1997.
[118] D. C. Moore, "A simplified maneuver for transarterial approach to axillary block for use by a single anesthesiologist—needs more explanation!," *Regional Anesthesia*, vol. 22, no. 3, pp. 293–294, 1997.
[119] F. C. Liu, J. T. Liou, Y. F. Tsai et al., "Efficacy of ultrasound-guided axillary brachial plexus block: a comparative study with nerve stimulator-guided method," *Chang Gung Medical Journal*, vol. 28, no. 6, pp. 396–402, 2005.
[120] D. Chayen, H. Nathan, and M. Chayen, "The psoas compartment block," *Anesthesiology*, vol. 45, no. 1, pp. 95–99, 1976.
[121] X. Capdevila, P. Macaire, C. Dadure et al., "Continuous psoas compartment block for postoperative analgesia after total hip arthroplasty: new landmarks, technical guidelines, and clinical evaluation," *Anesthesia and Analgesia*, vol. 94, no. 6, pp. 1606–1613, 2002.
[122] S. Lopez, T. Gros, N. Bernard, C. Plasse, and X. Capdevila, "Fascia iliaca compartment block for femoral bone fractures in prehospital care," *Regional Anesthesia and Pain Medicine*, vol. 28, no. 3, pp. 203–207, 2003.
[123] B. Dalens, G. Vanneuville, and A. Tanguy, "Comparison of the fascia iliaca compartment block with the 3-in-1 block in children," *Anesthesia and Analgesia*, vol. 69, no. 6, pp. 705–713, 1989.
[124] O. Paut, M. Sallabery, E. Schreiber-Deturmeny, C. Rémond, B. Bruguerolle, and J. Camboulives, "Continuous fascia iliaca compartment block in children: a prospective evaluation of plasma bupivacaine concentrations, pain scores, and side effects," *Anesthesia and Analgesia*, vol. 92, no. 5, pp. 1159–1163, 2001.
[125] C. Cauhepe, M. Olivier, R. Colombani, and N. Railhac, "The '3 in 1' block: myth or reality?" *Annales Francaises d'Anesthesie et de Reanimation*, vol. 8, no. 4, pp. 376–378, 1989.
[126] P. Marhofer, C. Našel, C. Sitzwohl, and S. Kapral, "Magnetic resonance imaging of the distribution of local anesthetic during the three-in-one block," *Anesthesia and Analgesia*, vol. 90, no. 1, pp. 119–124, 2000.
[127] S. A. Lang, R. W. Yip, P. C. Chang, and M. A. Gerard, "The femoral 3-in-1 block revisited," *Journal of Clinical Anesthesia*, vol. 5, no. 4, pp. 292–296, 1993.
[128] O. Choquet, X. Capdevila, K. Bennourine, J. L. Feugeas, S. Bringuier-Branchereau, and J. C. Manelli, "A new inguinal approach for the obturator nerve block: anatomical and randomized clinical studies," *Anesthesiology*, vol. 103, no. 6, pp. 1238–1245, 2005.
[129] D. Macalou, S. Trueck, P. Meuret et al., "Postoperative analgesia after total knee replacement: the effect of an obturator nerve block added to the femoral 3-in-1 nerve block," *Anesthesia and Analgesia*, vol. 99, no. 1, pp. 251–254, 2004.
[130] R. Guardini, B. A. Waldron, and W. A. Wallace, "Sciatic nerve block: a new lateral approach," *Acta Anaesthesiologica Scandinavica*, vol. 29, no. 5, pp. 515–519, 1985.
[131] P. C. Chang, S. A. Lang, and R. W. Yip, "Reevaluation of the sciatic nerve block," *Regional Anesthesia*, vol. 18, no. 1, pp. 18–23, 1993.
[132] C. D. Franco, "Posterior approach to the sciatic nerve in adults: is Euclidean geometry still necessary?" *Anesthesiology*, vol. 98, no. 3, pp. 723–728, 2003.
[133] P. Di Benedetto, G. Fanelli, J. E. Chelly, A. Casati, F. V. Salinas, and S. S. Liu, "Continuous sciatic nerve block: how to choose among different proximal approaches? Gluteal or subgluteal continuous sciatic nerve block," *Anesthesia and Analgesia*, vol. 97, no. 1, pp. 296–297, 2003.
[134] M. J. Fredrickson, C. M. Ball, and A. J. Dalgleish, "Successful continuous interscalene analgesia for ambulatory shoulder surgery in a private practice setting," *Regional Anesthesia and Pain Medicine*, vol. 33, no. 2, pp. 122–128, 2008.
[135] J. J. Davis, J. D. Swenson, P. E. Greis, R. T. Burks, and R. Z. Tashjian, "Interscalene block for postoperative analgesia using only ultrasound guidance: the outcome in 200 patients," *Journal of Clinical Anesthesia*, vol. 21, no. 4, pp. 272–277, 2009.
[136] M. E. Slater, S. R. Williams, P. Harris et al., "Preliminary evaluation of infraclavicular catheters inserted using ultrasound guidance: through-the-catheter anesthesia is not inferior to through-the-needle blocks," *Regional Anesthesia and Pain Medicine*, vol. 32, no. 4, pp. 296–302, 2007.
[137] A. Z. Wang, L. Gu, Q. H. Zhou, W. Z. Ni, and W. Jiang, "Ultrasound-guided continuous femoral nerve block for analgesia after total knee arthroplasty: catheter perpendicular to the nerve versus catheter parallel to the nerve," *Regional Anesthesia and Pain Medicine*, vol. 35, no. 2, pp. 127–131, 2010.
[138] M. J. Fredrickson, C. M. Ball, and A. J. Dalgleish, "Posterior versus anterolateral approach interscalene catheter placement: a prospective randomized trial," *Regional Anesthesia and Pain Medicine*, vol. 36, no. 2, pp. 125–133, 2011.
[139] B. M. Ilfeld, M. J. Fredrickson, and E. R. Mariano, "Ultrasound-guided perineural catheter insertion: three approaches but few illuminating data," *Regional Anesthesia and Pain Medicine*, vol. 35, no. 2, pp. 123–126, 2010.
[140] G. J. van Geffen, M. Scheuer, A. Müller, J. Garderniers, and M. Gielen, "Ultrasound-guided bilateral continuous sciatic nerve blocks with stimulating catheters for postoperative pain relief after bilateral lower limb amputations," *Anaesthesia*, vol. 61, no. 12, pp. 1204–1207, 2006.
[141] A. Walker and S. Roberts, "Stimulating catheters: a thing of the past?" *Anesthesia and Analgesia*, vol. 104, no. 4, pp. 1001–1002, 2007.
[142] M. J. Fredrickson, "The sensitivity of motor response to needle nerve stimulation during ultrasound guided interscalene catheter placement," *Regional Anesthesia and Pain Medicine*, vol. 33, no. 4, pp. 291–296, 2008.
[143] A. Stojadinovic, A. Auton, G. E. Peoples et al., "Responding to challenges in modern combat casualty care: innovative use of advanced regional anesthesia," *Pain Medicine*, vol. 7, no. 4, pp. 330–338, 2006.
[144] A. R. Plunkett, D. S. Brown, J. M. Rogers, and C. C. Buckenmaier, "Supraclavicular continuous peripheral nerve block in a wounded soldier: when ultrasound is the only option," *British Journal of Anaesthesia*, vol. 97, no. 5, pp. 715–717, 2006.
[145] C. Heiring and B. B. Kristensen, "Sciatic nerve block performed with nerve stimulation technique in an amputee—a case study," *Ugeskrift for Laeger*, vol. 170, no. 6, p. 461, 2008.
[146] P. E. Bigeleisen, "Ultrasound-guided infraclavicular block in an anticoagulated and anesthetized patient," *Anesthesia and Analgesia*, vol. 104, no. 5, pp. 1285–1287, 2007.
[147] V. Minville, P. J. Zetlaoui, C. Fessenmeyer, and D. Benhamou, "Ultrasound guidance for difficult lateral popliteal catheter insertion in a patient with peripheral vascular disease,"

Regional Anesthesia and Pain Medicine, vol. 29, no. 4, pp. 368–370, 2004.

[148] S. H. Renes, G. J. Van Geffen, H. C. Rettig, M. J. Gielen, and G. J. Scheffer, "Ultrasound-guided continuous phrenic nerve block for persistent hiccups," *Regional Anesthesia and Pain Medicine*, vol. 35, no. 5, pp. 455–457, 2010.

[149] B. M. Ilfeld, V. J. Loland, and E. R. Mariano, "Prepuncture ultrasound imaging to predict transverse process and lumbar plexus depth for psoas compartment block and perineural catheter insertion: a prospective, observational study," *Anesthesia and Analgesia*, vol. 110, no. 6, pp. 1725–1728, 2010.

[150] B. M. K. Emanuelsson, D. Zaric, P. A. Nydahl, and K. H. Axelsson, "Pharmacokinetics of ropivacaine and bupivacaine during 21 hours of continuous epidural infusion in healthy male volunteers," *Anesthesia and Analgesia*, vol. 81, no. 6, pp. 1163–1168, 1995.

[151] N. Rawal, R. Allvin, K. Axelsson et al., "Patient-controlled regional analgesia (PCRA) at home: controlled comparison between bupivacaine and ropivacaine brachial plexus analgesia," *Anesthesiology*, vol. 96, no. 6, pp. 1290–1296, 2002.

[152] A. Borgeat, F. Kalberer, H. Jacob, Y. A. Ruetsch, and C. Gerber, "Patient-controlled interscalene analgesia with ropivacaine 0.2% versus bupivacaine 0.15% after major open shoulder surgery: the effects on hand motor function," *Anesthesia and Analgesia*, vol. 92, no. 1, pp. 218–223, 2001.

[153] A. Borgeat, B. Schäppi, N. Biasca, and C. Gerber, "Patient-controlled analgesia after major shoulder surgery: patient-controlled interscalene analgesia versus patient-controlled analgesia," *Anesthesiology*, vol. 87, no. 6, pp. 1343–1347, 1997.

[154] A. Borgeat, E. Tewes, N. Biasca, and C. Gerber, "Patient-controlled interscalene analgesia with ropivacaine after major shoulder surgery: PCIA vs PCA," *British Journal of Anaesthesia*, vol. 81, no. 4, pp. 603–605, 1998.

[155] A. Borgeat, H. Perschak, P. Bird, J. Hodler, and C. Gerber, "Patient-controlled interscalene analgesia with ropivacaine 0.2% versus patient-controlled intravenous analgesia after major shoulder surgery: effects on diaphragmatic and respiratory function," *Anesthesiology*, vol. 92, no. 1, pp. 102–108, 2000.

[156] F. J. Singelyn, S. Seguy, and J. M. Gouverneur, "Interscalene brachial plexus analgesia after open shoulder surgery: continuous versus patient-controlled infusion," *Anesthesia and Analgesia*, vol. 89, no. 5, pp. 1216–1220, 1999.

[157] M. J. Fredrickson, A. Abeysekera, D. J. Price, and A. C. Wong, "Patient-initiated mandatory boluses for ambulatory continuous interscalene analgesia: an effective strategy for optimizing analgesia and minimizing side-effects," *British Journal of Anaesthesia*, vol. 106, no. 2, pp. 239–245, 2011.

[158] B. M. Ilfeld, E. R. Mariano, S. J. Madison et al., "Continuous femoral versus posterior lumbar plexus nerve blocks for analgesia after hip arthroplasty: a randomized, controlled study," *Anesthesia & Analgesia*, vol. 113, no. 4, pp. 897–903, 2011.

[159] F. J. Singelyn, P. E. Vanderelst, and J. M. A. Gouverneur, "Extended femoral nerve sheath block after total hip arthroplasty: continous versus patient-controlled techniques," *Anesthesia and Analgesia*, vol. 92, no. 2, pp. 455–459, 2001.

[160] F. J. Singelyn and J. M. A. Gouverneur, "Extended "three-in-one" block after total knee arthroplasty: continuous versus patient-controlled techniques," *Anesthesia and Analgesia*, vol. 91, no. 1, pp. 176–180, 2000.

[161] J. J. Eledjam, P. Cuvillon, X. Capdevila et al., "Postoperative analgesia by femoral nerve block with ropivacaine 0.2% After major knee surgery: continuous versus patient-controlled techniques," *Regional Anesthesia and Pain Medicine*, vol. 27, no. 6, pp. 604–611, 2002.

[162] P. Di Benedetto, A. Casati, and L. Bertini, "Continuous subgluteus sciatic nerve block after orthopedic foot and ankle surgery: comparison of two infusion techniques," *Regional Anesthesia and Pain Medicine*, vol. 27, no. 2, pp. 168–172, 2002.

[163] J. Steinmetz, K. S. Funder, B. T. Dahl, and L. S. Rasmussen, "Depth of anaesthesia and post-operative cognitive dysfunction," *Acta Anaesthesiologica Scandinavica*, vol. 54, no. 2, pp. 162–168, 2010.

[164] L. Evered, D. A. Scott, B. Silbert, and P. Maruff, "Postoperative cognitive dysfunction is independent of type of surgery and anesthetic," *Anesthesia and Analgesia*, vol. 112, no. 5, pp. 1179–1185, 2011.

[165] Z. Wajima, Y. Nakajima, C. Kim et al., "I.v. compared with brachial plexus infusion of butorphanol for postoperative analgesia," *British Journal of Anaesthesia*, vol. 74, no. 4, pp. 392–395, 1995.

[166] P. R. Picard, M. R. Tramèr, H. J. McQuay, and R. Andrew Moore, "Analgesic efficacy of peripheral opioids (all except intra-articular): a qualitative systematic review of randomised controlled trials," *Pain*, vol. 72, no. 3, pp. 309–318, 1997.

[167] B. L. Partridge and D. Phil, "The effects of local anesthetics and epinephrine on rat sciatic nerve blood flow," *Anesthesiology*, vol. 75, no. 2, pp. 243–251, 1991.

[168] D. M. Pöpping, N. Elia, E. Marret, M. Wenk, and M. R. Tramèr, "Clonidine as an adjuvant to local anesthetics for peripheral nerve and plexus blocks: a meta-analysis of randomized trials," *Anesthesiology*, vol. 111, no. 2, pp. 406–415, 2009.

[169] B. M. Ilfeld, T. E. Morey, L. J. Thannikary, T. W. Wright, and F. K. Enneking, "Clonidine added to a continuous interscalene ropivacaine perineural infusion to improve postoperative analgesia: a randomized, double-blind, controlled study," *Anesthesia and Analgesia*, vol. 100, no. 4, pp. 1172–1178, 2005.

[170] A. Casati, F. Vinciguerra, G. Cappelleri et al., "Adding clonidine to the induction bolus and postoperative infusion during continuous femoral nerve block delays recovery of motor function after total knee arthroplasty," *Anesthesia and Analgesia*, vol. 100, no. 3, pp. 866–872, 2005.

[171] B. M. Ilfeld, V. J. Loland, J. C. Gerancher et al., "The effects of varying local anesthetic concentration and volume on continuous popliteal sciatic nerve blocks: a dual-center, randomized, controlled study," *Anesthesia and Analgesia*, vol. 107, no. 2, pp. 701–707, 2008.

[172] L. T. Le, V. J. Loland, E. R. Mariano et al., "Effects of local anesthetic concentration and dose on continuous interscalene nerve blocks: a dual-center, randomized, observer-masked, controlled study," *Regional Anesthesia and Pain Medicine*, vol. 33, no. 6, pp. 518–525, 2008.

[173] B. M. Ilfeld, T. E. Morey, T. W. Wright, L. K. Chidgey, and F. K. Enneking, "Interscalene perineural ropivacaine infusion: a comparison of two dosing regimens for postoperative analgesia," *Regional Anesthesia and Pain Medicine*, vol. 29, no. 1, pp. 9–16, 2004.

[174] B. M. Ilfeld, L. K. Moeller, E. R. Mariano et al., "Continuous peripheral nerve blocks: is local anesthetic dose the only factor, or do concentration and volume influence infusion effects as well?" *Anesthesiology*, vol. 112, no. 2, pp. 347–354, 2010.

[175] B. M. Ilfeld, L. T. Le, J. Ramjohn et al., "The effects of local anesthetic concentration and dose on continuous

infraclavicular nerve blocks: a multicenter, randomized, observer-masked, controlled study," *Anesthesia and Analgesia*, vol. 108, no. 1, pp. 345–350, 2009.

[176] G. Brodner, H. Buerkle, H. Van Aken et al., "Postoperative analgesia after knee surgery: a comparison of three different concentrations of ropivacaine for continuous femoral nerve blockade," *Anesthesia and Analgesia*, vol. 105, no. 1, pp. 256–262, 2007.

[177] B. M. Ilfeld, L. J. Thannikary, T. E. Morey, R. A. Vander Griend, and F. K. Enneking, "Popliteal sciatic perineural local anesthetic infusion: a comparison of three dosing regimens for postoperative analgesia," *Anesthesiology*, vol. 101, no. 4, pp. 970–977, 2004.

[178] B. M. Ilfeld, K. B. Duke, and M. C. Donohue, "The association between lower extremity continuous peripheral nerve blocks and patient falls after knee and hip arthroplasty," *Anesthesia and Analgesia*, vol. 111, no. 6, pp. 1552–1554, 2010.

[179] P. H. Rosenberg, B. T. Veering, and W. F. Urmey, "Maximum recommended doses of local anesthetics: a multifactorial concept," *Regional Anesthesia and Pain Medicine*, vol. 29, no. 6, pp. 564–575, 2004.

[180] L. L. Bleckner, S. Bina, K. H. Kwon, G. McKnight, A. Dragovich, and C. C. Buckenmaier, "Serum ropivacaine concentrations and systemic local anesthetic toxicity in trauma patients receiving long-term continuous peripheral nerve block catheters," *Anesthesia and Analgesia*, vol. 110, no. 2, pp. 630–634, 2010.

[181] G. Ekatodramis, A. Borgeat, G. Huledal, L. Jeppsson, L. Westman, and J. Sjövall, "Continuous interscalene analgesia with ropivacaine 2 mg/ml after major shoulder surgery," *Anesthesiology*, vol. 98, no. 1, pp. 143–150, 2003.

[182] B. M. Ilfeld, "Continuous peripheral nerve blocks in the hospital and at home," *Anesthesiology Clinics*, vol. 29, no. 2, pp. 193–211, 2011.

[183] E. A. Skryabina and T. S. Dunn, "Disposable infusion pumps," *American Journal of Health-System Pharmacy*, vol. 63, no. 13, pp. 1260–1268, 2006.

[184] X. Capdevila, P. Macaire, P. Aknin, C. Dadure, N. Bernard, and S. Lopez, "Patient-controlled perineural analgesia after ambulatory orthopedic surgery: a comparison of electronic versus elastomeric pumps," *Anesthesia and Analgesia*, vol. 96, no. 2, pp. 414–417, 2003.

[185] J. Aguirre, B. Baulig, C. Dora et al., "Continuous epicapsular ropivacaine 0.3% infusion after minimally invasive hip arthroplasty: a prospective, randomized, double-blinded, placebo-controlled study comparing continuous wound infusion with morphine patient-controlled analgesia," *Anesthesia and Analgesia*, vol. 114, no. 2, pp. 456–461, 2012.

[186] F. Martin, V. Martinez, J. X. Mazoit et al., "Antiinflammatory effect of peripheral nerve blocks after knee surgery: clinical and biologic evaluation," *Anesthesiology*, vol. 109, no. 3, pp. 484–490, 2008.

[187] A. Chudinov, H. Berkenstadt, M. Salai, A. Cahana, and A. Perel, "Continuous psoas compartment block for anesthesia and perioperative analgesia in patients with hip fractures," *Regional Anesthesia and Pain Medicine*, vol. 24, no. 6, pp. 563–568, 1999.

[188] G. J. Mar, M. J. Barrington, and B. R. McGuirk, "Acute compartment syndrome of the lower limb and the effect of postoperative analgesia on diagnosis," *British Journal of Anaesthesia*, vol. 102, no. 1, pp. 3–11, 2009.

[189] D. J. G. Johnson and G. A. Chalkiadis, "Does epidural analgesia delay the diagnosis of lower limb compartment syndrome in children?" *Paediatric Anaesthesia*, vol. 19, no. 2, pp. 83–91, 2009.

[190] B. M. Ilfeld, T. E. Morey, R. D. Wang, and F. K. Enneking, "Continuous popliteal sciatic nerve block for postoperative pain control at home: a randomized, double-blinded, placebcontrolled study," *Anesthesiology*, vol. 97, no. 4, pp. 959–965, 2002.

[191] J. D. Swenson, N. Bay, E. Loose et al., "Outpatient management of continuous peripheral nerve catheters placed using ultrasound guidance: an experience in 620 patients," *Anesthesia and Analgesia*, vol. 103, no. 6, pp. 1436–1443, 2006.

[192] B. A. Williams, M. L. Kentor, and M. T. Bottegal, "The incidence of falls at home in patients with perineural femoral catheters: a retrospective summary of a randomized clinical trial," *Anesthesia and Analgesia*, vol. 104, no. 4, p. 1002, 2007.

[193] J. Aguirre and A. Borgeat, "Anesthesia for shoulder surgery," Anesthesia International 2010.

[194] S. Lehtipalo, L. O. D. Koskinen, G. Johansson, J. Kolmodin, and B. Biber, "Continuous interscalene brachial plexus block for postoperative analgesia following shoulder surgery," *Acta Anaesthesiologica Scandinavica*, vol. 43, no. 3, pp. 258–264, 1999.

[195] S. M. Klein, S. A. Grant, R. A. Greengrass et al., "Interscalene brachial plexus block with a continuous catheter insertion system and a disposable infusion pump," *Anesthesia and Analgesia*, vol. 91, no. 6, pp. 1473–1478, 2000.

[196] J. Kean, C. A. Wigderowitz, and D. M. Coventry, "Continuous interscalene infusion and single injection using levobupivacaine for analgesia after surgery of the shoulder," *Journal of Bone and Joint Surgery B*, vol. 88, no. 9, pp. 1173–1177, 2006.

[197] B. M. Ilfeld, T. E. Morey, T. W. Wright, L. K. Chidgey, and F. K. Enneking, "Continuous interscalene brachial plexus block for postoperative pain control at home: a randomized, double-blinded, placebo-controlled study," *Anesthesia and Analgesia*, vol. 96, no. 4, pp. 1089–1095, 2003.

[198] K. Hofmann-Kiefer, T. Eiser, D. Chappell, S. Leuschner, P. Conzen, and D. Schwender, "Does patient-controlled continuous interscalene block improve early functional rehabilitation after open shoulder surgery?" *Anesthesia and Analgesia*, vol. 106, no. 3, pp. 991–996, 2008.

[199] E. R. Mariano, R. Afra, V. J. Loland et al., "Continuous interscalene brachial plexus block via an ultrasound-guided posterior approach: a randomized, triple-masked, placebo-controlled study," *Anesthesia and Analgesia*, vol. 108, no. 5, pp. 1688–1694, 2009.

[200] M. J. Fredrickson, C. M. Ball, and A. J. Dalgleish, "Analgesic effectiveness of a continuous versus single-injection interscalene block for minor arthroscopic shoulder surgery," *Regional Anesthesia and Pain Medicine*, vol. 35, no. 1, pp. 28–33, 2010.

[201] S. Goebel, J. Stehle, U. Schwemmer, S. Reppenhagen, B. Rath, and F. Gohlke, "Interscalene brachial plexus block for open-shoulder surgery: a randomized, double-blind, placebo-controlled trial between single-shot anesthesia and patient-controlled catheter system," *Archives of Orthopaedic and Trauma Surgery*, vol. 130, no. 4, pp. 533–540, 2010.

[202] B. M. Ilfeld, T. E. Morey, and F. K. Enneking, "Continuous infraclavicular brachial plexus block for postoperative pain control at home: a randomized, double-blinded, placebo-controlled study," *Anesthesiology*, vol. 96, no. 6, pp. 1297–1304, 2002.

[203] M. H. A. Salonen, "Evaluation of efficacy and plasma concentrations of ropivacaine in continuous axillary brachial plexus block: high dose for surgical anesthesia and low dose

for postoperative analgesia," *Regional Anesthesia and Pain Medicine*, vol. 25, no. 1, pp. 47–51, 2000.

[204] E. R. Mariano, N. S. Sandhu, V. J. Loland et al., "A randomized comparison of infraclavicular and supraclavicular continuous peripheral nerve blocks for postoperative analgesia," *Regional Anesthesia and Pain Medicine*, vol. 36, no. 1, pp. 26–31, 2011.

[205] P. B. Cornish, C. J. Leaper, G. Nelson, F. Anstis, C. Mcquillan, and R. Stienstra, "Avoidance of phrenic nerve paresis during continuous supraclavicular regional anaesthesia," *Anaesthesia*, vol. 62, no. 4, pp. 354–358, 2007.

[206] H. Bagry, J. C. de la Cuadra Fontaine, J. F. Asenjo, D. Bracco, and F. Carli, "Effect of a continuous peripheral nerve block on the inflammatory response in knee arthroplasty," *Regional Anesthesia and Pain Medicine*, vol. 33, no. 1, pp. 17–23, 2008.

[207] F. J. Singelyn, T. Ferrant, M. F. Malisse, and D. Joris, "Effects of intravenous patient-controlled analgesia with morphine, continuous epidural analgesia, and continuous femoral nerve sheath block on rehabilitation after unilateral total-hip arthroplasty," *Regional Anesthesia and Pain Medicine*, vol. 30, no. 5, pp. 452–457, 2005.

[208] M. W. Watson, D. Mitra, T. C. McLintock, and S. A. Grant, "Continuous versus single-injection lumbar plexus blocks: comparison of the effects on morphine use and early recovery after total knee arthroplasty," *Regional Anesthesia and Pain Medicine*, vol. 30, no. 6, pp. 541–547, 2005.

[209] W. T. Long, S. R. Ward, L. D. Dorr, J. Raya, M. Boutary, and L. E. Sirianni, "Postoperative pain management following total knee arthroplasty: a randomized comparison of continuous epidural versus femoral nerve infusion," *The journal of knee surgery*, vol. 19, no. 2, pp. 137–143, 2006.

[210] C. B. Johnson and S. K. Steele-Moses, "The use of continuous femoral nerve blocks versus extended release epidural morphine: a study comparing outcomes in total knee arthroplasty procedures," *Orthopaedic Nursing*, vol. 30, no. 1, pp. 44–53, 2011.

[211] B. M. Ilfeld, L. T. Le, R. S. Meyer et al., "Ambulatory continuous femoral nerve blocks decrease time to discharge readiness after tricompartment total knee arthroplasty: a randomized, triple-masked, placebo-controlled study," *Anesthesiology*, vol. 108, no. 4, pp. 703–713, 2008.

[212] J. T. Wegener, B. Van Ooij, C. N. Van Dijk, M. W. Hollmann, B. Preckel, and M. F. Stevens, "Value of single-injection or continuous sciatic nerve block in addition to a continuous femoral nerve block in patients undergoing total knee arthroplasty: a prospective, randomized, controlled trial," *Regional Anesthesia and Pain Medicine*, vol. 36, no. 5, pp. 481–488, 2011.

[213] G. Mistraletti, J. C. De La Cuadra-Fontaine, F. J. Asenjo et al., "Comparison of analgesic methods for total knee arthroplasty: metabolic effect of exogenous glucose," *Regional Anesthesia and Pain Medicine*, vol. 31, no. 3, pp. 260–269, 2006.

[214] A. M. Morin, C. D. Kratz, L. H. J. Eberhart et al., "Postoperative analgesia and functional recovery after total-knee replacement: comparison of a continuous posterior lumbar plexus (Psoas Compartment) block, a continuous femoral nerve block, and the combination of a continuous femoral and sciatic nerve block," *Regional Anesthesia and Pain Medicine*, vol. 30, no. 5, pp. 434–445, 2005.

[215] J. E. Paul, A. Arya, L. Hurlburt et al., "Femoral nerve block improves analgesia outcomes after total knee arthroplasty: a meta-analysis of randomized controlled trials," *Anesthesiology*, vol. 113, no. 5, pp. 1144–1162, 2010.

[216] F. V. Salinas, S. S. Liu, and M. F. Mulroy, "The effect of single-injection femoral nerve block versus continuous femoral nerve block after total knee arthroplasty on hospital length of stay and long-term functional recovery within an established clinical pathway," *Anesthesia and Analgesia*, vol. 102, no. 4, pp. 1234–1239, 2006.

[217] A. Hadzic, T. T. Houle, X. Capdevila, and B. M. Ilfeld, "Femoral nerve block for analgesia in patients having knee arthroplasty," *Anesthesiology*, vol. 113, no. 5, pp. 1014–1015, 2010.

[218] M. J. Barrington, D. J. Olive, and R. Kluger, "Inappropriate conclusion from meta-analysis of randomized controlled trials," *Anesthesiology*, vol. 114, no. 6, pp. 1494–1495, 2011.

[219] L. Collins, A. Halwani, and H. Vaghadia, "Impact of a regional anesthesia analgesia program for outpatient foot surgery," *Canadian Journal of Anaesthesia*, vol. 46, no. 9, pp. 840–845, 1999.

[220] S. M. Klein, R. Pietrobon, K. C. Nielsen, D. S. Warner, R. A. Greengrass, and S. M. Steele, "Peripheral nerve blockade with long-acting local anesthetics: a survey of the Society for Ambulatory Anesthesia," *Anesthesia and Analgesia*, vol. 94, no. 1, pp. 71–76, 2002.

[221] D. Zaric, K. Boysen, J. Christiansen, U. Haastrup, H. Kofoed, and N. Rawal, "Continuous popliteal sciatic nerve block for outpatient foot surgery—a randomized, controlled trial," *Acta Anaesthesiologica Scandinavica*, vol. 48, no. 3, pp. 337–341, 2004.

[222] P. F. White, T. Issioui, G. D. Skrivanek, J. S. Early, and C. Wakefield, "The use of a continuous popliteal sciatic nerve block after surgery involving the foot and ankle: does it improve the quality of recovery?" *Anesthesia and Analgesia*, vol. 97, no. 5, pp. 1303–1309, 2003.

[223] J. E. Chelly, J. Greger, A. Casati, T. Al-Samsam, W. McGarvey, and T. Clanton, "Continuous lateral sciatic blocks for acute postoperative pain management after major ankle and foot surgery," *Foot and Ankle International*, vol. 23, no. 8, pp. 749–752, 2002.

[224] K. Rongstad, R. A. Mann, D. Prieskorn, S. Nichelson, and G. Horton, "Popliteal sciatic nerve block for postoperative analgesia," *Foot and Ankle International*, vol. 17, no. 7, pp. 378–382, 1996.

[225] D. H. McLeod, D. H. W. Wong, R. J. Claridge, and P. M. Merrick, "Lateral popliteal sciatic nerve block compared with subcutaneous infiltration for analgesia following foot surgery," *Canadian Journal of Anaesthesia*, vol. 41, no. 8, pp. 673–676, 1994.

[226] D. M. Grosser, M. J. Herr, R. J. Claridge, and L. G. Barker, "Preoperative lateral popliteal nerve block for intraoperative and postoperative pain control in elective foot and ankle surgery: a prospective analysis," *Foot and Ankle International*, vol. 28, no. 12, pp. 1271–1275, 2007.

[227] B. M. Ilfeld, T. W. Wright, F. K. Enneking, and T. E. Morey, "Joint range of motion after total shoulder arthroplasty with and without a continuous interscalene nerve block: a retrospective, case-control study," *Regional Anesthesia and Pain Medicine*, vol. 30, no. 5, pp. 429–433, 2005.

[228] M. L. De Ruyter, K. E. Brueilly, B. A. Harrison, R. A. Greengrass, J. D. Putzke, and M. P. Brodersen, "A pilot study on continuous femoral perineural catheter for analgesia after total knee arthroplasty: the effect on physical rehabilitation and outcomes," *Journal of Arthroplasty*, vol. 21, no. 8, pp. 1111–1117, 2006.

[229] C. Raimer, K. Priem, A. A. Wiese et al., "Continuous psoas and sciatic block after knee arthroplasty: good effects compared to epidural analgesia or i.v. opioid analgesia: a

prospective study of 63 patients," *Acta Orthopaedica*, vol. 78, no. 2, pp. 193–200, 2007.

[230] F. J. Singelyn, M. Deyaert, D. Joris, E. Pendeville, and J. M. Gouverneur, "Effects of intravenous patient-controlled analgesia with morphine, continuous epidural analgesia, and continuous three-in-one block on postoperative pain and knee rehabilitation after unilateral total knee arthroplasty," *Anesthesia and Analgesia*, vol. 87, no. 1, pp. 88–92, 1998.

[231] F. Carli, A. Clemente, J. F. Asenjo et al., "Analgesia and functional outcome after total knee arthroplasty: periarticular infiltration vs continuous femoral nerve block," *British Journal of Anaesthesia*, vol. 105, no. 2, pp. 185–195, 2010.

[232] B. M. Ilfeld, S. T. Ball, P. F. Gearen et al., "Health-related quality of life after hip arthroplasty with and without an extended-duration continuous posterior lumbar plexus nerve block: a prospective, 1-year follow-up of a randomized, triple-masked, placebo-controlled study," *Anesthesia and Analgesia*, vol. 109, no. 2, pp. 586–591, 2009.

[233] L. Kadic, M. C. Boonstra, M. C. De Waal Malefijt, S. J. Lako, J. Van Egmond, and J. J. Driessen, "Continuous femoral nerve block after total knee arthroplasty?" *Acta Anaesthesiologica Scandinavica*, vol. 53, no. 7, pp. 914–920, 2009.

[234] B. A. Williams, Q. Dang, J. E. Bost et al., "General health and knee function outcomes from 7 days to 12 weeks after spinal anesthesia and multimodal analgesia for anterior cruciate ligament reconstruction," *Anesthesia and Analgesia*, vol. 108, no. 4, pp. 1296–1302, 2009.

[235] B. M. Ilfeld, R. S. Meyer, L. T. Le et al., "Health-related quality of life after tricompartment knee arthroplasty with and without an extended-duration continuous femoral nerve block: a prospective, 1-year follow-up of a randomized, triple-masked, placebo-controlled study," *Anesthesia and Analgesia*, vol. 108, no. 4, pp. 1320–1325, 2009.

[236] B. M. Ilfeld, J. J. Shuster, D. W. Theriaque et al., "Long-term pain, stiffness, and functional disability after total knee arthroplasty with and without an extended ambulatory continuous femoral nerve block: a prospective, 1-year follow-up of a multicenter, randomized, triple-masked, placebo-controlled trial," *Regional Anesthesia and Pain Medicine*, vol. 36, no. 2, pp. 116–120, 2011.

[237] C. F. Shum, N. N. Lo, S. J. Yeo, K. Y. Yang, H. C. Chong, and S. N. Yeo, "Continuous femoral nerve block in total knee arthroplasty: immediate and two-year outcomes," *Journal of Arthroplasty*, vol. 24, no. 2, pp. 204–209, 2009.

[238] S. E. Mason, A. Noel-Storr, and C. W. Ritchie, "The impact of general and regional anesthesia on the incidence of post-operative cognitive dysfunction and post-operative delirium: a systematic review with meta-analysis," *Journal of Alzheimer's Disease*, vol. 22, no. 3, pp. S67–S79, 2010.

[239] A. Ganesh, J. B. Rose, L. Wells et al., "Continuous peripheral nerve blockade for inpatient and outpatient postoperative analgesia in children," *Anesthesia and Analgesia*, vol. 105, no. 5, pp. 1234–1242, 2007.

[240] B. M. Ilfeld and F. K. Enneking, "Continuous peripheral nerve blocks at home: a review," *Anesthesia and Analgesia*, vol. 100, no. 6, pp. 1822–1833, 2005.

[241] D. D. Denson, P. P. Raj, and F. Saldahna, "Continuous perineural infusion of bupivacaine for prolonged analgesia: pharmacokinetic considerations," *International Journal of Clinical Pharmacology Therapy and Toxicology*, vol. 21, no. 12, pp. 591–597, 1983.

[242] C. Gonano, S. C. Kettner, M. Ernstbrunner, K. Schebesta, A. Chiari, and P. Marhofer, "Comparison of economical aspects of interscalene brachial plexus blockade and general anaesthesia for arthroscopic shoulder surgery," *British Journal of Anaesthesia*, vol. 103, no. 3, pp. 428–433, 2009.

[243] B. A. Williams, M. L. Kentor, M. T. Vogt et al., "Economics of nerve block pain management after anterior cruciate ligament reconstruction: potential hospital cost savings via associated postanesthesia care unit bypass and same-day discharge," *Anesthesiology*, vol. 100, no. 3, pp. 697–706, 2004.

[244] A. Hadzic, B. A. Williams, P. E. Karaca et al., "For outpatient rotator cuff surgery, nerve block anesthesia provides superior same-day recovery over general anesthesia," *Anesthesiology*, vol. 102, no. 5, pp. 1001–1007, 2005.

[245] A. Hadzic, P. E. Karaca, P. Hobeika et al., "Peripheral nerve blocks result in superior recovery profile compared with general anesthesia in outpatient knee arthroscopy," *Anesthesia and Analgesia*, vol. 100, no. 4, pp. 976–981, 2005.

[246] M. J. Fredrickson and A. W. Stewart, "Continuous interscalene analgesia for rotator cuff repair: a retrospective comparison of effectiveness and cost in 205 patients from a multi-provider private practice setting," *Anaesthesia and Intensive Care*, vol. 36, no. 6, pp. 786–791, 2008.

[247] B. M. Ilfeld, E. R. Mariano, B. A. Williams, J. N. Woodard, and A. Macario, "Hospitalization costs of total knee arthroplasty with a continuous femoral nerve block provided only in the hospital versus on an ambulatory basis: a retrospective, case-control, cost-minimization analysis," *Regional Anesthesia and Pain Medicine*, vol. 32, no. 1, pp. 46–54, 2007.

[248] M. C. Pourtales, H. Kuntzmann, F. Bertrand, T. Pottecher, S. Gouzou, and P. Liverneaux, "Continuous at-home postoperative analgesia using a catheter in the case of hand surgery: preliminary study about 40 cases," *Chirurgie de la Main*, vol. 29, no. 2, pp. 82–87, 2010.

[249] B. M. Ilfeld, T. W. Wright, F. K. Enneking et al., "Total shoulder arthroplasty as an outpatient procedure using ambulatory perineural local anesthetic infusion: a pilot feasibility study," *Anesthesia and Analgesia*, vol. 101, no. 5, pp. 1319–1322, 2005.

[250] B. M. Ilfeld, P. F. Gearen, F. K. Enneking et al., "Total hip arthroplasty as an overnight-stay procedure using an ambulatory continuous psoas compartment nerve block: a prospective feasibility study," *Regional Anesthesia and Pain Medicine*, vol. 31, no. 2, pp. 113–118, 2006.

[251] J. E. Bost, B. A. Williams, M. T. Bottegal, Q. Dang, and D. M. Rubio, "The 8-item Short-Form Health Survey and the physical comfort composite score of the quality of recovery 40-item scale provide the most responsive assessments of pain, physical function, and mental function during the first 4 days after ambulatory knee surgery with regional anesthesia," *Anesthesia and Analgesia*, vol. 105, no. 6, pp. 1693–1700, 2007.

[252] X. Capdevila, P. Pirat, S. Bringuier et al., "Continuous peripheral nerve blocks in hospital wards after orthopedic surgery: a multicenter prospective analysis of the quality of postoperative analgesia and complications in 1,416 patients," *Anesthesiology*, vol. 103, no. 5, pp. 1035–1045, 2005.

[253] M. Neuburger, J. Breitbarth, F. Reisig, D. Lang, and J. Büttner, "Complications and adverse events in continuous peripheral regional anesthesia. Results of investigations on 3,491 catheters," *Anaesthesist*, vol. 55, no. 1, pp. 33–40, 2006.

[254] S. Ganapathy, R. A. Wasserman, J. T. Watson et al., "Modified continuous femoral three-in-one block for postoperative pain after total knee arthroplasty," *Anesthesia and Analgesia*, vol. 89, no. 5, pp. 1197–1202, 1999.

[255] B. M. Ilfeld, S. T. Ball, P. F. Gearen et al., "Ambulatory continuous posterior lumbar plexus nerve blocks after hip arthroplasty: a dual-center, randomized, triple-masked, placebo-controlled trial," *Anesthesiology*, vol. 109, no. 3, pp. 491–501, 2008.

[256] B. A. Williams, M. A. Bolland, S. L. Orebaugh, M. T. Bottegal, and M. L. Kentor, "Skin reactions at the femoral perineural catheter insertion site: retrospective summary of a randomized clinical trial," *Anesthesia and Analgesia*, vol. 104, no. 5, pp. 1309–1310, 2007.

[257] M. K. Tuominen, P. Pere, and P. H. Rosenberg, "Unintentional arterial catheterization and bupivacaine toxicity associated with continuous interscalene brachial plexus block," *Anesthesiology*, vol. 75, no. 2, pp. 356–358, 1991.

[258] V. Souron, Y. Reiland, A. De Traverse, L. Delaunay, and L. Lafosse, "Interpleural migration of an interscalene catheter," *Anesthesia and Analgesia*, vol. 97, no. 4, pp. 1200–1201, 2003.

[259] J. Rodríguez, M. Taboada, M. Blanco, J. Oliveira, M. Bárcena, and J. Alvarez, "Intraneural catheterization of the sciatic nerve in humans: a pilot study," *Regional Anesthesia and Pain Medicine*, vol. 33, no. 4, pp. 285–290, 2008.

[260] A. Faust, R. Fournier, O. Hagon, P. Hoffmeyer, and Z. Gamulin, "Partial sensory and motor deficit of ipsilateral lower limb after continuous interscalene brachial plexus block," *Anesthesia and Analgesia*, vol. 102, no. 1, pp. 288–290, 2006.

[261] B. Lekhak, C. Bartley, I. D. Conacher, and S. M. Nouraei, "Total spinal anaesthesia in association with insertion of a paravertebral catheter," *British Journal of Anaesthesia*, vol. 86, no. 2, pp. 280–282, 2001.

[262] R. M. Pousman, Z. Mansoor, and D. Sciard, "Total spinal anesthetic after continuous posterior lumbar plexus block," *Anesthesiology*, vol. 98, no. 5, pp. 1281–1282, 2003.

[263] R. J. Litz, O. Vicent, D. Wiessner, and A. R. Heller, "Misplacement of a psoas compartment catheter in the subarachnoid space," *Regional Anesthesia and Pain Medicine*, vol. 29, no. 1, pp. 60–64, 2004.

[264] C. R. Jenkins and M. K. Karmakar, "An unusual complication of interscalene brachial plexus catheterization: delayed catheter migration," *British Journal of Anaesthesia*, vol. 95, no. 4, pp. 535–537, 2005.

[265] W. Harrop-Griffiths, N. Denny, H. Jutzi et al., "Migration of interscalene catheter—not proven," *British Journal of Anaesthesia*, vol. 96, no. 2, pp. 266–267, 2006.

[266] V. Compère, J. F. Legrand, P. G. Guitard et al., "Bacterial colonization after tunneling in 402 perineural catheters: a prospective study," *Anesthesia and Analgesia*, vol. 108, no. 4, pp. 1326–1330, 2009.

[267] P. Cuvillon, J. Ripart, L. Lalourcey et al., "The continuous femoral nerve block catheter for postoperative analgesia: bacterial colonization, infectious rate and adverse effects," *Anesthesia and Analgesia*, vol. 93, no. 4, pp. 1045–1049, 2001.

[268] M. Neuburger, J. Büttner, S. Blumenthal, J. Breitbarth, and A. Borgeat, "Inflammation and infection complications of 2285 perineural catheters: a prospective study," *Acta Anaesthesiologica Scandinavica*, vol. 51, no. 1, pp. 108–114, 2007.

[269] X. Capdevila, S. Bringuier, and A. Borgeat, "Infectious risk of continuous peripheral nerve blocks," *Anesthesiology*, vol. 110, no. 1, pp. 182–188, 2009.

[270] G. Ekatodramis and A. Borgeat, "Subcutaneous tunneling of the interscalene catheter," *Canadian Journal of Anaesthesia*, vol. 47, no. 7, pp. 716–717, 2000.

[271] S. R. Clendenen, C. B. Robards, R. D. Wang, and R. A. Greengrass, "Continuous interscalene block associated with neck hematoma and postoperative sepsis," *Anesthesia and Analgesia*, vol. 110, no. 4, pp. 1236–1238, 2010.

[272] X. Capdevila, S. Jaber, P. Pesonen, A. Borgeat, and J. J. Eledjam, "Acute neck cellulitis and mediastinitis complicating a continuous interscalene block," *Anesthesia and Analgesia*, vol. 107, no. 4, pp. 1419–1421, 2008.

[273] A. Borgeat, G. Ekatodramis, F. Kalberer, and C. Benz, "Acute and nonacute complications associated with interscalene block and shoulder surgery," *Anesthesiology*, vol. 95, no. 4, pp. 875–880, 2001.

[274] M. Wiegel, U. Gottschaldt, R. Hennebach, T. Hirschberg, and A. Reske, "Complications and adverse effects associated with continuous peripheral nerve blocks in orthopedic patients," *Anesthesia and Analgesia*, vol. 104, no. 6, pp. 1578–1582, 2007.

[275] A. Dullenkopf, P. Zingg, A. Curt, and A. Borgeat, "Persistent neurological deficit of the upper extremity after a shoulder operation under general anaesthesia combined with a preoperatively placed interscalene catheter," *Anaesthesist*, vol. 51, no. 7, pp. 547–551, 2002.

[276] J. R. Hebl, J. A. Dilger, D. E. Byer et al., "A pre-emptive multimodal pathway featuring peripheral nerve block improves perioperative outcomes after major orthopedic surgery," *Regional Anesthesia and Pain Medicine*, vol. 33, no. 6, pp. 510–517, 2008.

[277] B. D. Bergman, J. R. Hebl, J. Kent, and T. T. Horlocker, "Neurologic complications of 405 consecutive continuous axillary catheters," *Anesthesia and Analgesia*, vol. 96, no. 1, pp. 247–252, 2003.

[278] S. Dhir, S. Ganapathy, P. Lindsay, and G. S. Athwal, "Case report: ropivacaine neurotoxicity at clinical doses in interscalene brachial plexus block," *Canadian Journal of Anesthesia*, vol. 54, no. 11, pp. 912–916, 2007.

[279] V. Compère, N. Rey, O. Baert et al., "Major complications after 400 continuous popliteal sciatic nerve blocks for postoperative analgesia," *Acta Anaesthesiologica Scandinavica*, vol. 53, no. 3, pp. 339–345, 2009.

[280] Q. Hogan, R. Dotson, S. Erickson, R. Kettler, and K. Hogan, "Local anesthetic myotoxicity: a case and review," *Anesthesiology*, vol. 80, no. 4, pp. 942–947, 1994.

[281] R. Werdehausen, S. Fazeli, S. Braun et al., "Apoptosis induction by different local anaesthetics in a neuroblastoma cell line," *British Journal of Anaesthesia*, vol. 103, no. 5, pp. 711–718, 2009.

[282] J. S. Kroin, A. Buvanendran, D. K. Williams et al., "Local anesthetic sciatic nerve block and nerve fiber damage in diabetic rats," *Regional Anesthesia and Pain Medicine*, vol. 35, no. 4, pp. 343–350, 2010.

[283] B. A. Williams and B. B. Murinson, "Diabetes mellitus and subclinical neuropathy: a call for new paths in peripheral nerve block research," *Anesthesiology*, vol. 109, no. 3, pp. 361–362, 2008.

[284] S. Blumenthal, A. Borgeat, K. Maurer et al., "Preexisting subclinical neuropathy as a risk factor for nerve injury after continuous ropivacaine administration through a femoral nerve catheter," *Anesthesiology*, vol. 105, no. 5, pp. 1053–1056, 2006.

[285] H. M. Nguyen and A. L. Goldin, "Sodium channel carboxyl-terminal residue regulates fast inactivation," *Journal of Biological Chemistry*, vol. 285, no. 12, pp. 9077–9089, 2010.

[286] S. England, "Voltage-gated sodium channels: the search for subtype-selective analgesics," *Expert Opinion on Investigational Drugs*, vol. 17, no. 12, pp. 1849–1864, 2008.

[287] J. Lai, F. Porreca, J. C. Hunter, and M. S. Gold, "Voltage-gated sodium channels and hyperalgesia," *Annual Review of Pharmacology and Toxicology*, vol. 44, pp. 371–397, 2004.

[288] E. A. Shipton, "New formulations of local anaesthetics-Part i," *Anesthesiology Research and Practice*, vol. 2012, Article ID 546409, 11 pages, 2012.

[289] S. A. Grant, "The Holy Grail: long-acting local anaesthetics and liposomes," *Best Practice and Research: Clinical Anaesthesiology*, vol. 16, no. 2, pp. 345–352, 2002.

[290] P. Mura, F. Maestrelli, M. L. González-Rodríguez, I. Michelacci, C. Ghelardini, and A. M. Rabasco, "Development, characterization and in vivo evaluation of benzocaine-loaded liposomes," *European Journal of Pharmaceutics and Biopharmaceutics*, vol. 67, no. 1, pp. 86–95, 2007.

[291] C. F. Weiniger, M. Golovanevski, M. Sokolsky-Papkov, and A. J. Domb, "Review of prolonged local anesthetic action," *Expert Opinion on Drug Delivery*, vol. 7, no. 6, pp. 737–752, 2010.

[292] G. J. Grant, Y. Barenholz, E. M. Bolotin et al., "A novel liposomal bupivacaine formulation to produce ultralong-acting analgesia," *Anesthesiology*, vol. 101, no. 1, pp. 133–137, 2004.

[293] J. G. Boogaerts, N. D. Lafont, A. G. Declercq et al., "Epidural administration of liposome-associated bupivacaine for the management of postsurgical pain: a first study," *Journal of Clinical Anesthesia*, vol. 6, no. 4, pp. 315–320, 1994.

[294] B. R. Swenson, A. Gottschalk, L. T. Wells et al., "Intravenous lidocaine is as effective as epidural bupivacaine in reducing ileus duration, hospital stay, and pain after open colon resection: a randomized clinical trial," *Regional Anesthesia and Pain Medicine*, vol. 35, no. 4, pp. 370–376, 2010.

[295] G. S. De Oliveira, S. Ahmad, J. C. Schink, D. K. Singh, P. C. Fitzgerald, and R. J. McCarthy, "Intraoperative neuraxial anesthesia but not postoperative neuraxial analgesia is associated with increased relapse-free survival in ovarian cancer patients after primary cytoreductive surgery," *Regional Anesthesia and Pain Medicine*, vol. 36, no. 3, pp. 271–277, 2011.

11

A Study to Compare the Analgesic Efficacy of Intrathecal Bupivacaine Alone with Intrathecal Bupivacaine Midazolam Combination in Patients undergoing Elective Infraumbilical Surgery

Anirban Chattopadhyay,[1] Souvik Maitra,[2] Suvadeep Sen,[2] Sulagna Bhattacharjee,[3] Amitava Layek,[3] Sugata Pal,[3] and Kakali Ghosh[4]

[1] *Lilavati Hospital & Research Center, Mumbai 400050, India*
[2] *Department of Anaesthesiology and Intensive Care, AIIMS, New Delhi 110029, India*
[3] *Department of Anaesthesiology, IPGME&R and SSKM Hospital, Kolkata 700020, India*
[4] *Department of Cardiac Anaesthesiology, IPGME&R and SSKM Hospital, Kolkata 700020, India*

Correspondence should be addressed to Suvadeep Sen; s.sen2011@hotmail.com

Academic Editor: D. John Doyle

Spinal anaesthesia, which is one of the techniques for infraumbilical surgeries, is most commonly criticized for limited duration of postoperative analgesia. Several adjuvants have been tried along with local anesthetic for prolonging the duration of analgesia. In this study, we have observed the effect of midazolam as an adjuvant in patients undergoing infraumbilical surgery. In this prospective, randomized, double blinded, and parallel group and open label study of 90 adult patients aged 18–60 years, of American Society of Anaesthesiologists (ASA) status I and II, scheduled for elective infraumbilical surgery, were randomly allocated in two groups. Each patient in group "B" received hyperbaric bupivacaine 12.5 mg along with 0.4 mL of normal saline in the subarachnoid block, and patients of group "BM" received 12.5 mg hyperbaric bupivacaine along with preservative free midazolam 0.4 mL (2 mg). We found that use of midazolam as adjuvant with the local anesthetic in spinal anaesthesia significantly increases the duration of analgesia (median 320 min versus 220 min) and motor block (median 255 min versus 195 min) but decreases the incidence of postoperative nausea-vomiting (PONV).

1. Introduction

Spinal subarachnoid block is one of the most versatile regional anesthesia techniques available today. Regional anesthesia offers several advantages over general anesthesia—blunts stress response to surgery, decreases intraoperative blood loss, lowers the incidence of postoperative thromboembolic events, and provides analgesia in early postoperative period. Subarachnoid block provides adequate anesthesia for patients undergoing infraumbilical surgery.

Among the local anesthetics, 0.5% hyperbaric bupivacaine is the most commonly used drug for spinal anesthesia [1]. The most important disadvantage of single injection SAB is the limited duration. Adjuvants have long been used along with local anesthetics to prolong the duration of anesthesia and analgesia. Prolongation of pain relief by various adjuvants like opioids (like morphine [2], fentanyl [3]), ketamine [4], clonidine [5], and neostigmine [6] were investigated by various investigators. However, each drug has its limitations and side effects, and the need for an alternative methods and drugs always exist.

Discovery of benzodiazepine receptors in spinal cord in 1977 [7] triggered the use of intrathecal midazolam for prolongation of spinal anesthesia. In vitro autoradiography has shown that there is a high density of benzodiazepine (GABA-A) receptors in Lamina II of the dorsal horn in the human spinal cord, suggesting a possible role in pain modulation [8].

So far different animal studies have revealed no damage to the spinal cord, nerve roots, or meninges and in vitro studies suggested that clinically useful doses of intrathecal midazolam are unlikely to be neurotoxic [9–12].

2. Aims and Objective

In this study, intrathecal analgesia with 0.5% hyperbaric bupivacaine 2.5 mL with 0.4 mL 0.9% normal saline has been compared with 0.5% hyperbaric bupivacaine 2.5 mL plus 0.4 mL (2 mg) preservative free midazolam in a predetermined dose, and two groups will be compared in terms of duration of effective analgesia by time interval between the onset of intrathecal block to time for request for first rescue analgesia and by VAS pain score. Perioperative sedation, hemodynamic changes, peak height of block, time for regression of motor block to sacral dermatome, and any obvious side effect were also assessed.

3. Specific Objectives of This Study

(1) To compare duration of effective analgesia between the two groups.

(2) To assess the perioperative hemodynamic changes.

(3) To observe perioperative sedation and any obvious adverse effects.

4. Methodology

After obtaining institutional ethics committee clearance and written informed consent from the patients, 90 adult patients of ASA physical status I and II and aged 18–60 years undergoing elective infraumbilical (gynecologic/urologic) under spinal subarachnoid block anesthesia were included into the study. Patients refusing to participate, with known allergic to local anaesthetic and midazolam, suffering from chronic pain, and pregnant women were excluded from the study. Patients having the level of sensory block below T10 after 15 minutes of subarachnoid block or having VAS pain score greater than 40 at any point of time during intraoperative period were offered general anesthesia for the rest of the procedure. This subset of patients were planned to regard as "incomplete block" category and planned to exclude from the final data analysis.

4.1. Calculation of Sample Size. Sample size estimation was done using power and sample size calculation software (version 2.1.30, DuPont & Plummer, February 2003). Based on clinical experience and review of the literature an educated guess was made that a 30-minute difference of mean duration of analgesia between two groups would be statistically significant. Within group standard deviation was assumed to be 60. Using this data and assuming a study power of 90% and probability of type I error of 5%, a sample size of 85 patients was found to be required for obtaining statistically significant mean difference of mean duration of analgesia in two groups. So assuming equal distribution of patients in both groups a total number of 90 patients were incorporated in the study (n = 90), with 45 patients in each group (n = 45).

4.2. Randomization and Blinding. A computer-generated randomization table (Microsoft Excel 2007 software) was used to assign each patient into either group "BM" (patients receiving bupivacaine and midazolam during subarachnoid block) or group "B" (patient receiving bupivacaine only). For ensuring blinding, randomly allocated coded syringes of drugs were prepared by an anesthesiologist who did not perform subarachnoid block or record the outcome intraoperative and postoperative period. The investigator and the anaesthesiologist performing the study were blinded to the content of the drugs contained in the syringes. The solution intended for group BM contained 2.5 mL hyperbaric bupivacaine (0.5%) plus 0.4 mL (2 mg) preservative free midazolam, and solution intended for group B contained 2.5 mL hyperbaric bupivacaine (0.5%) plus 0.4 mL normal saline (0.9%). The total volume of subarachnoid injection in either group was 2.9 mL.

4.3. Study Protocol. Explanation regarding the procedure and study, education regarding VAS score, and necessary written informed consent were taken during the preoperative checkup ad visit. Standard ASA fasting guidelines were followed in all patients. Patients were not given any premedication.

On arrival at the operation theatre, intravenous access was established with an 18G intravenous cannula in a large vein of forearm, and coloading was done with prewarmed ringer's lactate solution 15 mL/kg body weight, that was infused over 15 minutes.

4.3.1. Procedure of Intrathecal Injection. Under strict aseptic precautions a 25G Quincke spinal needle was introduced into L3-L4 or L4-L5 intervertebral space in midline approach in lateral posture, and, after confirming free flow of CSF, predetermined 2.9 mL of drug solution was injected. The rate of injection was kept 0.2 mL/second. At the end of the injection, a small sterile dressing was applied and patients were placed supine with a pillow under the head and neck soon after administration of intrathecal drugs.

Oxygen (2 L/min) was administered throughout the procedure via nasal cannula. Intraoperative fluid management was done in relation to body weight of the patient, vital signs, and intraoperative losses. At the end of the surgery, the patients were shifted to the postoperative ward for clinical monitoring of vital signs, appropriate fluid therapy, and other treatment.

Assessments of parameters include the following.

(i) Height of sensory block (by the ability to perceive cold sensation with spirit soaked blunt tipped cotton swab in midaxillary line bilaterally) every 5 minutes for first 30 minutes and then at 15-minute interval till the end of surgery and hourly thereafter till rescue analgesic was required. Duration of sensory analgesia was calculated with two dermatome regression from peak block height for each patient.

(ii) Motor block was assessed using a 6-point-modified Bromage scale [13] (1 = complete motor block; 2 = almost complete blockade, the patient is able to move feet only; 3 = partial motor blockade, the patient is able to move the knees; 4 = detectable weakness of hip flexion, the patient is able to raise the leg but is unable to keep it raised; 5 = no detectable weakness of hip flexion; 6 = no weakness at all). These measurements were performed at 5, 10, and 15 min after intrathecal injection and then every 15 min after surgery until no motor blockade regressed to sacral dermatome. Duration of motor block was calculated till modified Bromage value reached six for each patient.

(iii) Hemodynamic changes—heart rate, blood pressures every 5 minutes for first 30 minutes and then at 10-minute interval till the end of surgery and hourly there after till rescue analgesic are required. Only hemodynamic changes that require treatment as described below were considered significant.

(iv) Visual analogue scale (VAS) score is a tool for assessment of analgesia in the intraoperative and postoperative period. VAS pain score is a linear pain scoring tool ranging from 0 to 100 mm where patients marked a circle around a point (0, 10, 20, 30, etc.) on a 100 mm scale. Duration of analgesia was defined from the administration of subarachnoid block till patient demanded for rescue analgesia or VAS greater than 40 which ever earlier.

(v) Level of sedation (assessed by four-point ordinal scale 0 = awake, alert; 1 = drowsy, responds to call; 2 = drowsy, responds to tactile stimulus; 3 = deep sedation, unresponsive) 5 minutes for first 30 minutes and then at 10-minute interval till the end of surgery and hourly there after till rescue analgesic was required.

(vi) Side effects such as nausea and vomiting, pruritus, and respiratory depression were observed in the intraoperative period and in the postoperative period till requirement of rescue analgesic.

Episodes of intraoperative side effects such as hypotension (a decrease in systolic blood pressure of more than 20% from baseline) and bradycardia (HR < 45/min) were recorded. Hypotension was treated with bolus of ringer lactate and incremental doses of mephentermine 6 mg IV, and bradycardia was treated with atropine sulphate 0.6 mg IV bolus.

Rescue analgesia was administered postoperatively when VAS score >40 or when patient requested for analgesia with diclofenac sodium 1 mg/kg body weight intramuscularly. Time from institution of successful subarachnoid block to request for first rescue analgesia was recorded. The study was terminated when patient requested for first rescue analgesia or VAS reached greater than 40 which ever earlier.

4.4. Analysis of Data. All raw data of study parameters were entered into a Microsoft excel spread sheet and analyzed using IBM SPSS v17.0. The categorical variables were analyzed using Mantel-Haenszel chi-square test or Fischer exact test as appropriate. Parametrical numerical valuables were analyzed using independent sample t-test. All statistical analysis was two tailed, and a P value of <0.05 was considered statistically significant.

TABLE 1: Demographic profiles of the patients in two groups.

	Group B ($n = 45$)	Group BM ($n = 45$)	Significance
Age (year)	46.56 ± 12.63	42.71 ± 11.75	NS
Height (cm)	160.71 ± 5.59	161.89 ± 6.25	NS
Weight (kg)	58.37 ± 5.95	58.91 ± 6.25	NS
Sex (male/female)	30/15	31/14	NS
ASA PS (I/II)	24/21	25/20	NS
Duration of surgery (min)	79.78 ± 31.5	83.22 ± 31.10	NS
Types of surgery (myomectomy/vaginal hysterectomy/TURP/TURBT)	8/7/15/15	7/7/16/15	$P = 0.99^{\#}$

[#] Fisher exact probability test.
TURP: transurethral resection of prostate, TURBT: transurethral resection of bladder tumor.

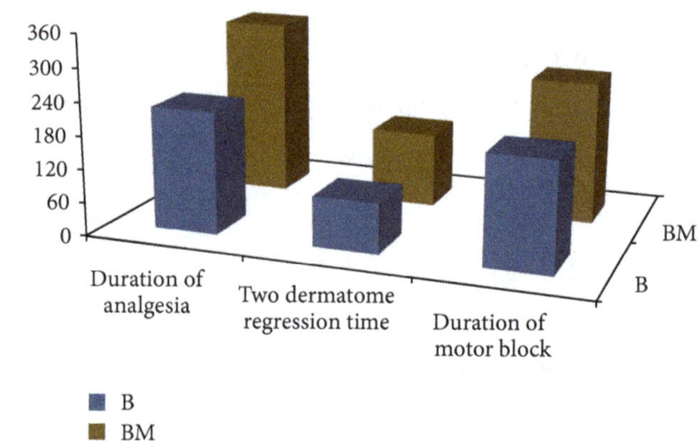

FIGURE 1: Comparison of median duration of analgesia, two dermatome regression time, and duration of motor block in two groups.

5. Results

The patients in both groups were comparable in terms of demographic profile, that is, age, height, weight, sex, ASA PS distribution, duration of surgery, and types of surgeries (Table 1).

Twenty eight patients in group B and thirty one patients in group BM had at least one episode of hypotension requiring fluid bolus or vasopressor; however, no statistical difference has been found. Three patients in group B and two patients in group BM had one episode of bradycardia and required intravenous atropine injection.

Median peak height of sensory block was up to T4 dermatome in both groups. However, duration of motor block as defined above (median 255 min versus 195 min) and two dermatome regression time of sensory block (median 135 min versus 90 min) have been found to be significantly higher in BM group (Table 2, Figure 1).

Incidence of intraoperative sedation was higher in patients who received midazolam, but the incidence of intraoperative nausea-vomiting and incomplete sensory block (Table 3) was similar between two groups.

TABLE 2: Characteristics of subarachnoid block in patients of two groups.

	Group B ($n = 45$)	Group BM ($n = 45$)	Significance
Peak height of sensory block	T4	T4	NS
Two dermatome regression time of sensory block (in minute)	90 (60–135)	135 (105–165)	$P = 0.000^*$
Duration of motor block (in minute)	195 (165–225)	255 (210–285)	$P = 0.000^*$
Duration of effective analgesia (in minute)	220 (165–265)	320 (250–450)	$P = 0.000^*$

*Mann-Whitney U test.

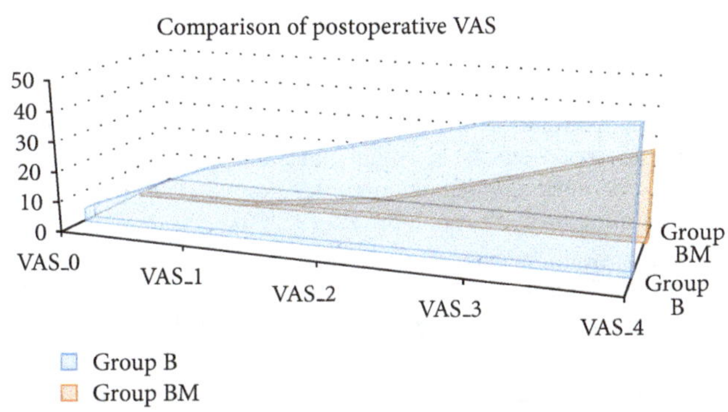

FIGURE 2: Area under curve of VAS-hr in two groups.

The duration of analgesia was significantly higher in patients receiving bupivacaine and midazolam in comparison to bupivacaine alone (median 320 min versus 220 min) (Figure 1). VAS score was found to be significantly higher ($P < 0.05$) among the patients who received only bupivacaine in 0 (immediately in the postoperative recovery room), 1st, 2nd, 3rd, and 4th hours in the postoperative period. After 4th hour, the comparison was not possible because all patients in group B had received rescue analgesia by that time. Area under curve for the postoperative VAS score-time (mm-hr) is also significantly higher in group B (119.8 versus 37.48) (Figure 2). Incidence of PONV is significantly lower in patients who received intrathecal midazolam; however, sedation score was similar in the postoperative period and none of the patients experienced pruritus or respiratory depression in the postoperative period (Table 4).

6. Discussion

The baseline characteristics in either group were similar from statistical standpoint. Considering the intraoperative hemodynamic variables the result of our study is comparable with studies done by Batra et al. [14], Kim and Lee [15], Agrawal et al. [16], and Gupta et al. [17] who also did not find statistically significant difference in heart rate, arterial blood pressure in their studies. Incidence of hypotension and bradycardia is found to be similar in both groups.

TABLE 3: Comparison of intraoperative events in patients of two groups.

	Group B ($n = 45$)	Group BM ($n = 45$)	Significance
Hypotension	28/45	31/45	NS*
Bradycardia	3/45	2/45	NS*
Nausea-vomiting	5/45	2/45	NS*
Respiratory depression	0/45	0/45	NS*
Sedation (0/1/2/3)	43/2/0/0	35/6/4/0	$P = 0.017^+$
Incomplete block	0/45	0/45	NS

*Mantel-Haenszel chi-square.
+Fisher exact probability test.

TABLE 4: Comparison of postoperative complications in two groups.

	Group B ($n = 45$)	Group BM ($n = 45$)	Significance
PONV	9/45	2/45	$P = 0.025^*$
Sedation (0/1/2/3)	44/1/0/0	42/2/1/0	NS
Respiratory depression	0/45	0/45	NS
Pruritus	0/45	0/45	NS

*Mantel-Haenszel chi-square.

The most significant finding of our study is a significant prolongation of sensory blockade which is reflected as the time to request first rescue analgesic and two dermatome regression time of sensory block, both of which were significantly higher in patients receiving midazolam as adjuvant. Batra et al. [14] in 1999 reported a similar finding; they concluded that intrathecal administration of midazolam along with bupivacaine produces better postoperative analgesia and a prolonged sensory blockade; however, they used a much smaller sample size. Kim and Lee [15] in 2001 in a meta-analysis concluded that addition of 1 or 2 mg of intrathecal midazolam prolonged the postoperative analgesic effect of bupivacaine by approximately 2 h and 4.5 h, respectively, compared with controls after hemorrhoidectomy, and this finding suggested a dose-dependent action of intrathecal midazolam. However, we should keep in mind that hemorrhoidectomy pain can be alleviated only by sacral sensory nerves. Our patients were undergoing infraumbilical gynecologic or urologic surgeries, and, for effective analgesia, these patients require blockade of lower thoracic and lumber dermatomes as well. However, we also found that intrathecal midazolam at a dose of 2 mg significantly prolongs the duration of motor block also which may be an important consideration where early ambulation is desirable. Bharti et al. [18] in 2003 reported a prolonged sensory and motor block following midazolam administration as adjuvant with bupivacaine in lower abdominal surgery.

We have found significant difference in sedation level in intraoperative period but not in the postoperative period. Whether intrathecal midazolam causes clinically significant sedation or not is a debatable issue; Yegin et al. [19] found that 2 mg intrathecal midazolam causes significant sedation, but others did not [14, 20]. We think that intraoperative sedation may be a desirable property of intrathecal midazolam.

We also have found that there is a decrease in the incidence of PONV in patients who received intrathecal midazolam. Prakash et al. [21] also reported similar findings in patients undergoing cesarean section. However, it should be interpreted with caution as none of the studies have adequate power to detect a difference in the incidence of PONV.

7. Conclusion

We conclude that the addition of 2 mg preservative free midazolam to 0.5% hyperbaric bupivacaine for subarachnoid block in infraumbilical surgery prolongs the duration of effective analgesia as compared to bupivacaine alone and delays the need for postoperative rescue analgesics without having any sedative effect, pruritus, or respiratory depression. The use of intrathecal midazolam also decreases the incidence of postoperative nausea-vomiting (PONV). Intrathecal midazolam in a dose of 2 mg does not have any clinically significant effect on perioperative hemodynamics.

Disclosure

The study has been registered under CTRI India, with registration number CTRI/2013/04/003600.

Conflict of Interests

The authors declare that they have no conflict of interests.

References

[1] G. E. Morgan Jr., M. S. Mikhail, M. J. Murray, and C. P. Larson Jr., *Clinical Anaesthesiology*, Lange, New York, NY, USA, 4th edition, 2002.

[2] P. H. Tan, Y. Y. Chia, Y. Lo, K. Liu, L. C. Yang, and T. H. Lee, "Intrathecal bupivacaine with morphine or neostigmine for postoperative analgesia after total knee replacement surgery," *Canadian Journal of Anesthesia*, vol. 48, no. 6, pp. 551–556, 2001.

[3] C. O. Hunt, J. S. Naulty, A. M. Badder et al., "Peri operative analgesia with subarachnoid fentanyl-bupivacaine for caesarian section," *Anaesthesiology*, vol. 71, no. 4, pp. 535–540, 1989.

[4] S. Karthival, SdhasivamS, A. Saxena, T. R. Kannah, and P. Ganjoop, "Effects of intrathecal ketamine added to bupivacaine for spinal anesthesia," *Anarsthesia*, vol. 55, no. 9, pp. 899–904, 2001.

[5] DobrydjnovI, K. Axelsson, J. Samarutel, and B. Holmstrom, "Post operative pain relief following intrathecal bupivcaine with intrathecal or oral clonidine," *Acta Anaesthesiologica Scandinavica*, vol. 46, no. 7, pp. 806–814, 2002.

[6] S. Liu, "Dose-response effects of spinal neostigmine added to bupivacaine spinal anesthesia in volunteers," *Anesthesiology*, vol. 90, no. 3, pp. 710–717, 1999.

[7] H. Mohler and T. Okada, "Benzodiazepine receptor: demonstration in the central nervous system," *Science*, vol. 198, no. 4319, pp. 849–851, 1977.

[8] R. L. M. Faull and J. W. Villiger, "Benzodiazepine receptors in the human spinal cord: a detailed anatomical and pharmacological study," *Neuroscience*, vol. 17, no. 3, pp. 791–802, 1986.

[9] M. E. Crawford, F. Molke Jensen, D. B. Toftdahl, and J. B. Madsen, "Direct spinal effect of intrathecal and extradural midazolam on visceral noxious stimulation in rabbits," *British Journal of Anaesthesia*, vol. 70, no. 6, pp. 642–646, 1993.

[10] T. Nishiyama, T. Matsukawa, and K. Hanoaka, "Acute phase histopathological study of spinally administered midazolamin cats," *Anesthesia and Analgesia*, vol. 89, no. 3, pp. 717–720, 1999.

[11] T. Nishiyama, N. Sugai, and K. Hanaoka, "*In vitro* changes in the transparency and pH of cerebrospinal fluid caused by adding midazolam," *European Journal of Anaesthesiology*, vol. 15, no. 1, pp. 27–31, 1998.

[12] A. P. Tucker, C. Lai, R. Nadeson, and C. S. Goodchild, "Intrathecal midazolam I: a cohort study investigation safety," *Anesthesia and Analgesia*, vol. 98, no. 6, pp. 1512–1520, 2004.

[13] T. W. Breen, T. Shapiro, B. Glass, D. Foster-Payne, and N. E. Oriol, "Epidural anesthesia for labor in an ambulatory patient," *Anesthesia and Analgesia*, vol. 77, no. 5, pp. 919–924, 1993.

[14] Y. K. Batra, K. Jain, P. Chari, M. S. Dhillon, B. Shaheen, and G. M. Reddy, "Addition of intrathecal midazolam to bupivacaine produces better post-operative analgesia without prolonging recovery," *International Journal of Clinical Pharmacology and Therapeutics*, vol. 37, no. 10, pp. 519–523, 1999.

[15] M. H. Kim and Y. M. Lee, "Intrathecal midazolam increases the analgesic effects of spinal blockade with bupivacaine in patients undergoing haemorrhoidectomy," *British Journal of Anaesthesia*, vol. 86, no. 1, pp. 77–79, 2001.

[16] N. Agrawal, Aushani, R. Sehgal, R. Kumar, and P. Bhadoria, "Effect of intrathecal midazolam bupivacaine on post-operative analgesia," *Indian Journal of Anaesthesia*, vol. 49, pp. 37–39, 2005.

[17] A. Gupta, S. Prakash, S. Deshpande, and K. S. Kale, "The effects of intrathecal midazolam 2.5 mg with hyperbaric bupivacaine on post operative pain relief in patient undergoing orthopaedic surgery," *The Internet Journal of Anesthesiology*, vol. 14, no. 2, pp. 189–192, 2007.

[18] N. Bharti, R. Madan, P. R. Mohanty, and H. L. kaul, "Intrathecal midazolam added to bupivacaine improves the duration and quality of spinal anaesthesia," *Acta Anaesthesiologica Scandinavica*, vol. 47, no. 9, pp. 1101–1105, 2003.

[19] A. Yegin, S. Sanli, L. Dosemeci, N. Kayacan, M. Akbas, and B. Karsli, "The analgesic and sedative effects of intrathecal midazolam in perianal surgery," *European Journal of Anaesthesiology*, vol. 21, no. 8, pp. 658–662, 2004.

[20] B. K. Shadangi, R. Garg, R. Pandey, and T. Das, "Effects of intrathecal midazolam in spinal anaesthesia: a prospective randomised case control study," *Singapore Medical Journal*, vol. 52, no. 6, pp. 432–435, 2011.

[21] S. Prakash, N. Joshi, A. R. Gogia, S. Prakash, and R. Singh, "Analgesic efficacy of twodoses of intrathecal midazolam with bupivacaine in patients undergoing cesarean delivery," *Regional Anesthesia and Pain Medicine*, vol. 31, no. 3, pp. 221–226, 2006.

12

Clinical Implications of the Transversus Abdominis Plane Block in Adults

Mark J. Young,[1] Andrew W. Gorlin,[2] Vicki E. Modest,[1,3] and Sadeq A. Quraishi[1,3]

[1] *Department of Anesthesiology, Critical Care and Pain Medicine, Massachusetts General Hospital, Boston, MA 02114, USA*
[2] *Department of Anesthesiology, Perioperative and Pain Medicine, Brigham and Women's Hospital, Boston, MA 02115, USA*
[3] *Harvard Medical School, Boston, MA 02115, USA*

Correspondence should be addressed to Sadeq A. Quraishi, squraishi@partners.org

Academic Editor: D. John Doyle

The transversus abdominis plane (TAP) block is a relatively new regional anesthesia technique that provides analgesia to the parietal peritoneum as well as the skin and muscles of the anterior abdominal wall. It has a high margin of safety and is technically simple to perform, especially under ultrasound guidance. A growing body of evidence supports the use of TAP blocks for a variety of abdominal procedures, yet, widespread adoption of this therapeutic adjunct has been slow. In part, this may be related to the limited sources for anesthesiologists to develop an appreciation for its sound anatomical basis and the versatility of its clinical application. As such, we provide a brief historical perspective on the TAP block, describe relevant anatomy, review current techniques, discuss pharmacologic considerations, and summarize the existing literature regarding its clinical utility with an emphasis on recently published studies that have not been included in other systematic reviews or meta-analyses.

1. Introduction

The transversus abdominis plane (TAP) block is a regional anesthesia technique that provides analgesia to the parietal peritoneum as well as the skin and muscles of the anterior abdominal wall [1]. First described just a decade ago, it has undergone several modifications, which have highlighted its potential utility for an increasing array of surgical procedures [2]. Despite a relatively low risk of complications and a high success rate using modern techniques, TAP blocks remain overwhelmingly underutilized [3]. Although the block is technically straightforward, there is inertia regarding its adoption into clinical practice. In part, this may be related to limited sources for anesthesiologists to develop a comprehensive understanding of the transversus abdominis plane. As such, we provide a brief historical perspective on the TAP block, describe relevant anatomy, review current techniques, discuss pharmacologic considerations, and summarize the existing literature regarding its clinical utility.

2. History

Rafi first described the TAP block in 2001 [2]. He portrayed it as a refined abdominal field block, with a targeted single shot anesthetic delivery into the TAP, a site traversed by relevant nerve branches. This was a significant advance from earlier strategies that required multiple injections [4]. In this approach, utilizing surface anatomical landmarks, the TAP was reached by first identifying the lumbar triangle of Petit (Figure 1), an area enclosed medially by the external oblique, posteriorly by the latissimus dorsi, and inferiorly by the iliac crest [2]. A 24-gauge, blunt-tipped, 2-inch needle was then advanced perpendicular to the skin through a preceding skin incision until a single confirmatory "pop" was appreciated. This sensation was thought to indicate proper needle depth for anesthetic delivery. In 2004, McDonnell et al. presented preliminary work on TAP blocks in cadavers and in healthy volunteers at the scientific meeting of the American Society of Anesthesiologists [5]. Although referred to as the

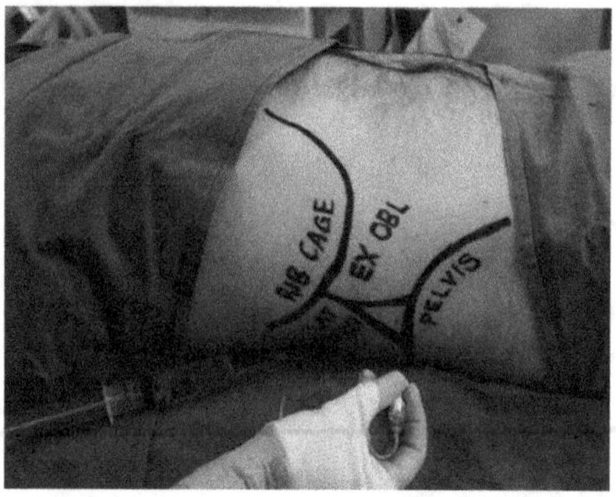

Figure 1: Surface anatomical landmarks can be utilized to identify the triangle of Petit [9]. Reproduced with permission.

regional abdominal field infiltration (RAFI) technique, the authors brought forward preliminary evidence to support the anatomical basis for TAP blocks and demonstrated sensory loss spanning the xiphoid to the pubic symphysis following delivery of local anesthetic to the TAP via the triangle of Petit. By the time the study was completed and published in 2007, McDonnell and his colleagues had already adopted the term TAP block and had demonstrated its analgesic utility in patients undergoing open retropubic prostatectomy [6–8].

3. Anatomy

The musculature of the lateral abdomen has three layers (Figure 2). From superficial to deep, they are the external oblique, the internal oblique, and the transversus abdominis muscles. On its course from medial to lateral, the internal oblique muscle slopes upward and creates a small gap above the iliac crest. It is this sloping edge, above the iliac crest, that defines the medial aspect of the lumbar triangle of Petit (Figure 1). Based on cadaveric dissections, Jankovic et al. noted that the location of the medial edge of the triangle varies significantly between individuals, but is always located at a point posterior to the midaxillary line [10]. The posterior edge of the triangle is the latissimus dorsi muscle. It is not uncommon for the triangle to be quite small or poorly defined. Often, the external oblique may overlap the medial edge of the latissimus dorsi muscle. The inferior aspect of the triangle is the iliac crest, and the peritoneum rests directly deep to the innermost muscle. The TAP is the fascial layer between the internal oblique and the transversus abdominis muscles. It exists as a continuous plane located at any point on the abdomen where the two innermost muscle layers exist. Anterior rami of thoracolumbar nerves that innervate the anterior abdominal wall pass through this plane as small, but well-defined neurovascular bundles. Furthermore, Rozen et al. described an extensive fascial layer, nonadherent to the deep surface of the internal oblique that bind down the nerves on its deep surface, superficial to the transversus abdominis muscle [11]. They also observed that, while nerve segments from T6-L1 reliably innervate the abdominal wall, individual nerve segments branch and communicate extensively with other nerve segments as they travel in the TAP. Moreover, they noted that nerve segments entered the TAP from the costal margin in an inferolateral distribution such that segments from T6 entered adjacent to the linea alba whereas segments from T9 entered near the anterior axillary line (Figure 3). Along the anterior axillary line, between the costal margin and the ileum, near the triangle of Petit, nerves running in the TAP originate strictly from T9-L1.

4. Technique

4.1. Anatomical Landmark-Based Approaches. In Rafi's classic description of the TAP block, surface anatomic landmarks were used to determine the needle insertion site within the lumbar triangle of Petit, and a single "pop" sensation served as an endpoint for appropriate needle depth [2]. Patients were placed in the supine position, and a finger was walked from the anterior superior iliac spine along the top of the iliac crest until it dipped slightly inward. On further posterior movement, the finger tip was felt to slip over the lateral border of the latissimus dorsi, where it is attached to the external lip of the iliac crest. At this location, the skin was first pierced anterior to the finger tip with an 18-gauge cutting needle at the level of the external lip, and then followed by a 24-guage, blunt-tipped, 2-inch needle, which was inserted perpendicular to the skin until it touched the bone of the external lip. The needle was then slowly advanced over the intermediate zone of the iliac crest until the definite "pop" was felt. This single "pop" method differs from the "double pop" method described by O'Donnell et al. in which the needle was inserted cephalad to the iliac crest and advanced until two distinct "pops" were appreciated [8]. The authors explained that a "double pop" resulted from the blunt needle passing through the "fascial extensions of the abdominal wall muscles (external and internal obliques) within the floor of the triangle of Petit [12]." All anatomical landmark-based approaches to the TAP make use of blunt-tipped needles to improve tactile sensitivity and appreciation for distinct "pop" sensations.

4.2. Ultrasound-Guided Approaches. An ultrasound-guided approach was first described in 2007 by Hebbard et al. [13]. The authors applied a transversely orientated ultrasound probe to the anterolateral abdominal wall where the three muscle layers are most distinct. After identification of the TAP between the internal oblique and transversus abdominis muscles, the probe was moved posterolaterally to lie across the midaxillary line just superior to the iliac crest (i.e., over the triangle of Petit). The block needle was then introduced anteriorly and advanced in an in-plane approach (Figure 4). Real-time ultrasonography facilitates easy needle visualization as it approaches and reaches the target fascial plane. A hypoechoic layer, created by injection of local anesthetic, is also easily visualized (Figure 5). Hebbard et al. also noted that the "pop" sensations in the classic approach could be imprecise due to anatomic variability,

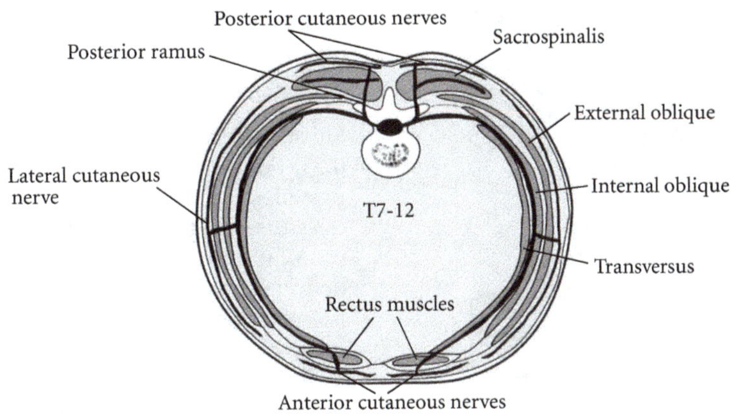

FIGURE 2: Transverse section of the abdominal wall demonstrating the relevant muscular structures and course of nerves (T7-T12) within the TAP [9]. Reproduced with permission.

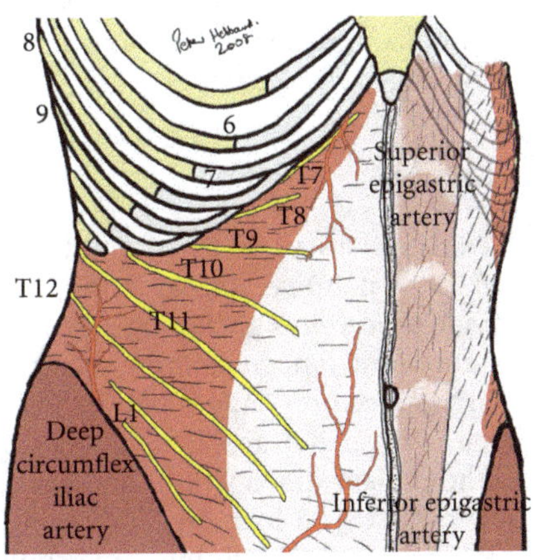

FIGURE 3: Typical distribution of nerves in the TAP. Generously shared from the personal files of Prof. P. Hebbard.

especially in patients with large BMI and, as such, concluded that real-time visualization of local anesthetic spread was likely to be a more definitive endpoint, as is often the case with other regional block techniques. This ultrasound-guided technique is commonly referred to as the posterior approach. In 2008, Hebbard described another ultrasound-guided TAP block technique designed for upper abdominal surgery referred to as the oblique subcostal approach [14]. In this variation, the needle entered the skin in an area near the xyphoid and was advanced inferolaterally such that local anaesthetic is delivered to the TAP along the costal margin (Figure 6). Importantly, the lateral abdominal muscle layers give way to an aponeurosis medially so that the TAP is defined by different muscle layers in this area. In some patients, the transversus abdominis muscle extended medially, and the roof of the TAP was formed by the rectus abdominis muscle. In other patients, the transversus abdominis muscle did not extend to the site of local injection, so the plane between the rectus abdominis and the rectus sheath was targeted. Børglum et al. recently described an ultrasound-guided, four-point, single-shot technique that combines the posterior and oblique subcostal techniques in an effort to provide wider bilateral analgesic coverage [15]. The subcostal TAP block was performed in a manner similar to that described by Hebbard when the transversus abdominis extended medially beneath the rectus abdominis [14]. This method was referred to as the medial intercostal TAP block. When the transversus abdominis terminated laterally at the linea semilunaris, the subcostal block was instead performed within the TAP at the lateral most extent of the transversus abdominis. This method was referred to as the lateral intercostal TAP block. In addition, the posterior TAP block was performed between the costal margin and the iliac crest at the anterior axillary line. It is important to note that the triangle of Petit is posterior to the midaxillary line, and, as a consequence, the posterior TAP as described in this study was performed in a location anterior to the original description [2].

4.3. Surgeon-Assisted Approaches. While the majority of published literature on TAP blocks is purely from the perspective of anesthesiologists, a growing number of reports have demonstrated that surgeons can help to facilitate these blocks. Chetwood et al. described a laparoscopic-assisted technique wherein a classic TAP block (based on anatomical landmarks) was performed while the injection area is observed with an intra-abdominal laparoscopic camera [16]. A peritoneal bulge at the area of injection was seen after local anesthetic was delivered within the TAP, and this visual served as the desired endpoint for this technique. Such direct visualization may help to avoid intraperitoneal injection, one of the major potential risks of the TAP block. More recently, a surgical TAP block utilizing a transperitoneal approach was also described. Performed intraoperatively, a blunt-tipped block needle was advanced from inside the abdominal wall through the parietal peritoneum, then the transversus abdominis muscle, and into the TAP as indicated by a single pop sensation [17, 18]. In addition, Araco et al. described a surgical TAP block in which blunt dissection through the external and internal oblique muscles leads to injection of local anesthetic into the TAP under direct visualization [19].

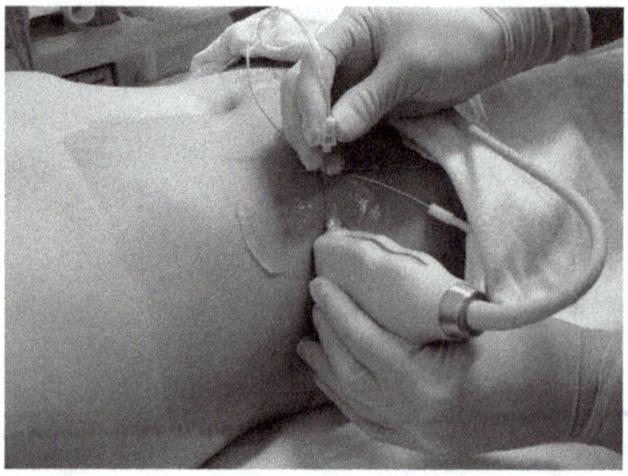

FIGURE 4: Ultrasound-guided TAP block showing needle alignment and ultrasound transducer placement on skin using an in-plane technique [20]. Reproduced with permission.

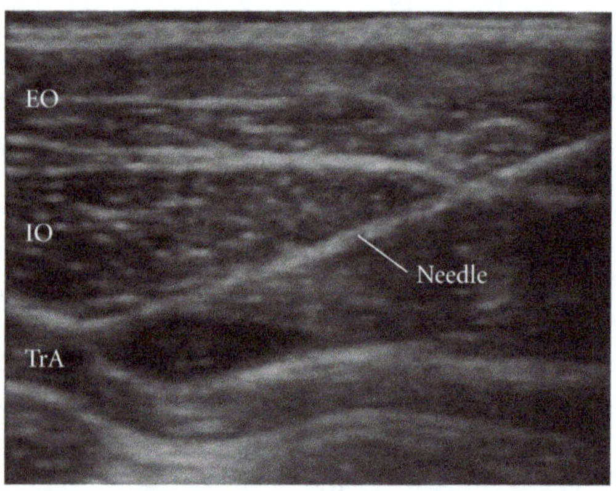

FIGURE 5: Ultrasound image during initial injection of a small amount of local anesthetic [9]. Reproduced with permission. EO: external oblique, IO: internal oblique, TrA: transversus abdominis.

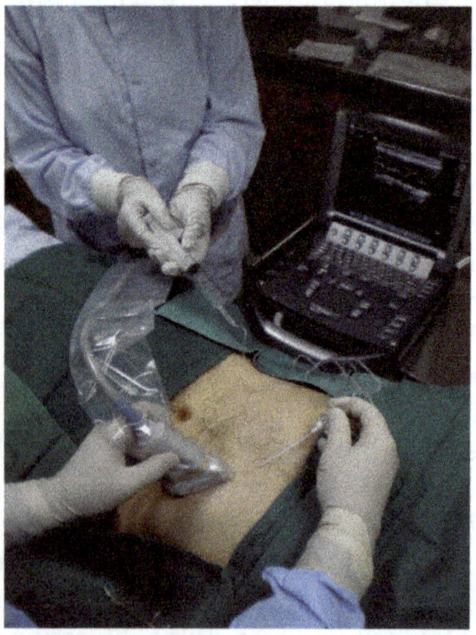

FIGURE 6: Placement of ultrasound probe for subcostal TAP blocks. Generously shared from the personal files of Prof. P. Hebbard.

5. Local Anesthetic Dosing

In his original report, Rafi described the use of 20 mL of "a local anaesthetic agent" for each side requiring analgesia [3]. Subsequently, McDonnell et al. reported the use of 20 mL of 0.5% lidocaine for each side in healthy volunteers [5]. Table 1 provides a current summary of the various agents and related doses used in published clinical studies.

While local anesthetic agent, volume, concentration, and delivery method differ between studies, these regimens have not yet been compared against each other. Therefore, there is insufficient evidence to support any particular combination in lieu of another. When duration of analgesia is an issue, there is good evidence to support using TAP catheters. This technique was first described in 2009 in a small case series [42]. Two years later, the same group showed similar pain control between epidural and TAP catheter analgesia in a randomized study [26]. In both reports, an intermittent bolus protocol was used. It remains unclear whether the use of a continuous infusion offers any advantage over intermittent blousing for TAP catheters.

6. Clinical Use

TAP blocks have been described as an effective component of multimodal postoperative analgesia for a wide variety of abdominal procedures including large bowel resection, open/laparoscopic appendectomy, cesarean section, total abdominal hysterectomy, laparoscopic cholecystectomy, open prostatectomy, renal transplant surgery, abdominoplasty with/without flank liposuction, and iliac crest bone graft [8, 15–19, 21–48]. Most reports demonstrate the efficacy of TAP blocks by highlighting some combination of reduced postoperative opioid requirement, lower pain scores, and/or reduction in opioid-related side effects.

Petersen et al. reviewed 7 randomized, double-blinded, clinical trials of both landmark-based ($n = 3$) and ultrasound-guided ($n = 4$) TAP blocks for managing postoperative pain after abdominal surgery with incisions below the level of the umbilicus [49]. All 7 studies compared pain-related outcomes with TAP blocks as part of a multimodal postoperative analgesic regimen. Morphine PCA ± acetaminophen ± nonsteroidal anti-inflammatory drugs was most commonly used to complement TAP blocks. In one study, intrathecal morphine was also part of the analgesic regimen. A meta-analysis of these 7 studies (180 cases and 184 controls) demonstrated an average reduction in 24-hour morphine consumption of 22 mg (95% confidence interval: −31 mg to −13 mg) in favor of TAP block patients compared with standard management. Furthermore, TAP blocks were associated with reduced early postoperative visual analog scores (VAS) both at rest and during mobilization in 4 of the 7 studies (1 study did not record VAS scores). Postoperative sedation, as well as postoperative nausea and vomiting (PONV), was marginally reduced in patients with TAP blocks. In a separate meta-analysis using 4 of the 7 studies reviewed by Petersen et al., Siddiqui et al. also demonstrated a morphine-sparing effect of TAP blocks in the first 24 hours after surgery [20]. Similarly, another meta-analysis

TABLE 1: List of published clinical studies on the use of TAP blocks. Single patient case reports have been excluded. (*) 20 patients were randomized to receive TAP block and spinal block with plain bupivacaine, while 20 patients were randomized to receive TAP block, bupivacaine spinal block, and intrathecal morphine. (**) Volume includes some local anesthetic used to perform ilioinguinal block in conjunction with TAP block. US-guided: ultrasound-guided. L-bupivacaine: Levobupivacaine.

Reference	Study sample	Local anesthetic	Block operator	Surgical procedure	Outcome
Sforza et al., 2011 [21]	14 cases 14 controls	10 mL/side of 0.5% bupivacaine with 10 mL/side lidocaine + 1 : 200,000 epinephrine	Surgical team	Abdominoplasty	Superior analgesia compared to IV/PO medications
Kadam and Moran 2011 [22]	15 cases 15 controls	8 mL/hr/side (continuous bilateral catheters) of 0.2% ropivacaine	Anesthesia team	Variety of upper and/or lower abdominal surgery	Noninferior outcome compared to epidural analgesia
Hivelin et al., 2011 [23]	15 cases 15 controls	1.5 mg/kg/side of 0.475% ropivacaine	Surgical team	Breast reconstruction with deep inferior epigastric perforator flap	Superior analgesia compared to IV/PO medications
McMorrow et al., 2011 [24]	40 cases 40 controls*	1 mg/kg/side of 0.375% bupivacaine	Anesthesia team	C-section	Inferior analgesia compared to intrathecal morphine
Mei et al., 2011 [25]	4 cases	20 mL/side** of 0.5% ropivacaine	Anesthesia team (US-guided)	C-section	Superior analgesia compared to local infiltration
Bharti et al., 2011 [17]	20 cases 20 controls	20 mL/side of 0.25% bupivacaine	Surgical team	Colorectal surgery	Superior analgesia compared to IV/PO medications
Børglum et al. 2011 [15]	25 cases	30 mL/side of 0.25% bupivacaine	Anesthesia team (US-guided)	Various upper and/or lower abdominal surgery	Significant reduction in pain and anticipated need for IV/PO analgesics
Niraj et al., 2011 [26]	29 cases 33 controls	1 mg/kg/side/8 hr (intermittent dosing through bilateral catheters) of 0.375% bupivacaine	Anesthesia team (US-guided)	Open hepatobiliary or renal surgery	Noninferior outcome compared to epidural analgesia
Aveline et al., 2011 [27]	134 cases 139 controls	1.5 mg/kg (unilateral block) of 0.5% L-bupivacaine	Anesthesia team (US-guided)	Open inguinal hernia repair	Superior analgesia compared to landmark-based ilioinguinal/iliohypogastric nerve block
Owen et al., 2011 [18]	16 cases 18 controls	20 mL/side of 0.25% bupivacaine	Surgical team	C-section	Superior analgesia compared to IV/PO medications
Gravante et al., 2011 [28]	51 cases	1 mg/kg/side of 0.5% bupivacaine	Surgical team	Abdominoplasty	Superior analgesia compared to IV/PO medications
Allcock et al., 2010 [29]	2 cases	20 mL/side bolus with 0.5% bupivacaine + 1 : 400,000 epinephrine followed by 8 mL/hr bilateral continuous infusion of 0.125% bupivacaine	Anesthesia team (US-guided)	Major thorax/abdominal trauma	Superior outcomes compared to expected results with IV/PO medications
Baaj et al., 2010 [30]	20 cases 20 controls	20 mL/side of 0.25% bupivacaine	Anesthesia team (US-guided)	C-section	Superior analgesia compared to IV/PO medications
Heil et al., 2010 [31]	3 cases	30 mL unilateral bolus of 1.5% mepivacaine followed by 8 mL/hr continuous unilateral infusion of 0.2% ropivacaine	Anesthesia team (US-guided)	Open inguinal hernia repair	Superior outcome compared to anticipated results with IV/PO medications
Chiono et al., 2010 [32]	33 cases	15 mL (unilateral block) of 0.33% ropivacaine	Anesthesia team (US-guided)	Iliac crest bone graft	Superior outcome compared to anticipated results with IV/PO medications

Table 1: Continued.

Reference	Study sample	Local anesthetic	Block operator	Surgical procedure	Outcome
Araco et al., 2010 [19]	34 cases 41 controls	1 mg/kg/side of 0.5% bupivacaine	Surgical team	Abdominoplasty	Superior analgesia compared to IV/PO medications
Griffiths et al., 2010 [33]	32 cases 33 controls	15 mL/side of 0.5% ropivacaine	Anesthesia team (US-guided)	Gynecological malignancy surgery	No benefit in analgesia compared to IV/PO medications
Lee et al., 2010 [34]	50 cases	20 mL of 1% ropivacaine for unilateral blocks and 20 mL/side of 0.5% ropivacaine for bilateral blocks	Anesthesia team (US-guided)	Dermatomal coverage of subcostal versus posterior approach	Most cephalad dermatome of T8 by subcostal approach versus T10 by posterior approach
Kanazi et al., 2010 [35]	29 cases 28 controls	20 mL/side of 0.375% bupivacaine + 1 : 200,000 epinephrine	Anesthesia team (US-guided)	C-section	Inferior analgesia compared to intrathecal morphine
Mukhtar and Khattak 2010 [36]	10 cases 10 controls	20 mL (unilateral block) of 0.5% bupivacaine	Anesthesia team	Renal transplant	Superior analgesia compared to IV/PO medications
Conaghan et al., 2010 [37]	40 cases 34 controls	20 mL/side of 0.25% L-bupivacaine	Anesthesia team (US-guided)	Laparoscopic colorectal surgery	Superior analgesia compared to IV/PO medications
Araco et al., 2010 [38]	24 cases	1 mg/kg/side of 0.5% bupivacaine	Surgical team	Abdominoplasty	Superior outcome compared to anticipated results with IV/PO medications
Asensio-Samper et al., 2010 [39]	2 cases	20 mL (unilateral block) of 0.5% ropivacaine	Anesthesia team (US-guided)	Morphine pump implantation	Superior outcome compared to anticipated results with IV/PO medications
Costello et al., 2009 [40]	47 cases 49 controls	20 mL/side of 0.375 Ropivacaine	Anesthesia team	C-section	Noninferior outcome compared to intrathecal morphine
Jankovic et al., 2009 [41]	7 cases 35 controls	20 mL unilateral bolus of 0.375% L-bupivacaine followed by 10 mL/hr continuous unilateral 0.15% Bupivacaine infusion	Surgical team	Renal transplant	Superior outcome compared to IV/PO medications
Niraj et al., 2009 [42]	3 cases	20 mL/side/12 hr of 0.5% or 0.375% bupivacaine for bilateral catheters and 25 mL/12 hr of 0.5% bupivacaine for unilateral catheter	Anesthesia team (US-guided)	Upper and/or lower abdominal surgeries	Superior outcome compared to anticipated results with IV/PO medications
Belavy et al., 2009 [43]	23 cases 24 controls	20 mL/side of 0.5% ropivacaine	Anesthesia team (US-guided)	C-section	Superior outcome compared to IV/PO medications
Niraj et al., 2009 [44]	3 cases	1 mg/kg/side of 0.375% bupivacaine	Anesthesia team (US-guided)	Upper abdominal surgery	Superior outcome compared to anticipated results with IV/PO medications
Niraj et al., 2009 [45]	26 cases 26 controls	20 mL (unilateral block) of 0.5% bupivacaine	Anesthesia team (US-guided)	Open appendectomy	Superior outcome compared to IV/PO medications
El-Dawlatly et al., 2009 [46]	21 cases 21 controls	15 mL/side of 0.5% bupivacaine	Anesthesia team (US-guided)	Laparoscopic cholecystectomy	Superior outcome compared to IV/PO medications

TABLE 1: Continued.

Reference	Study sample	Local anesthetic	Block operator	Surgical procedure	Outcome
Carney et al., 2008 [47]	24 cases 26 controls	1.5 mg/kg (max 20 mL)/side of 0.75% ropivacaine	Anesthesia team	Total abdominal hysterectomy	Superior outcome compared to IV/PO medications
McDonnell et al., 2008 [48]	25 cases 25 controls	1.5 mg/kg (max 20 mL)/side of 0.75% ropivacaine	Anesthesia team	C-section	Superior outcome compared to IV/PO medications
McDonnell et al., 2007 [12]	16 cases 16 controls	20 mL/side of 0.375% L-bupivacaine	Anesthesia team	Bowel resection	Superior outcome compared to IV/PO medications
O'Donnell 2006 [8]	12 cases	20 mL/side of 0.375% bupivacaine	Anesthesia team	Open retropubic prostatectomy	Superior outcome compared to anticipated results with IV/PO medications

by Charlton et al., which reviewed 236 participants from 5 studies (including landmark- and ultrasound-guided TAP blocks), demonstrated a significant reduction in 24-hour morphine requirements (average –22 mg, 95% confidence interval –38 mg to –6 mg) in TAP block patients compared to controls [1]. A significant difference in postoperative sedation, nausea, and vomiting was not appreciated between TAP-block and non-TAP block patients in this paper.

A number of new clinical studies utilizing TAP blocks have recently been published. Bharti et al. randomized 40 patients undergoing colorectal surgery to standard treatment (diclofenac and intravenous morphine) and bilateral intra-operative TAP block with either 0.25% bupivacaine (n = 20) or saline (n = 20) [17]. The bupivacaine group had a significant reduction in 24-hour morphine requirements (6.45 ± 3.26 mg versus 17.55 ± 5.78 mg; $P < 0.0001$) as well as a significant reduction in early postoperative pain scores both at rest and with coughing. Furthermore, early postoperative sedation scores were significantly lower in the bupivacaine group, and patient satisfaction was higher (6.8 ± 1.1 mg versus 3.5 ± 1.5 mg; $P < 0.001$). Although there was no difference between groups in the incidence of PONV, patients in the control group experienced significantly more severe PONV, requiring pharmacological intervention. Hivelin et al. studied the effect of TAP blocks for postoperative analgesia in patients with abdominal deep inferior epigastric perforator flaps for breast reconstruction [23]. The TAP block group (n = 15) required significantly less morphine (median and interquartile range: 28 mg (27 mg–38 mg) versus 42 mg (36 mg–46 mg); P = 0.0057) than controls (n = 15) in the first 24 hours after surgery. Early postoperative numerical pain scale scores were also significantly lower in the TAP block group compared to the non-TAP-block patients. However, no difference was observed between groups for postoperative sedation, PONV, and 48-hour satisfaction with pain management. Sforza et al. also studied the effect of TAP blocks on patients in the first 12 hours following abdominoplasty and reported significant postoperative morphine sparing, improved pain scores, and earlier ambulation in the TAP block group (n = 14) versus controls (n = 14) [21]. It is important to note that both groups received 10 mg of morphine and 1 gm of acetaminophen intraoperatively. Unfortunately, the information from this study is difficult to interpret and/or generalize, since data is reported without standard deviations or confidence intervals, and the follow-up time was abbreviated. However, not all reports demonstrate an analgesic benefit to TAP blocks when compared to standard therapy. Griffiths et al. randomized 65 patients undergoing surgery for presumed gynecologic malignancy to standard treatment (parecoxib, acetaminophen, and morphine) plus ultrasound-guided TAP block with either ropivacaine (n = 32) or saline (n = 33) [33]. No significant difference was found in the two groups for 24-hour morphine consumption (34 mg ± 27 mg versus 36 mg ± 27 mg; P = 0.76), VAS scores at rest (18 mm ± 19 mm versus 23 mm ± 22 mm; P = 0.33), VAS scores with coughing (39 mm ± 24 mm versus 48 mm ± 31 mm; P = 0.2), patient satisfaction (9 ± 2 versus 8 ± 3; P = 0.36), or incidence of nausea and pruritis. The authors speculated that the negative study may have been due to a combination of factors including a high incidence of obesity in the study population leading to potentially more technical failures, a wide age range, and the fact that 18 of the 65 patients had incisions that extended above the umbilicus (7 in the sham group versus 11 in the treatment group). The authors also hypothesized that the study population had a larger variation in "surgical insult;" that is, some cases involved more organ manipulation and dissection resulting in more visceral pain, for which TAP blocks would be less effective than those for parietal/incisional pain.

In another study, Baaj et al. randomized 40 women to receive either local anesthetic (n = 20) or saline (n = 20) TAP blocks in addition to a plain bupivacaine spinal block for elective cesarean section [30]. A significant reduction in 24-hour morphine requirement was observed in the local anesthetic TAP block group versus controls (26 mg ± 5 mg versus 63 mg ± 5 mg; $P < 0.05$). Although the authors report lower PONV, lower 24-hour VAS scores, and higher satisfaction in the local anesthetic TAP block group, no statistical measures were reported. These results are in line with previous reports by McDonnell et al. and Belavy et al. that demonstrated superior analgesia and significantly decreased 24-hour morphine consumption following C-section in patients who received TAP blocks in addition to plain local anesthetic spinal blocks when compared to patients with just local anesthetic spinal blocks [43, 48]. The use of intrathecal morphine, on the other hand, may minimize the analgesic advantage of TAP blocks when performed in addition to neuraxial blockade. McMorrow et al. randomized 80 patients to 4 equal groups ($n = 20$ in each arm) and reported that they found no overall analgesic advantage to TAP blocks and no incremental benefit of adding TAP blocks when patients receive intrathecal morphine [24]. They also reported similar overall patient satisfaction among groups despite more frequent pruritis in patients who received intrathecal morphine. These data are difficult to interpret since medians are reported without interquartile ranges (though box plots with whiskers are displayed) and comparisons are only performed between the highest and lowest scores in each category. Costello et al. also evaluated the incremental benefit of TAP blocks in addition to intrathecal morphine for C-section and found no difference in morphine requirements, VAS scores, or satisfaction in 96 patients (all received intrathecal morphine but were randomized to receive either local anesthetic or saline TAP blocks) [40]. Of note, the authors did not assess rates of nausea or pruritis. Similarly, Kanazi et al. compared TAP block without intrathecal morphine ($n = 30$) to sham TAP block with intrathecal morphine ($n = 30$) for c-sections and found a significantly longer time to first analgesic request as well as lower immediate postoperative VAS scores in the intrathecal morphine group [35]. However, the authors also reported significantly higher rates of both nausea and pruritis in the intrathecal morphine group as compared to the TAP block group. Patient satisfaction scores were similar between groups. Again, the data are difficult to interpret since only group medians and ranges are reported.

Few studies have compared TAP blocks to epidural analgesia. Recently, Kadam and Moran conducted a retrospective matched case-control study comparing continuous TAP block catheters (posterior and subcostal approaches; $n = 15$) to thoracic epidural analgesia ($n = 15$) [22]. Except for assessments in the postanesthesia care unit, there was no appreciable difference in pain scores between the two groups over a 3-day follow-up period. While patient satisfaction was similar between groups, the TAP block group required a significantly higher amount of breakthrough fentanyl over the study period. Therapeutic failure rate was higher in the epidural group (patchy block in 4 patients) versus the TAP catheter group (unilateral block in 2 patients). Hypotension was reported in 2 patients from the epidural group. As with a number of the previously discussed reports, these findings are difficult to interpret since the data tables do not provide sufficient information to perform a critical appraisal. In their prospective analysis, Niraj et al. compared continuous thoracic epidural analgesia to bilateral intermittent-bolus subcostal TAP catheters in open hepatobiliary and renal surgery patients [26]. The authors observed no significant difference in patient satisfaction as well as VAS scores at rest or with coughing at 8 hours to 72 hours after surgery. Rescue analgesia with tramadol, however, was significantly higher ($P = 0.002$) in the TAP catheter group (400 mg, interquartile range 300–500 mg) versus the epidural group (200 mg, interquartile range 100–350 mg) over 72 hours. Although a similar therapeutic failure rate was reported among the groups (22% versus 30% for epidural versus TAP), it should be noted that 8 of the TAP catheter patients had incisions or drains in locations not necessarily covered by subcostal TAP blocks. Data comparing hemodynamic consequences were not reported.

A number of case reports have also highlighted new potential clinical scenarios to integrate the use of TAP blocks. Singh et al. demonstrated that bilateral TAP blocks in addition to noninvasive positive pressure ventilation was effective in the management of a 74-year-old patient with impending respiratory failure resulting from excessive pain and narcosis following emergency laparotomy [50]. Similarly, Børglum et al. demonstrated that TAP blocks maybe an effective rescue therapy for patients with uncontrolled pain following major abdominal surgery [15]. The authors reported that their 4-point TAP block was effective in managing pain, decreasing opioid consumption, facilitating quicker postanesthesia care unit discharge, and improving mobilization. In addition, a growing number of reports suggest that TAP blocks may also be a safe alternative to neuraxial blockade in patients who are anti-coagulated, coagulopathic, or in patients who would not tolerate the hemodynamic sequelae often associated with profound neuraxial sympathectomy [29, 51, 52].

7. Complications

Complications of the TAP block are rare. To date, there are no published reports in the English language of local anesthetic toxicity following TAP blocks. Griffiths et al. reported a mean peak plasma ropivacaine level of 2.54 ± 0.75 mcg/mL using a total dose of 3 mg/kg to perform bilateral TAP blocks [53]. While this level is above previously established minimum toxic plasma levels of 2.2 mcg/mL, it is similar to levels achieved in other commonly utilized peripheral nerve blocks (e.g., 2.58 mcg/mL for axillary blocks). Kato et al. also suggested that toxic plasma levels maybe achieved when using 40 mL of 1% lidocaine [54]. Though direct intravascular injection of local anesthetics is very unlikely with TAP blocks, these studies do suggest that systemic toxicity is possible, and, as such, caution should be exercised throughout drug delivery.

Case reports of liver lacerations caused by right-sided TAP blocks can also be found in the literature. Farooq and Carey described a liver laceration after a landmark-based TAP block [55]. Upon laparotomy, the patient was subsequently found to have an enlarged liver that extended down to the iliac crest. As a consequence, the authors recommended routine palpation of the liver edge prior to landmark-based right-sided TAP blocks. Lancaster and Chadwick also reported a liver laceration after ultrasound-guided TAP block, which was likely as a result of failure to adequately visualize the needle during the procedure [56]. Furthermore, at least in theory, the spleen and kidneys are also at risk during TAP blocks. And although Jankovic et al.

observed a TAP catheter in the peritoneal cavity upon surgical exposure of the abdomen for an open nephrectomy, no reports of injury to these organs were found during a thorough literature search [57].

While the likelihood of needle placement misadventures may be minimized with the proper use of ultrasound guidance, the potential complication of femoral nerve blocks (partial or complete) may not be completely avoided. The transversalis fascia comprises the fascial plane deep to the rectus abdominis muscles. This fascial plane is continuous with the *fascia iliaca*. Local anesthetic injected into the TAP can theoretically track along the transversalis fascia to the *fascia iliaca* and, in doing so, may block the femoral nerve and place the patient at risk of a fall.

8. Conclusions

The TAP block is an effective and safe adjunct to multimodal postoperative analgesia for abdominal surgery. Multiple studies have demonstrated its superiority over standard medical therapy for postoperative pain control. Limited data also suggest, that in select patient populations, TAP blocks/catheters may provide comparable analgesia as well as patient satisfaction to epidural therapy. However, the data is less encouraging for patients who receive intrathecal morphine during c-section, where the addition of TAP blocks does not appear to improve postoperative pain control. Nonetheless, it may be a good alternative strategy for patients who are highly sensitive to opioids.

Absolute contraindications to TAP blocks include patient refusal, soft tissue infection of the abdominal wall and skin, or abnormality at the needle insertion site. Coagulation status is an area of uncertainty with the TAP block and will require further investigation. Optimal dosing schemes (i.e., single shot versus catheter, intermittent versus continuous catheter infusions, type of local anesthetic, use of adjuvants) will also need to be determined. Moreover, there remains considerable debate over which type of TAP block provides the best coverage for specific surgeries. While many believe that the posterior approach is ideal for incisions below the umbilicus, that the subcostal block is best suited for upper abdominal procedures, and that a combined approach provides the greatest analgesic coverage, supporting data is conflicting at best. Well-designed and adequately powered studies are needed to address these clinically relevant questions.

Funding

There is Harvard Anaesthesia Center (5T32GM007592-33) support for S. A. Quraishi.

References

[1] S. Charlton, A. M. Cyna, P. Middleton, and J. D. Griffiths, "Perioperative transversus abdominis plane (TAP) blocks for analgesia after abdominal surgery," *Cochrane Database of Systematic Reviews*, vol. 8, Article ID CD007705, 2010.

[2] A. N. Rafi, "Abdominal field block: a new approach via the lumbar triangle," *Anaesthesia*, vol. 56, no. 10, pp. 1024–1026, 2001.

[3] R. J. Kearns and S. J. Young, "Transversus abdominis plane blocks; a national survey of techniques used by UK obstetric anaesthetists," *International Journal of Obstetric Anesthesia*, vol. 20, no. 1, pp. 103–104, 2011.

[4] R. S. Atkinson, G. B. Rushman, and J. A. Lee, *A Synopsis of Anaesthesia*, Wright, Bristol, UK, 10th edition, 1987.

[5] J. G. McDonnell, B. D. O'Donnell, D Tuite, T. Farrell, and C. Power, "The Regional Abdominal Field Infiltration (R.A.F.I.) technique computerised tomographic and anatomical identification of a novel approach to the transversus abdominis neuro-vascular fascial plain," in *Proceedings of the American Society of Anesthesiologists Annual Meeting*, 2004, A-899. Abstract.

[6] J. G. McDonnell, B. D. O'Donnell, T. Farrell et al., "Transversus abdominis plane block: a cadaveric and radiological evaluation," *Regional Anesthesia and Pain Medicine*, vol. 32, no. 5, pp. 399–404, 2007.

[7] J. G. McDonnell and J. G. Laffey, "Transversus abdominis plane block," *Anesthesia and Analgesia*, vol. 105, no. 3, article 883, 2007.

[8] B. D. O'Donnell, J. G. McDonnell, and A. J. McShane, "The Transversus Abdominis Plane (TAP) block in open retropubic prostatectomy," *Regional Anesthesia and Pain Medicine*, vol. 31, no. 1, article 91, 2006.

[9] K. Webster, "The Transversus Abdominis Plane (TAP) block: abdominal plane regional anaesthesia," *Update in Anaesthesia*, vol. 24, no. 1, pp. 24–29, 2008.

[10] Z. B. Jankovic, F. M. du Feu, and P. McConnell, "An anatomical study of the transversus abdominis plane block: location of the lumbar triangle of petit and adjacent nerves," *Anesthesia and Analgesia*, vol. 109, no. 3, pp. 981–985, 2009.

[11] W. M. Rozen, T. M. N. Tran, M. W. Ashton, M. J. Barrington, J. J. Ivanusic, and G. I. Taylor, "Refining the course of the thoracolumbar nerves: a new understanding of the innervation of the anterior abdominal wall," *Clinical Anatomy*, vol. 21, no. 4, pp. 325–333, 2008.

[12] J. G. McDonnell, B. O'Donnell, G. Curley, A. Heffernan, C. Power, and J. G. Laffey, "The analgesic efficacy of transversus abdominis plane block after abdominal surgery: a prospective randomized controlled trial," *Anesthesia and Analgesia*, vol. 104, no. 1, pp. 193–197, 2007.

[13] P. Hebbard, Y. Fujiwara, Y. Shibata, and C. Royse, "Ultrasound-guided transversus abdominis plane (TAP) block," *Anaesthesia and Intensive Care*, vol. 35, no. 4, pp. 616–617, 2007.

[14] P. Hebbard, "Subcostal transversus abdominis plane block under ultrasound guidance," *Anesthesia and Analgesia*, vol. 106, no. 2, pp. 674–675, 2008.

[15] J. Børglum, C. Maschmann, B. Belhage, and K. Jensen, "Ultrasound-guided bilateral dual transversus abdominis plane block: a new four-point approach," *Acta Anaesthesiologica Scandinavica*, vol. 55, no. 6, pp. 658–663, 2011.

[16] A. Chetwood, S. Agrawal, D. Hrouda, and P. Doyle, "Laparoscopic assisted transversus abdominis plane block: a novel insertion technique during laparoscopic nephrectomy," *Anaesthesia*, vol. 66, no. 4, pp. 317–318, 2011.

[17] N. Bharti, P. Kumar, I. Bala, and V. Gupta, "The efficacy of a novel approach to transversus abdominis plane block for postoperative analgesia after colorectal surgery," *Anesthesia and Analgesia*, vol. 112, no. 6, pp. 1504–1508, 2011.

[18] D. J. Owen, I. Harrod, J. Ford, M. Luckas, and V. Gudimetla, "The surgical transversus abdominis plane block—a novel approach for performing an established technique," *British Journal of Obstetrics and Gynaecology*, vol. 118, no. 1, pp. 24–27, 2011.

[19] A. Araco, J. Pooney, F. Araco, and G. Gravante, "Transversus abdominis plane block reduces the analgesic requirements after abdominoplasty with flank liposuction," *Annals of Plastic Surgery*, vol. 65, no. 4, pp. 385–388, 2010.

[20] M. R.S. Siddiqui, M. S. Sajid, D. R. Uncles, L. Cheek, and M. K. Baig, "A meta-analysis on the clinical effectiveness of transversus abdominis plane block," *Journal of Clinical Anesthesia*, vol. 23, no. 1, pp. 7–14, 2011.

[21] M. Sforza, K. Andjelkov, R. Zaccheddu, H. Nagi, and M. Colic, "Transversus abdominis plane block anesthesia in abdominoplasties," *Plastic and Reconstructive Surgery*, vol. 128, no. 2, pp. 529–535, 2011.

[22] V.R. Kadam and J. L. Moran, "Epidural infusions versus transversus abdominis plane (TAP) block infusions: retrospective study," *Journal of Anesthesia*, vol. 25, no. 5, pp. 786–787, 2011.

[23] M. Hivelin, A. Wyniecki, B. Plaud, J. Marty, and L. Lantieri, "Ultrasound-guided bilateral transversus abdominis plane block for postoperative analgesia after breast reconstruction by DIEP flap," *Plastic and Reconstructive Surgery*, vol. 128, no. 1, pp. 44–55, 2011.

[24] R. C.N. McMorrow, R. J. Ni Mhuircheartaigh, K. A. Ahmed et al., "Comparison of transversus abdominis plane block vs spinal morphine for pain relief after Caesarean section," *British Journal of Anaesthesia*, vol. 106, no. 5, pp. 706–712, 2011.

[25] W. Mei, C. Jin, L. Feng et al., "Case report: bilateral ultrasound-guided transversus abdominis plane block combined with ilioinguinal-iliohypogastric nerve block for cesarean delivery anesthesia," *Anesthesia and Analgesia*, vol. 113, no. 1, pp. 134–137, 2011.

[26] G. Niraj, A. Kelkar, I. Jeyapalan et al., "Comparison of analgesic efficacy of subcostal transversus abdominis plane blocks with epidural analgesia following upper abdominal surgery," *Anaesthesia*, vol. 66, no. 6, pp. 465–471, 2011.

[27] C. Aveline, H. Le Hetet, A. Le Roux et al., "Comparison between ultrasound-guided transversus abdominis plane and conventional ilioinguinal/iliohypogastric nerve blocks for day-case open inguinal hernia repair," *British Journal of Anaesthesia*, vol. 106, no. 3, pp. 380–386, 2011.

[28] G. Gravante, F. Castrì, F. Araco, and A. Araco, "A comparative study of the transversus abdominis plane (TAP) block efficacy on post-bariatric vs aesthetic abdominoplasty with flank liposuction," *Obesity Surgery*, vol. 21, no. 3, pp. 278–282, 2010.

[29] E. Allcock, E. Spencer, R. Frazer, G. Applegate, and C. Buckenmaier III, "Continuous transversus abdominis plane (TAP) block catheters in a combat surgical environment," *Pain Medicine*, vol. 11, no. 9, pp. 1426–1429, 2010.

[30] J. M. Baaj, R. A. Alsatli, H. A. Majaj, Z. A. Babay, and A. K. Thallaj, "Efficacy of ultrasound-guided transversus abdominis plane (TAP) block for post-cesarean section delivery analgesia—a double-blind, placebo-controlled, randomized study," *Middle East Journal of Anesthesiology*, vol. 20, no. 6, pp. 821–826, 2010.

[31] J. W. Heil, B. M. Ilfeld, V. J. Loland, N. S. Sandhu, and E. R. Mariano, "Ultrasound-guided transversus abdominis plane catheters and ambulatory perineural infusions for outpatient inguinal hernia repair," *Regional Anesthesia and Pain Medicine*, vol. 35, no. 6, pp. 556–558, 2010.

[32] J. Chiono, N. Bernard, S. Bringuier et al., "The ultrasound-guided transversus abdominis plane block for anterior iliac crest bone graft postoperative pain relief: a prospective descriptive study," *Regional Anesthesia and Pain Medicine*, vol. 35, no. 6, pp. 520–524, 2010.

[33] J. D. Griffiths, J. V. Middle, F. A. Barron, S. J. Grant, P. A. Popham, and C. F. Royse, "Transversus abdominis plane block does not provide additional benefit to multimodal analgesia in gynecological cancer surgery," *Anesthesia and Analgesia*, vol. 111, no. 3, pp. 797–801, 2010.

[34] T. H. W. Lee, M. J. Barrington, T. M. N. Tran, D. Wong, and P. D. Hebbard, "Comparison of extent of sensory block following posterior and subcostal approaches to ultrasound-guided transversus abdominis plane block," *Anaesthesia and Intensive Care*, vol. 38, no. 3, pp. 452–460, 2010.

[35] G. E. Kanazi, M. T. Aouad, F. W. Abdallah et al., "The analgesic efficacy of subarachnoid morphine in comparison with ultrasound-guided transversus abdominis plane block after cesarean delivery: a randomized controlled trial," *Anesthesia and Analgesia*, vol. 111, no. 2, pp. 475–481, 2010.

[36] K. Mukhtar and I. Khattak, "Transversus abdominis plane block for renal transplant recipients," *British Journal of Anaesthesia*, vol. 104, no. 5, pp. 663–664, 2010.

[37] P. Conaghan, C. Maxwell-Armstrong, N. Bedforth et al., "Efficacy of transversus abdominis plane blocks in laparoscopic colorectal resections," *Surgical Endoscopy and Other Interventional Techniques*, vol. 24, no. 10, pp. 2480–2484, 2010.

[38] A. Araco, J. Pooney, L. Memmo, and G. Gravante, "The transversus abdominis plane block for body contouring abdominoplasty with flank liposuction," *Plastic and Reconstructive Surgery*, vol. 125, no. 4, pp. 181e–182e, 2010.

[39] J. M. Asensio-Samper, J. De Andrés-Ibáñez, G. Fabregat Cid, V. Villanueva Pérez, and L. L. Alarcón, "Ultrasound-guided transversus abdominis plane block for spinal infusion and neurostimulation implantation in two patients with chronic pain," *Pain Practice*, vol. 10, no. 2, pp. 158–162, 2010.

[40] J. F. Costello, A. R. Moore, P. M. Wieczorek, A. J. Macarthur, M. Balki, and J. C. A. Carvalho, "The transversus abdominis plane block, when used as part of a multimodal regimen inclusive of intrathecal morphine, does not improve analgesia after cesarean delivery," *Regional Anesthesia and Pain Medicine*, vol. 34, no. 6, pp. 586–589, 2009.

[41] Z. B. Jankovic, S. G. Pollard, and M. M. Nachiappan, "Continuous transversus abdominis plane block for renal transplant recipients," *Anesthesia and Analgesia*, vol. 109, no. 5, pp. 1710–1711, 2009.

[42] G. Niraj, A. Kelkar, and A. J. Fox, "Oblique sub-costal transversus abdominis plane (TAP) catheters: an alternative to epidural analgesia after upper abdominal surgery," *Anaesthesia*, vol. 64, no. 10, pp. 1137–1140, 2009.

[43] D. Belavy, P. J. Cowlishaw, M. Howes, and F. Phillips, "Ultrasound-guided transversus abdominis plane block for analgesia after Caesarean delivery," *British Journal of Anaesthesia*, vol. 103, no. 5, pp. 726–730, 2009.

[44] G. Niraj, A. Kelkar, and A. J. Fox, "Application of the transversus abdominis plane block in the intensive care unit," *Anaesthesia and Intensive Care*, vol. 37, no. 4, pp. 650–652, 2009.

[45] G. Niraj, A. Searle, M. Mathews et al., "Analgesic efficacy of ultrasound-guided transversus abdominis plane block in patients undergoing open appendicectomy," *British Journal of Anaesthesia*, vol. 103, no. 4, pp. 601–605, 2009.

[46] A. A. El-Dawlatly, A. Turkistani, S. C. Kettner et al., "Ultrasound-guided transversus abdominis plane block:

description of a new technique and comparison with conventional systemic analgesia during laparoscopic cholecystectomy," *British Journal of Anaesthesia*, vol. 102, no. 6, pp. 763–767, 2009.

[47] J. Carney, J. G. McDonnell, A. Ochana, R. Bhinder, and J. G. Laffey, "The transversus abdominis plane block provides effective postoperative analgesia in patients undergoing total abdominal hysterectomy," *Anesthesia and Analgesia*, vol. 107, no. 6, pp. 2056–2060, 2008.

[48] J. G. McDonnell, G. Curley, J. Carney et al., "The analgesic efficacy of transversus abdominis plane block after cesarean delivery: a randomized controlled trial," *Anesthesia and Analgesia*, vol. 106, no. 1, pp. 186–191, 2008.

[49] P. L. Petersen, O. Mathiesen, H. Torup, and J. B. Dahl, "The transversus abdominis plane block: a valuable option for postoperative analgesia? A topical review," *Acta Anaesthesiologica Scandinavica*, vol. 54, no. 5, pp. 529–535, 2010.

[50] M. Singh, K. J. Chin, and V. Chan, "Ultrasound-guided transversus abdominis plane (TAP) block: a useful adjunct in the management of postoperative respiratory failure," *Journal of Clinical Anesthesia*, vol. 23, no. 4, pp. 303–306, 2011.

[51] K. O'Connor and C. Renfrew, "Subcostal transversus abdominis plane block," *Anaesthesia*, vol. 65, no. 1, pp. 91–92, 2010.

[52] M. Forero, V. M. Neira, A. J. Heikkila, and J. E. Paul, "Continuous lumbar transversus abdominis plane block may spread to supraumbilical dermatome," *Canadian Journal of Anesthesia*, vol. 58, no. 10, pp. 948–951, 2011.

[53] J. D. Griffiths, F. A. Barron, S. Grant, A. R. Bjorksten, P. Hebbard, and C. F. Royse, "Plasma ropivacaine concentrations after ultrasound-guided transversus abdominis plane block," *British Journal of Anaesthesia*, vol. 105, no. 6, pp. 853–856, 2010.

[54] N. Kato, Y. Fujiwara, M. Harato et al., "Serum concentration of lidocaine after transversus abdominis plane block," *Journal of Anesthesia*, vol. 23, no. 2, pp. 298–300, 2009.

[55] M. Farooq and M. Carey, "A case of liver trauma with a blunt regional anesthesia needle while performing transversus abdominis plane block," *Regional Anesthesia and Pain Medicine*, vol. 33, no. 3, pp. 274–275, 2008.

[56] P. Lancaster and M. Chadwick, "Liver trauma secondary to ultrasound-guided transversus abdominis plane block," *British Journal of Anaesthesia*, vol. 104, no. 4, pp. 509–510, 2010.

[57] Z. Jankovic, N. Ahmad, N. Ravishankar, and F. Archer, "Transversus abdominis plane block: how safe is it?" *Anesthesia and Analgesia*, vol. 107, no. 5, pp. 1758–1759, 2008.

13

Regional Blockade of the Shoulder: Approaches and Outcomes

Clifford Bowens Jr. and Ramprasad Sripada

Department of Anesthesiology, Vanderbilt University School of Medicine, 1301 Medical Center Drive, 4648 The Vanderbilt Clinic, Nashville, TN 37232-5614, USA

Correspondence should be addressed to Clifford Bowens Jr., clifford.bowens@vanderbilt.edu

Academic Editor: Attila Bondar

The article reviews the current literature regarding shoulder anesthesia and analgesia. Techniques and outcomes are presented that summarize our present understanding of regional anesthesia for the shoulder. Shoulder procedures producing mild to moderate pain may be managed with a single-injection interscalene block. However, studies support that moderate to severe pain, lasting for several days is best managed with a continuous interscalene block. This may cause increased extremity numbness, but will provide greater analgesia, reduce supplemental opioid consumption, improve sleep quality and patient satisfaction. In comparison to the nerve stimulation technique, ultrasound can reduce the volume of local anesthetic needed to produce an effective interscalene block. However, it has not been shown that ultrasound offers a definitive benefit in preventing major complications. The evidence indicates that the suprascapular and/or axillary nerve blocks are not as effective as an interscalene block. However in patients who are not candidates for the interscalene block, these blocks may provide a useful alternative for short-term pain relief. There is substantial evidence showing that subacromial and intra-articular injections provide little clinical benefit for postoperative analgesia. Given that these injections may be associated with irreversible chondrotoxicity, the injections are not presently recommended.

1. Introduction

Common shoulder procedures include hemiarthroplasty, total shoulder arthroplasty, shoulder arthroscopy, subacromial decompression, and shoulder instability procedures such as rotator cuff repair. Anesthesia and analgesia for these surgical procedures are provided by general anesthesia, regional anesthesia, or the combination of general and regional anesthesia. Postoperative pain following shoulder surgery in many patients is severe and may be exacerbated by movement during rehabilitation [1]. Procedures done to help manage the dynamic pain of shoulder surgery include interscalene block, cervical paravertebral block, suprascapular nerve block, subacromial block, and intra-articular injections. Some of these techniques are performed as a single injection, while others are done as a single-injection or continuous infusion. There has been an increase in the number of surgical procedures done in the ambulatory environment. Single-injection and infusion systems utilizing portable, disposable elastomeric pumps help provide safe pain control in this environment. This paper will review the current literature regarding shoulder anesthesia and analgesia. For outcomes, when possible, procedures for shoulder analgesia are compared to the benchmark procedure, the interscalene block.

2. Research Method

Medline and PubMed searches were performed for relevant publications regarding shoulder anesthesia and analgesia. Keywords included the following: "shoulder anesthesia," "shoulder analgesia," "regional anesthesia," "interscalene block," "suprascapular block," "subacromial block," and "intra-articular injection." In addition, the MeSH headings "nerve block" was used. The search was limited to human studies with a concentration on articles occurring in the last five years, but references were included from 1970 to the present. The search identified 259 abstracts that were

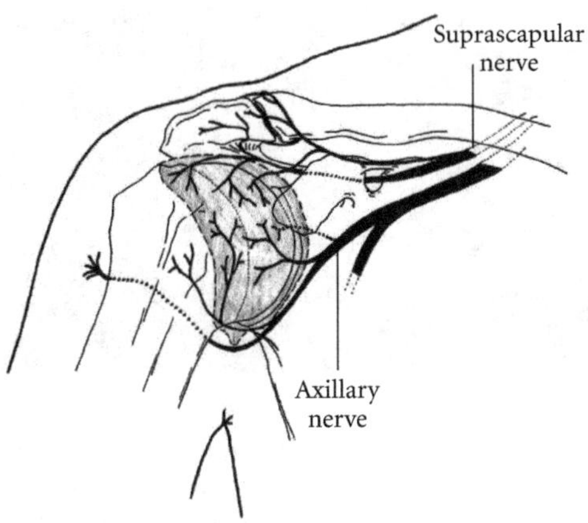

FIGURE 1: Anterior innervation of the shoulder joint. The suprascapular nerve and axillary nerve are the primary nerves supplying the capsule and the glenohumeral joint (Borgeat and Ekatodramis [1]). (Reprinted with permission from Elsevier.)

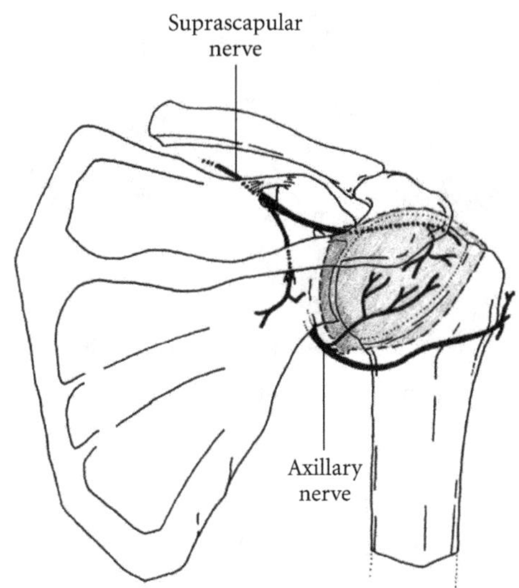

FIGURE 2: Posterior innervation of the shoulder joint. The suprascapular nerve and axillary nerve are the primary nerves supplying this region (Borgeat and Ekatodramis [1]). (Reprinted with permission from Elsevier.)

reviewed. The resulting publication list was then hand-searched, emphasizing randomized controlled trials. One hundred articles were read and reference lists reviewed.

3. Shoulder Anatomy and Innervation

The dynamic interaction of bones, joints, muscles, and ligaments establishes the foundation for the unique functions of the human shoulder. The bones which provide the framework for the shoulder girdle are the humerus, scapula, and clavicle. The shoulder girdle consists of three joints and one articulation: sternoclavicular joint, acromioclavicular joint, glenohumeral joint (shoulder joint), and scapulothoracic articulation. The muscles and ligaments of the shoulder allow and restrict movement along with providing active and passive stabilization of the shoulder. Biomechanically, the shoulder has three degrees of freedom and the muscles act at the shoulder to permit particularly free motion: flexion, extension, abduction, adduction, circumduction, internal rotation, and external rotation. Static stability of shoulder is provided by the labrum, capsule, and glenohumeral ligament while dynamic stability is provided by the rotator cuff, long head of the biceps tendon, and periscapular muscles [7].

The brachial plexus supplies all the motor and most of sensory functions of the shoulder, except the cephalad cutaneous areas of the shoulder, which are innervated by the supraclavicular nerves, originating from the superficial cervical plexus (C3-C4) [1]. Effective control of postoperative shoulder pain generally requires local anesthetic blockade of the nerve supply to the synovium, capsule, articular surfaces, periosteum, ligaments, and muscles of the shoulder [1, 3]. The terminal branches of the brachial plexus that supply the majority of the shoulder innervation are the suprascapular and axillary nerves (Figures 1 and 2).

The suprascapular nerve supplies sensory innervation to the subacromial bursa, acromioclavicular joint, coracoclavicular ligament, and 70% of the shoulder joint capsule [8]. This nerve arises from the superior trunk of the brachial plexus, C5-C6 and possibly C4. The suprascapular nerve descends posteriorly, passing through the scapular notch, innervating the supraspinatus and infraspinatus muscles. It provides sensation for the posterior shoulder capsule, acromioclavicular joint, subacromial bursa, and coracoclavicular ligament.

The axillary nerve originates from C5-C6 nerve roots, with occasional contribution from C4. It is derived from the posterior cord of the brachial plexus. The axillary nerve crosses the anteroinferior aspect of the subscapularis muscle where it crosses posteriorly through the quadrilateral space and divides into two trunks. The anterior trunk supplies the motor innervation to the anterior and middle deltoid muscle. The posterior trunk gives off a branch to the teres minor muscle and the posterior deltoid muscle before terminating as the superior lateral brachial cutaneous nerve, which supplies the cutaneous innervation to the skin overlying the deltoid muscle.

4. Interscalene Block

The interscalene block is the gold standard for shoulder anesthesia and the most commonly used block for shoulder procedures. This approach blocks the brachial plexus at the nerve root or trunk level. Local anesthetic is directed toward C5-C6 nerve roots or the superior trunk. Depending on the volume of local anesthetic used, C7 and even C8 nerve roots may be blocked. The block is especially useful for procedures involving the shoulder, including the lateral two-thirds of the clavicle, proximal humerus, and shoulder joint [1]. Ulnar sparing (C8 and T1 nerve roots) is often seen with this block which limits its usefulness for distal surgical procedures. The interscalene block is performed as a single-injection or continuous peripheral nerve block. The block is done using the paresthesia technique, nerve stimulation technique,

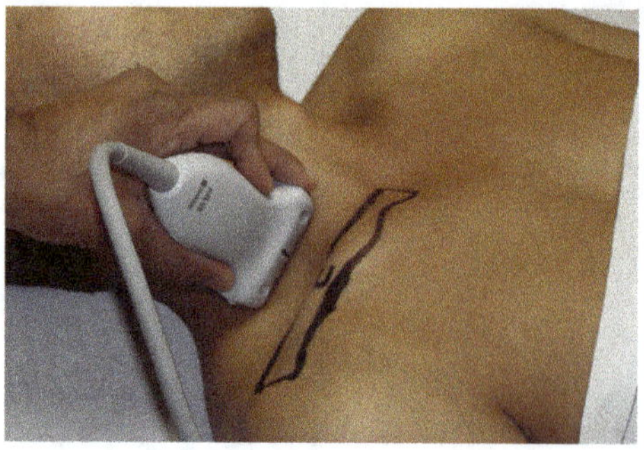

Figure 3: Ultrasound probe position for the interscalene brachial plexus block.

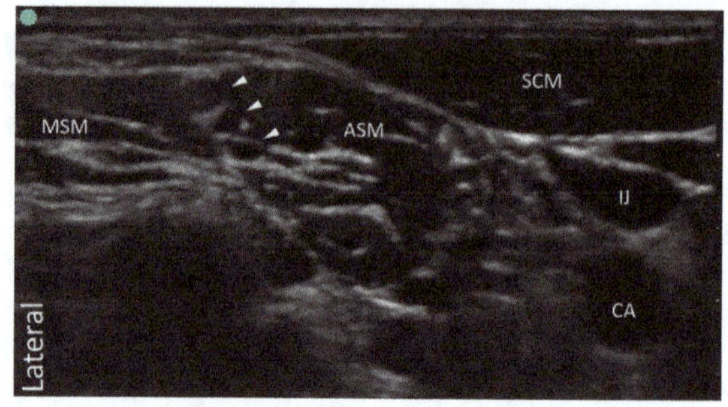

Figure 4: Transverse ultrasound image of interscalene brachial plexus. Arrowheads outline brachial plexus roots within the interscalene groove. SCM: sternocleidomastoid muscle, IJ: internal jugular vein, CA: carotid artery, ASM: anterior scalene muscle, MSM: middle scalene muscle.

ultrasound guidance, or nerve stimulation-ultrasound combination.

4.1. Classic Approaches. The classic approach of Winnie, which is considered the anterior approach, is still commonly performed, especially for single-injection blockade [9]. The technique is performed by palpating the interscalene groove at the level of the cricoid cartilage (C6 vertebra). The needle is directed medially, slightly caudal, and slightly posterior (toward the contralateral elbow) while seeking to elicit a paresthesia in the C5-C6 nerve distribution as the endpoint for injection. The nerve stimulation technique is more commonly used with this approach today, with a relevant motor twitch being the endpoint for injection. Winnie's technique was modified by Meier et al. to reduce complications and to facilitate placement of catheters [10]. Meier used the same landmarks, but enters the skin at 30 degrees and 2-3 cm cephalad to the Winnie approach. The needle is directed toward the middle to lateral third of the clavicle. Borgeat and Ekatodramis also modified the Winnie approach [1]. In this case, the needle is inserted approximately 0.5 cm below the level of the cricoid and directed 45–60 degrees toward the interscalene groove. The Meier and Borgeat modifications, considered lateral approaches to the interscalene block, use the nerve stimulation technique to identify the endpoint for injection. Chan used ultrasound to directly visualize the nerve roots of the brachial plexus in the interscalene groove at the level of cricoid (Figures 3 and 4) [11]. Using ultrasound, the needle is either inserted using an in-plane technique (alignment with the long axis of the probe) or an out-of-plane technique (alignment with the short axis of the probe). While the in-plane technique allows better visualization of the needle, the out-of-plane technique provides a shorter path to target tissues.

4.2. Posterior Approaches. The posterior approach to the interscalene blockade has had renewed interest. The cervical paravertebral block was first described by Pippa et al. [12]. Boezaart et al. modified this technique by passing the needle between the levator scapulae and the trapezius muscle to reduce neck pain, which was thought to be due to the needle entering the extensor musculature (Figure 5) [13]. Using the landmarks described by Pippa et al., van Geffen et al. used

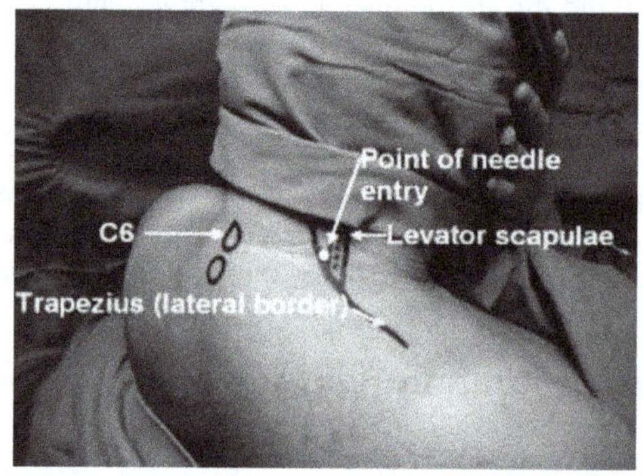

Figure 5: Cervical paravertebral block. Needle entry is at the level of C6, anterolateral to the trapezius muscle and posteromedial to the levator scapulae muscle (Boezaart [2]). (Reprinted with permission from Elsevier.)

ultrasound to perform a single-injection interscalene block and Antonakakis et al. used ultrasound to place a catheter for a continuous interscalene block [12, 14, 15]. When using the cervical paravertebral approach, the catheter is better anchored because it passes through multiple layers of muscle and vital anterior structures have less risk of being injured. The major disadvantage of the cervical paravertebral approach is the distance the needle must travel to reach target. The needle must pass through multiple muscle layers which may be painful to the patient. Also, the needle passes through the middle scalene muscle where injury to the long thoracic and dorsal scapular nerves could occur.

4.3. Interscalene Block Outcomes

4.3.1. Single-Injection versus Continuous Infusion. Mariano et al. conducted a randomized trial with 30 patients who underwent shoulder surgery that caused moderate-to-severe pain [16]. All patients had a posterior approach, nerve stimulation/ultrasound-guided catheter placement, and a bolus injection of 40 mL of 0.5% ropivacaine. Postoperatively, the patients were discharged with oral analgesics and a portable infusion pump containing either 0.2% ropivacaine or normal saline. The ropivacaine infusion group compared to the normal saline infusion group had greater pain relief, lower supplemental opioid requirements, improved sleep quality, and increased patient satisfaction. Fredrickson et al. performed a randomized study with 68 patients who underwent minor arthroscopic surgery: arthroscopic subacromial decompression, excision of the lateral clavicle, or stabilization [17]. Sixty-one patients included in the study received an ultrasound-guided catheter placement with a bolus of 0.5% ropivacaine. Thirty patients had this catheter removed at the end of the procedure. The other 31 patients received an elastomeric infusion consisting of 0.2% ropivacaine 2 mL/h with a bolus option of 5 mL/h. The continuous infusion group had less pain at rest and with movement during the first 24 hours and lower consumption of Tramadol, but a higher rate of extremity numbness. Kean et al. conducted a clinical trial comparing a single-injection interscalene block to a continuous interscalene infusion [18]. This study only consisted of 16 patients, but revealed that the continuous interscalene infusion group consumed less morphine, had lower visual analogue scores, and overall had higher satisfaction after major surgery of the shoulder. Trompeter et al. assessed 100 patients who underwent shoulder surgery that caused moderate pain [19]. The patients were administered a single-injection interscalene block, followed by general anesthesia for the operation. At discharge, the patients were given a pain diary and followed for 5 days. Fifteen percent of patients experienced severe pain at some point over the first 3 days, but this percentage decreased to 7% by day 5. Ninety-seven percent of the patients were satisfied with their postoperative oral analgesia management and less than 5% contacted their primary care provider for additional analgesia. The authors concluded that a continuous infusion may not be justified for shoulder surgery causing moderate pain.

4.3.2. Neurostimulation versus Ultrasound. Since the arrival of ultrasound as an alternative to performing peripheral nerve blocks, there has been the question, what is better, the nerve stimulation technique or ultrasound? When an accurate image is obtained, ultrasound permits direct visualization of target tissues and surrounding structures. This potentially reduces complications, enhances success rates, and reduces local anesthetic volumes. However, the nerve stimulation technique done for the interscalene block has a high success rate and low complication rate. Furthermore, the nerve stimulation technique is less expensive, more portable and requires less setup time.

Liu et al. performed a randomized trial with 230 patients comparing ultrasound-guided to nerve-stimulation-guided interscalene blocks [20]. Ultrasound reduced the number of needle passes needed to perform the interscalene block and enhanced motor blockade at the 5-minute assessment period; however, there were no differences in block failure, patient satisfaction, or the incidence or severity of postoperative neurological symptoms. Kapral et al. evaluated the success rate of ultrasound compared to nerve stimulation in 160 randomized patients [21]. Surgical anesthesia was achieved in 99% of patients in the ultrasound group compared to 91% of patients in the nerve stimulation group ($P < 0.01$). Furthermore, sensory, motor, and extent of blockade were significantly better in the ultrasound group. Fredrickson et al. conducted a prospective, randomized study in 83 patients comparing ultrasound-guided to nerve-stimulation-guided interscalene catheter placement [22]. The ultrasound group had less needle under the skin time, less need for catheter manipulation after surgery and improved pain scores on the first day, but no difference on the second day.

4.3.3. Local Anesthetic Volumes. One of the advantages of ultrasound-guided nerve blockade is the capacity to place local anesthetic under direct visualization and observe the spread, which allows local anesthetic administration to be adjusted in real time. Since less total volume of local anesthetic may be required to produce an effective block, this could reduce the risk of local anesthetic systemic toxicity [23]. McNaught et al. performed a randomized study with 40 patients comparing ultrasound to nerve stimulation to determine the minimum volume of local anesthetic needed for a successful interscalene block [24]. The minimum effective analgesic volume for the ultrasound group was 0.9 mL compared to 5.4 mL for the nerve stimulation group ($P = 0.034$). Fredrickson et al. conducted a three-staged study that estimated the volume and concentration of interscalene ropivacaine that would prevent recovery room pain after shoulder surgery under general anesthesia [25]. Comparing 20 mL of 0.375% ropivacaine (new, experimental dose) to 30 mL of 0.5% ropivacaine (standard dose), there was no difference in pain or grip strength, but satisfaction was slightly higher with the lower dose. Riazi et al. studied 40 patients randomized to receive an ultrasound-guided single-injection interscalene block using either 5 or 20 mL of 0.5% ropivacaine [26]. The incidence of hemidiaphragmatic paresis was significantly lower in the low-volume group compared to the standard-volume group (45% versus 100%). Postoperative oxygen saturation was higher in the low-volume group (−1.50 versus −5.85, $P = 0.004$). There were no differences in pain scores, sleep quality, and total morphine consumption during the first 24 hours after surgery. Renes et al. studied 30 patients that received a low (C7 level) interscalene block by ultrasound guidance or nerve stimulation [27]. In each group, 10 mL of 0.75% ropivacaine was administered. The incidence of hemidiaphragmatic paresis was lower in the ultrasound group (13% versus 93%, $P < 0.0001$). However, Sinha et al. randomized 30 patients to receive either 20 mL or 10 mL of 0.5% ropivacaine for an ultrasound-guided interscalene block performed at the level of the cricoid cartilage (C5-C6 roots) [28]. The reduction in local anesthetic volume did not reduce the incidence of hemidiaphragmatic paresis, which occurred in 93% of patients in each group.

4.4. Complications. Common complications of the interscalene nerve block include phrenic nerve blockade (hemidiaphragmatic paresis), Horner's syndrome, recurrent laryngeal nerve blockade, and vasculature puncture (hematoma). Rarer, but potentially devastating, complications include carotid artery puncture and intervertebral artery injection, pneumothorax, subdural injection, intervertebral foramina injection resulting in spinal or epidural anesthesia, and nerve injury. In addition, indwelling catheters may become infected, kinked, knotted, or entrapped [29, 30]. The risk for most of these complications is minimized by awareness of the location of the needle and surrounding structures. This is facilitated with ultrasound guidance, but even with landmark techniques, the clinician should be aware of areas that are at high risk.

Interscalene blocks and perineural catheters have a risk of complications, but most of these are minor and resolve without sequelae [31–36]. However, the possibility of catastrophic complications exists especially since the interscalene brachial plexus block brings the needle so close to neuraxial structures. Voermans et al. reported a case of permanent loss of cervical spinal cord function associated with the posterior approach to the interscalene block [37]. This was thought to be due to a direct intrathecal and intramedullary injection. Aramideh et al. reported a case in which a patient remained conscious, but developed total paralysis and Horner's syndrome after a brachial plexus block utilizing a posterior approach [38]. Finally, Benumof reported four cases in which the performance of interscalene block during general anesthesia was followed by total spinal anesthesia and extensive permanent loss of bilateral cervical spinal cord function [39].

4.5. Summary. Shoulder procedures producing mild-to-moderate pain may be managed with a single-injection interscalene block. However, studies support that moderate-to-severe pain, lasting for several days, is best managed with a continuous interscalene block. This may cause increased extremity numbness, but will provide greater analgesia, reduce supplemental opioid consumption, and improve sleep quality and patient satisfaction. Nerve stimulation is still a good technique for performing an interscalene block. Ultrasound may improve the efficiency of performing blocks since studies reveal less need to manipulate the needle. Also, some studies have shown an improved success rate and faster interscalene block onset with ultrasound. Ultrasound can reduce the volume of local anesthetic needed to produce an effective interscalene block. Blockade performed at the C6 level did not lead to a decrease in hemidiaphragmatic paresis. However, a block performed at the C7 level and volumes less than 10 mL did show a substantial decrease in hemidiaphragmatic paresis, but did not eliminate this problem. Major complications with the interscalene block are rare, but the capacity to view the needle with ultrasound may be beneficial in reducing complications. Presently, it has not been shown that ultrasound offers a definitive benefit in preventing major complications when compared to the nerve stimulation technique.

5. Suprascapular Nerve Block

The suprascapular nerve block combined with an axillary nerve block may provide an efficacious alternative to the interscalene nerve block for shoulder anesthesia. The axillary nerve block as described in this section refers to blockade of a terminal branch of the brachial plexus, the axillary nerve. As previously mentioned, the majority of the nerve supply to the shoulder is provided by the suprascapular and axillary nerves (Figures 1 and 2). When these nerves are blocked separately, there may be fewer complications and side effects than the traditional interscalene block [3, 4]. The phrenic nerve is not blocked; therefore, these blocks may be used for patients that are not candidates for an interscalene block, for example, severe chronic obstructive pulmonary disease or contralateral hemidiaphragmatic paresis. This technique may also be used as a rescue block for unsuccessful interscalene blocks. A disadvantage of these blocks is that branches proximal to the injection site or regions not innervated by these nerves are not blocked. This may leave analgesia to the surgical region incomplete, requiring supplementation by intravenous analgesics, local anesthetic infiltration, or general anesthesia.

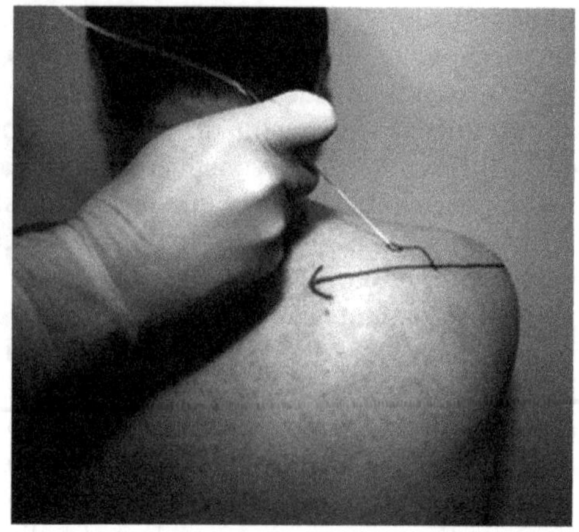

FIGURE 6: Meier technique for the suprascapular nerve block. Needle insertion is 2 cm cephalad and 2 cm medial to the midpoint of a line connecting the lateral acromion and medial border of the spine of the scapula. The needle is angled 45° in the coronal plane, with 30° of ventral inclination (Price [3]). (Reprinted with permission.)

5.1. Approaches. For the suprascapular nerve block, the ideal approach ensures blockade of the more proximal branches to the acromion and the subacromial region to maximize coverage. This may be achieved by blocking the nerve in the suprascapular notch; however, this location is associated with a small risk of pneumothorax [3, 40]. Price described a technique for this block that was adopted from Meier et al. in which the suprascapular nerve is blocked as it travels across the supraspinous fossa (Figures 6 and 7) [3, 41]. In addition, Price described a technique to block the axillary nerve immediately after it passes through the quadrilateral space as it lies just posterior to the humerus (Figures 8 and 9) [3]. Checcucci et al. also described techniques for blocking the suprascapular and axillary nerves [4]. The suprascapular nerve is blocked by eliciting a supraspinatus and infraspinatus motor response (arm abduction and external rotation) after inserting a nerve-stimulating needle at a point 2 cm medial to the medial border of the acromion and approximately 2 cm cephalad to the superior margin of the scapular

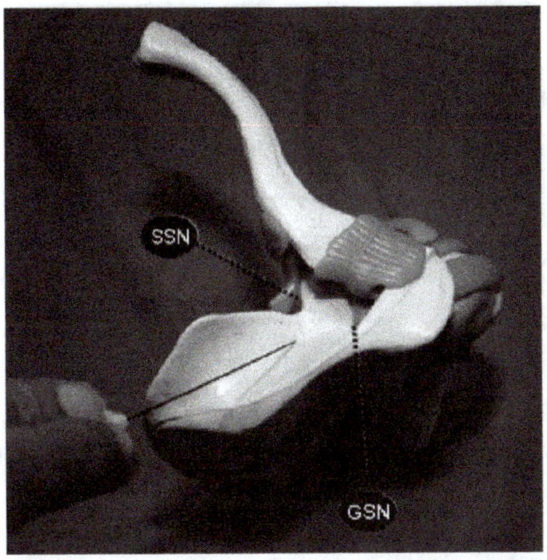

Figure 7: Anatomic representation of the superior view of the Meier technique. Note the needle is in the supraspinous fossa, demonstrating the 30° of ventral inclination. The suprascapular nerve enters the groove at the suprascapular notch (SSN) and winds laterally around the greater scapular notch (GSN) (Price [3]). (Reprinted with permission.)

spine (Figure 10). The axillary nerve is blocked by drawing a line between the lateral-posterior angle of the acromion and the olecranon tip of the elbow. A perpendicular line is drawn from this line to the axillary fold. A nerve-stimulating needle is inserted 2 cm cephalad to the intersection of the lines and a deltoid muscle motor response is sought to identify the axillary nerve (Figure 11). Matsumoto et al. developed a technique for performing the suprascapular nerve block based upon cadaveric anatomy (Figures 12 and 13) [5]. The insertion point is the midpoint of the anterolateral angle of the acromion and the medial edge of the scapular spine. The needle is inclined at a 30-degree angle dorsal to the coronal plane (axis of the body) and inserted until it reaches the base of the coracoid process. Finally, Harmon and Hearty described an ultrasound technique for blocking the suprascapular nerve (Figures 14 and 15) [6]. The ultrasound probe, oriented transversely to the scapula spine, is moved cephalad and lateral to directly visualized and inject around the nerve in the suprascapular notch.

5.2. Suprascapular Nerve Block Outcomes. Singelyn et al. conducted a randomized trial of 120 patients comparing an interscalene nerve block to a suprascapular nerve block, intra-articular injection, and control group [42]. There was no difference between the intra-articular injection group and the control group. The suprascapular and interscalene block groups had lower pain scores compared to the intra-articular injection and control groups. The interscalene group had better pain relief with movement than suprascapular group. Overall, the interscalene group had decreased opioid consumption and better patient satisfaction. Jerosch et al. performed a randomized trial of 260 patients who had shoulder operations which caused moderate-to-severe pain [43]. The patients either had a suprascapular nerve block or no block

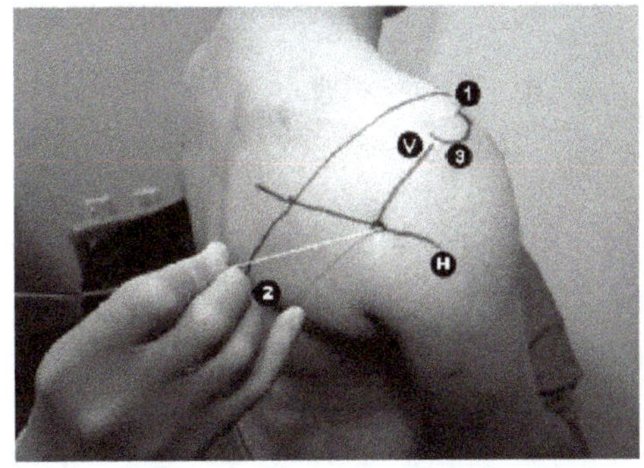

Figure 8: Price technique for the axillary nerve block. A line connects the anterior acromion (1) with the inferior angle of the scapula (2). The midpoint of the line represents the level of the horizontal axis (H) of the quadrilateral space. The line representing the vertical axis (V) is drawn down from the posterolateral aspect of the acromion (3) (Price [3]). (Reprinted with permission.)

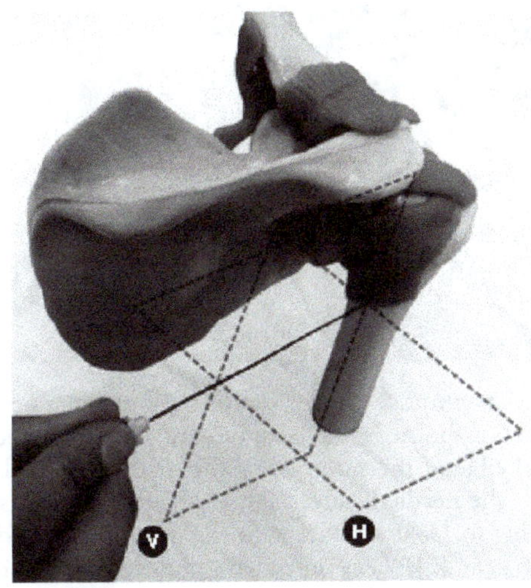

Figure 9: Anatomic representation of the Price technique. The horizontal axis (H) lies at the level of the quadrilateral space, where the axillary nerve passes beneath the glenohumeral joint capsule. The interception of the vertical axis (V) with the horizontal axis (H) allows location of the axillary nerve as it crossing the posterior neck of the humerus (Price [3]). (Reprinted with permission.)

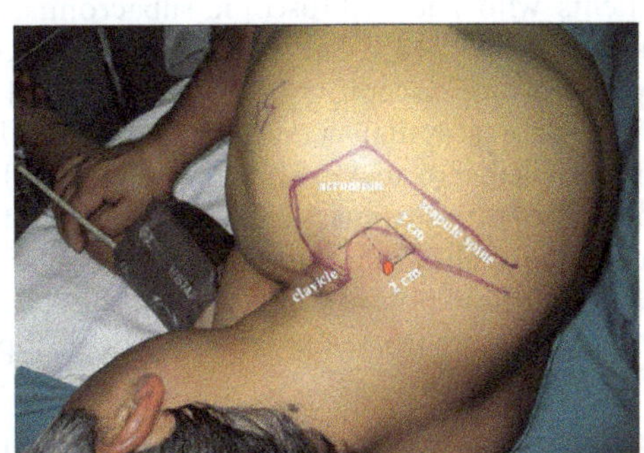

Figure 10: Checcucci technique for the suprascapular nerve block. Needle insertion is 2 cm medial to the medial border of the acromion and 2 cm cephalad to the superior margin of the scapular spine (Checcucci et al. [4]). (Reprinted with permission from Elsevier.)

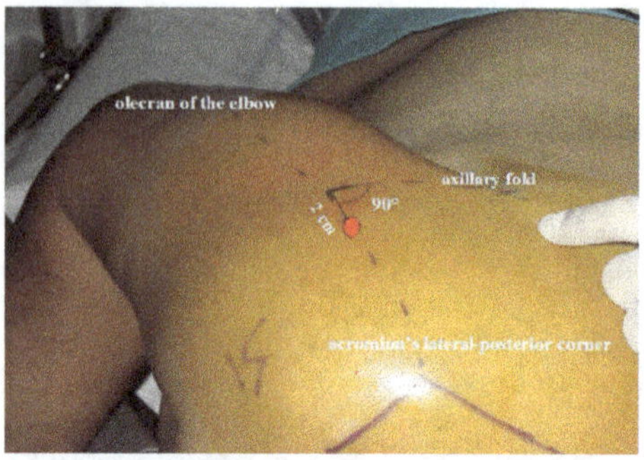

Figure 11: Checcucci technique for the axillary nerve block. A line is drawn between the posterolateral angle of the acromion and the olecranon tip of the elbow. The needle insertion is 2 cm cephalad to the convergence of this line with the perpendicular line originating from the axillary fold (Checcucci et al. [4]). (Reprinted with permission from Elsevier.)

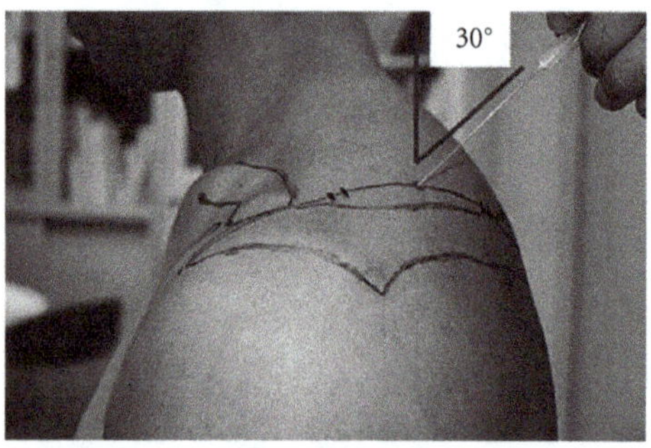

Figure 12: Matsumoto technique for the suprascapular nerve block. Needle insertion point is the midpoint of a line connecting the anterolateral edge of the acromion and the superomedial angle of the scapula. The needle is advanced, at an angle 30° dorsal to the coronal plane, to make contact with the base of coracoid process (Matsumoto et al. [5]). (Reprinted with permission from Elsevier.)

(control). The results showed that from day 1 to day 3 the suprascapular group had significantly better pain scores; however, pain score differences between the groups were relatively small. Jeske et al. conducted a randomized study of 45 patients who had arthroscopic subacromial decompressions performed [44]. The patients were placed in 3 groups: placebo (suprascapular nerve block with 10 mL of 0.9% saline), suprascapular nerve block with 10 mL of 1% ropivacaine, or subacromial infiltration with 20 mL of 1% ropivacaine. The suprascapular group had significantly lower pain scores at 6 h and 24 h, better range of motion, and patient satisfaction. Reported pain scores in the subacromial infiltration group were worse than the placebo group.

5.3. Complications. The suprascapular or the axillary nerve blocks have the basic risks of any peripheral nerve block: nerve injury, intravascular injection, and vascular puncture. In addition, the suprascapular block may have a small risk of a pneumothorax.

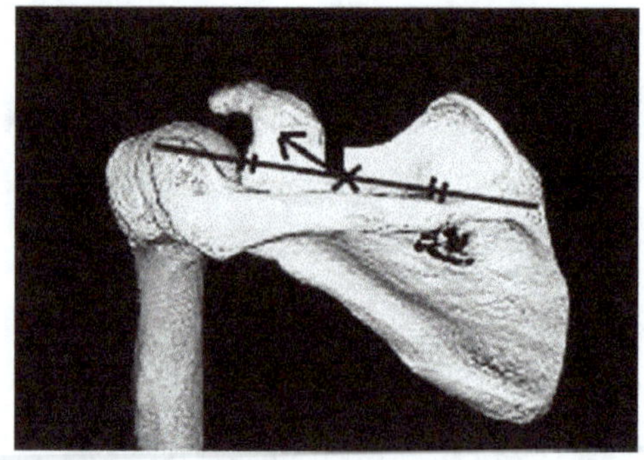

Figure 13: Anatomic representation of the Matsumoto technique (Matsumoto et al. [5]). (Reprinted with permission from Elsevier.)

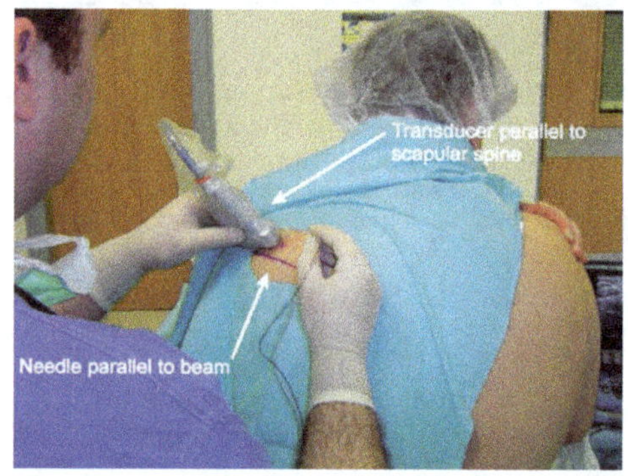

Figure 14: Ultrasound probe and needle position for suprascapular nerve block (Harmon and Hearty [6]). (Reprinted with permission.)

5.4. Summary. The evidence indicates that the suprascapular and/or axillary nerve blocks are not as effective as an interscalene block. Also, these blocks are performed as single injections and have limited use for prolonged postoperative analgesia. However in patients who are not candidates for the interscalene block, these blocks may provide a useful alternative for short-term pain relief.

6. Supraclavicular Block

Supraclavicular block provides anesthesia of the entire upper extremity in the most consistent, time-efficient manner of any brachial plexus technique [45]. The "divisions" of the brachial plexus are blocked. Similar to the interscalene nerve block, the block is done between the anterior and middle scalene muscles. The popularity of this approach was limited in the past due to the risk of pneumothorax when using landmark-based techniques [46, 47]. However, ultrasound has rejuvenated interest in this block by providing real-time visualization of the target tissues and surrounding structures, potential reducing complications such as pneumothorax and nerve injury [48, 49]. The block is frequently used for elbow, forearm, wrist, and hand surgery. Since it is performed above the clavicle, it can also provide shoulder analgesia. The concern with using this block for shoulder surgery is that

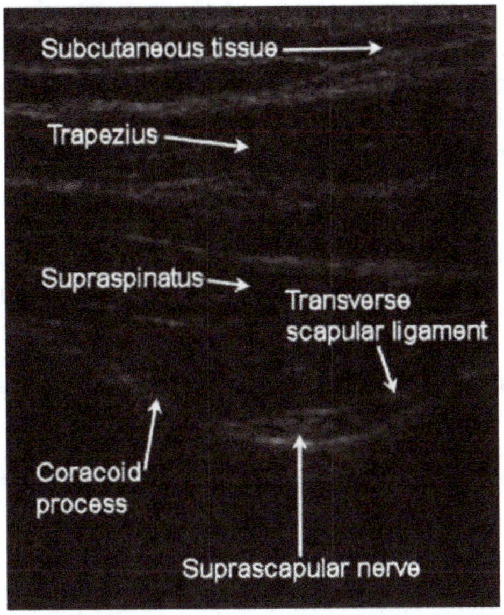

FIGURE 15: Transverse view of suprascapular fossa and suprascapular notch (Harmon and Hearty [6]). (Reprinted with permission.)

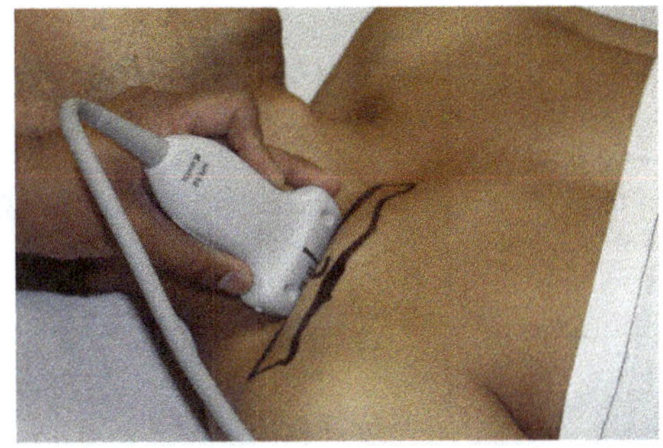

FIGURE 16: Ultrasound probe position for the supraclavicular brachial plexus block.

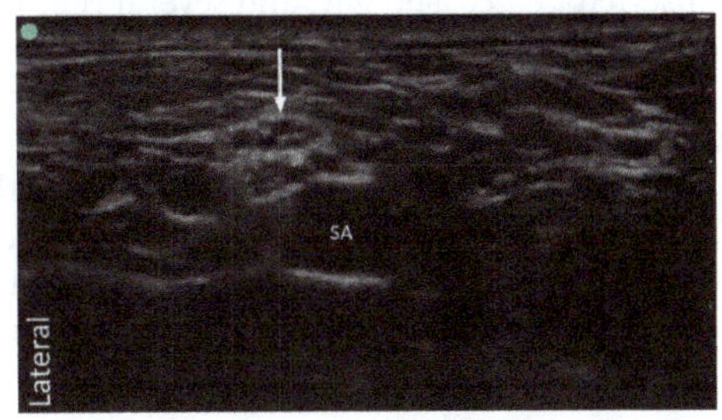

FIGURE 17: Transverse ultrasound image of supraclavicular brachial plexus. Arrow points toward the divisions of the brachial plexus. The location of the brachial plexus is posterolateral to the subclavian artery (SA).

proximal nerves and nerve branches that supply the shoulder may be missed.

6.1. Approaches. The supraclavicular block can be performed by two landmark-based techniques, classic approach and plumb-bob approach [45]. Using the classic approach, the needle entry point is 1 cm superior to the clavicle, at the midpoint of the clavicle. It is advanced approximately parallel to the patient's neck and head, from cephalad to caudad toward the first rib. The plumb-bob technique uses an anterior-to-posterior trajectory of the needle to reduce the risk for pneumothorax. With either method, the paresthesia technique or nerve stimulation technique may be used to determine the endpoint for injection. When utilizing ultrasound guidance, a linear probe is placed above and parallel to the clavicle to produce a transverse image of the brachial plexus as it passes just posterolateral to the subclavian artery (Figures 16 and 17) [49]. An in-plane technique (long axis) permits visualization of the entire needle, which allows the provider to direct the needle toward targeted tissues.

6.2. Supraclavicular Block Outcomes. Liu et al. conducted a prospective clinical registry of 1,169 patients who underwent shoulder arthroscopy with either an interscalene ($n = 515$) or supraclavicular block ($n = 654$) performed at the discretion of the clinical team [50]. Success rate was excellent for both blocks: interscalene (100%) and supraclavicular (99.7%). The incidence of hoarseness in the postanesthesia care unit was significantly less for the supraclavicular group (22%) compared to interscalene group (31%). The incidence of dyspnea was similar: interscalene (10%) and supraclavicular (7%). There was no clinical evidence of a pneumothorax, and the incidence of postoperative neurological symptoms was low, 0.4%. The authors concluded that ultrasound-guided interscalene and supraclavicular blocks are effective and safe for shoulder arthroscopy.

6.3. Complications. Complications of supraclavicular block include pneumothorax (0.6%–6.1%), vascular puncture, intravascular injection, Horner's syndrome, recurrent laryngeal nerve blockade, nerve injury, and phrenic nerve blockade with transient hemidiaphragmatic paresis [51–55].

6.4. Summary. There is not enough evidence to support the use of the supraclavicular block for shoulder surgery. The supraclavicular block, similar to the low interscalene block, has a lower incidence of hemidiaphragmatic paresis. Further clinical trials may show the usefulness of the supraclavicular or low interscalene block as an effective alternative to the traditional interscalene block.

7. Subacromial Block/Intra-Articular Injections

The subacromial block is generally used for arthroscopic shoulder procedures including subacromial decompression and rotator cuff repair [56, 57]. The pain for these procedures can vary from mild to severe. Therefore, single-injection or continuous infusions are employed depending on the anticipated intensity of the pain. Single-injection and continuous infusions of local anesthetic in the subacromial space have been shown to provide superior pain relief compared to placebo [58–60]. The advantages of subacromial injection (infusion) compared to an interscalene block (infusion) include easy and rapid catheter placement, direct visualization to facilitate proper placement, and little to no extremity numbness or weakness.

Intra-articular injections have many of the same advantages as a subacromial block. However, the efficacy of these injections for postoperative pain management has recently been questioned [42].

7.1. Approaches. A subacromial continuous infusion catheter is placed intraoperatively by the surgeon [56]. At the end of the arthroscopy, the posterior portal is used to visualize the subacromial space. Under direct visualization, the catheter sheath is inserted posterolaterally, and several centimeters of catheter are placed in the subacromial space. An elastomeric pump is connected to the catheter for outpatient use. The patient discontinues the pump at home by removing the dressing and catheter. Single injections are done in the same manner without placing the catheter. In the case of intra-articular injections, the glenohumeral joint is directly injected with a local anesthetic, opioid, or combination. This is easily done with direct visualization during arthroscopy.

7.2. Subacromial/Intra-Articular Injection Outcomes. Delaunay et al. conducted a randomized trial in 30 patients, who had undergone arthroscopic rotator cuff repair. A subacromial continuous infusion was compared to an interscalene continuous infusion [61]. Both groups received a single-injection interscalene block as their primary anesthetic for the surgery. While the interscalene group had an indwelling catheter placed after the single injection, the subacromial group had a subacromial catheter placed at the end of the surgery. Postoperatively, each patient received a 0.2% ropivacaine continuous infusion (5 mL/h) with a patient-controlled bolus option (5 mL/30 min). The patients were followed for 48 hours. The interscalene group had lower pain scores at rest and with passive motion, decreased morphine consumption, and fewer extra ropivacaine boluses over the 48-hour period. Eleven patients in the interscalene group compared to one in the subacromial group complained of numbness and weakness. Patient satisfaction was comparable between the two groups. Nisar et al. performed a randomized controlled trial of 60 patients who underwent arthroscopic subacromial decompression [62]. The groups consisted of a single-injection interscalene block, single-injection subacromial block, or no block (control). Postoperative pain management was with patient-controlled analgesia (PCA) and oral pain medications. The pain scores in the interscalene and subacromial groups were lower than those in the control group in the first 12 hours postoperatively. The control group consumed more morphine (mean, 32.3 mg) compared with the subacromial group (mean, 21.2 mg) and interscalene group (mean, 14.0 mg) ($P < 0.001$). Winkler et al. conducted a randomized clinical trial in 40 patients who underwent arthroscopic acromioplasty [63]. A subacromial continuous infusion was compared to an interscalene continuous infusion with 0.2% ropivacaine (2 mL/h). The interscalene infusion group had significantly reduced pain scores at rest and during exercise and lower incidence of night pain. Finally, Fontana et al. conducted a clinical trial with 120 patients scheduled for arthroscopy and randomized them to one of five groups: intra-articular injection, subacromial block, interscalene block, intra-articular injection/subacromial block, or control group [64]. All patients underwent general anesthesia. Postoperatively, PCA bolus injections of fentanyl, pain scores, and patient satisfaction were compared. Mean bolus injections and pain scores were as follows: control > intra-articular > subacromial > intra-articular/subacromial > interscalene. However, the patient satisfaction between the intra-articular/subacromial and interscalene block groups was comparable. The authors concluded that a combination of an intra-articular and subacromial block may be a good alternative to an interscalene block.

7.3. Complications. One of the advantages of the subacromial injection or infusion may be a lower complication rate in comparison to the interscalene nerve block. Also, there is less risk of extremity numbness or weakness. Busfield et al. conducted a prospective, consecutive study with 583 patients evaluating the short-term complication rate of subacromial infusion pumps [56]. There were no cases of infection, internal catheter breakage, pump failure, or hospital admission for pain control. They concluded that subacromial pain pumps used for arthroscopic shoulder procedures are safe in the short term. Recently, there has been concern about chondrolysis or rapid articular cartilage destruction related to intra-articular injections. Local anesthetics have been shown to induce chondrotoxicity in animal studies, especially when bupivacaine is used in high doses [65]. This is a devastating complication in a young patient and difficult to manage. Even though the cases series by Bailie and Ellenbecker concluded that the etiology of chondrolysis was most likely multifactorial, there was a strong recommendation against the use of large doses of intra-articular local anesthetics [66].

7.4. Summary. There is substantial evidence showing that subacromial and intra-articular injections provide little clinical benefit for postoperative analgesia, especially for open and/or rotator cuff procedures. Given that these injections may be associated with irreversible chondrotoxicity, the injections are not presently recommended [8].

8. Conclusion

The interscalene brachial plexus block remains the mainstay for shoulder surgery. It is especially beneficial for shoulder surgery causing moderate-to-severe pain. For cases in which pain is anticipated to last for several days, a continuous interscalene block is appropriate. In all the outcome studies in this paper, the interscalene block produced superior analgesia to other techniques. For mild pain, other methods may be considered, but it is still unclear how much benefit these techniques offer in comparison to oral analgesics. When an interscalene block is contraindicated, the suprascapular and axillary nerve blocks offer a reasonable alternative. Since these techniques have not gained widespread use, providers may be less familiar with how to perform them. The suprascapular and axillary nerve blocks appear safe and should be added to the anesthesia provider's skill set. The use of ultrasound in the last five years has enhanced regional anesthesia. Ultrasound-guided upper extremity blockade often provides faster block performance, faster block onset, and greater block success compared to the nerve stimulation technique, while providing a similar safety profile [67]. Finally, intra-articular injection of local anesthetic is not recommended because of the association with chondrolysis.

References

[1] A. Borgeat and G. Ekatodramis, "Anaesthesia for shoulder surgery," *Best Practice and Research*, vol. 16, no. 2, pp. 211–225, 2002.

[2] A. P. Boezaart, "Continuous interscalene block for ambulatory shoulder surgery," *Best Practice and Research*, vol. 16, no. 2, pp. 295–310, 2002.

[3] D. J. Price, "The shoulder block: a new alternative to interscalene brachial plexus blockade for the control of postoperative shoulder pain," *Anaesthesia and Intensive Care*, vol. 35, no. 4, pp. 575–581, 2007.

[4] G. Checcucci, A. Allegra, P. Bigazzi, L. Gianesello, M. Ceruso, and G. Gritti, "A new technique for regional anesthesia for arthroscopic shoulder surgery based on a suprascapular nerve block and an axillary nerve block: an evaluation of the first results," *Arthroscopy*, vol. 24, no. 6, pp. 689–696, 2008.

[5] D. Matsumoto, N. Suenaga, N. Oizumi, Y. Hisada, and A. Minami, "A new nerve block procedure for the suprascapular nerve based on a cadaveric study," *Journal of Shoulder and Elbow Surgery*, vol. 18, no. 4, pp. 607–611, 2009.

[6] D. Harmon and C. Hearty, "Ultrasound-guided suprascapular nerve block technique," *Pain Physician*, vol. 10, no. 6, pp. 743–746, 2007.

[7] A. P. Boezaart, *Anesthesia and Orthopaedic Surgery*, Mac-Graw Hill, New York, NY, USA, 2006.

[8] M. J. Fredrickson, S. Krishnan, and C. Y. Chen, "Postoperative analgesia for shoulder surgery: a critical appraisal and review of current techniques," *Anaesthesia*, vol. 65, no. 6, pp. 608–624, 2010.

[9] A. P. Winnie, "Interscalene brachial plexus block," *Anesthesia and Analgesia*, vol. 49, no. 3, pp. 455–466, 1970.

[10] G. Meier, C. Bauereis, and C. Heinrich, "The interscalene brachial plexus catheter for anaesthesia and postoperative pain management. Experience with a modified technique," *Anaesthesist*, vol. 46, no. 8, pp. 715–719, 1997.

[11] V. W. S. Chan, "Applying ultrasound imaging to interscalene brachial plexus block," *Regional Anesthesia and Pain Medicine*, vol. 28, no. 4, pp. 340–343, 2003.

[12] P. Pippa, E. Cominelli, C. Marinelli, and S. Aito, "Brachial plexus block using the posterior approach," *European Journal of Anaesthesiology*, vol. 7, no. 5, pp. 411–420, 1990.

[13] A. P. Boezaart, R. Koorn, and R. W. Rosenquist, "Paravertebral approach to the brachial plexus: an anatomic improvement in technique," *Regional Anesthesia and Pain Medicine*, vol. 28, no. 3, pp. 241–244, 2003.

[14] J. G. Antonakakis, B. D. Sites, and J. Shiffrin, "Ultrasound-guided posterior approach for the placement of a continuous interscalene catheter," *Regional Anesthesia and Pain Medicine*, vol. 34, no. 1, pp. 64–68, 2009.

[15] G. J. van Geffen, H. C. Rettig, T. Koornwinder, S. Renes, and M. J. M. Gielen, "Ultrasound-guided training in the performance of brachial plexus block by the posterior approach: an observational study," *Anaesthesia*, vol. 62, no. 10, pp. 1024–1028, 2007.

[16] E. R. Mariano, R. Afra, V. J. Loland et al., "Continuous interscalene brachial plexus block via an ultrasound-guided posterior approach: a randomized, triple-masked, placebo-controlled study," *Anesthesia and Analgesia*, vol. 108, no. 5, pp. 1688–1694, 2009.

[17] M. J. Fredrickson, C. M. Ball, and A. J. Dalgleish, "Analgesic effectiveness of a continuous versus single-injection interscalene block for minor arthroscopic shoulder surgery," *Regional Anesthesia and Pain Medicine*, vol. 35, no. 1, pp. 28–33, 2010.

[18] J. Kean, C. A. Wigderowitz, and D. M. Coventry, "Continuous interscalene infusion and single injection using levobupivacaine for analgesia after surgery of the shoulder," *Journal of Bone and Joint Surgery B*, vol. 88, no. 9, pp. 1173–1177, 2006.

[19] A. Trompeter, G. Camilleri, K. Narang, W. Hauf, and R. Venn, "Analgesia requirements after interscalene block for shoulder arthroscopy: the 5 days following surgery," *Archives of Orthopaedic and Trauma Surgery*, vol. 130, no. 3, pp. 417–421, 2010.

[20] S. S. Liu, V. M. Zayas, M. A. Gordon et al., "A prospective, randomized, controlled trial comparing ultrasound versus nerve stimulator guidance for interscalene block for ambulatory shoulder surgery for postoperative neurological symptoms," *Anesthesia and Analgesia*, vol. 109, no. 1, pp. 265–271, 2009.

[21] S. Kapral, M. Greher, G. Huber et al., "Ultrasonographic guidance improves the success rate of interscalene brachial plexus blockade," *Regional Anesthesia and Pain Medicine*, vol. 33, no. 3, pp. 253–258, 2008.

[22] M. J. Fredrickson, C. M. Ball, and A. J. Dalgleish, "A prospective randomized comparison of ultrasound guidance versus neurostimulation for interscalene catheter placement," *Regional Anesthesia and Pain Medicine*, vol. 34, no. 6, pp. 590–594, 2009.

[23] J. M. Neal, C. M. Bernards, J. F. Butterworth et al., "ASRA practice advisory on local anesthetic systemic toxicity," *Regional Anesthesia and Pain Medicine*, vol. 35, no. 2, pp. 152–161, 2010.

[24] A. McNaught, U. Shastri, N. Carmichael et al., "Ultrasound reduces the minimum effective local anaesthetic volume compared with peripheral nerve stimulation for interscalene block," *British Journal of Anaesthesia*, vol. 106, no. 1, pp. 124–130, 2011.

[25] M. J. Fredrickson, K. R. Smith, and A. C. Wong, "Importance of volume and concentration for ropivacaine interscalene block in preventing recovery room pain and minimizing motor block after shoulder surgery," *Anesthesiology*, vol. 112, no. 6, pp. 1374–1381, 2010.

[26] S. Riazi, N. Carmichael, I. Awad, R. M. Holtby, and C. J. L. McCartney, "Effect of local anaesthetic volume (20 verses 5 ml) on the efficacy and respiratory consequences of ultrasound-guided interscalene brachial plexus block," *British Journal of Anaesthesia*, vol. 101, no. 4, pp. 549–556, 2008.

[27] S. H. Renes, H. C. Rettig, M. J. Gielen, O. H. Wilder-Smith, and G. J. van Geffen, "Ultrasound-guided low-dose interscalene brachial plexus block reduces the incidence of hemidiaphragmatic paresis," *Regional Anesthesia and Pain Medicine*, vol. 34, no. 5, pp. 498–502, 2009.

[28] S. K. Sinha, J. H. Abrams, J. T. Barnett et al., "Decreasing the local anesthetic volume from 20 to 10 mL for ultrasound-guided interscalene block at the cricoid level does not reduce the incidence of hemidiaphragmatic paresis," *Regional*

Anesthesia and Pain Medicine, vol. 36, no. 1, pp. 17–20, 2011.

[29] C. Bowens Jr., E. R. Briggs, and R. J. Malchow, "Brachial plexus entrapment of interscalene nerve catheter after uncomplicated ultrasound-guided placement," *Pain Medicine*, vol. 12, no. 7, pp. 1117–1120, 2011.

[30] X. Capdevila, S. Jaber, P. Pesonen, A. Borgeat, and J. J. Eledjam, "Acute neck cellulitis and mediastinitis complicating a continuous interscalene block," *Anesthesia and Analgesia*, vol. 107, no. 4, pp. 1419–1421, 2008.

[31] J. M. Bert, E. Khetia, and D. A. Dubbink, "Interscalene block for shoulder surgery in physician-owned community ambulatory surgery centers," *Arthroscopy*, vol. 26, no. 9, pp. 1149–1152, 2010.

[32] J. Y. Bishop, M. Sprague, J. Gelber et al., "Interscalene regional anesthesia for shoulder surgery," *Journal of Bone and Joint Surgery A*, vol. 87, no. 5, pp. 974–979, 2005.

[33] A. Borgeat, G. Ekatodramis, F. Kalberer, and C. Benz, "Acute and nonacute complications associated with interscalene block and shoulder surgery," *Anesthesiology*, vol. 95, no. 4, pp. 875–880, 2001.

[34] N. A. Bryan, J. D. Swenson, P. E. Greis, and R. T. Burks, "Indwelling interscalene catheter use in an outpatient setting for shoulder surgery: technique, efficacy, and complications," *Journal of Shoulder and Elbow Surgery*, vol. 16, no. 4, pp. 388–395, 2007.

[35] K. D. Candido, R. Sukhani, R. Doty Jr. et al., "Neurologic sequelae after interscalene brachial plexus block for shoulder/upper arm surgery: the association of patient, anesthetic, and surgical factors to the incidence and clinical course," *Anesthesia and Analgesia*, vol. 100, no. 5, pp. 1489–1495, 2005.

[36] M. J. Fredrickson, "The sensitivity of motor response to needle nerve stimulation during ultrasound guided interscalene catheter placement," *Regional Anesthesia and Pain Medicine*, vol. 33, no. 4, pp. 291–296, 2008.

[37] N. C. Voermans, B. J. Crul, B. de Bondt, M. J. Zwarts, and B. G. M. van Engelen, "Permanent loss of cervical spinal cord function associated with the posterior approach," *Anesthesia and Analgesia*, vol. 102, no. 1, pp. 330–331, 2006.

[38] M. Aramideh, H. L. A. van den Oever, G. J. Walstra, and M. Dzoljic, "Spinal anesthesia as a complication of brachial plexus block using the posterior approach," *Anesthesia and Analgesia*, vol. 94, no. 5, pp. 1338–1339, 2002.

[39] J. L. Benumof, "Permanent loss of cervical spinal cord function associated with interscalene block performed under general anesthesia," *Anesthesiology*, vol. 93, no. 6, pp. 1541–1544, 2000.

[40] J. M. Neal, S. B. McDonald, K. L. Larkin, and N. L. Polissar, "Suprascapular nerve block prolongs analgesia after nonarthroscopic shoulder surgery but does not improve outcome," *Anesthesia and Analgesia*, vol. 96, no. 4, pp. 982–986, 2003.

[41] G. Meier, C. Bauereis, and H. Maurer, "The modified technique of continuous suprascapular nerve block. A safe technique in the treatment of shoulder pain," *Anaesthesist*, vol. 51, no. 9, pp. 747–753, 2002.

[42] F. J. Singelyn, L. Lhotel, and B. Fabre, "Pain relief after arthroscopic shoulder surgery: a comparison of intraarticular analgesia, suprascapular nerve block, and interscalene brachial plexus block," *Anesthesia and Analgesia*, vol. 99, no. 2, pp. 589–592, 2004.

[43] J. Jerosch, M. Saad, M. Greig, and T. Filler, "Suprascapular nerve block as a method of preemptive pain control in shoulder surgery," *Knee Surgery, Sports Traumatology, Arthroscopy*, vol. 16, no. 6, pp. 602–607, 2008.

[44] H.-C. Jeske, F. Kralinger, M. Wambacher et al., "A randomized study of the effectiveness of suprascapular nerve block in patient satisfaction and outcome after arthroscopic subacromial decompression," *Arthroscopy*, vol. 27, no. 10, pp. 1323–1328, 2011.

[45] D. L. Brown, *Atlas of Regional Anesthesia*, Elsevier Saunders, Philadelphia, Pa, USA, 3rd edition, 2006.

[46] D. L. Brown, D. R. Cahill, and L. D. Bridenbaugh, "Supraclavicular nerve block: anatomic analysis of a method to prevent pneumothorax," *Anesthesia and Analgesia*, vol. 76, no. 3, pp. 530–534, 1993.

[47] M. E. Guzeldemir, "Pneumothorax and supraclavicular block," *Anesthesia and Analgesia*, vol. 76, no. 3, article 685, 1993.

[48] M. L. Beach, B. D. Sites, and J. D. Gallagher, "Use of a nerve stimulator does not improve the efficacy of ultrasound-guided supraclavicular nerve blocks," *Journal of Clinical Anesthesia*, vol. 18, no. 8, pp. 580–584, 2006.

[49] V. W. S. Chan, A. Perlas, R. Rawson, and O. Odukoya, "Ultrasound-guided supraclavicular brachial plexus block," *Anesthesia and Analgesia*, vol. 97, no. 5, pp. 1514–1517, 2003.

[50] S. S. Liu, M. A. Gordon, P. M. Shaw, S. Wilfred, T. Shetty, and J. T. YaDeau, "A prospective clinical registry of ultrasound-guided regional anesthesia for ambulatory shoulder surgery," *Anesthesia and Analgesia*, vol. 111, no. 3, pp. 617–623, 2010.

[51] A. Bhatia, J. Lai, V. W. S. Chan, and R. Brull, "Pneumothorax as a complication of the ultrasound-guided supraclavicular approach for brachial plexus block," *Anesthesia and Analgesia*, vol. 111, no. 3, pp. 817–819, 2010.

[52] A. Perlas, G. Lobo, N. Lo, R. Brull, V. W. S. Chan, and R. Karkhanis, "Ultrasound-guided supraclavicular block. Outcome of 510 consecutive cases," *Regional Anesthesia and Pain Medicine*, vol. 34, no. 2, pp. 171–176, 2009.

[53] W. Reiss, S. Kurapati, A. Shariat, and A. Hadzic, "Nerve injury complicating ultrasound/electrostimulation-guided supraclavicular brachial plexus block," *Regional Anesthesia and Pain Medicine*, vol. 35, no. 4, pp. 400–401, 2010.

[54] S. H. Renes, H. H. Spoormans, M. J. Gielen, H. C. Rettig, and G. J. van Geffen, "Hemidiaphragmatic paresis can be avoided in ultrasound-guided supraclavicular brachial plexus block," *Regional Anesthesia and Pain Medicine*, vol. 34, no. 6, pp. 595–599, 2009.

[55] D. Q. H. Tran, L. Muñoz, C. Zaouter, G. Russo, and R. J. Finlayson, "A prospective, randomized comparison between single-and double-injection, ultrasound-guided supraclavicular brachial plexus block," *Regional Anesthesia and Pain Medicine*, vol. 34, no. 5, pp. 420–424, 2009.

[56] B. T. Busfield, G. H. Lee, M. Carrillo, R. Ortega, and F. D. Kharrazi, "Subacromial pain pump use with arthroscopic shoulder surgery: a short-term prospective study of complications in 583 patients," *Journal of Shoulder and Elbow Surgery*, vol. 17, no. 6, pp. 860–862, 2008.

[57] J. A. Coghlan, A. Forbes, D. McKenzie, S. N. Bell, and R. Buchbinder, "Efficacy of subacromial ropivacaine infusion for rotator cuff surgery: a randomized trial," *Journal of Bone and Joint Surgery A*, vol. 91, no. 7, pp. 1558–1567, 2009.

[58] G. P. Harvey, J. E. Chelly, T. Al Samsam, and K. Coupe, "Patient-controlled ropivacaine analgesia after arthroscopic subacromial decompression," *Arthroscopy*, vol. 20, no. 5, pp. 451–455, 2004.

[59] W. J. Mallon and C. W. Thomas, "Patient-controlled lidocaine analgesia for acromioplasty surgery," *Journal of Shoulder and Elbow Surgery*, vol. 9, no. 2, pp. 85–88, 2000.

[60] F. H. Savoie, L. D. Field, R. N. Jenkins, W. J. Mallon, and R. A. Phelps II, "The pain control infusion pump for postoperative pain control in shoulder surgery," *Arthroscopy*, vol. 16, no. 4, pp. 339–342, 2000.

[61] L. Delaunay, V. Souron, L. Lafosse, E. Marret, and B. Toussaint, "Analgesia after arthroscopic rotator cuff repair: subacromial versus interscalene continuous infusion of ropivacaine," *Regional Anesthesia and Pain Medicine*, vol. 30, no. 2, pp. 117–122, 2005.

[62] A. Nisar, M. W. J. Morris, J. V. Freeman, J. M. Cort, P. R. Rayner, and S. A. Shahane, "Subacromial bursa block is an effective alternative to interscalene block for postoperative pain control after arthroscopic subacromial decompression: a randomized trial," *Journal of Shoulder and Elbow Surgery*, vol. 17, no. 1, pp. 78–84, 2008.

[63] T. Winkler, A. J. Suda, R. V. Dumitrescu et al., "Interscalene versus subacromial continuous infusion of ropivacaine after arthroscopic acromioplasty: a randomized controlled trial," *Journal of Shoulder and Elbow Surgery*, vol. 18, no. 4, pp. 566–572, 2009.

[64] C. Fontana, A. Di Donato, G. D. Giacomo et al., "Postoperative analgesia for arthroscopic shoulder surgery: a prospective randomized controlled study of intraarticular, subacromial injection, interscalenic brachial plexus block and intraarticular plus subacromial injection efficacy," *European Journal of Anaesthesiology*, vol. 26, no. 8, pp. 689–693, 2009.

[65] A. H. Gomoll, R. W. Kang, J. M. Williams, B. R. Bach, and B. J. Cole, "Chondrolysis after continuous intra-articular bupivacaine infusion: an experimental model investigating chondrotoxicity in the rabbit shoulder," *Arthroscopy*, vol. 22, no. 8, pp. 813–819, 2006.

[66] D. S. Bailie and T. S. Ellenbecker, "Severe chondrolysis after shoulder arthroscopy: a case series," *Journal of Shoulder and Elbow Surgery*, vol. 18, no. 5, pp. 742–747, 2009.

[67] C. J. McCartney, L. Lin, and U. Shastri, "Evidence basis for the use of ultrasound for upper-extremity blocks," *Regional Anesthesia and Pain Medicine*, vol. 35, no. 2, pp. S10–S15, 2010.

14

A Comparative Study of 0.25% Levobupivacaine, 0.25% Ropivacaine, and 0.25% Bupivacaine in Paediatric Single Shot Caudal Block

Jagdeep Sharma,[1] Ruchi Gupta,[2] Anita Kumari,[2] Lakshmi Mahajan,[3] and Jasveer Singh[4]

[1]*Senior Resident, Dept. of Anaesthesia & Intensive Care, Govt. Medical College & Hospital, Sector-32, Chandigarh, India*
[2]*Professor, Dept. of Anaesthesia & Intensive Care, Shri Guru Ram Das Institute of Medical Sciences and Research, Vallah, Amritsar, India*
[3]*Assistant Professor, Dept. of Anaesthesia & Intensive Care, Shri Guru Ram Das Institute of Medical Sciences and Research, Vallah, Amritsar, India*
[4]*Associate Professor, Dept. of Anaesthesia & Intensive Care, Govt. Medical College & Hospital, Sector-32, Chandigarh, India*

Correspondence should be addressed to Jasveer Singh; drjassy18@gmail.com

Academic Editor: Ronald G. Pearl

Aim. There are limited data comparing levobupivacaine, ropivacaine, and bupivacaine in paediatric patients. So, this study was performed to evaluate the caudal effectiveness of all the three drugs in paediatric patients undergoing infraumbilical surgeries and associated complications with these drugs. *Material and Methods.* 90 patients of ASA grade I and II posted for elective infraumbilical surgeries were randomly divided into three groups of 30 each. A standardized anaesthetic protocol was used. Patients received 0.25% levobupivacaine in group 1, 0.25% ropivacaine in group 2, and 0.25% bupivacaine in group 3. The effectiveness of block was assessed using caudal effectiveness score. Postoperative pain relief was assessed with modified Hannallah pain score. Haemodynamic parameter monitoring was done. The duration of analgesia and associated complications were studied. Statistical analysis was done using the chi-square test for nonparametric data. Parametric data were analysed using ANOVA for intergroup comparison and Tukey's HSD for intragroup comparison. *Results.* Demographic data were comparable. Haemodynamic parameters remained within normal range. Mean caudal effectiveness score in all the three groups was statistically insignificant ($p > 0.05$). The duration of analgesia provided by bupivacaine (145.31 ± 26.17 min) was longer than levobupivacaine (126.15 ± 15.15 min) and ropivacaine (114.68 ± 11.32 min) ($p < 0.01$). Mean postoperative pain scores were lower in group 3 as compared to group 1 and group 2. *Conclusion.* We conclude that levobupivacaine and ropivacaine provide similar intraoperative quality with minimal haemodynamic variability and shorter duration of postoperative analgesia without any significant complications when compared with racemic bupivacaine. This trial is registered with CTRI/2018/03/012402.

1. Introduction

Anaesthesia for paediatric patients is highly specialised because of the physiological, pharmacological, and psychological differences between children and adults [1]. Regional anaesthesia techniques have become routine interventions in children and infants [2, 3]. Paediatric regional anaesthesia is an excellent technique for balanced intraoperative and postoperative analgesia [4]. Most frequently used technique is epidural block through a caudal approach [5, 6]. It is a useful adjunct during general anaesthesia and for providing postoperative analgesia after genital, lower abdominal, and lower limb operations [7]. It can reduce the inhaled and intravenous anaesthetic requirement, attenuate the stress response to surgery, facilitate a rapid smooth recovery, and provide good immediate postoperative analgesia [8, 9]. Racemic bupivacaine is the most commonly used local anaesthetic. Various single enantiomeric drugs such as levobupivacaine and ropivacaine are now being used, with concerns regarding cardiac toxicity of racemic bupivacaine. Very few studies in the literature had compared all the three drugs together, so this study was planned. It was conducted to compare the caudal effectiveness of the three drugs as the primary outcome and duration of analgesia, associated complications, and haemodynamic variables as secondary outcome.

2. Material and Methods

A prospective randomized, double blind study was conducted on 90 patients of ASA grade I and II of either sex aged 1 to 10 years, undergoing infraumbilical surgery as circumcision, herniotomies, orchidopexies, etc. after approval from the hospital ethics committee.

After taking informed written consent, the patients were randomly divided into three groups of 30 each. Randomisation was performed by the computer-generated random number table. For having a power of study more than 80%, the required sample size was calculated to be approximately 90 patients through a pilot study. It was calculated using the number of groups, mean difference of the caudal effectiveness scores and duration of analgesia, standard deviation, and Z power table.

Group 1: the patients received 1 ml/kg of 0.25% levobupivacaine

Group 2: the patients received 1 ml/kg of 0.25% ropivacaine

Group 3: the patients received 1 ml/kg of 0.25% bupivacaine

2.1. Exclusion Criteria. Patients with following problems were excluded from the study: refusal by parents or guardian, preexisting neurological disease, hypersensitivity to local anaesthetics under study, bleeding diathesis or coagulation disorder, local sepsis at the site of puncture, and technical problems such as persistent paresthesias or bloody/CSF tap.

The haemodynamic parameters were noted in the preoperative room. All children were premedicated with syrup midazolam 0.5 mg/kg half an hour before surgery. On arrival in the operating room after attaching standard monitoring, all patients were induced with oxygen, nitrous oxide, and sevoflurane, an appropriate sized cannula was inserted, and the intravenous line was started with Isolyte P. The patients were kept on spontaneous ventilation on bag and mask. Lateral decubitus position was made in patients, and caudal block was given after confirming the space with the "Whoosh" test. The study drug was injected. The patients were made to lie in supine position with spontaneous ventilation and anesthesia maintained with oxygen, nitrous oxide, and sevoflurane. Caudal effectiveness score was assessed intraoperatively before beginning of the surgical procedure (Table 1). Surgery was allowed after achieving caudal efficacy.

This would be graded as follows:

Table 1: Caudal effectiveness score.

Score	Definition
1	Able to reduce sevoflurane concentration, heart rate >20% of baseline, along with limb movements
2	Able to reduce sevoflurane concentration, heart rate >20% baseline, with no movements
3	Sevoflurane concentration stopped, minimal or no change in heart rate, no movement on stimulation

1 = ineffective block

2 = partial block

3 = complete block

Continuous intraoperative monitoring will be done, and haemodynamic parameters were recorded every 5 minutes. The patients were shifted to the postanaesthesia care unit. The pain relief was assessed with modified Hannallah pain score [10] (Table 2) in the recovery room and ward every 15 minutes. The duration of absolute analgesia was taken as time from injection of local anaesthetic to modified Hannallah pain score of more than or equal to 4. Injectable paracetamol 10 mg/kg was given as rescue analgesia as required.

Postoperatively vitals in the form of heart rate, respiratory rate, systolic and diastolic blood pressure, and oxygen saturation were monitored. The presence of other adverse events such as bradycardia, respiratory depression, urinary retention, retching, vomiting, and fever was evaluated.

At the end of study, decoding of groups and the data compilation was done. Statistical analysis was done using the chi-square test for nonparametric data. Parametric data were analysed using ANOVA for intergroup comparison and Tukey's HSD for intragroup comparison. p value of less than 0.05 was considered significant and less than 0.001 as highly significant. All statistical data analysis was performed using SPSS software (Version 22).

3. Results

There was no statistically significant difference in all the three groups with regard to age, sex, weight, ASA physical status, and duration of surgery as shown in (Table 3). Mean baseline vitals like heart rate, systolic and diastolic blood pressure, respiratory rate, and oxygen saturation were comparable in all the three groups (Table 3). The mean duration of surgery in all the three groups was comparable. Haemodynamic parameters, namely, heart rate, systolic and diastolic blood pressure, respiratory rate, and oxygen saturation, remained within normal range during the observation period, and the difference in all the three groups was statistically insignificant. The difference in mean caudal effectiveness score (CES) in all the three groups was statistically insignificant ($p > 0.05$). 21 patients in group 1 (levobupivacaine), 19 patients in group 2 (ropivacaine), and 22 patients in group 3 (bupivacaine) had a caudal effectiveness score of 3 (Figure 1). Mean postoperative pain scores as assessed with modified Hannallah pain score were lower in the bupivacaine group as compared

TABLE 2: Modified Hannallah pain score (MHPS) [10].

Observation	Criteria	Points
Blood pressure	±10% preop	0
	>20% preop	1
	>30% preop	2
Crying	Not crying	0
	Crying but responds to tender loving care (TLC)	1
	Crying and does not responds to TLC	2
Movement	None	0
	Restless	1
	Thrashing	2
Agitation	Patient asleep or calm	0
	Mild	1
	Hysterical	2
Posture	No special posture	0
	Flexing legs and thighs	1
	Holding scrotum or groin	2
Complains of pain (where appropriate by age)	Asleep or states no pain	0
	Cannot localize	1
	Can localize	2

TABLE 3: Demographic distribution and baseline vitals.

	Group 1	Group 2	Group 3	Statistical analysis
Age (years)	3.78 ± 3.02	4.48 ± 3.24	4.04 ± 3.24	0.631
Sex (F : M)	1 : 29	1 : 29	3 : 27	0.429
Weight (kg)	12.33 ± 5.66	12.96 ± 5.39	11.50 ± 5.39	0.656
Duration of surgery	48.83 ± 19.14	45.83 ± 19.14	48.60 ± 19.92	0.745
Heart rate	116.57 ± 14.31	115.97 ± 10.96	115.87 ± 15.89	0.45
Systolic blood pressure	104.37 ± 3.13	104.27 ± 3.47	103.87 ± 3.44	0.51
Diastolic blood pressure	59.43 ± 3.97	57.47 ± 5.89	59.99 ± 5.37	0.34

Data are mean ± SD. $p > 0.05$ insignificant; $p < 0.05$ significant.

to the levobupivacaine and ropivacaine groups during 1st hour postoperatively (Figure 2). The duration of postoperative analgesia in group 1 (levobupivacaine) was 126.15 ± 15.15 min (2.10 ± 0.25 hr), group 2 (ropivacaine) was 114.68 ± 11.32 min (1.91 ± 0.18 hr), and group 3 (bupivacaine) was 145.31 ± 15.15 min (2.42 ± 0.43 hr). The difference in duration of postoperative analgesia was statistically highly significant ($p < 0.001$). Levobupivacaine and ropivacaine provided similar duration of postoperative analgesia. Bupivacaine provided longer duration of analgesia than levobupivacaine and ropivacaine.

Three patients, one in each, had laryngospasm intraoperatively. It was managed adequately. Two patients in group 3 (bupivacaine) had bradycardia intraoperatively, which was managed with intravenous atropine. None of the patients in all the three groups had any significant postoperative complications. No neurological sequelae were seen in any patient in all the three groups (Figure 3).

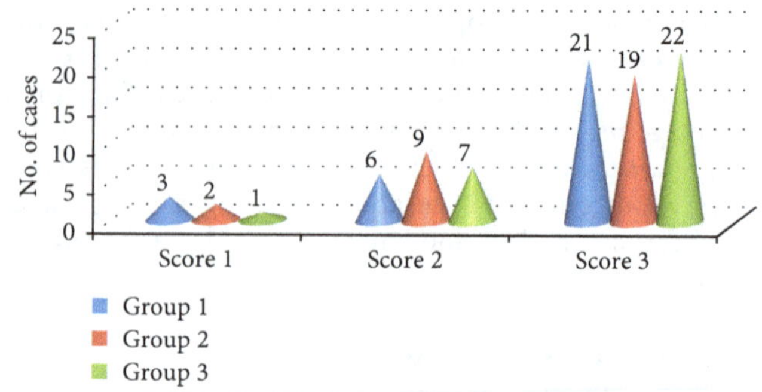

FIGURE 1: Caudal effectiveness score of the three drugs: group 1 (levobupivacaine); group 2 (ropivacaine); group 3 (bupivacaine).

4. Discussion

In paediatric patients, although general anaesthesia is the commonly used technique, regional anaesthesia has gained considerable popularity. The primary advantage of regional supplementation is lowering the requirement of general anaesthesia intraoperatively and providing good post-operative pain relief. Caudal anaesthesia is considered as one of the most popular regional blocks performed in children for infraumbilical surgeries. It is safe, reliable, easy to administer, and not associated with any significant complications.

Intraoperative analgesic efficacy of the block was assessed with caudal effectiveness score which include the autonomic component in the form of heart rate and motor component as limb movements [11]. In children undergoing infraumbilical surgery, caudal levobupivacaine 0.25% produced similar intraoperative analgesic efficacy compared to ropivacaine 0.25% and bupivacaine 0.25% [12] similar to this study. Bupivacaine, an amino amide local anaesthetic, is the most commonly used drug in single shot caudal block. It causes more prolonged caudal blockade as compared to single en-antiomers like ropivacaine and levobupivacaine. It also causes more prolonged motor blockade as compared to the single enantiomeric drugs [11, 12]. Ropivacaine causes least motor blockade because of its differential action on A delta-fibres than A beta-fibres responsible for motor activity. Bupivacaine tends to be having more cardio depressant effects at similar doses as compared to levobupivacaine and ropivacaine. The three drugs cause minimal variation on haemodynamic parameters. Bupivacaine has an average duration of action of 3.5 to 6 hr given in peridural block. Ivani et al. in their study found the duration of analgesia provided by bupivacaine was 233 min (3.80 hr) [13]. But others have found it to be 2-3 hr as was in this study [12]. Praveen et al. compared 0.25% levobupivacaine and 0.25% ropivacaine for caudal epidural analgesia in paediatric patients. The duration of analgesia provided by both the drugs is statistically similar in both the groups, as in our study, although with longer duration (330 ± 9.54 min in levobupivacaine and 312.67 ± 5.56 min in ropivacaine) as compared with ours [14]. The difference in results among these study results can be due to difference in study age groups involved and induction/maintenance techniques of anaesthesia intraoperatively. Ropivacaine produces 3 to 6 hr of analgesia [15], whereas some authors have reported it to be 1 to 2 hr [11].

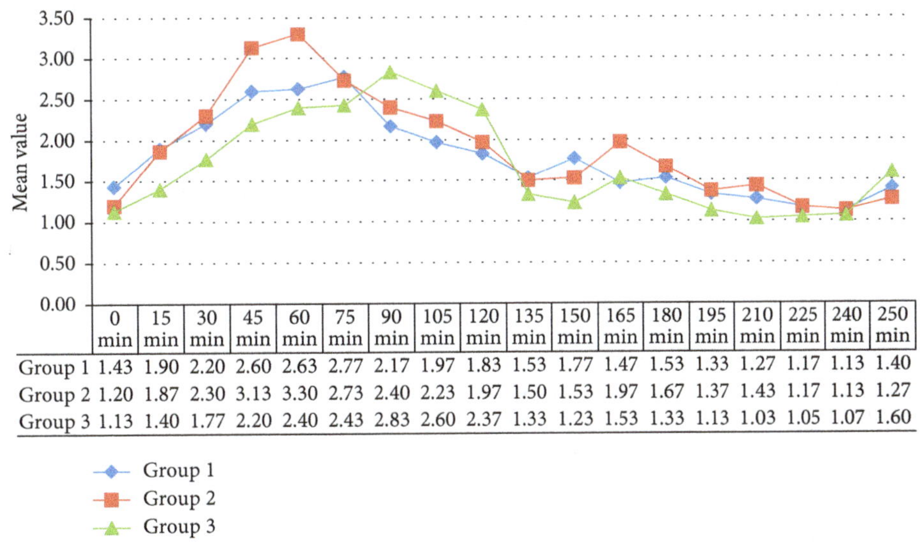

	0 min	15 min	30 min	45 min	60 min	75 min	90 min	105 min	120 min	135 min	150 min	165 min	180 min	195 min	210 min	225 min	240 min	250 min
Group 1	1.43	1.90	2.20	2.60	2.63	2.77	2.17	1.97	1.83	1.53	1.77	1.47	1.53	1.33	1.27	1.17	1.13	1.40
Group 2	1.20	1.87	2.30	3.13	3.30	2.73	2.40	2.23	1.97	1.50	1.53	1.97	1.67	1.37	1.43	1.17	1.13	1.27
Group 3	1.13	1.40	1.77	2.20	2.40	2.43	2.83	2.60	2.37	1.33	1.23	1.53	1.33	1.13	1.03	1.05	1.07	1.60

FIGURE 2: Mean modified Hannallah pain scores of the three drugs: group 1 (levobupivacaine); group 2 (ropivacaine); group 3 (bupivacaine) over the observation period.

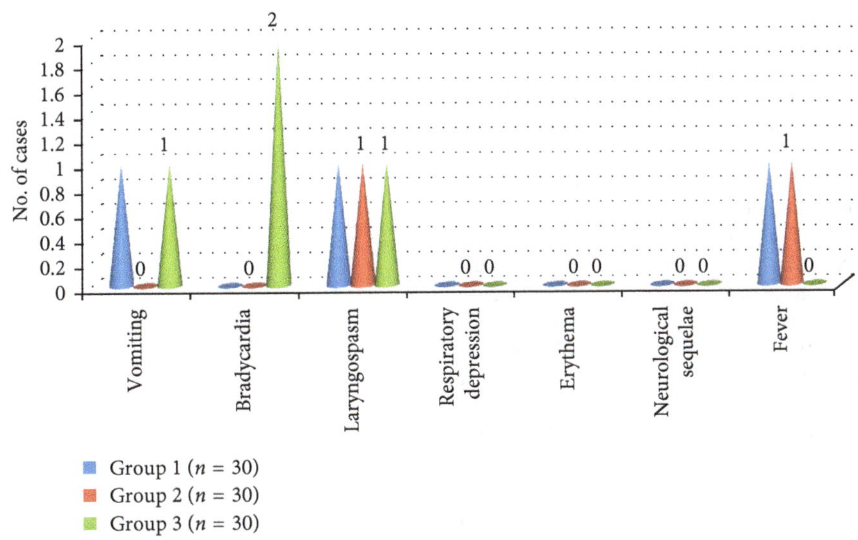

FIGURE 3: Various complications encountered in all the three groups: group 1 (levobupivacaine); group 2 (ropivacaine); group 3 (bupivacaine).

Levobupivacaine provide 3 to 6 hr of analgesia [15], whereas others have reported it to be 1 to 2 hr [11] similar to this study. On literature review, the majority of studies have shown the duration of analgesia provided by all the three drugs is quite similar, contrary to our study. The rate of serious complications reported had been 1/40,000 and the total complication rate 1.5/1000. During caudal block, the most frequent complications (due to the technique) encountered were vessel perforation (1.6%–10.6%) and subcutaneous infiltration (5%–19%). Although the local anaesthetics use is quite safe and effective, they may produce systemic toxic reactions affecting the brain and heart. Various complications such as allergic reactions, urinary retention, nausea and vomiting, headache, and dizziness can occur.

We did not encounter any such complications. We had three patients who developed intraoperative laryngospasm which can be due to stimulation in light plane of anaesthesia. Two patients had bradycardia in group 3 which can be attributed to the cardiac effect of systemic absorption of bupivacaine. None of the three drugs were associated with any significant complications. Limitation of our study was that we did not use the awareness monitoring under anesthesia (BIS).

5. Conclusion

Thus to conclude, levobupivacaine, bupivacaine, and ropivacaine were effective and safe in terms of stable haemodynamic profile, intraoperative quality, and no significant complications when they were given to patients undergoing infraumbilical surgery under caudal block. Contrary to other studies where these three drugs have shown similar effects, we found that bupivacaine provides longer duration of analgesia than levobupivacaine and ropivacaine, so it needs further studies to substantiate this.

Conflicts of Interest

The authors declare that they have no conflicts of interest.

References

[1] C. J. Cote, "Pediatric anesthesia," in *Miller's Anesthesia*, R. D. Miller, L. I. Eriksson, L. A. Fleisher, J. P. Wiener-Kronish, and W. L. Young, Eds., pp. 2559-2560, Churchill Livingstone,Philadelphia, PA, USA, 7th edition., 2009.

[2] A. K. Ross, J. B. Eck, and J. D. Tobias, "Pediatric regional anesthesia: beyond the caudal," *Anesthesia & Analgesia*, vol. 91, no. 1, pp. 16–26, 2000.

[3] D. A. Markakis, "Regional anesthesia in pediatrics," *Anesthesiology Clinics of North America*, vol. 18, no. 2, pp. 355–381, 2000.

[4] D. A. Rowney and E. Doyle, "Epidural and subarachnoid blockade in children," *Anaesthesia*, vol. 53, no. 10, pp. 980-981, 1998.

[5] M. Ansermino, R. Basu, C. Vandebeek, and C. Montgomery, "Nonopioid additives to local anaesthetics for caudal blockade in children: a systematic review," *Pediatric Anesthesia*, vol. 13, no. 7, pp. 561–573, 2003.

[6] J. D. Tobias, "Caudal epidural block: a review of test dosing and recognition of systemic injection in children," *Anesthesia & Analgesia*, vol. 93, no. 5, pp. 1156–1161, 2001.

[7] P. Silvani, A. Camporesi, M. R. Agostino, and I. Salvo, "Caudal anesthesia in pediatrics: an update," *Minerva Anestesiologica*, vol. 72, no. 6, pp. 453–459, 2006.

[8] G. Schuepfer, C. Konrad, J. Schmeck, G. Poortmans, B. Staffelbach, and M. Jöhr, "Generating a learning curve for pediatric caudal epidural blocks: an empirical evaluation of technical skills in novice and experienced anesthetists," *Regional Anesthesia and Pain Medicine*, vol. 25, no. 4, pp. 385–388, 2000.

[9] L. Mather and J. Mackie, "The incidence of postoperative pain in children," *Pain*, vol. 15, no. 1, pp. 271–282, 1983.

[10] R. S. Hannallah, L. M. Broadman, A. B. Belman, M. D. Abramowitz, and B. S. Epstein, "Comparison of caudal and ilioinguinal/iliohypogastric nerve blocks for control of postorchidopexy pain in pediatric ambulatory surgery," *Anesthesiology*, vol. 66, no. 6, pp. 832–834, 1987.

[11] B. Locatelli, P. Ingelmo, V. Sonzogni et al., "Randomized, double blind phase III, controlled trial comparing levobupivacaine 0.25%, ropivacaine 0.25% and bupivacaine 0.25% by the caudal route in children," *British Journal of Anaesthesia*, vol. 94, no. 3, pp. 366–371, 2005.

[12] M. J. Da Conceicao, L. Coelho, and M. Khalil, "Ropivacaine 0.25% compared with bupivacaine 0.25% by the caudal route," *Paediatric Anaesthesia*, vol. 9, no. 3, pp. 229–233, 1999.

[13] G. Ivani, E. Lampugnani, M. Torre, G. Calevo Maria, P. De Negri, and F. Borrometti, "Comparison of ropivacaine and bupivacaine for paediatric caudal block," *British Journal of Anaesthesia*, vol. 81, no. 2, pp. 247-248, 1998.

[14] P. Praveen, R. Remadevi, and N. Pratheeba, "Caudal epidural analgesia in pediatric patients: comparison of 0.25% levobupivacaine and 0.25% ropivacaine in terms of motor blockade and postoperative analgesia," *Anesthesia: Essays and Researches*, vol. 11, no. 1, pp. 223–227, 2017.

[15] C. B. Berde and G. R. Strichartz, "Local anesthetics," in *Miller's Anesthesia*, R. D. Miller, L. I. Eriksson, L. A. Fleisher, J. P. Wiener-Kronish, and W. L. Young, Eds., p. 928, Churchill Livingstone, Philadelphia, PA, USA, 7th edition, 2009.

15

Transient Neurologic Symptoms following Spinal Anesthesia with Isobaric Mepivacaine: A Decade of Experience at Toronto Western Hospital

Ashwin Sankar,[1] **Minou Behboudi**,[2] **Faraj W. Abdallah**,[3] **Alan Macfarlane**,[4,5] **and Richard Brull**[2]

[1]*Department of Anesthesia, University of Toronto, Toronto, ON, Canada*
[2]*Department of Anesthesia and Pain Management, Toronto Western Hospital, University Health Network, Toronto, ON, Canada*
[3]*Department of Anesthesia and Keenan Research Centre, Li Ka Shing Knowledge Institute, St. Michael's Hospital, Toronto, ON, Canada*
[4]*Department of Anaesthesia, Glasgow Royal Infirmary, Glasgow, UK*
[5]*Department of Anaesthesia, Critical Care and Pain Medicine, University of Glasgow, Glasgow, UK*

Correspondence should be addressed to Richard Brull; richard.brull@uhn.ca

Academic Editor: Enrico Camporesi

Background. Transient neurologic symptoms (TNSs) can be distressing for patients and providers following uneventful spinal anesthesia. Spinal mepivacaine may be less commonly associated with TNS than lidocaine; however, reported rates of TNS with intrathecal mepivacaine vary considerably. *Materials and Methods.* We conducted a retrospective cohort study reviewing the internal medical records of surgical patients who underwent mepivacaine spinal anesthesia at Toronto Western Hospital over the last decade to determine the rate of TNS. We defined TNS as new onset back pain that radiated to the buttocks or legs bilaterally. *Results.* We found one documented occurrence of TNS among a total of 679 mepivacaine spinal anesthetics (0.14%; CI: 0.02–1.04%) that were performed in 654 patients. *Conclusion.* Our retrospective data suggest that the rate of TNS associated with mepivacaine spinal anesthesia is lower than that previously reported in the literature.

1. Introduction

Transient neurologic symptoms (TNSs), characterized by low back pain that radiates to the buttocks or legs after recovering from spinal anesthesia [1, 2], can be distressing to patients and providers. TNS typically appears within 24 hours of spinal anesthesia, lasts 2–5 days, and resolves completely without sequelae [2]. Because TNS is traditionally associated with intrathecal lidocaine, mepivacaine has been the local anesthetic of choice for short-acting spinal anesthesia at our institution for over a decade. While TNS following mepivacaine occurs less frequently compared to similar doses of lidocaine [3, 4], varied rates of TNS have been reported following mepivacaine spinal anesthesia. Previous small randomized trials examining patients undergoing isobaric intrathecal mepivacaine anesthesia for knee arthroscopy surgery have reported rates of TNS as high as 7.5% [3, 5–8]; however, intraoperative positioning for this procedure has been associated with an increased risk of TNS [1, 9]. It is our anecdotal experience that TNS following intrathecal mepivacaine is rare, occurring far less than the 6.4% incidence reported in one large prospective cohort of knee arthroscopy patients [9]. Therefore, we undertook this retrospective cohort study to understand the rate of TNS reported among surgical patients who underwent spinal anesthesia with isobaric mepivacaine at Toronto Western Hospital (TWH) over the last 10 years. We hypothesized that TNS following isobaric mepivacaine spinal anesthesia is rare.

2. Materials and Methods

Following the University Health Network ethics approval, we conducted a retrospective cohort study of consecutive patients who received spinal anesthesia with 1.5% or 2% isobaric mepivacaine for elective surgery at TWH between January 1, 2006 and March 31, 2017. We adhered to the STROBE recommendations for the design and reporting of observational studies [10].

We identified all mepivacaine spinal anesthetics by searching our regional anesthesia database, which captures data for all neuraxial blocks performed in the block procedure room at our institution. Patients who received multiple mepivacaine spinal anesthetics for more than one operative procedure in separate encounters during the study period and patients who received rescue spinal anesthesia using mepivacaine following failed spinal anesthesia with bupivacaine during the same encounter were both included.

All spinal anesthetics were performed by a regional anesthesia resident or fellow under direct supervision of the attending anesthesiologist or by the attending anesthesiologist. The dose and concentration of mepivacaine, along with any additives, were administered at the discretion of the attending anesthesiologist. Since 1.5% mepivacaine is not commercially available in Canada, this concentration was achieved by diluting 2% mepivacaine hydrochloride (Carbocaine® 2%, Hospira, Montreal, Canada) with preservative-free normal saline.

It is our institutional practice that any patient who develops neurologic symptoms following neuraxial anesthesia, including TNS, postdural puncture headache, and meningeal, neuropathic, or radicular symptoms, is referred to our anesthesiology department for immediate evaluation and management. Severe cases or patients at risk of acute deterioration are referred to the emergency department and/or for urgent neurosurgical consultation.

For each mepivacaine spinal anesthetic administered, the corresponding patient's internal medical record was reviewed for any documented indication of TNS postoperatively. We defined TNS as new onset back pain radiating to the buttocks or legs bilaterally [1, 2]. Specifically, we reviewed the initial surgical service postoperative follow-up note (hospital visit typically scheduled 2–6 weeks postoperatively); any postoperative anesthetic, medical, or surgical consultations; and any postoperative emergency room visit records. For patients who were unanticipatedly admitted to the hospital, the inpatient surgical service notes were reviewed for evidence of TNS. Patients for whom the medical record did not include any postoperative follow-up notes, consultation entries, or emergency records were excluded from the analyses.

2.1. Analysis. Descriptive statistics were generated for the entire sample using counts and frequencies for categorical variables and means, medians, standard deviations, and interquartile ranges for continuous variables. The distribution of continuous variables was assessed using the Shapiro–Wilk test of normality; none of the continuous variables were normally distributed, and medians with interquartile ranges are therefore reported. We describe the cases developing the outcome, and the absolute risk of developing the outcome with 95% confidence intervals is reported. In a secondary analysis, the characteristics of excluded patients were descriptively compared with those comprising the primary cohort. Statistical analyses were performed using SAS University Edition 9.4 (Cary, NC, USA).

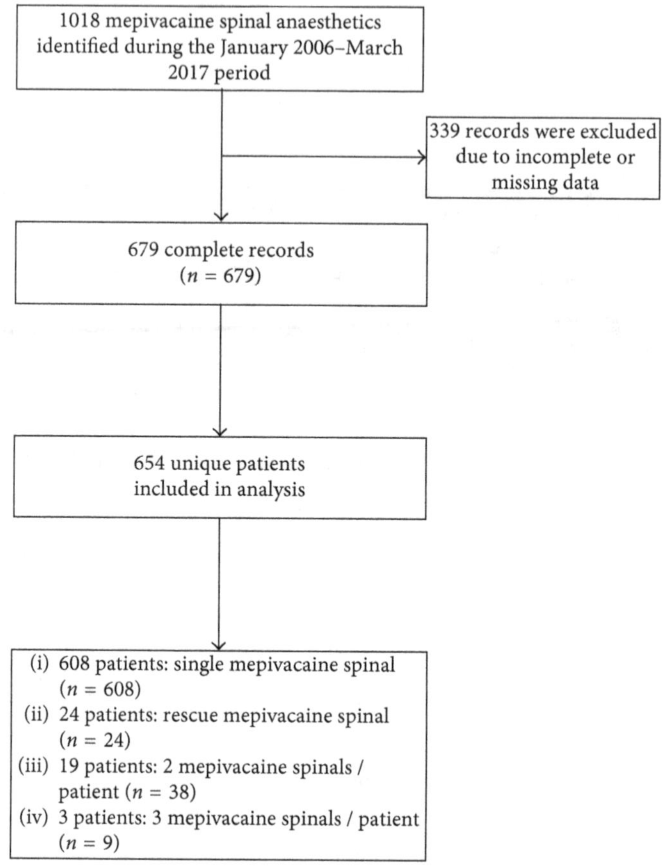

Figure 1: Flow diagram detailing the identification process for the present cohort of mepivacaine spinal anesthetics.

3. Results

A total of 679 mepivacaine spinal anesthetics were performed in 654 patients. Twenty-two patients (3.3%) underwent multiple mepivacaine spinal anesthetics, among whom 19 (2.9%) received two mepivacaine spinal anesthetics and 3 (0.4%) received three mepivacaine spinal anesthetics, each in separate encounters. Twenty-four patients (3.6%) received a rescue spinal anesthetic using isobaric mepivacaine following a failed spinal anesthetic with isobaric bupivacaine (5–15 mg) during the same encounter. Figure 1 details the identification process for the present cohort.

Our cohort characteristics are presented in Table 1. Among the 679 spinal anesthetics, 606 (89%) were performed using 2% mepivacaine and the remaining 73 (11%) were performed with 1.5% mepivacaine. 220 (32%) and six (0.9%) spinal anesthetics included intrathecal fentanyl (5–25 mcg) or morphine (50 mcg), respectively, in an admixture with isobaric mepivacaine. Four (0.6%) spinal anesthetics included hyperbaric bupivacaine (3.75–7.5 mg) in an admixture with isobaric mepivacaine for added baricity.

The spinal anesthesia procedures were most commonly performed in the sitting position ($n = 671$, 99%), using a midline approach ($n = 660$, 97%) with a 25 gauge ($n = 641$,

Table 1: Cohort characteristics ($n = 679$ mepivacaine spinal anesthetics).

Age (in years; median, IQR)	61	71
Sex (*n* male, %)	336	49%
Height (cm; median, IQR)	168	161–177
Weight (kg; median, IQR)	86	71–100
BMI (kg/m^2; median, IQR)	29	25–35
Mepivacaine volume (mL; *n*, %)		
≤1.5	81	13%
1.6–2.0	64	9%
2.1–2.5	178	26%
2.6–3.0	336	49%
>3	20	3%
Spinal position (*n*, %)		
Sitting	670	99%
Lateral	9	1%
Spinal approach (*n*, %)		
Midline	660	97%
Paramedian	19	3%
Spinal level (*n*, %)		
L2-L3	58	8%
L3-L4	466	69%
L4-L5	153	23%
Not defined	2	0%
Spinal needle type (*n*, %)		
Quincke	6	1%
Sprotte	10	1%
Whitacre	663	98%
Spinal needle Gauge (*n*, %)		
<24	26	4%
25	641	94%
27	11	2%
Not defined	1	0%
Surgical procedure (*n*, %)		
General surgery		
Inguinal hernia repair	4	1%
Orthopedics		
Ankle		
Arthroscopy	29	4%
Fusion	2	0%
Hardware removal	56	8%
ORIF	45	7%
Tendon repair	24	4%
Foot		
1st MTP surgery	36	5%
Reconstruction	60	9%
Hip		
Arthroplasty	4	0%
Arthroscopy	6	1%
Knee		
Arthroplasty	68	10%
Arthroscopy		
Bilateral	31	5%
Unilateral	226	33%
Hardware removal	39	6%
ORIF	13	2%
Plastic surgery		
Soft tissue surgery*	10	1%
Urology		
Cystoscopy or cystolithopaxy	12	2%
TURP or TURBT	14	2%
Intraoperative position (*n*, %)		
Knee arthroscopy	257	38%
Lateral	17	2%
Lithotomy	27	4%
Prone	7	1%
Supine	371	55%

BMI = body mass index; MTP = metatarsal-phalangeal joint; ORIF = open reduction internal fixation; TURBT = transurethral resection of bladder tumor; TURP = transurethral resection of the prostate; *carcinoma excision, hematoma evacuation, and skin graft excision.

94%) Whitacre needle ($n = 663$, 98%). Paresthesia during intrathecal injection was reported during a single spinal anesthetic, while pain upon intrathecal injection was not reported during any spinal anesthetic. No patients experienced any new postoperative motor deficits.

The median time to the initial postoperative surgical visit was 20 days (IQR 13–47 days). One patient was referred to our anesthesia department for consultation regarding postoperative neurological symptoms. None of the remaining 653 patients (who underwent 677 mepivacaine spinal anesthetics in total) received postoperative consultation by any medical or surgical service at our institution, none were referred to our emergency room, and none were readmitted postoperatively.

3.1. Primary Outcome: TNS. Among the 679 mepivacaine spinal anesthetics performed, a single occurrence of TNS (0.14%; CI: 0.02–1.04%) was found in a 75-year-old female patient (BMI 27) undergoing ankle hardware removal surgery, who received spinal anesthesia with 2.5 mL of 2% mepivacaine at the L4-L5 level. No pain or paresthesia was reported during intrathecal injection. Of note, this patient appeared in our dataset twice, as she received a mepivacaine spinal anesthetic in a separate encounter for knee arthroscopy 43 months prior with no complications, but developed TNS following second exposure.

In secondary analyses (Table 2), the characteristics of excluded patients did not qualitatively differ from the primary study cohort.

4. Discussion

Our single-institution retrospective cohort study suggests that the reported rate of TNS following spinal anesthesia with isobaric mepivacaine is very low. Our large cohort of mepivacaine spinal anesthetics allowed for addressing some important shortcomings in previous small randomized trials, wherein a wide range of 0–7.5% rates of TNS have been observed [3, 5–8]. The majority of previously published studies were small, each including less than 100 patients [3, 5–8]; and several of these studies employed a combined spinal-epidural technique which may have obscured the relationship between spinal mepivacaine and TNS [6–9]. Further, almost all previous studies investigating the association between spinal mepivacaine and TNS were conducted in patients undergoing arthroscopic knee surgery [3, 5–9], the intraoperative surgical position for which has been associated with an increased risk of TNS [9]. In our study, 38% of mepivacaine spinal anesthetics were performed for knee arthroscopy procedures; the remaining spinal anesthetics were performed for lower extremity orthopedic and lower abdominal procedures. This variety of surgical procedures may have contributed to the low rate of TNS observed herein. Our low rate of TNS may also have been impacted by contemporary anesthetic practice, including the adoption of multimodal analgesia and prophylactic antiemetic medications as evidence supporting their use became available. It is possible that the increasingly routine use of nonsteroidal antiinflammatory drugs such as ketorolac administered for preventive analgesia and the inherent antiinflammatory properties of dexamethasone administered for postoperative nausea and vomiting may prevent and/or mask symptoms of TNS, and at least partially account for our low reported rates of TNS. The latter notwithstanding, the results of this retrospective review underscore that TNS following mepivacaine spinal anesthesia has not posed a clinical challenge to our regional anesthesia teaching program over the last decade.

Under the conditions for detection of TNS in the present study, a single case was identified. The single observed case of TNS occurred in an elderly patient who received mepivacaine spinal anesthesia for ankle hardware removal after 43 months of having received mepivacaine spinal anesthesia for knee arthroscopy. While advanced age is independently associated with TNS [9], the effect of multiple exposures to intrathecal mepivacaine or rescue mepivacaine spinal anesthesia has not been extensively investigated. Unfortunately, although our cohort captured the greatest number of patients receiving multiple isobaric mepivacaine spinal anesthetics to date, the single observed occurrence of TNS precluded examining statistical associations of previously identified risk factors for TNS such as age [9] or novel considerations such as multiple exposures.

Our results are subject to several limitations. First, our study comprised all mepivacaine spinal anesthetics conducted in a single-academic tertiary care hospital in a manner reflective of institutional clinical practice. Similar studies at centres with differing case mixes are necessary to generalize our findings to other practice settings. Second, due to the retrospective nature of our study, there is considerable potential for underreporting. It is possible that minor episodes resolved spontaneously and may not have been recalled, reported, and/or documented. Given that TNS is routinely discussed and disclosed during our informed consent process prior to performing spinal anesthesia using mepivacaine, it is also possible that even moderate-or-severe TNS symptoms were appropriately disregarded and unreported by patients. Further, we excluded 339 mepivacaine spinal anesthetics from our analyses due to incomplete or missing postoperative data, most likely because follow-up occurred in a private clinic. However, none of these patients were referred to our anesthesia department for consultation, none received any other medical or surgical consultation, none were readmitted, and none visited our emergency room postoperatively. It is also noteworthy that the characteristics of excluded patients (Table 2) did not appreciably differ from the present study cohort. In addition, though our dataset includes patients undergoing several surgical procedures, given the single case of TNS

Table 2: Characteristics of excluded records (n = 339 mepivacaine spinal anesthetics).

Age (in years; median, IQR)	54	44–63
Sex (*n* male, %)	190	56%
Height (cm; median, IQR)	171	164–179
Weight (kg; median, IQR)	93	74–110
BMI (kg/m^2; median, IQR)	31	25–38
Mepivacaine volume (mL; *n*, %)		
≤1.5	22	7%
1.6–2.0	17	5%
2.1–2.5	82	24%
2.6–3.0	213	63%
>3	5	1%
Spinal position (*n*, %)		
Sitting	338	100%
Lateral	1	0%
Spinal approach (*n*, %)		
Midline	331	98%
Paramedian	8	2%
Spinal level (*n*, %)		
L2-L3	25	7%
L3-L4	232	68%
L4-L5	79	24%
Not defined	3	1%
Spinal needle type (*n*, %)		
Quincke	2	0%
Sprotte	6	2%
Whitacre	331	98%
Spinal needle Gauge (*n*, %)		
<24	13	4%
25	323	95%
27	1	0%
Not defined	2	1%
Surgical procedure (*n*, %)		
General Surgery		
Inguinal hernia repair	3	1%
Orthopedics		
Ankle		
Arthroscopy	40	12%
Fusion	7	2%
Hardware removal	26	8%
ORIF	36	11%
Tendon repair	11	3%
Foot		
1st MTP surgery	6	2%
Reconstruction	10	3%
Hip		
Arthroplasty	0	0%
Arthroscopy	4	1%
Knee		
Arthroplasty	33	10%
Arthroscopy		
Bilateral	7	2%
Unilateral	122	36%
Hardware removal	11	3%
ORIF	10	3%
Plastic Surgery		
Soft tissue surgery*	5	2%
Urology		
Cystoscopy or cystolithopaxy	2	0%
TURP or TURBT	6	2%
Intraoperative position (*n*, %)		
Knee arthroscopy	129	38%
Lateral	8	2%

Table 2: Continued.

Lithotomy	7	2%
Prone	3	1%
Supine	192	57%

BMI = body mass index; MTP = metatarsal-phalangeal joint; ORIF = open reduction internal fixation; TURBT = transurethral resection of bladder tumor; TURP = transurethral resection of the prostate; *carcinoma excision, hematoma evacuation, and skin graft excision.

observed, we are unable to statistically verify known risk factors for TNS, such as lithotomy position and obesity [1].

5. Conclusion

A large cohort comprising a decade of experience with isobaric mepivacaine for short-acting spinal anesthesia at our institution suggests that the rate of TNS is lower than that previously reported in the literature. Practically, TNS following mepivacaine spinal anesthesia has not posed a clinical challenge to our regional anesthesia teaching program over the last decade.

Conflicts of Interest

The authors declare that they have no conflicts of interest.

Acknowledgments

Drs. Faraj Abdallah and Richard Brull received support from the Merit Award Program, Department of Anesthesia, University of Toronto.

References

[1] J. M. Freedman, D. K. Li, K. Drasner, M. C. Jaskela, B. Larsen, and S. Wi, "Transient neurologic symptoms after spinal anesthesia: an epidemiologic study of 1,863 patients," *Anesthesiology*, vol. 89, no. 3, pp. 633–641, 1998.

[2] J. E. Pollock, "Transient neurologic symptoms: etiology, risk factors, and management," *Regional Anesthesia and Pain Medicine*, vol. 27, no. 6, pp. 581–586, 2002.

[3] G. A. Liguori, V. M. Zayas, and M. F. Chisholm, "Transient neurologic symptoms after spinal anesthesia with mepivacaine and lidocaine," *Anesthesiology*, vol. 88, no. 3, pp. 619–623, 1998.

[4] D. Zaric and N. L. Pace, "Transient neurologic symptoms (TNS) following spinal anaesthesia with lidocaine versus other local anaesthetics," *Cochrane Database of Systematic Reviews*, vol. 2, p. Cd003006, 2009.

[5] D. O'Donnell, B. Manickam, A. Perlas et al., "Spinal mepivacaine with fentanyl for outpatient knee arthroscopy surgery: a randomized controlled trial," *Canadian Journal of Anesthesia*, vol. 57, no. 1, pp. 32–38, 2010.

[6] J. Pawlowski, K. Orr, K. M. Kim, A. L. Pappas, R. Sukhani, and W. S. Jellish, "Anesthetic and recovery profiles of lidocaine versus mepivacaine for spinal anesthesia in patients undergoing outpatient orthopedic arthroscopic procedures," *Journal of Clinical Anesthesia*, vol. 24, no. 2, pp. 109–115, 2012.

[7] J. Pawlowski, R. Sukhani, A. L. Pappas et al., "The anesthetic and recovery profile of two doses (60 and 80 mg) of plain mepivacaine for ambulatory spinal anesthesia," *Anesthesia and Analgesia*, vol. 91, no. 3, pp. 580–584, 2000.

[8] V. M. Zayas, G. A. Liguori, M. F. Chisholm, M. H. Susman, and M. A. Gordon, "Dose response relationships for isobaric spinal mepivacaine using the combined spinal epidural technique," *Anesthesia and Analgesia*, vol. 89, no. 5, pp. 1167–1171, 1999.

[9] J. T. YaDeau, G. A. Liguori, and V. M. Zayas, "The incidence of transient neurologic symptoms after spinal anesthesia with mepivacaine," *Anesthesia and Analgesia*, vol. 101, no. 3, pp. 661–665, 2005.

[10] E. von Elm, D. G. Altman, M. Egger, S. J. Pocock, P. C. Gøtzsche, and J. P. Vandenbroucke, "Strengthening the reporting of observational studies in epidemiology (STROBE) statement: guidelines for reporting observational studies," *BMJ*, vol. 335, pp. 806–808, 2007.

16

Efficacy of Bilateral Transversus Abdominis Plane and Ilioinguinal-Iliohypogastric Nerve Blocks for Postcaesarean Delivery Pain Relief under Spinal Anesthesia

Seid Adem Ahemed, Zewditu Abdissa Denu, Habtamu Getinet Kassahun, and Demeke Yilikal Fentie

Department of Anesthesia, College of Medicine and Health Sciences, University of Gondar, Gondar, Ethiopia

Correspondence should be addressed to Zewditu Abdissa Denu; zewditudenuabdissa@gmail.com

Academic Editor: Ronald G. Pearl

Background. Caesarean delivery can be associated with considerable postoperative pain. While the benefits of transversus abdominis plane (TAP) and ilioinguinal-iliohypogastric (II-IH) nerve blocks on pain after caesarean delivery via Pfannenstiel incision have been demonstrated, no enough investigations on the comparison of these blocks on pain after caesarean delivery have been conducted in our setup. *Method.* An institutional-based prospective observational cohort study was conducted to compare the analgesic efficacy of those blocks. We observed 102 postoperative parturients. The outcome measure was the severity of pain measured using a numeric rating scale. *Result.* Twenty-four hours after surgery, the NRS score at rest was (0.90 ± 0.80) versus (0.67 ± 0.58) and at movement (1.2 ± 1.07) versus (0.88 ± 0.76) for the TAP and II-IH groups, respectively. Twenty-four hours after surgery, the mean tramadol consumption was (55.45 ± 30.51) versus (37.27 ± 27.09) mg in TAP and II-IH groups, respectively ($p = 0.009$). The mean first analgesic requirement time was also prolonged in the II-IH group. *Conclusion and Recommendations.* There was no statically significant difference between TAP and II-IH blocks regarding postoperative pain score, but the II-IH block significantly reduced the total tramadol consumption and prolonged the time to first analgesic request than TAP. Thus, we recommend the II-IH nerve block.

1. Introduction

Pain management is crucially important in the postoperative period as it increases patient comfort and satisfaction [1]. Caesarean delivery (CD) has been one of the most frequently performed major surgical interventions and causes severe postoperative pain [2]. Caesarean delivery and subsequent manipulation performed through Pfannenstiel incision are associated commonly with a significant degree of pain in the postoperative period; 79% of women experience pain at the incision site that can last for up to 2 months [3].

Inadequate postoperative analgesia is one of the most common causes for poor patient satisfaction following caesarean delivery [3, 4].

Childbirth is an emotion-filled event, and the mother wants to bond with her newborn as early as possible. Inadequate postoperative pain relief after CD can negatively impact ambulation, breastfeeding, and even maternal bonding [2, 5].

Poor pain control in the postoperative period can lead to chronic pain syndromes and poor quality of life [2, 5].

The provision of effective postoperative analgesia is a key to facilitate early mobilization of the mother, infant care, and prevention of postoperative morbidity. Improvement in postoperative analgesia may not only increase patient satisfaction but also diminish the duration of hospital stay and reduce the risk of complications [6, 7].

The ideal form of postoperative analgesia is unknown, but many procedures are carried out under spinal anesthesia, and currently, opioids are commonly used for relief of postoperative pain after caesarean section, either by intrathecal administration prior to section or by postoperative parenteral administration as a component of multimodal analgesia during the postoperative period [6, 8].

Even if opioids are available to be administered via the spinal or systemic route, they had adverse effects such as nausea, vomiting, sedation, itching, and risk of delayed maternal respiratory depression, all of which reduce overall patient satisfaction [2, 3, 8].

Additionally, these opioid-related adverse effects can produce other problems for new mothers such as delayed initiation of breastfeeding and impairment of mother/infant bonding [3].

An ideal method of pain relief after caesarean delivery should be cost-effective, safe for the mother, require minimal monitoring, and use drugs that are not secreted into breast milk. Moreover, the mother should not be sedated by the drugs that prevent her from moving freely and caring for the newborn.

Minor side effects, such as pruritus and shivering, may interfere with care of the newborn, leading to less maternal satisfaction. Drug availability, maternal health conditions, patient preferences, and availability of medical expertise and trained support staff also play a role in choice of the analgesic method.

Many scholars have been studying to find the safest and effective way of interventions for postoperative CD pain management, and they suggest methods like opioid or local anesthetic skin infiltration, epidural analgesia, intrathecal or intravenous opioids, and abdominal field blocks like TAP and II-IH.

Among the above-listed ways of pain management, intravenous opioids and regional nerve blocks are the mainstay of treatment for postcaesarean pain here in the study area.

Epidural analgesia, which is the gold standard for control of labour pain and postoperative pain, is not commonly practiced in our setup due to lack of the epidural kit.

Abdominal field blocks like TAP and II-IH are the mainstay of treatment for postcaesarean pain for both the midline and Pfannenstiel incision because of the opioid sparing effect, prolonged pain relief, and technical simplicity, and also, it does not need repeated injection for optimal pain relief [3, 9].

TAP and II-IH nerve blocks are well known and easy to perform, and currently, these blocks are done in the study area for post-CD pain management.

There are no enough data concerning the efficacy of TAP versus II-IH nerve blocks in the management of postoperative pain in parturients undergoing caesarean section.

Most of the studies that have been done to determine the efficacy of those blocks in post-CD pain management are done in western countries, but there is no published literature in Ethiopia.

The presence of racial, cultural, genetic, and sociodemographic differences in the perception of pain has been well documented [10, 11].

There is also controversy regarding the efficacy of the two blocks [12, 13], so comparing the effectiveness of TAP blocks with that of II-IH nerve blocks will help us to have a best practice to the study area, and knowing the efficacy of these blocks will allow anesthetists to choose the most effective one to manage postoperative CD pain.

The aim of this study was to compare the efficacy of the TAP block and II-IH block in controlling postcaesarean section pain.

2. Methods

An institutional-based observational cohort study was conducted from April 1 to May 30, 2017, at Gondar University Teaching Hospital after we secured ethical approval from the University of Gondar Ethical Review Board. The minimum sample size calculated for this study was 102, and the sample size calculation was done based on the two population proportion principles:

$$\frac{p_1(1-p_1)+p_2(1-p_2)}{(p_2-p_1)^2}\times f(\alpha,\beta). \tag{1}$$

(i) Hence, the incidence of moderate-to-severe pain after CD without intervention was 87%, and we got pain reduction after clients received bilateral TAP and II-IH blocks 40% and 70%, respectively. And we calculated p_1 by reducing 40% of 87% from 87% ($p_1 = 0.87-0.348 = 0.522$) and p_2 by reducing 70% of 87% from 87% ($0.87-0.69 = 0.261$) since we need only pain reduction after the block from the incidence of pain (87%) by taking $\dot{f}(\alpha, \beta) = 7.85$ with a power of 80% and 0.05 significance.

(ii) Since $f(\alpha, \beta) = 7.85$ or 10.5 for 80% or 90% power, respectively, with 5% significance, the significance (risk of type I error) is almost always set at 5%.

So per group, we have 51 participants.

We included ASA I and ASA II patients. Finally, we selected every consecutive parturient for whom the above-mentioned nerve blocks were done and who also volunteered to give consent to participate in the study till the required sample is achieved. Our primary outcome measure was the severity of pain which was measured using the numeric rating scale. The secondary outcomes were the total analgesic consumption and time for the first analgesic request. As to the data collection procedure, two trained anesthetists collect all the required information based on the checklist prepared in English. The investigators had no power to decide which type of block would be given for the mother (only the responsible anesthesiologist had this right, i.e., he/she did the block as he/she wishes, either TAP or II-IH).

But the investigator stayed in the operating theater and saw the type of block that the responsible anesthesiologist had done and put the code on the chart. The type of block was not clearly recorded on the chart except the code so that data collectors are blinded to the type of block done for each mother.

The relative proportion of these blocks in our institution looks equal (1 : 1) because everybody is doing these blocks randomly as they wish for transverse incision, but for vertical incision, they do only TAP.

The block was done by using the landmark technique for both types, and a total of 32 ml of 0.25% bupivacaine for II-IH block (8 ml in each side) and 40 ml of 0.25% bupivacaine for TAP block (20 ml in each side) were given.

Pain assessment was performed at 0 hr, 4 hr, 6 hr, 8 hr, 12 hr, and 24 hr in the ward by blinded data collectors who were unaware of the type of the nerve block done. And the total analgesic consumption within 24 hours was also recorded.

Data were coded, entered, cleaned, and cross-checked with SPSS version 20 statistical package. The data were tested for normality using the Shapiro–Wilk normality test. Normally distributed data were analyzed using Student's t-test.

All data other than categorical parameters were analyzed using Student's t-test.

The comparisons of categorical parameters were analyzed using the chi-square test or Fisher's exact test as required and expressed in % and numbers. Data were presented as mean ± SD. p value < 0.05 was considered statistically significant.

3. Results

A total of hundred and two clients were enrolled in the current study with a response rate of 100%. The age of participants was 26.98 with a standard deviation of 2.4 years. Assessment of the ASA physical status showed that 78% of the TAP and 76% of the II-IH groups were ASA I and 21.56% of the TAP and 23.5% of the II-IH groups were ASA II (Table 1).

Postoperative vital signs (postoperative pulse rate and mean arterial blood pressure) were comparable between the two groups (Tables 2 and 3).

3.1. Postoperative Pain Scores using Numerical Rating Scale. With regard to the postoperative pain score, there was no difference between the two groups. We assessed the pain score at rest, on coughing, and at movement. The result shows no statistically significant difference between the two groups (Tables 4 and 5).

The mean tramadol consumption for the TAP group was 52.45 with a standard deviation of 30.5, and for the II IH group, it was 37.25 ± 27.09 mg; the mean first analgesic consumption time in this study was 10.71 ± 7.67 hr for the TAP group and 14.09 ± 8.20 hr for the II-IH group, with a p value of 0.03 (Table 6)

4. Discussion

We found that there was no statistically significant difference between TAP and II-IH blocks in the numeric pain rating score both at rest and at movement for the first postoperative 24 hours, but the II-IH nerve block significantly reduced total tramadol consumption and prolonged the time for the first analgesic request.

Studies comparing the two blocks are rare, so we compare our results separately for each block.

Table 1: Sociodemographic and other characteristics of study participants from April 1 to May 30, 2017, in Northwest Ethiopia.

Character	TAP (n = 51)	II-IH (n = 51)	p value
Age (years)	27.27 ± 2.88	26.69 ± 1.79	0.219
Height (meter)	1.67 ± 0.04	1.65 ± 0.04	0.077
Weight (kg)	63.10 ± 7.69	64.88 ± 9.45	0.299
BMI (kg/m^2)	22.63 ± 2.01	23.29 ± 2.97	0.192
ASA I	40 (78.51%)	39 (76.34%)	0.814
ASA II	11 (21.56%)	12 (23.52 %)	
Parity			
Nulliparous	28 (54.90%)	27 (52.90%)	0.843
Multiparous	23 (45.09%)	24 (47.05%)	
Number of previous c/s			
0	39 (76.47%)	38 (74.50%)	
1	11 (21.56%)	9 (17.64%)	0.529
2	1 (1.96%)	3 (5.88%)	
3	0 (0%)	1 (1.96%)	
Level of sensory block			
T6-T4	7 (13.72%)	8 (15.68%)	0.780
T7-T10	44 (86.27%)	43 (84.31%)	
Duration of surgery (min)	45.29 ± 9.24	48.33 ± 7.85	0.077

Table 2: Postoperative pulse rate (beats per minute) in both groups who underwent caesarean delivery under spinal anesthesia in Gondar University Hospital from April 1 to May 30, 2017, in Northwest Ethiopia.

Postoperative time	TAP group (n = 51)	II-IH group (n = 51)	p value
0 hour	77.29 ± 4.11	75.20 ± 7.91	0.96
4 hours	76.00 ± 5.21	77.27 ± 5.37	0.22
6 hours	76.02 ± 5.98	77.35 ± 2.99	0.15
8 hours	76.04 ± 6.09	76.16 ± 6.76	0.92
12 hours	76.41 ± 3.00	76.53 ± 2.36	0.82
24 hours	76.53 ± 3.85	75.16 ± 3.63	0.06

Data are mean ± SD.

Table 3: Postoperative mean arterial blood pressure (mmHg) in both groups who underwent caesarean delivery under spinal anesthesia in Gondar University Hospital from April 1 to May 30, 2017, in Northwest Ethiopia.

Postoperative time	TAP group (n = 51)	II-IH group (n = 51)	p value
0 hour	78.43 ± 5.45	76.42 ± 5.59	0.06
4 hours	84.33 ± 8.29	84.25 ± 7.62	0.96
6 hours	85.05 ± 6.18	85.01 ± 6.47	0.97
8 hours	87.23 ± 5.43	88.08 ± 3.88	0.36
12 hours	84.77 ± 6.66	86.22 ± 6.02	0.25
24 hours	89.03 ± 3.24	89.41 ± 3.84	0.58

Data are mean ± SD.

Table 4: Postoperative NRS scores at rest over the first 24 postoperative hours among parturients who underwent caesarean delivery under spinal anesthesia in Gondar University Hospital from April 1 to May 30, 2017, in Northwest Ethiopia.

Character	TAP group	II-IH group	p value
NRS score at 0 hr	0.00	0.00	
NRS score at 4 hr	0.69 ± 1.46	0.41 ± 1.00	0.27
NRS score at 6 hr	0.67 ± 0.136	0.41 ± 1.09	0.30
NRS score at 8 hr	0.65 ± 1.18	0.35 ± 0.79	0.14
NRS score at 12 hr	0.49 ± 0.857	0.16 ± 0.46	0.22
NRS score at 24 hr	0.90 ± 0.80	0.67 ± 0.58	0.95

Data are mean ± SD.

Table 5: Postoperative NRS scores at movement or on coughing in the postoperative 24 hours of parturients who underwent caesarean delivery under spinal anesthesia in Gondar University Hospital from April 1 to May 30, 2017, in Northwest Ethiopia.

Character	TAP group	II-IH group	p value
NRS score at 0 hr	0.00	0.00	
NRS score at 4 hr	1.63 ± 2.12	0.96 ± 1.52	0.07
NRS score at 6 hr	1.84 ± 1.88	1.24 ± 1.53	0.07
NRS score at 8 hr	1.39 ± 1.53	1.00 ± 1.09	0.14
NRS score at 12 hr	1.39 ± 1.49	0.92 ± 1.197	0.08
NRS score at 24 hr	1.20 ± 1.07	0.88 ± 0.76	0.09

Data are mean ± SD.

Table 6: Postoperative total opioid consumption and first analgesic request time over the first 24 postoperative hours of parturients who underwent caesarean delivery under spinal anesthesia in Gondar University Hospital from April 1 to May 30, 2017, in Northwest Ethiopia.

Character	TAP group	II-IH group	p value
Total tramadol consumption (mg)	52.45 ± 30.51	37.25 ± 27.09	0.009
First analgesic request time (hr)	10.71 ± 7.67	14.09 ± 8.20 hr	0.03

Data are mean ± SD.

Our result was comparable with the randomized controlled study done in Russia which showed that there was no statistically significant VAS (visual analogue score) difference between TAP and II-IH blocks after caesarean delivery via Pfannenstiel incision within 24 hours postoperatively [14].

A randomized comparative study done in New Zealand showed that the II-IH nerve block reduced the pain score significantly and postoperative total tramadol consumption ($p = 0.03$) than the TAP block after inguinal surgery [12]. This is consistent with our result regarding tramadol consumption.

A systematic review and meta-analysis done by Abdallah et al. in Canada demonstrated that the TAP block enhances analgesia after caesarean delivery with detectable analgesic effects for the entire 24 hours [5].

Another review and meta-analysis done by Mishriky et al. concluded that the TAP block improved postoperative analgesia and reduced the pain score in women undergoing CD [4]. These two are in agreement with our results.

A meta-analysis done by Champaneria et al. in 2016 showed that the TAP block provided effective analgesia and reduced the postoperative pain score after caesarean section [15]. This is comparable to our result.

Our result is comparable with a randomized control trial study done in Saudi Arabia that showed the NRS score was significantly lower in the TAP group than the control up to 24 hr both at rest and at movement after caesarean delivery via Pfannenstiel incision [15].

On the other hand, a study done by Sakalli et al. showed that the II-IH nerve block decreased the mean VAS score both at rest and at movement within 24 hours after CD [2]. This is comparable with our finding.

Similarly, a study done in Jordan showed a significant reduction in the mean VAS score after the II-IH nerve block when compared with the placebo group in parturients who underwent caesarean delivery under general anesthesia [16, 17].

Our study demonstrated that II-IH reduced the NRS pain score which is consistent with a study done by Bunting and McConachie and Ganta and colleagues, who analyzed the mean VAS score, and they found it to be less with the II-IH block as compared with the placebo group in parturients who underwent caesarean delivery [18]. A study of Bell and colleagues also demonstrated that the VAS score was reduced with the II IH nerve block [3].

A study done in Turkey by Yucel and colleagues showed that the II-IH nerve block reduced the VAS score for the first 24 hr postoperatively than the control group. This is comparable with the current study [19].

In this study, the mean time for the first analgesic request was significantly prolonged in the II-IH group ($p = 0.03$). This is consistent with the finding of the previous comparative study done in Russia which showed that the II-IH block prolonged the time to first analgesic requirement in a statistically significant fashion than the TAP block following CD [14].

We found that the total amount of tramadol consumption over the first 24-hour postoperative time was lower in the II-IH group than that in the TAP group. This result is comparable with the previous study [14]. One study done in New Zealand was also in line with this study [12].

Our finding was also comparable with the studies conducted by Yucel et al. and Naghshineh et al. where they have found that postoperative analgesic consumption was significantly lower in the parturients who received the II-IH block as compared with the control group [20].

5. Conclusion and Recommendation

There was no statistically significant difference between TAP and II-IH nerve blocks regarding the postoperative pain score in each time point both at rest and at movement, but the II-IH block significantly reduced total tramadol consumption and prolonged the time to first analgesic request than TAP.

We recommend the II-IH nerve block for postcaesarean delivery pain management via Pfannenstiel incision.

Conflicts of Interest

The authors declare no conflicts of interest.

Authors' Contributions

All authors contributed equally to this work.

Acknowledgments

The authors would like to acknowledge the University of Gondar, Research and Community Service Vice President Office, for their support. The authors would also like to appreciate data collectors, our participants, and Gondar University Hospital.

References

[1] L. Eslamian, M. Kabiri-Nasab, M. Agha-Husseini, O. Azimaraghi, G. Barzin, and A. Movafegh, "Adding sufentanil to TAP block hyperbaric bupivacaine decreases post-cesarean delivery morphine consumption," *Acta medica Iranica*, vol. 54, no. 3, pp. 185–190, 2016.

[2] M. Sakalli, A. Ceyhan, H. Y. Uysal, I. Yazici, and H. Başar, "The efficacy of ilioinguinal and iliohypogastric nerve block for postoperative pain after caesarean section," *Journal of Research in Medical Sciences*, vol. 15, no. 1, pp. 6–13, 2010.

[3] E. A. Bell, B. P. Jones, A. J. Olufolabi et al., "Iliohypogastric-ilioinguinal peripheral nerve block for post-Cesarean delivery analgesia decreases morphine use but not opioid-related side effects," *Canadian Journal of Anaesthesia*, vol. 49, no. 7, pp. 694–700, 2002.

[4] B. M. Mishriky, R. B. George, and A. S. Habib, "Transversus abdominis plane block for analgesia after Cesarean delivery: a systematic review and meta-analysis," *Canadian Journal of Anesthesia*, vol. 59, no. 8, pp. 766–778, 2012.

[5] F. W. Abdallah, S. H. Halpern, and C. B. Margarido, "Transversus abdominis plane block for postoperative analgesia after Caesarean delivery performed under spinal anaesthesia? A systematic review and meta-analysis," *British Journal of Anaesthesia*, vol. 109, no. 5, pp. 679–687, 2012.

[6] N. Nguyen, A. Landais, A. Barbaryan et al., "Analgesic efficacy of Pfannenstiel incision infiltration with ropivacaine 7.5 mg/mL for caesarean section," *Anesthesiology Research and Practice*, vol. 2010, pp. 1–7, 2010.

[7] L. Buhagiar, O. A. Cassar, M. P. Brincat et al., "Predictors of post-caesarean section pain and analgesic consumption," *Journal of Anaesthesiology Clinical Pharmacology*, vol. 27, no. 2, p. 185, 2011.

[8] X. Li, M. Zhou, X. Shi, et al., "Local anaesthetic wound infiltration used for caesarean section pain relief: a meta-analysis," *International Journal of Clinical and Experimental Medicine*, vol. 8, no. 6, pp. 10213–10224, 2015.

[9] W. Mei, C. Jin, L. Feng et al., "Bilateral ultrasound-guided transversus abdominis plane block combined with ilioinguinal-iliohypogastric nerve block for cesarean delivery anesthesia," *Anesthesia and Analgesia*, vol. 113, no. 1, pp. 134–137, 2011.

[10] D. Belavy, P. Cowlishaw, M. Howes, and F. Phillips, "Ultrasound-guided transversus abdominis plane block for analgesia after caesarean delivery," *British Journal of Anaesthesia*, vol. 103, no. 5, pp. 726–730, 2009.

[11] M. C. Vallejo, T. L. Steen, B. T. Cobb, et al., "Efficacy of the bilateral ilioinguinal-iliohypogastric block with intrathecal morphine for postoperative cesarean delivery analgesia," *The Scientific World Journal*, vol. 2012, Article ID 107316, 6 pages, 2012.

[12] M. J. Fredrickson, C. Paine, and J. Hamill, "Improved analgesia with the ilioinguinal block compared to the transversus abdominis plane block after pediatric inguinal surgery: a prospective randomized trial," *Pediatric Anesthesia*, vol. 20, no. 11, pp. 1022–1027, 2010.

[13] C. Aveline, H. Le Hetet, A. Le Roux et al., "Comparison between ultrasound-guided transversus abdominis plane and conventional ilioinguinal/iliohypogastric nerve blocks for day-case open inguinal hernia repair," *British Journal of Anaesthesia*, vol. 106, no. 3, pp. 380–386, 2011.

[14] A. E. Bessmertnyj, E. E Antipin, D. N Uvarov, S. V Sedyh, and E. V Nedashkovsky, "Comparison of the effectiveness of ilioinguinal-iliohypogastric blockade and transversus abdominis plane block for analgesia after cesarean section," *Anesteziologiia i Reanimatologiia*, vol. 60, no. 2, pp. 51–54, 2015.

[15] R. Champaneria, L. Shah, M. J. Wilson, and J. P. Daniels, "Clinical effectiveness of transversus abdominis plane (TAP) blocks for pain relief after caesarean section: a meta-analysis," *International Journal of Obstetric Anesthesia*, vol. 28, pp. 45–60, 2016.

[16] G. Al-Dehayat and M. Al-Momany, "Ilioinguinal-iliohypogastric peripheral nerve block for analgesia after caesarean section," *Journal of the Ramanujan Mathematical Society*, vol. 15, no. 2, pp. 70–72, 2008.

[17] J. G. McDonnell, G. Curley, J. Carney et al., "The analgesic efficacy of transversus abdominis plane block after cesarean delivery: a randomized controlled trial," *Anesthesia and Analgesia*, vol. 106, no. 1, pp. 186–191, 2008.

[18] P. Bunting and I. McConachie, "Ilioinguinal nerve blockade for analgesia after caesarean section," *British Journal of Anaesthesia*, vol. 61, no. 6, pp. 773–775, 1988.

[19] E. Yucel, I. O. Kol, C. Duger, K. Kaygusuz, S. Gursoy, and C. Mimaroglu, "Ilioinguinal-iliohypogastric nerve block with intravenous dexketoprofen improves postoperative analgesia in abdominal hysterectomies," *Brazilian Journal of Anesthesiology*, vol. 63, no. 4, pp. 334–339, 2013.

[20] E. Naghshineh, S. Shiari, and M. Jabalameli, "Preventive effect of ilioinguinal nerve block on postoperative pain after cesarean section," *Advanced Biomedical Research*, vol. 4, p. 229, 2015.

17

Objective Evaluation of a New Epidural Simulator by the CompuFlo® Epidural Instrument

Giorgio Capogna,[1] **Alessandra Coccoluto**,[1,2] **Emanuele Capogna**,[1] **and Angelica Del Vecchio**[1]

[1]*European School of Obstetric Anesthesia (EESOA), Maternal Neonatal Simulation Centre, Roma, Italy*
[2]*Policlinico Casilino Hospital, Roma, Italy*

Correspondence should be addressed to Giorgio Capogna; capogna.eesoa@gmail.com

Academic Editor: Enrico Camporesi

Background. In this study, we describe a custom-made new epidural simulator, created by modifying the inner structure of a commercially available one, in the attempt to make it adequately realistic. To validate and evaluate the realism of our device, we used the Computerized Epidural Instrument CompuFlo. *Method.* The Compuflo CompuFlo curves obtained from 64 experiments on the epidural simulator were compared to 64 curves obtained from a previous human study, from consecutive laboring parturients requesting epidural analgesia. *Results.* Epidural simulator and human pressure curves were very similar. There was a significant difference between the drop of pressure due to false and true loss of resistance (LOR) in both the groups. *Discussion.* Our simulator can realistically reproduce the anatomical layers the needle must pass as demonstrated by the similarity between the simulator and human pressure curves and the small differences of pressure values recorded. CompuFlo may be used as an objective tool to create and assess and compare objectively the epidural task trainers.

1. Introduction

Manikin epidural simulators are based upon dummy models made from plastic or rubber. They are portable and easy to set up and use. One major limitation of these models is that they do not reproduce the anatomical features of all the layers the needle must pass (skin, subcutaneous fat, supraspinous and interspinous ligament, and ligamenta flava) and sometimes the solid plastic structure to represent the vertebare do not accurately reproduce the vertebral arch and the other possible bony parts which may be encountetred during needle insertion. The average impression of the users of the commercially available simulators, based on subjective scales, has been reported to be largely variable, usually achieving medium or low scores [1, 2].

In one recent study, four commercially available different epidural puncture training simulators were evaluated in a single-blinded, randomised controlled manikin study by expert consultant anesthesiologists, and none of the simulators tested reached a high enough score to indicate that they provided an experience close to a real patient [3].

In this study, we describe a custom-made new epidural simulator, created by modifying the inner structure of a commercially available one, and using some materials of our own design in the attempt to make it adequately realistic. The aim of the study was to validate and evaluate the realism of our device by using a Computerized Epidural Instrument (CompuFlo) [4].

2. Methods

After having removed the inner length of plastic of a commercially available epidural simulator (P61, 3B Scientific, 3B Italy, Ozzano Bologna), we inserted in its place a modified solid rigid polyurethane foam spinal column model (SKU #1323-3, Sawbones, Europe). The spinal column model was sawn to obtain vertebral segments from L5 to T11. Each vertebra was modified by cutting the transverse processes

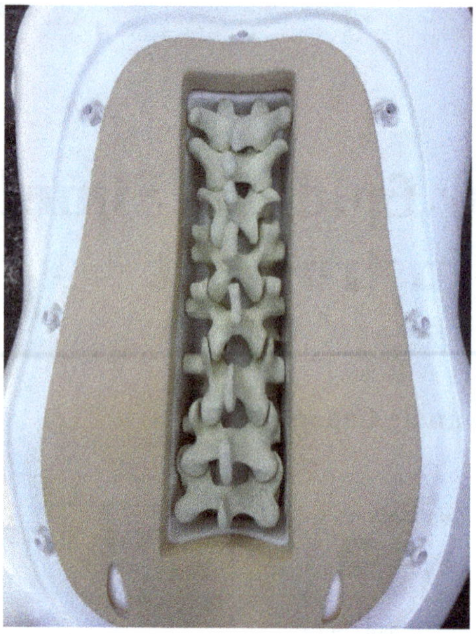

Figure 1: After having removed the inner length of plastic of a commercially available epidural simulator (P61, 3B Scientific), we inserted in its place a modified solid rigid polyurethane foam spinal column model. This way the vertebral arch and the other possible bony parts which may be encountered during needle insertion were present into the model in a life-like dimension and structure.

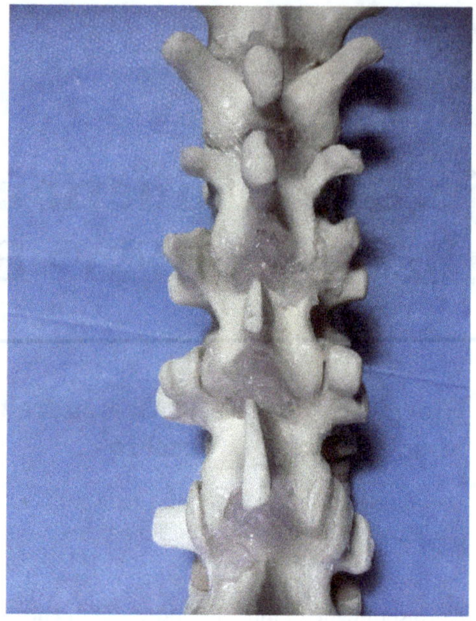

Figure 2: A layer of clear, transparent sealant silicone was modelled from the inferior edge and anteroinferior surface of cranial vertebra to the superior edge and posterosuperior surface of caudal vertebra to mimic the ligamenta flava.

and the dorsal part of the model in order to adapt it to the inside of the plastic torso. This way the vertebral arch and the other possible bony parts which may be encountered during needle insertion were present into the model in a life-like dimension and structure (Figure 1).

A layer of clear, transparent sealant silicone (Bostik, UHU Bostik, Milano, Italy) was modelled from the inferior edge and anteroinferior surface of cranial vertebra to the superior edge and posterosuperior surface of caudal vertebra to mimic the ligamenta flava (Figure 2).

The silicone rubber exhibits tactile sensation similar to that of ligamentum flavum, providing hard texture for needle insertion and gives a tactile sensation when penetrated [5].

A standard closed-cell neoprene pipe insulation tube (Cestaro, Padova, Italy) has been reduced to pieces of the size, on the average, of 1 cm of diameter and mixed with the transparent sealant silicone in a ratio of 3 : 1 to mimic the ligamentum sovraspinosus. The same neoprene-silicone mixture was used for ligamentum interspinous and paravertebral muscles (multifidus), but in this case, the average diameter of the neoprene pieces was 1.5–2 cm in order to obtain a less-dense material capable to be crossed by the needle in a low resistant fashion.

The dough taken was molded on the spine model to replace ligaments and muscles (Figure 3).

We completed the set with the standard artificial skin and the tubing and connectors representing the fluid-filled dural sac originally provided by the manufacturer (P61, 3B Scientific, Ozzano Bologna, Italy). This dura-simulating latex tube provides a distinct "pop" sensation when breached, indicating the tip of the needle has reached the subarachnoid space. When the stylet is withdrawn from the needle water which mimics "cerebrospinal fluid" that appears at the hub of the needle indicating the success of spinal puncture. The dura-simulating tube is self sealing allowing for repeated use.

We also modified the base body of the standard 3M Scientific simulator to better collect and drain the water used for loss of resistance to saline.

The CompuFlo Epidural Instrument (Milestone Scientific, Inc., Livingston, New Jersey, USA) [6] is a computer-controlled drug delivery system that can precisely measure the pressure of human tissues in real time at the tip of the needle. It is capable of distinguishing different tissue types by providing continuously real-time "exit-pressure" data at the needle tip when placed in-situ. The instrument uses an algorithm to determine the pressure at the tip of the needle via a continuous fluid path. This system is unique in that pressure is a feedback loop and controller to the system, thus regulating the electromechanical motor which controls flow-rate and the fluid dispensed by the system. An audible and visual graphic of exit-pressure is provided to the health care practitioner enabling the operator to focus on the injection site.

Using the CompuFlo, entry of the needle into the ligamentum flavum is indicated by a great increase in pressure with a simultaneous increase of the audible tone, while the entry of the needle into the epidural space results in a brisk drop in pressure on the visual display as well as a distinct fall in the tone of the audio output [4]. A drop in pressure sustained for more than 5 seconds is deemed consistent with entry into the epidural space. Typical curves can be obtained from epidural insertion, as reported in human studies [4, 7].

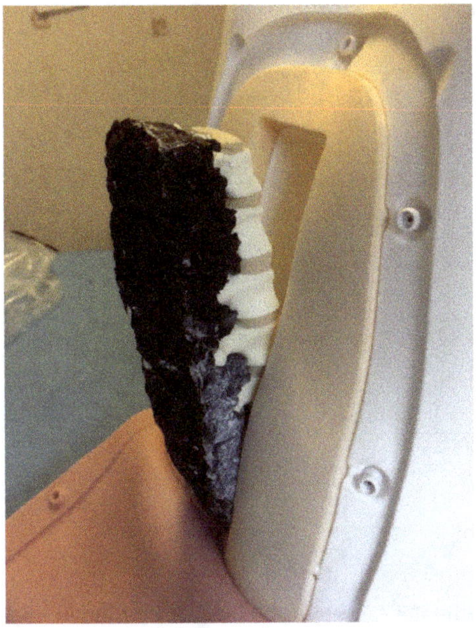

FIGURE 3: The neoprene-silicone mixture used for ligamentum interspinosus and paravertebral muscles (multifidus).

3. Experiment

For the purpose of the study, we used the same epidural technique and CompuFlo setting procedure previously used for one of our human studies [7].

The CompuFlo device was set to deliver normal saline at a rate of 0.05 mL/s with a maximum pressure limited to 200 mmHg, and the 0 point of pressure calibration was checked by positioning the needle at the level of the site of puncture.

In accordance with the standard anesthesia textbooks, the epidural needle (with stylet) should be placed into the ligamentum flavum before attaching the syringe, allowing an improved appreciation of epidural anatomy for the operator. However, in clinical practice, the epidural needle is frequently introduced in the lumbar area to a depth of approximately 2-3 cm to avoid accidental epidural space puncture. In this case, the needle may be inserted into the supraspinous or interspinous ligament, in the paraspinous muscles or subcutaneous tissue before the LOR with syringe is achieved, creating sometimes a pseudo or false LOR.

To evaluate both the LOR and the false LOR, we decided to introduce the epidural needle after skin puncture and to track the needle until the epidural space.

A Tuohy epidural needle 16G previously connected to the computerized injection pump via the arterial line extension tubing was introduced in the phantom and the CompuFlo instrument was started (Figure 4).

The Tuohy needle was then advanced very slowly, and pressures were recorded continuously.

An increase in pressure followed by a sudden drop in pressure (typically greater than 50% of the maximum pressure) lasting for at least 5 seconds, resulting in the formation of a low and stable pressure plateau, was considered as definite epidural space identification (Figure 5).

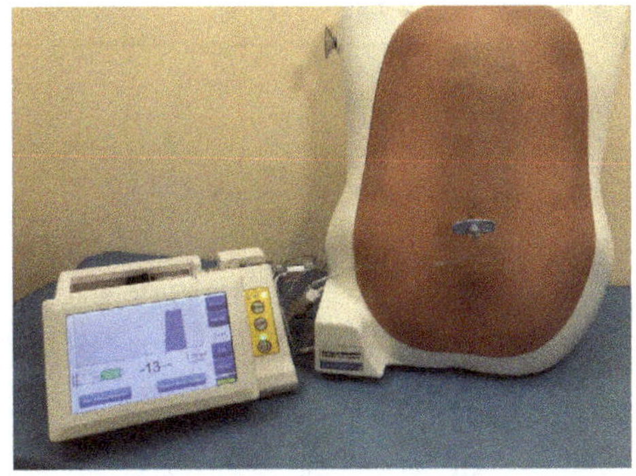

FIGURE 4: Connection of the CompuFlo instrument to the epidural simulator.

If both these criteria were not fulfilled, and a small increase of delta of pressure followed by a transient drop of a lesser degree was observed, the result was considered as "false loss of resistance," and the epidural needle was further advanced and/or repositioned until a true loss of resistance was obtained.

A sample size of 64 observations for each group was required to set 80% test power and a 95% significance level. The CompuFlo curves obtained from 64 experiments on the epidural simulator were compared to 64 curves obtained from a previous human study, from consecutive laboring parturients requesting epidural analgesia [7].

The differences between the mean of the two curves (the CompuFlo analysis in vivo and in simulation) were analyzed by using the R software. Differences in pressure drop were compared using unpaired two samples *t*-test.

4. Results

Epidural simulator and human pressure curves were very comparable (Figure 6).

As expected, we observed more variability in the plateau values indicating the epidural space in the control group as compared to those obtained with the simulator. This is obvious since epidural pressure is variable in humans, being approximately 15–20 mmHg in pregnancy, while the "epidural pressure" in the simulator is always equal to the atmospheric pressure, and comparable to that reported in nonpregnant subjects [8].

There was a significant difference in percentage of drop of pressure between the drop of pressure due to false loss of resistance (LOR) and that due to the entry of the needle in the epidural space in both the groups (Table 1).

5. Discussion

In this study, we reported the description of a new custom-made simulator and demonstrated its realism by the similarity between the simulator and human pressure curves objectively obtained with the CompuFlo Epidural instrument.

In a large review, Stunt et al. [9] reported that there are, on the average, more than 400 commercially available simulators for medical training, but 93.5% percent of these are not known to be tested for validity. The majority of

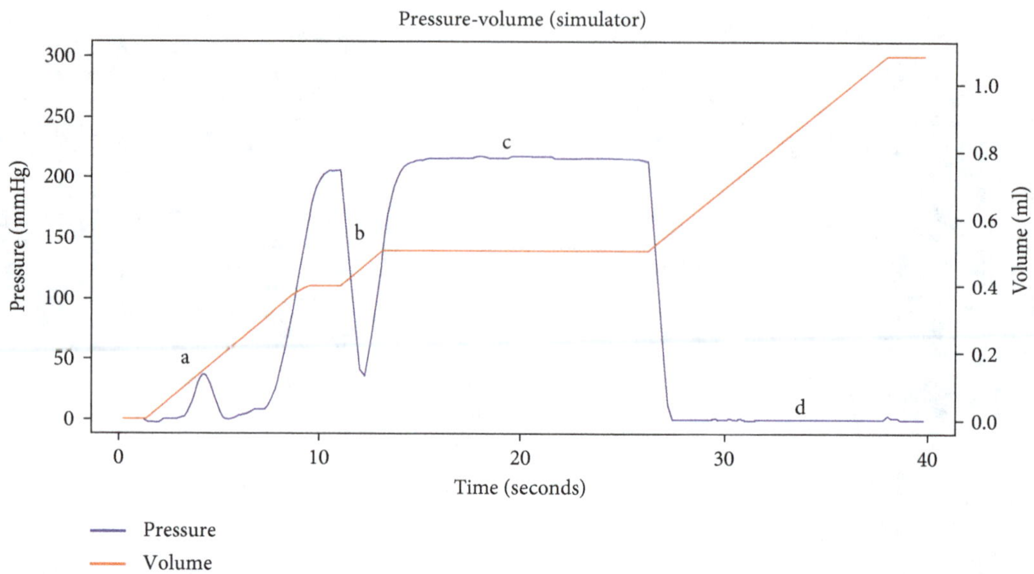

FIGURE 5: Typical pressure-volume infused curve during identification of the epidural space with Compuflo: a, supraspinous ligament (first small peak); b, false loss of resistance (first dip); c, legamentum flavum (increase in resistance); and d, final identification of the epidural space (sudden drop in pressure lasting for at least 5 seconds, resulting in the formation of a low and stable pressure plateau).

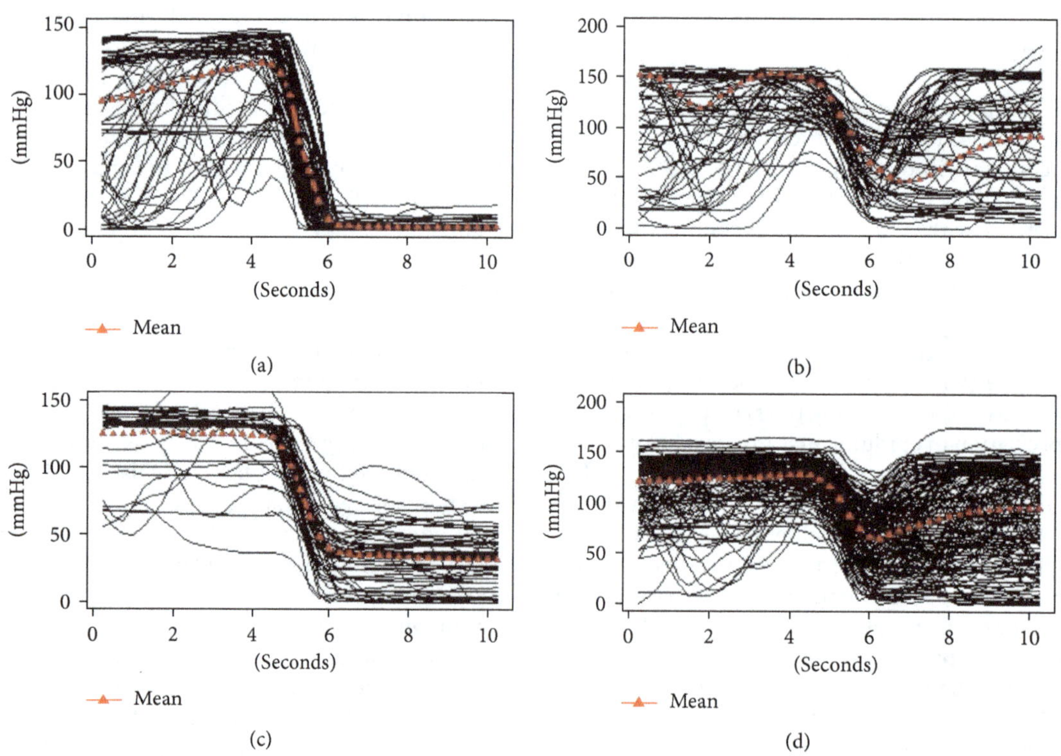

FIGURE 6: Epidural simulator and human pressure curves immediately before and after the needle have entered the epidural space. (a) LOR ES simulator, (b) false LOR simulator, (c) LOR ES, and (d) false LOR. LOR ES = loss of resistance in the epidural space, False LOR = false loss of resistance (needle not in the epidural space).

TABLE 1: Differences in the mean values of false and true LOR (loss of resistance) between the drop of pressure observed with the simulator when compared to those of the controls.

Mean % of drop of pressure (mean, CI)	False LOR	True LOR (epidural space)	P
Simulator	9 (0.04–23)	97 (96–98)	0.04
Control	5.5 (2–13)	65 (63–75)	0.03

studies on medical simulators did not describe a power analysis and lacked standardized assessment methods and blinded assessors.

To guarantee patient safety, it is important that simulators designed for each type of training demonstrate high levels of validity.

In particular, the major problems with epidural simulator assessment is that they are usually evaluated by subjective Likert like scales reported by physicians, and this kind of scales may have some disadvantages and are subjected to a large variability of ratings [1–3]. Due to the nature of this subjective evaluation, results of previous studies on epidural simulators are controversial.

In one study [2], the simulator was thought to be borderline for life-likeness for the "feel" of the supraspinous ligament and ligamentum flavum, and in another study, none of the commercially available simulators tested were considered to provide an experience close to a real patient [3].

The limits of the subjective physicians' evaluation are witnessed by one blinded study [3] that compared the identification of landmarks by palpation to select the point of puncture in different epidural simulators and reported that some participants felt that the palpation of landmarks with the banana were highly realistic, despite the fact that there were no vertebrae-like structures to feel.

To overcome such subjective nature of human evaluation, we decided to use the Computerized Epidural Instrument CompuFlo as an assessment tool to more impartially evaluate the realism of our simulator.

The results of this study suggest that our simulator can realistically reproduce the anatomical features of the layers the needle must pass through to reach the epidural space as demonstrated by the similarity between the simulator and human pressure curves.

Naemura et al. [10] studied the force of penetration waveforms of the epidural needle into a porcine model, reporting two peaks representing the needle penetrating in the supraspinous ligament and/or the muscle fiber and in the ligamentum flavum. Conventional simulators have been reported to be able to show only the simple increase up to peak when the needle is in the ligamentum flavum, followed by a plateau when the needle reaches the epidural space.

The biphasic curve observed in our simulator confirms the capability of our new device to reproduce even the subtle pressure changes due to the passage of the needle through the supraspinous ligamentum. In addition, it was able to identify the false loss of resistance due to the position of needle into the interspinous ligament, in the paraspinous muscles or in the subcutaneous tissue before the LOR with syringe is achieved. These features may positively contribute to improve the realism of the simulator.

We are certainly aware that our preliminary evaluation should be confirmed by clinical follow-up to investigate the training efficacy of such instrument in clinical teaching practice, and studies on this matter are in progress.

For correct medical psychomotor skills training and to provide objective and correct feedback, it is essential to have a realistic training environment. Scientific testing of simulators is an important way to prove and validate the training method. To guarantee effective training skills and patient safety, it is important that epidural simulators designed for this type of training demonstrate high levels of validity. We believe that the method we used to assess the realism of our simulator may be useful in future studies to better evaluate validity of a device as condition to guarantee proper acquisition of psychomotor skills.

In conclusion, our results suggest that our simulator can realistically reproduce the anatomical features of the layers the needle must pass through to reach the epidural space as demonstrated by the similarity between the simulator and human pressure curves and the small differences of pressure values recorded during the needle insertion. Our simulator may be a promising, realistic device in teaching epidural needle-handling skills for epidural technique. CompuFlo may be used as an objective tool to create and assess and compare objectively the epidural task trainers.

Conflicts of Interest

The authors declare that they have no conflicts of interest.

References

[1] R. A. Lee, T. C. van Zundert, J. J. van Koesveld et al., "Evaluation of the Mediseus epidural simulator," *Anaesthesia and Intensive Care*, vol. 40, no. 2, pp. 311–318, 2012.

[2] V. Uppal, R. Kearns, and E. McGrady, "Evaluation of M43B lumbar puncture simulator-II as a training tool for identification of the epidural space and lumbar puncture," *Anaesthesia*, vol. 66, no. 6, pp. 493–496, 2011.

[3] T. H. Pedersen, J. Meuli, E. J. Plazikowski et al., "Loss of resistance. A randomised controlled trial assessing four low-fidelity epidural puncture simulators," *European Journal of Anaesthesiology*, vol. 34, no. 9, pp. 602–608, 2017.

[4] O. Ghelber, R. E. Gebhard, S. Vora, C. A. Hagberg, and P. Szmuk, "Identification of the epidural space using pressure measurement with the compuflo injection pump—a pilot study," *Regional Anesthesia and Pain Medicine*, vol. 33, no. 4, pp. 346–352, 2008.

[5] E. C. S. Chen, G. Ameri, R. V. Sondekoppam, S. Ganapathy, and T. Peters, "Navigated simulator for spinal needle interventions," in *Medicine Meets Virtual Reality*, J. D. Westwood, S. W. Westwood, L. Fellander-Tsai et al., Eds., p. 59, IOS Press, Amsterdam, Netherlands, 2014.

[6] M. N. Hochman, M. J. Friedman, W. Williams, and C. Hochman, "Interstitial tissue pressure associated with dental injections: a clinical study," *Quintessence International*, vol. 37, no. 6, pp. 469–476, 2006.

[7] A. Coccoluto, F. Chiarenza, M. Camorcia, and G. Capogna, "Identification of the epidural space: a double blind comparison between the CompuFlo® epidural computer controlled system and the standard LOR to saline technique in obstetrics," *European Journal of Anaesthesiology*, vol. 34, article 04AP03-11, 2017.

[8] J. E. Usubiaga, F. Moya, and L. E. Usubiaga, "Effect of thoracic and abdominal pressure changes on the epidural space

pressure," *British Journal of Anaesthesia*, vol. 39, no. 8, pp. 612–618, 1967.

[9] J. J. Stunt, P. H. Wulms, G. M. Kerkhoffs, J. Dankelman, C. N. van Dijk, and G. J. M. Tuijthof, "How valid are commercially available medical simulators?," *Advances in Medical Education and Practice*, vol. 5, pp. 385–395, 2014.

[10] K. Naemura, A. Sakai, T. Hayashi, and H. Saito, "Epidural insertion simulator of higher insertion resistance and drop rate after puncture," in *Proceedings of the 30th Annual International IEE EMBS Conference*, pp. 3249–3252, Vanvouver, BC, Canada, August 2008.

18

Comparison between Vapocoolant Spray and Eutectic Mixture of Local Anesthetics Cream in Reducing Pain during Spinal Injections

Riyadh Firdaus, Besthadi Sukmono, Annemarie Chrysantia Melati, and Berial Dewin Marzaini

Department of Anesthesiology and Intensive Care, Cipto Mangunkusumo National Central Hospital and Faculty of Medicine, Universitas Indonesia, Jakarta 10430, Indonesia

Correspondence should be addressed to Riyadh Firdaus; riyadh116@gmail.com

Academic Editor: Yukio Hayashi

Background. Eutectic mixture of local anesthetics (EMLA) cream is often used for local anesthesia during spinal injections. However, this agent has delayed onset of action while vapocoolant spray serves more advantages. The vapocoolant spray containing ethyl chloride has fast onset and is safe, low cost, and widely available. This study aimed at comparing the effectiveness of vapocoolant spray and EMLA cream in reducing pain for spinal injections. *Methods.* This was an experimental study on 94 subjects with 47 subjects treated with EMLA cream and 47 subjects treated with vapocoolant spray. The effectiveness of anesthesia was assessed by using Numeric Pain Rating Scale (NPRS) and patient movement during the surgery. *Results.* This study found that the pain scale was NPRS 0 (0–3) for the EMLA group and NPRS 0 (0–4) for the vapocoolant spray group. There was no significant difference between two groups for pain scale according to the Mann–Whitney *U* test. For patient movement, the movement was reported only in one (2.1%) patient in the EMLA group and one (2.1%) patient in the vapocoolant spray group. Based on Fisher's test, there was no significant difference between the two groups for patient movement. *Conclusions.* Both EMLA cream and vapocoolant spray were equally effective in reducing pain during spinal injection. There was no difference in degree of pain reduction and patient movement between the EMLA cream group and the vapocoolant spray group during spinal injection.

1. Background

Pain during any medical procedures, including spinal anesthesia, should be managed carefully as this would affect the perception and comfort of the patients [1, 2]. Kim et al. mentioned that pain during spinal injections had mean pain scale of 3.9 based on Numeric Pain Rating Scale (NPRS). Additionally, the diameter of the needle was correlated with the pain during injections: 32 G needle generated pain in 31% of patients, 27 G needle generated pain in 53% of patients, and 23 G needle generated pain in 63% of patients [3]. Reduced pain during spinal injection would increase the quality of anesthesia. Additionally, the patient would have positive experience during the anesthesia procedure.

Local anesthetic agents may be administered to relieve the pain during any injections. Anesthetic agents often used are eutectic mixture of local anesthetics (EMLA) cream, ethyl chloride, nonsteroidal anti-inflammatory drugs (NSAIDs), lidocaine, and opioid [4–6]. EMLA cream is often used to decrease the pain during spinal injections. However, this agent has longer onset of action, up to 30 minutes, before the peak of action [7].

The vapocoolant spray contains ethyl chloride which serves as topical anesthetic agents. The vapocoolant spray generates cooling effect on the skin surface. There are many advantages of this agent, including fast onset of action, its safety profile, and low cost, and it is widely available [8]. The mechanism of action is that the vapors create sudden decrease of the skin temperature and disrupt the ion channel activation. Therefore, this would impair the pain reception [9]. This agent is often used in minor medical procedures, including arterial/venous cannulation [10].

Past studies have mentioned the wide indications of vapocoolant spray for many medical procedures. Celik et al. have compared the administration of vapocoolant spray, EMLA cream, and placebo cream during venous cannulation among patients undergoing hemodialysis. The result showed that both vapocoolant spray and EMLA cream significantly decreased the pain intensity during injections [11].

Based on the preliminary study conducted during February 2016 in Cipto Mangunkusumo Hospital, there were 94.3% of respondents who had movements during spinal injections by using 27 G needle. Additionally, there were 5.7% respondents with pain score of 5, 25.7% respondents with pain scale of 3, 51.4% respondents with pain scale of 2, and 17.1% respondents with pain score of 1. The mean pain score for all respondents undergoing spinal injections was 2.3.

In Indonesia, currently there is no study regarding the use of vapocoolant spray as local anesthetic agent during spinal injections. However, this agent is cheaper and widely available in the daily practice in comparison with EMLA cream. This study aimed to compare the effectiveness between vapocoolant spray and EMLA cream as the local anesthetic agent during spinal injections.

2. Methods

2.1. Research Design. This was an experimental study conducted in a stereotactic operating room of Cipto Mangunkusumo Hospital from October 2016 to January 2017. Research subjects were divided into two groups with administration of vapocoolant spray containing ethyl chloride for the treatment group and EMLA cream for the control group.

2.2. Inclusion and Exclusion Criteria. Inclusion criteria were adult subjects over the age of 18 undergoing first brachytherapy procedure and planned for spinal anesthesia and having physical status of the American Society of Anesthesiologist (ASA) I–III. Exclusion criteria were subjects with allergy to anesthetic drugs, hemodynamically unstable, contraindications to spinal injection, unwilling to sign informed consent, and current consumption of psychiatric drug. Drop-out criteria were subjects with allergic reaction during injection, refractory hypotension (decreased blood pressure >20%) despite of administration of ephedrine, and refractory desaturation (peripheral oxygen saturation <92%) despite of positive ventilation pressure.

2.3. Research Protocol. There were 94 subjects with 47 subjects for each group consecutively. Following the ethical clearance, and registered in clinicaltrials.gov (NCT 03134391), research subjects were randomized by using block randomization into control and experimental group. All subjects had 22 G intravenous cannula with ringer acetate fluid administration. Mean arterial pressure (MAP), pulse rate, respiratory rate, and peripheral capillary oxygen saturation (SpO_2) were recorded. Patients were positioned in sitting position with the head flexed and back arched posteriorly. Spinal injection site was identified in the L4-5 intervertebral space.

In the EMLA group, research subjects received 2 ml of EMLA cream containing a mixture of 2.5% lidocaine and 2.5% prilocaine in oil/water emulsion and further covered by clear dressing for 45–60 minutes. In the vapocoolant spray group, the patient received a spray from a vapocoolant pressure pack with a distance of about 10 cm from the surface for two seconds and at least 10 seconds for the vapocoolant spray to vaporize.

Spinal injection was conducted by using 27 G spinal needle with pointed tip with the bevel parallel to the durafiber. Spinal injection was conducted by a final year anesthesiologist resident. Pain intensity was measured by using NPRS, and patient movement was recorded to measure the success of anesthesia. Vital signs were observed every three minutes for the first 15 minutes and every five minutes until completion of the procedure.

2.4. Statistical Analysis. Data analysis was performed by using the Statistical Package for the Social Sciences (SPSS) for Windows version 20.0. NPRS score and patient movement was analyzed by using the independent T-test and chi-squared test if data had normal distribution and Mann–Whitney U test and Fisher's exact test if data had nonnormal distribution.

3. Results

There were no subjects that dropped out during the study (Figure 1). Baseline characteristics of study subjects are shown in Table 1. Demographic data were comparable between the EMLA cream group and the vapocoolant spray group. There was no significant difference in anthropometrical status such as weight, height, and body mass index between the two groups.

Data on pain intensity using NPRS and patient movement in both groups are shown in Tables 2 and 3. There was no significant difference in both groups for patient intensity and also movement.

There were no allergic reactions occurred during the study. There was no occurrence of desaturation/apnea events, bradycardia, nausea, vomiting, respiratory depression, hypotension, and agitation in both groups. Analysis of hemodynamic profile (MAP, pulse rate, respiratory rate, and SpO_2) according to time is shown in Figure 2. Based on unpaired T-test results, there were no significant differences for hemodynamic profile in the form of MAP, pulse rate, respiratory rate, and SpO_2.

4. Discussion

This study aimed to compare the effectiveness of vapocoolant spray and EMLA cream in reducing pain for spinal injections. Based on pain assessment in this study generated, there was no statistically significant pain scale difference between these two. This was similar with previous study by Cohen et al., in which found there were no significant

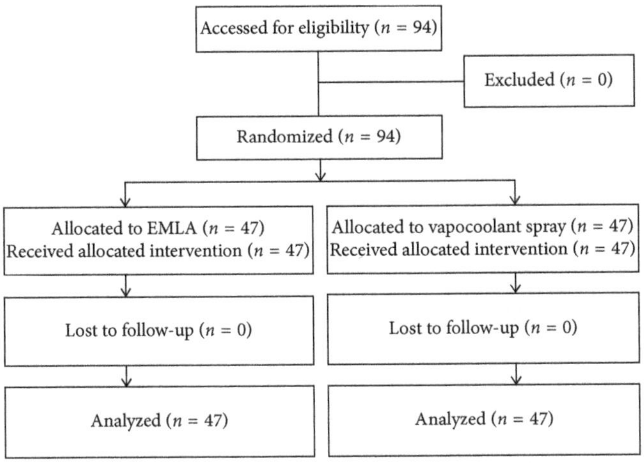

Figure 1: Study flow according to the Consolidated Standards of Reporting Trials (CONSORT) diagram.

Table 1: Baseline characteristic of both groups.

Characteristics	EMLA cream N = 47	Vapocoolant spray N = 47	p value
Age (years)	52.43 ± 10.37	53.81 ± 8.78	0.488[a]
Occupation			0.144[b]
Housewife	33 (70.2%)	39 (83.0%)	—
Non-housewife	14 (29.8%)	8 (17.0%)	—
Education			0.539[b]
None	3 (6.4%)	3 (6.4%)	—
Elementary school	18 (38.3%)	16 (34.0%)	—
Junior high school	8 (17.0%)	7 (14.9%)	—
Senior high school	14 (29.8%)	11 (23.4%)	—
University	4 (8.5%)	10 (21.3%)	—
Weight (kilogram)	55.70 ± 14.23	54.52 ± 10.11	0.645[a]
Height (centimeter)	150.34 ± 6.01	151.0 ± 682	0.619[a]
Body mass index	23.56 (14.79–52.07)	23.68 (17.10–36.89)	0.922[c]
ASA physical status			1.000[d]
I	0 (0%)	2 (4.3%)	—
II	45 (95.7%)	43 (91.5%)	—
III	2 (4.3%)	2 (4.3%)	—
Diagnosis			1.000[d]
Cervical cancer	45 (95.7%)	46 (97.9%)	—
Vagina cancer	1 (2.1%)	1 (2.1%)	—
Endometrium cancer	1 (2.1%)	0 (0%)	—

Numerical data were presented as mean ± standard deviation if distribution was normal and median (minimum-maximum) if distribution was not normal; categorical data were presented as N (percentage). [a]Independent T-test; [b]chi-squared test; [c]Mann–Whitney U test; [d]Kolmogorov–Smirnov test.

differences in the duration of crying, pain-related behavior, and pain based on child-scored faces scale and parent-scored faces scale [12]. Conversely, Celik et al. found that the pain intensity based on NPRS with EMLA cream is significantly lower than that with vapocoolant spray. This contradictory result might be due to differences in study population. In a study by Çelik et al., as many as 24.4% of subjects had diabetes mellitus as the etiology of renal failure; thus, it may also be accompanied by peripheral neuropathy [11]. Moon

Table 2: Comparison of pain intensity during spinal injection between the EMLA cream group and the vapocoolant spray group.

NPRS[a]	EMLA cream (N = 47)	Vapocoolant spray (N = 47)	p value
NPRS 0	30	25	1.000[b]
NPRS 1	13	17	
NPRS 2	3	4	
NPRS 3	1	0	
NPRS 4	0	1	

[a]NPRS, numeric pain rating scale; [b]Mann–Whitney U test, significant if p value < 0.05.

Table 3: Comparison of patient movement during spinal injection between the EMLA cream group and the vapocoolant spray group.

Group	N	Patient movement		p value
		No movement	Movement	
EMLA cream	47	46 (97.9%)	1 (2.1%)	1.000[a]
Vapocoolant spray	47	46 (97.9%)	1 (2.1%)	

[a]Fisher's exact test, significant if p value < 0.05.

et al. also showed different results, in which the vapocoolant spray was more effective in reducing pain compared with topical anesthetic cream for needle electromyography in the extremities region [13].

The ability to reduce pain following spinal injections between EMLA cream and vapocoolant spray was comparable. Both anesthetic agents might be utilized to reduce pain during regional anesthesia, including spinal injections. However, this study could not generate the similar finding for other medical procedures that required larger diameter of cannula. Further study should be conducted with different medical procedures.

Allergic reaction and other adverse event related with the procedure, such as desaturation/apnea events, bradycardia, nausea, vomiting, respiratory depression, hypotension, and agitation, were recorded in this study. However, there was no such finding in this study. The literature showed that the side effects associated with vapocoolant spray and EMLA cream anesthetic were quite rare. Çelik et al. mentioned only one subject suffered from allergic reaction following the administration of EMLA cream [11]. Any topical anesthetic agents should be absorbed locally. Therefore, it has minimal to no systemic effects. This study generated no significant hemodynamic profile differences between two groups.

This study found that in both groups, majority of patients moved during spinal injection similar to the preliminary study in which more than 90% of patients moved during the spinal injection. Therefore, the presence of local anesthetic during spinal injection did not affect any movement during spinal injection [14]. Movement during spinal injection might be contributed by many factors, such as nervousness, jitteriness, or fear. This movement did not necessarily mean that the patient felt any pain during injection.

Both anesthetic agents were widely available in the daily practice with excellent safety profile. EMLA cream is

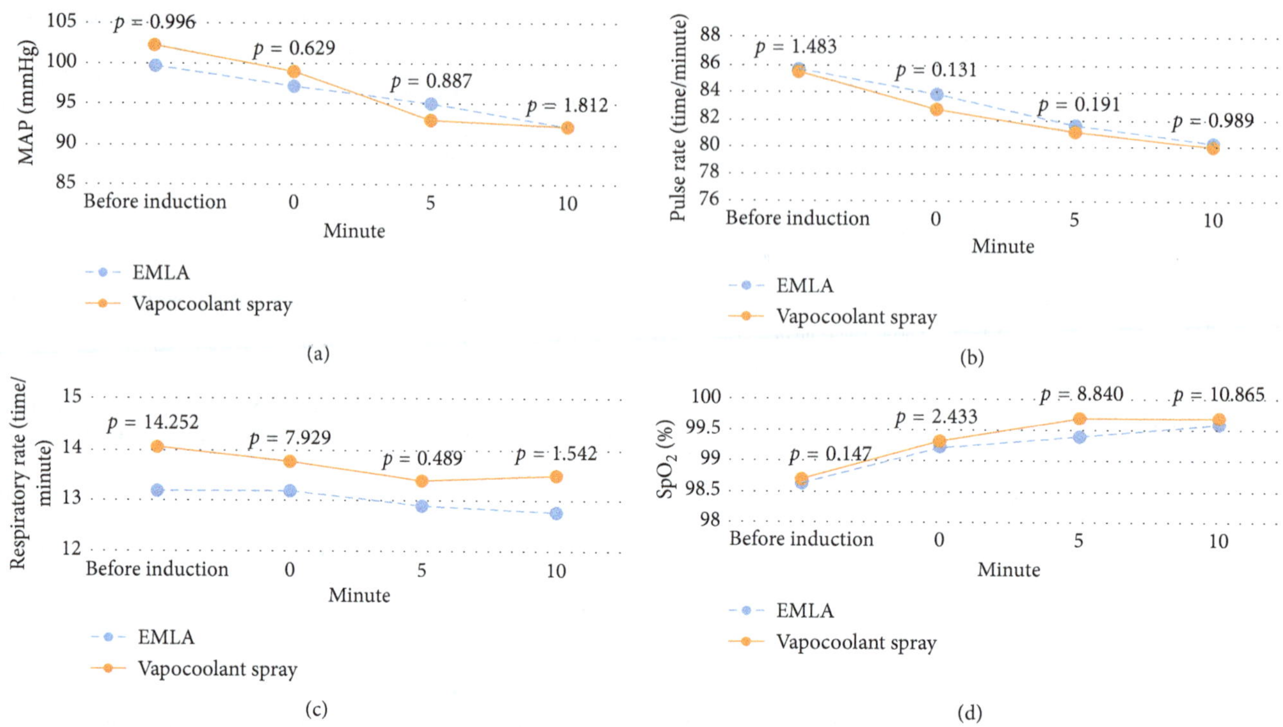

FIGURE 2: Analysis of hemodynamic profile. (a) Mean arterial pressure analysis by time. (b) Pulse rate analysis by time. (c) Respiratory rate analysis by time. (d) Peripheral capillary oxygen saturation analysis by time.

commonly used for local anesthesia in spinal injection. This study has shown that with regard to the ability to reduce pain during spinal injection, there was no significant difference between these two agents. However, one of the disadvantages of EMLA cream is its delayed onset of action; the patients should wait up to 60 minutes before injection after the administration of the EMLA cream. On the contrary, the vapocoolant spray showed that it has a rapid onset of action in which the patient only needed to wait for ten seconds before injection. This difference was clinically significant so that the vapocoolant spray was more suitable for any procedure that required shorter preparation time, such as emergency procedure. Additionally, both surgeons and patients did not have to wait an hour before starting the anesthesia procedure. Therefore, this was the main advantage of the vapocoolant spray.

There was some limitation in this study. Due to the preparation of both agents, it was difficult to do blinding for both researcher and subjects. Additionally, pain scale by using NPRS was a subjective assessment even though pain perception is subjective for each patient. However, this could create bias in this study. This study did not measure the difference in duration of the spinal anesthesia procedure. Reduced pain might affect the duration as well as the success rate of the spinal injection.

5. Conclusion

Administration of EMLA cream and vapocoolant spray was equally effective in reducing pain during spinal injection. There was no difference in terms of pain reduction between the EMLA cream group and the vapocoolant spray group during spinal injection.

Conflicts of Interest

The authors declare that they have no conflicts of interest.

References

[1] C. I. Ripamonti, "Pain management," *Annals of Oncology*, vol. 23, no. 10, pp. x294–x301, 2012.

[2] N. Wells, C. Pasero, and M. McCaffery, "Improving the quality of care through pain assessment and management," in *Patient Safety and Quality: An Evidence-Based Handbook for Nurses*, R. G. Hughes, Ed., pp. 469–497, Agency for Healthcare Research and Quality, Rockville, MD, USA, 2008.

[3] Y. J. Kim, M. H. Jung, Y. R. Choi et al., "The analgesic efficacy of a 5% eutectic mixture of lidocaine and prilocaine prior to insertion of spinal and epidural block," *Korean Journal of Anesthesiology*, vol. 54, no. 4, pp. 395–399, 2008.

[4] S. H. Kim, D. H. Jeon, C. H. Chang, S. J. Lee, and Y. S. Shin, "Spinal anesthesia with isobaric tetracaine in patients with previous lumbar spinal surgery," *Yonsei Medical Journal*, vol. 50, no. 2, pp. 252–256, 2009.

[5] B. M. Bujedo, "Current evidence for spinal opioid selection in postoperative pain," *Korean Journal of Pain*, vol. 27, no. 3, pp. 200–209, 2014.

[6] B. M. Bujedo, S. G. Santos, and A. U. Azpiazu, "A review of epidural and intrathecal opioids used in the management of postoperative pain," *Journal of Opioid Management*, vol. 8, no. 3, pp. 177–192, 2012.

[7] Medscape, *Topical Anesthesia Use in Children*, Medscape, New York, NY, USA, 2016, http://www.medscape.com.

[8] Medscape, *Vapocoolant Spray vs Subcutaneous Lidocaine Injection in IV Cannulation*, Medscape, New York, NY, USA, 2016, http://www.medscape.com.

[9] M. R. Waterhouse, D. R. Liu, and V. J. Wang, "Cryotherapeutic topical analgesics for pediatric intravenous catheter placement: ice versus vapocoolant spray," *Pediatric Emergency Care*, vol. 29, no. 1, pp. 8–12, 2013.

[10] K. J. Farion, K. L. Splinter, K. Newhook, I. Gaboury, and W. M. Splinter, "The effect of vapocoolant spray on pain due to intravenous cannulation in children: a randomized controlled trial," *Canadian Medical Association Journal*, vol. 179, no. 1, pp. 31–36, 2008.

[11] G. Çelik, O. Özbek, M. Yılmaz, I. Duman, S. Özbek, and S. Apiliogullari, "Vapocoolant spray vs lidocaine/prilocaine cream for reducing the pain of venipuncture in hemodialysis patients: a randomized, placebo-controlled, crossover study," *International Journal of Medical Sciences*, vol. 8, no. 7, pp. 623–627, 2011.

[12] E. C. Reis and R. Holubkov, "Vapocoolant spray is equally effective as EMLA cream in reducing immunization pain in school-aged children," *Pediatrics*, vol. 100, no. 6, p. E5, 1997.

[13] Y.-E. Moon, S.-H. Kim, and W.-H. Choi, "Comparison of the effects of vapocoolant spray and topical anesthetic cream on pain during needle electromyography in the medial gastrocnemius," *Archives of Physical Medicine and Rehabilitation*, vol. 94, no. 5, pp. 919–924, 2013.

[14] B. D. Marzaini, "Perbandingan vapocoolant spray dan krim campuran eutektik (EMLA) dalam menurunkan nyeri saat penyuntikan jarum spinal," Thesis, Universitas Indonesia, Jakarta, Indonesia, 2017.

19

Feasibility of Cervical Epidural Anesthesia for Breast Cancer Surgery

Manuel Wenk,[1] Christina Massoth,[1] Daniel M. Pöpping,[1] and Michael Möllmann[2]

[1] *Department of Anesthesiology, Intensive Care and Pain Medicine, University Hospital Muenster, Muenster, Germany*
[2] *Department of Anesthesiology and Intensive Care, St. Franziskus Hospital, Muenster, Germany*

Correspondence should be addressed to Manuel Wenk; manuelwenk@uni-muenster.de

Academic Editor: Enrico Camporesi

Background. Effects of perioperative cervical level neuraxial blocks on the dissemination of cancer metastases have become a matter of substantial interest. However, experience with these catheters has been limited and data on feasibility and efficacy is sparse. *Methods.* Data from 39 patients scheduled to undergo breast cancer surgery while awake with a cervical epidural alone was retrospectively analyzed. *Results.* In 26 patients (66,7%, 95% CI 51,7–81,7) the cervical epidural catheter was sufficient for surgery. In one patient (2.6%, 95% CI 0–7.6) identification of the epidural space was not possible. Four patients (10.3%, 95% CI 0,7–19,9) had an insufficient sensory block. Seven patients (17.9%, 95% CI 5,7–30,1) had a partially insufficient sensory block. Rates of failed epidural blocks were not significantly different between different insertion levels. 21 patients (80.8%, 95% CI 65,4–96,1) developed hypotension and required an intravenous vasopressor. One patient developed nausea. In one patient the dura was accidentally punctured. No neurological damage was observed. No other major complications were observed. *Discussion.* Epidural punctures in the cervical region are feasible but do bear potential for major complications. Anesthesiologists should familiarize themselves with high epidural block techniques.

1. Introduction

Cancer remains one of the leading causes of death in developed countries. While lung cancer is predominant in men (17%), women suffer most frequently from breast cancer (23%) [1]. While the primary tumor can be removed in almost all cases, the dilemma is that 90% of all cancer patients die from metastatic disease [2]. Over the last couple of years the role of a perioperatively compromised immune system leading to easier dissemination of tumor cells and accelerated growth of micrometastases has been extensively discussed [3–5]. It appears that reduced perioperative stress might transfer into a better immune response of the patient; hence anesthetic techniques per se have become a significant field of research [6–9]. Particularly the effects of epidural anesthesia have been the center of attention since neuraxial blocks generally provide excellent analgesia and potentially reduce perioperative stress resulting in an overall reduction of the requirement for other anesthetic and analgesic agents in the postoperative period [10–12]. However, despite intensified research, clinical evidence for a potentially protective effect of regional anesthetic and analgesic techniques with respect to cancer recurrence and the incidence of metastases after tumor surgery is still inconclusive [13].

Consequently, with no effect of regional anesthetic techniques known to promote the growth of tumor or metastases, it appears that these techniques should be widely employed whenever possible. However, particularly in the case of breast cancer surgery, a sufficient epidural technique requires the insertion of a cervical epidural catheter at the C6/C7/T1 level. In stark contrast to the high volume of breast cancer surgery performed in many hospitals stands the relatively rarely performed anesthetic technique of cervical epidural catheter insertion, which both can be challenging for the anesthetist and involves potentially devastating sequelae for the patient. Traditionally, cervical epidural catheters have only been used in selected centers performing cardiac or other high risk surgery; hence the familiarity of anesthetists with this technique is not necessarily ubiquitous. The available data on feasibility and efficacy of cervical epidural anesthesia is sparse, consisting mainly of case reports reporting complications and a few studies from the field of pain medicine [14, 15].

In this retrospective study we sought to verify the feasibility in terms of success/failure rates and investigated complications in a series of patients undergoing breast cancer surgery while awake with a cervical epidural catheter.

2. Methods and Materials

After approval from the Ethics Committee of the University of Muenster and the Medical Board of North-Rhine Westphalia (protocol number 2012415fN), data from 39 consecutive women planning to undergo breast cancer surgery while awake with only a cervical epidural catheter and no general anesthesia was retrospectively analyzed.

Briefly, patients with a normal coagulation profile (INR < 1.4, aPTT < 41 sec, and platelets > 80.000 per microliter of blood) were connected to standardized anesthetic monitoring, including electrocardiogram, noninvasive blood pressure with a 3 min cycle period, and peripheral oxygen saturation. An invasive blood pressure monitoring was used based on the patient's individual risk factors. All patients received a standardized cervical epidural catheter insertion by the same anesthesiologist preoperatively. Patients were placed in the lateral position with their heads anteflexed. The seventh cervical vertebra was marked as an orientation landmark and the area was thoroughly cleaned and disinfected. Operator was using sterile gloves, gown, and face mask for all procedures. The area was covered with sterile draping and the skin and subcutaneous tissue were infiltrated with 2–5 ml prilocaine 1% (Xylonest 1%, Astra Zeneca, Germany). The epidural space was punctured at the vertebrae level C6/C7 or C7/T1 or T1/T2 with a standard 18-gauge Tuohy needle (B. Braun, Melsungen, Germany) using a midline approach with a loss of resistance to air technique. An epidural catheter was then inserted via the Tuohy needle and advanced cranially in the epidural space for 2 cm. The Tuohy needle was then removed and the catheter was fixated and covered with sterile dressings. A bolus of 10 ml ropivacaine 0.75% (Astra Zeneca, Hamburg, Germany) was administered. Patients were then turned supine and after 7–10 minutes a further 3–5 ml ropivacaine 0.75% was given. Sufentanil (Actavis, Munich, Germany) was available to be used for epidural application at the anesthetist's discretion. Surgery was then started following a 20- to 30-minute wait. Postoperatively, the catheter was removed and after fading of the effects of the epidural anesthesia, patients were discharged from recovery and followed up two hourly for 12 postoperative hours.

Data with regard to patient and surgical characteristics, operator experience, site of insertion, and complications as well as the use of cardiovascular drugs was collected. Complications were divided into none, minor, major, or failed attempt. The following complications were defined as minor ones: inability to reach the epidural space, multiple attempts, change of insertion site or a second operator, bleeding from the epidural needle or blood in the epidural catheter, and difficulties advancing the epidural catheter as well as nausea, vomiting, or vertigo.

Table 1: Demographic data.

Age (yrs)	71.5 ± 16.0
Weight (kg)	71.8 ± 12.8
Height (cm)	165 ± 6
BMI (kg/m^2)	25.0 ± 7.5
Mastectomy (number of patients)	24
Breast conserving surgery (number of patients)	12
Secondary breast reconstruction (number of patients)	3
Number of epidural punctures at level	
C6/C7	27
C7/T1	9
T1/T2	3
Invasive blood pressure monitoring (number of patients)	15

Dural puncture, nerve injury or any other neurological complications, dyspnea or difficulty in breathing as well as significant hemodynamic depression (systolic blood pressure < 90 mmHg and/or heart rate < 50 or >120 beats per minute after injection of local anesthetic), or any other significant events were considered major complications.

All data was entered into a customized database. Statistical analysis was performed using SPSS Statistics 18.0 (SPSS Inc., Chicago, IL). Categorical variables are expressed as frequency and percentage, whereas continuous variables are represented as means with standard deviation. The nonparametric patients' baseline characteristics were assessed using the Kruskal-Wallis test. Differences were considered statistically significant at $p < 0.05$.

3. Results

39 patients aged 72 years (range: 29–92) underwent breast cancer surgery while awake using a cervical epidural catheter as the sole method of anesthesia. Demographic and surgery-related data of the patient population is shown in Table 1.

In 26 patients (66,7%, 95% CI 51,7–81,7) the cervical epidural catheter was sufficient as the sole method of anesthesia to perform breast cancer surgery.

In one patient (2.6%, 95% CI 0–7.6) identification of the epidural space was not possible and the procedure was aborted. Four patients (10.3%, 95% CI 0,7–19,9) had an insufficient sensory block leading to a conversion of anesthetic method from cervical epidural catheter to general anesthesia. Seven patients (17.9%, 95% CI 5,7–30,1) had a partially insufficient sensory block and anesthesia had to be supplemented with intermittent IV application of S-ketamine and/or midazolam.

Rates of total and partially insufficient epidural blocks were not significantly different between the three catheter insertion levels (C6/7 versus C7/T1 versus T1/T2).

To investigate the effect of a possible operator learning curve, the first 20 cervical epidural punctures were compared with the following 19 punctures. No significant changes in success/failure rates were observed.

21 of the 26 patients (80.8%, 95% CI 65,4–96,1) with a sufficient cervical epidural received at least one dose of an IV vasopressor after epidural puncture due to hypotension. 16 patients received fractionated doses of 20 mg cafedrine and 1 mg theodrenaline (Akrinor®; AWD.pharma, Dresden, Germany), three patients received intermittent doses of 5–10 μg nor-epinephrine (Arterenol®, Sanofi-Aventis, Frankfurt, Germany), and two patients received a combination of the two drugs. Reflex bradycardia was observed but no intervention was necessary. No patient developed a significant isolated bradycardia.

One patient received an epidural injection of 5 μg sufentanil in addition to the local anesthetic and rapidly developed severe nausea and vomiting. No other patient received any additional opioids. One patient developed late (>6 hrs) postoperative nausea and vomiting.

In one patient the dura was accidentally punctured at the C7/T1 level and the procedure was aborted. No neurological damage or any other sequelae were observed.

No other major complications were observed; particularly, no nerve or other neurological damage was seen during the observation period. No patient suffered from respiratory complications such as dyspnea or apnea.

4. Discussion

Our study has shown that cervical epidural anesthesia is a feasible technique with an acceptable success rate that offers sufficient and profound analgesia for breast cancer surgery while patients are awake.

With increasing evidence that neuraxial blocks such as epidural or paravertebral anesthesia may influence the degree of dissemination of metastatic disease [3, 6, 7, 12, 16, 17] anesthesiologists should no longer consider these techniques as rare methods performed in highly specialized centers. Even if the scientific evidence regarding the precise role of these techniques on cancer recurrence is still questioned by some experts [18], there is no known effect where these methods would in any way promote the spread of cancer cells. Hence the potential benefits in reducing postoperative pain alone appear to outweigh the risks of the method; hence anesthesiologists today find themselves in a situation where they need to discuss why they are not liberally employing these techniques. One obvious reason, particularly in breast cancer surgery, is the requirement of a high cervical level block which can be technically challenging and usually only few anesthesiologists would have had previous exposure to these techniques since they are usually restricted to selected centers. With breast cancer surgery being performed in many hospitals this gives rise to a significant discrepancy between the demand for cervical epidurals and the ability of the staff to perform these techniques.

In our study we were able to site a cervical epidural correctly in 67% of all patients. Although a failure rate of 32% may appear high at first glance it should be noted that this reflects epidural catheters that were sufficient to perform a surgical procedure without any further anesthesia necessary. 28% of patients had a partial block that needed either conversion to general anesthesia or supplementation with other analgesics/hypnotics. As such, the complete failure rate was rather low and since epidural blocks and general anesthesia are usually performed in combination it can be speculated that many partially working epidurals would have been considered fully functioning. The combined partial and total failure rates of epidural catheters are comparable to published data. Studies as well as a recent review have highlighted failure rates as high as 32% for thoracic and 27% for lumbar epidural catheters, which not only were total failures but also involved partial failures [19, 20]. This raises the important but yet unanswered question whether full or partial blocks do have different effects in their potential influence on intraoperative stress levels as well as on the spread of cancer cells during surgery. Differentiating between a fully and a partially functional neuraxial block may also be an important limitation for all prospective clinical trials currently underway.

Neuraxial anesthesia for breast surgery remains the gold standard in terms of providing postoperative analgesia with some studies even suggesting a reduction in the incidence of postoperative persistent pain, though the quantity of available evidence remains severely limited [21]. As an alternative to cervical epidural anesthesia, thoracic paravertebral block (TPVB) appears like a viable option that has shown some beneficial effects on postoperative pain intensity, perioperative opioid consumption, and prevention of chronic postsurgical pain for patients undergoing breast surgery; however, results vary substantially across studies and there is hardly any data available on the use of TPVB as the sole method of anesthesia for performing breast surgery while patients are awake [22].

We did observe some minor and one major complication. One patient developed severe nausea and vomiting after the epidural application of sufentanil. Close proximity to the area postrema of the brainstem may be a possible cause for this [23]. In one patient the epidural space could not be identified and the procedure was aborted. In one patient the dura was accidentally punctured at the C7/T1 level. Although an unfortunate and stressful event for the anesthetist, no neurological sequelae or other complications were observed. With just one millimeter the epidural space in the cervical region is significantly narrower as compared with the thoracic (4-5 mm) or lumbar (5-6 mm) region. However, since most of the available data being case reports there is a paucity of studies systematically investigating the use of cervical epidural injections and catheters at the cervical level. Some data is available from the field of interventional pain medicine where fluoroscopically guided (cervical) epidural injections are used for managing chronic spinal pain [24]. Although a higher rate of local hematoma was observed as compared to thoracic or lumbar epidurals, no major complications were reported. Injuries to the dural sac were not separately reported. A possible approach to increasing safety of cervical injections may be a prepuncture anatomy check using ultrasound or live puncturing under ultrasound guidance. A study by Kim et al. showed that a prepuncture anatomy check using ultrasound may provide valuable information about skin-space distance and potentially lead to increased safety [25].

Our study has limitations. Firstly, limitations of the retrospective nature of the data apply. Secondly, although this is currently the biggest study investigating cervical epidural blocks in patients undergoing breast cancer surgery, the number of patients is still too small to reliably assess safety. Larger prospective trials and data acquisition through network databases are necessary. Thirdly, we did not investigate the effects of varying local anesthetics or other supplements.

It is conceivable that once these techniques are employed more liberally we will see a significant increase in major complications. Therefore, a systematic in-hospital approach to detecting complications is highly recommended and agreements between anesthesia, neurosurgery, radiology, and neurology should be in place to provide sufficient emergency services in case of catastrophic sequelae. Furthermore, all data derived from these patients should be added to a national or international regional anesthesia network database to ensure that we as anesthesiologists get a better understanding of what risks these techniques may hold once they are employed more liberally.

5. Conclusions

Based on our data and previously published data from the field of pain medicine, epidural punctures in the cervical region are feasible methods with a failure rate comparable to thoracic or lumbar epidural punctures. Based on the available data they appear to be relatively safe since major complications such as nerve or spinal cord damage are rarely reported events. However, these are rarely performed techniques and it remains questionable whether safety concerns will change once these techniques are employed more liberally on a wider basis by heterogeneous operators. Data from prospective trials and regional anesthesia network databases are necessary.

Nevertheless, in the light of the current evidence regarding the effects of regional block on cancer recurrence anesthesiologists should be concerned with high epidural and other neuraxial techniques. It may still be too early to tell but if there is any relevant effect on cancer recurrence these anesthetic techniques will become the gold standard and it may become difficult to argue why these techniques should not be employed.

Conflicts of Interest

The authors declare that they have no conflicts of interest.

Authors' Contributions

Manuel Wenk designed the study, interpreted the data, and drafted the manuscript. Christina Massoth contributed to the design of the study and analyzed the data from the databases. Daniel M. Pöpping designed the study, analyzed the data, and participated in drafting the manuscript. Michael Möllmann initiated and coordinated the study and participated in interpretation of the data. All authors read and approved the final manuscript.

References

[1] A. Jemal, F. Bray, M. M. Center, J. Ferlay, E. Ward, and D. Forman, "Global cancer statistics," *CA: A Cancer Journal for Clinicians*, vol. 61, no. 2, pp. 69–90, 2011.

[2] G. P. Gupta and J. Massagué, "Cancer metastasis: building a framework," *Cell*, vol. 127, no. 4, pp. 679–695, 2006.

[3] S. Ben-Eliyahu, "The promotion of tumor metastasis by surgery and stress: immunological basis and implications for psychoneuroimmunology," *Brain, Behavior, and Immunity*, vol. 17, supplement 1, pp. S27–S36, 2003.

[4] G. L. Snyder and S. Greenberg, "Effect of anaesthetic technique and other perioperative factors on cancer recurrence," *British Journal of Anaesthesia*, vol. 105, no. 2, pp. 106–115, 2010.

[5] I. J. Fidler, "The pathogenesis of cancer metastasis: the "seed and soil" hypothesis revisited," *Nature Reviews Cancer*, vol. 3, no. 6, pp. 453–458, 2003.

[6] G. S. De Oliveira Jr., S. Ahmad, J. C. Schink, D. K. Singh, P. C. Fitzgerald, and R. J. McCarthy, "Intraoperative neuraxial anesthesia but not postoperative neuraxial analgesia is associated with increased relapse-free survival in ovarian cancer patients after primary cytoreductive surgery," *Regional Anesthesia and Pain Medicine*, vol. 36, no. 3, pp. 271–277, 2011.

[7] A. Gottschalk, J. G. Ford, C. C. Regelin et al., "Association between epidural analgesia and cancer recurrence after colorectal cancer surgery," *Anesthesiology*, vol. 113, no. 1, pp. 27–34, 2010.

[8] A. Gottschalk, "Continuous wound infusion of local anesthetics: importance in postoperative pain therapy," *Anaesthesist*, vol. 59, no. 12, pp. 1076–1082, 2010.

[9] M. Tylman, R. Sarbinowski, J. P. Bengtson, A. Kvarnström, and A. Bengtsson, "Inflammatory response in patients undergoing colorectal cancer surgery: the effect of two different anesthetic techniques," *Minerva Anestesiologica*, vol. 77, no. 3, pp. 275–282, 2011.

[10] G. S. Cheng and B. M. Ilfeld, "A review of postoperative analgesia for breast cancer surgery," *Pain Management*, vol. 6, no. 6, pp. 603–618, 2016.

[11] M. A. Palomero Rodríguez, L. Suarez Gonzalo, F. Villar Alvarez, C. Varela Crespo, I. Moreno Gomez Limon, and A. Criado Jimenez, "Thoracic epidural anesthesia decreases C-reactive protein levels in patients undergoing elective coronary artery bypass graft surgery with cardiopulmonary bypass," *Minerva Anestesiologica*, vol. 74, no. 11, pp. 619–626, 2008.

[12] J. Greisen, D. V. Nielsen, E. Sloth, and C.-J. Jakobsen, "High thoracic epidural analgesia decreases stress hyperglycemia and insulin need in cardiac surgery patients," *Acta Anaesthesiologica Scandinavica*, vol. 57, no. 2, pp. 171–177, 2013.

[13] K. Byrne, K. J. Levins, and D. J. Buggy, "Can anesthetic-analgesic technique during primary cancer surgery affect recurrence or metastasis?" *Canadian Journal of Anesthesia*, vol. 63, no. 2, pp. 184–192, 2016.

[14] B. Stauber, L. Ma, and R. Nazari, "Cardiopulmonary arrest following cervical epidural injection," *Pain Physician*, vol. 15, no. 2, pp. 147–152, 2012.

[15] D. S. Kloth, A. K. Calodney, R. Derby, F. P. Lagattuta, C. O'Neill, E. Yurth et al., "Improving the safety of transforaminal epidural steroid injections in the treatment of cervical radiculopathy," *Pain Physician*, vol. 14, no. 3, pp. 285–293, 2011.

[16] A. K. Exadaktylos, D. J. Buggy, D. C. Moriarty, E. Mascha, and D. I. Sessler, "Can anesthetic technique for primary breast cancer surgery affect recurrence or metastasis?" *Anesthesiology*, vol. 105, no. 4, pp. 660–664, 2006.

[17] A. Gottschalk, S. Sharma, J. Ford, M. E. Durieux, and M. Tiouririne, "The role of the perioperative period in recurrence after cancer surgery," *Anesthesia and Analgesia*, vol. 110, no. 6, pp. 1636–1643, 2010.

[18] G. Haller and P. S. Myles, "Regional block and cancer recurrence: too early to tell," *Anesthesiology*, vol. 107, no. 2, p. 354, 2007.

[19] J. Hermanides, M. W. Hollmann, M. F. Stevens, and P. Lirk, "Failed epidural: causes and management," *British Journal of Anaesthesia*, vol. 109, no. 2, pp. 144–154, 2012.

[20] L. B. Ready, "Acute pain: lessons learned from 25,000 patients," *Regional Anesthesia and Pain Medicine*, vol. 24, no. 6, pp. 499–505, 1999.

[21] A. S. Terkawi, S. Tsang, D. I. Sessler et al., "Improving analgesic efficacy and safety of thoracic paravertebral block for breast surgery: a mixed-effects meta-analysis," *Pain Physician*, vol. 18, no. 5, pp. E757–E780, 2015.

[22] A. Schnabel, S. U. Reichl, P. Kranke, E. M. Pogatzki-Zahn, and P. K. Zahn, "Efficacy and safety of paravertebral blocks in breast surgery: a meta-analysis of randomized controlled trials," *British Journal of Anaesthesia*, vol. 105, no. 6, pp. 842–852, 2010.

[23] P. R. Bromage, E. M. Camporesi, P. A. C. Durant, and C. H. Nielsen, "Rostral spread of epidural morphine," *Anesthesiology*, vol. 56, no. 6, pp. 431–436, 1982.

[24] L. Manchikanti, Y. Malla, B. W. Wargo, K. A. Cash, V. Pampati, and B. Fellows, "Complications of fluoroscopically directed facet joint nerve blocks: a prospective evaluation of 7,500 episodes with 43,000 nerve blocks," *Pain Physician*, vol. 15, no. 2, pp. E143–E150, 2012.

[25] S. H. Kim, K. H. Lee, K. B. Yoon, W. Y. Park, and D.-M. Yoon, "Sonographic estimation of needle depth for cervical epidural blocks," *Anesthesia and Analgesia*, vol. 106, no. 5, pp. 1542–1547, 2008.

20

The Effect of Dexmedetomidine on Lumbar Epidural Injection for Failed Back Surgery Syndrome

Ashraf Eskandr and Sadik Abdel Maseeh

Department of Anaesthesia, ICU and Pain Therapy, Faculty of Medicine, Menoufiya University, Shibin El-Koom 32518, Egypt

Correspondence should be addressed to Ashraf Eskandr; ameskandr@yahoo.com

Academic Editor: Yukio Hayashi

Purpose. Failed back surgery syndrome is a chronic pain condition requiring rapid, effective, and efficient management. This study evaluates the effect of adding dexmedetomidine to lumbar epidural steroids in patients with failed back surgery syndrome. *Methods*. Fifty patients suffering from failed back surgery syndrome were randomly assigned to one of two groups, receiving an epidural injection of 20 mL of either a mixture of betamethasone (14 mg) and bupivacaine 0.5 mg (group C) or a mixture of betamethasone (14 mg), bupivacaine 0.5 mg, and dexmedetomidine (0.5 μg/kg) (group D) adjusted to the volume with normal saline. The effect was evaluated using visual analogue scale (VAS), analgesic requirement, and Oswestry disability index 2 weeks, 4 weeks, 8 weeks, and 12 weeks after injection. *Results*. VAS and ibuprofen consumption showed a significant reduction in group D. The Oswestry disability index was significantly improved in group D. There were no records of hypotension, bradycardia, sedation, or hypoxemia in both groups. *Conclusion*. The present study demonstrated potential safe and effective usage of adding dexmedetomidine to epidural steroid to control pain in patients with failed back surgery syndrome.

1. Introduction

Failed back surgery syndromes (FBSS) occur in 5–40% of patients that underwent a back surgery [1] due to spinal stenosis, spinal segment degeneration, disc ruptures, recurred disc herniation, disc fragments remaining after surgery, epidural scars, facet joint pain, sacroiliac joint pain, spinal segment instability, and so forth [2]. Failed back surgery syndrome is a chronic pain condition which has a considerable effect on the patient and health care system [3]. So, finding an effective, rapid, and efficient method for pain control and treatment is highly desirable [4]. Lumbar epidural injection of long-acting steroids is commonly used to alleviate low back pain. The duration of analgesia varies among patients with FBSS and ranges from 15 days up to 180 days [4]. The mechanism of action of steroids in pain reduction following epidural injection is not well understood. However, the anti-inflammatory effects are the most probable mechanism, wherein the levels of tissue phospholipase and prostaglandins are decreased by steroids [5]. Alpha-2 agonists had been shown to reduce chronic allodynia in rat animal models [6], most probably through blocking pre- and postsynaptic α-2 receptors [7]. The addition of clonidine (α-2 agonist) to epidural steroid has been used to treat chronic intractable postthoracotomy pain [8].

We designed the present double-blind and randomized study using dexmedetomidine as an adjunct to epidural steroids to examine the effect of dexmedetomidine on pain, amount of analgesics, and activity of patients suffering FBSS.

2. Materials and Methods

After obtaining approval from the institutional ethics committee and written informed consent, 50 patients, 40–70 years old of both sexes, ASA physical status I–III, suffering from FBSS were included in this prospective, double-blind, randomized controlled study at the Menoufiya University outpatient pain clinic. The study protocol was registered with the Pan-African Clinical Trial Registry (http://www.pactr.org/). Patients were excluded if they suffered from a sacroiliac joint disease, facet joint arthritis revealed by magnetic resonant imaging, severe cardiopulmonary disease, uncontrolled diabetes, morbid obesity (body mass index ≥ 40 Kg/m^2), addiction, infection, and coagulation disorders and if patients were on opioid medications for pain management before or during the study period. After explaining study protocol and visual analogue score (VAS) graduated from zero (no pain) to 10 cm (worst pain) to the patients, they were randomly assigned by using closed envelope technique to one of two groups. Group C (control group) received an epidural injection of 20 mL of a mixture of betamethasone (14 mg) and bupivacaine (0.5 mg) adjusted to the volume with normal saline. Group D (dexmedetomidine group) received an epidural injection of 20 mL of a mixture of betamethasone (14 mg), bupivacaine (0.5 mg), and dexmedetomidine (0.5 μg/kg) adjusted to the volume with normal saline. The epidural injection was administered with the patient in a lateral recumbent position, while his/her neck, pelvis, and knees were bent. The skin and subcutaneous tissues were anesthetized by injecting 1-2 mL of lidocaine 2% between L2 and L5 spinous processes (identified by fluoroscopy) and a 20-gauge Touhy needle was inserted approximately 2-3 cm so that the needle went into the interspinal ligament. Then, a syringe containing air was attached to the needle and the needle was inserted slowly, 1-2 mm at a time until no resistance was felt. Afterward, 2 mL of nonionic radiocontrast was injected into the location of the needle to identify that the contrast was diffusing in the shape of thin strings toward the top of the image. When the needle was identified in the epidural space through the interspinal ligament approach method, the study drugs were injected. The patients were then transferred to the Peri-Anesthesia Care Unit (PACU) for monitoring vital signs, pain levels, and possible neurological and other adverse events for 60–90 minutes. They were then discharged home (4 hours after the procedure) in the care of a responsible adult and advised not to drive for 24 hours. The pain intensity was evaluated by visual analogue scale scores. As per the patient's request to analgesia when VAS was greater than or equal to 4, oral 200 mg ibuprofen tablet was given and the total amount of nonsteroidal anti-inflammatory drug (NSAID) per week was calculated and recorded. The effects of the procedures were evaluated by measuring the visual analogue scale (VAS) and Oswestry disability index (ODI) before the procedures then 2 weeks, 4 weeks, 8 weeks, and 12 weeks after the procedure. The incidence of complications was recorded, including the occurrence of hypotension (systolic blood pressure < 90 mmHg), bradycardia (pulse rate < 50/minute), extensive sedation (any sedation score above 1; 1 = sedated, but easily to be aroused), or hypoxemia (oxygen saturation below 90%). In a case of marked hypotension, rapid infusion of 500 mL crystalloids and ephedrine 5 mg was given, and heart rate less than 50 beats/min was treated with 0.3 mg atropine.

2.1. Statistical Analysis. The sample size was calculated based on results of previous studies, using a power of 85% and an α value 0.05. We assumed that the minimum difference of back pain score was 20% and 95% confidence interval. The sample size was calculated to be 23 patients so we decided to include 25 patients in each group in this study. We used GraphPad Stat-Mate version 2 statistics program for power analysis.

Table 1: Demographic data.

Character	Group C (n = 25)	Group D (n = 25)	P value
Age (years)	52 ± 7.36	52.52 ± 8.36	0.816
Sex (F/M)	14/11	16/9	0.773
Weight (kg)	86.56 ± 7.84	87.32 ± 7.69	0.731
Height (cm)	163.96 ± 5.99	163.2 ± 6.12	0.659

Group C: control group; group D: dexmedetomidine group; n = number of patients; M: male; F: female. Data were expressed as mean ± standard deviation and number of patients.

Table 2: Visual analogue scale of back pain.

Time	Group C (n = 25)	Group D (n = 25)	P value
Before	5 (4–8)	5 (4–8)	0.973
Week 2	4 (3–7)	3 (1–5)*	0.028
4	4 (3–7)	3 (2–6)*	0.049
8	4 (3–7)	4 (2–6)*	0.045
12	4 (3–7)	4 (2–6)*	0.023

Group C: control group; group D: dexmedetomidine group; n = number of patients. Data were expressed as median (interquartile range). $^*P < 0.05$: significant.

The collected data were analyzed by Statistical Package for Social Science (SPSS) version 16. Parametric data were expressed as mean ± SD. The comparison of the mean ± SD of two groups was done using the paired and unpaired Student's t-test (analgesic requirement, Oswestry disability index, age, weight, and height). Nonparametric data was expressed as a number of patients or median (interquartile range). Determining the extent of a single observed series of proportions and difference from a theoretical or expected distribution was done using the Chi-square test (sex) and Mann-Whitney U test (VAS). P value < 0.05 was considered statistically significant.

3. Results

The study was performed on 50 patients randomly divided into 2 equal groups. Patients characteristics were similar in the 2 groups regarding the demographic data (age, sex, height, and weight) (Table 1). For VAS of pain, there was a significant decrease in dexmedetomidine group compared to control group at 2, 4, 8, and 12 weeks after the procedure (Table 2). The mean consumption of NSAID during the study period was also significantly lower in dexmedetomidine group more than in control group (Table 3). Furthermore, there was a significant improvement in the quality of life and the levels of personal activity in the dexmedetomidine group as shown by the significant reduction of ODI in the group during the study period (Table 4). As regards side effects of dexmedetomidine injection, there was no recorded incident of hypotension, bradycardia, sedation, and hypoxemia.

TABLE 3: Ibuprofen (NSAID) consumption (mg/week).

Time	Group C ($n = 25$)	Group D ($n = 25$)	P value
Before	1412 ± 358.77	1408 ± 358.14	0.969
2	1220 ± 320.16	1032 ± 260.83*	0.027
4	1268 ± 321.85	1064 ± 288.71*	0.013
8	1286 ± 322.02	1056 ± 262.01*	0.008
12	1290 ± 322.38	1020 ± 260.66*	0.002

Group C: control group; group D: dexmedetomidine group; n = number of patients. Data were expressed as mean ± standard deviation. *$P < 0.05$: significant.

TABLE 4: Oswestry disability index (ODI).

Time	Group C ($n = 25$)	Group D ($n = 25$)	P value
Before	24.16 ± 8.74	23.12 ± 8.66	0.674
2	22.01 ± 7.93	16.11 ± 7.93*	0.011
4	19.93 ± 7.19	15.54 ± 8.01*	0.047
8	19.87 ± 7.12	15.1 ± 7.42*	0.025
12	19.52 ± 6.19	15.33 ± 7.41*	0.035

Group C: control group; group D: dexmedetomidine group; n = number of patients. Data were expressed as mean ± standard deviation. *$P < 0.05$: significant.

4. Discussion

FBSS is a major concern in pain therapy. Although the exact incidence remains unknown, it is estimated to be as high as 60% of patients who have had back surgeries [9]. In this study, we used dexmedetomidine as a novel adjuvant to epidural steroids to control pain in patients with failed back surgery. The study showed that addition of dexmedetomidine to epidural steroids results in superior pain control. This is evidenced by the decrease in VAS of back pain, along with a decrease in the total required dose of NSAID and a better lifestyle as documented by reduced ODI in patients suffering FBSS.

Due to the fact that dexmedetomidine has a high selectivity to $\alpha 2$ adrenergic receptor binding, it is widely used as a systemic analgesic adjuvant [10]. Furthermore, dexmedetomidine has been investigated as an adjuvant to local anesthetics in regional anesthesia and analgesia [11, 12]. Since the analgesic effect of $\alpha 2$-AR agonists is mostly mediated at the spinal level, neuraxial administration was chosen for the dexmedetomidine adjuvant. Moreover, its high lipophilicity allows for rapid absorption into the cerebrospinal fluid and binding to the spinal cord $\alpha 2$-AR [13].

Many studies have used dexmedetomidine safely in a dose of 1-2 μg/kg administered either epidurally [14–16] or caudally [12, 17–19] for the management of postoperative pain. In the present study, we used dexmedetomidine in a dose of 0.5 μg/kg added to epidural betamethasone due to short term follow-up of the patients as they were discharged home 4 hours after the procedure.

In the current study, we evaluated the effectiveness of the analgesic effect of long-acting steroid preparation, betamethasone, mixed with dexmedetomidine. The primary efficacy outcome parameters were a reduction in the intensity of pain after treatment with the epidural injection. Also, NSAID doses were significantly reduced when dexmedetomidine was added to the epidural steroid. Life style was improved in dexmedetomidine group as reported by the significant decrease in SDI. These results are consistent with the results of other studies using dexmedetomidine as an adjunct in the treatment of chronic pain syndromes in human [20–22], such as Lee and colleagues [20] who reported the antihyperalgesic effect of dexmedetomidine on patients undergoing a laparoscopic assisted vaginal hysterectomy. Additionally, Jain and others [21] found that the perioperative infusion of dexmedetomidine has a pivotal role in attenuating the incidence and severity of chronic pain and improving the quality of life in cases undergoing breast cancer surgery. Nama Sharanya et al. [22] reported the use of dexmedetomidine as an adjuvant with subanesthetic intravenous ketamine was effective in managing complex regional pain syndrome. This also agrees with the experimental work of Li and coworkers [23] who studied the analgesic effect of dexmedetomidine on naturopathic pain, as well as with Farghaly and colleagues [24] who studied the effects of intraperitoneal dexmedetomidine alone and in combination with tramadol or amitriptyline in a neuropathic pain model.

The same results of the present study were found by other studies performed by using another $\alpha 2$-AR agonist clonidine administered epidurally to control chronic pain. Lavand'homme and De Kock found that epidural or intrathecal clonidine added to local anesthetic may also prevent the development of chronic postsurgical pain and hyperalgesia after major abdominal surgery [25]. Lauretti et al. reported the similar efficacy of epidural clonidine and ketamine in chronic cancer pain [26]. Moreover, Ayad and El Masry [8] reported in a pilot study that a combination of epidural steroid and clonidine may provide pain relief in chronic postthoracotomy pain.

No significant adverse effects in the form of hypotension, bradycardia, sedation, or hypoxemia occurred and did not affect the time of hospital discharge of patients. All patients were discharged after 4 hours of the injection.

In conclusion, the present study demonstrated a potential safe and effective usage of adding dexmedetomidine to epidural steroid to control pain in patient with failed back surgery syndrome, as reflected by the significant reduction of pain intensity, reduction of NSID doses, and better quality of life with no significant adverse effects.

Competing Interests

Ashraf Eskandr and Sadik Abdel Maseeh have no conflict of interests.

Acknowledgments

Thanks go to Mohamed Ebied, Bachelor Degree Candidate in Biomedical Engineering, for proofreading and language review.

References

[1] S. B. Kim, K. W. Lee, J. H. Lee, M. A. Kim, and B. W. An, "The effect of hyaluronidase in interlaminar lumbar epidural injection for failed back surgery syndrome," *Annals of Rehabilitation Medicine*, vol. 36, no. 4, pp. 466–473, 2012.

[2] H. S. Yang, S. H. Lee, C. H. Ryu, J. Y. Lee, and J. H. Bae, "Correlation of the clinical factors and gait parameters in failed back surgery syndrome," *Journal of Korean Academy of Rehabilitation Medicine*, vol. 28, pp. 371–378, 2004.

[3] C.-W. Chan and P. Peng, "Failed back surgery syndrome," *Pain Medicine*, vol. 12, no. 4, pp. 577–606, 2011.

[4] P. Rahimzadeh, V. Sharma, F. Imani et al., "Adjuvant hyaluronidase to epidural steroid improves the quality of analgesia in failed back surgery syndrome: a prospective randomized clinical trial," *Pain Physician*, vol. 17, no. 1, pp. E75–E82, 2014.

[5] J. W. Geurts, J.-W. Kallewaard, J. Richardson, and G. J. Groen, "Targeted methylprednisolone acetate/hyaluronidase/clonidine injection after diagnostic epiduroscopy for chronic sciatica: a prospective, 1-year follow-up study," *Regional Anesthesia and Pain Medicine*, vol. 27, no. 4, pp. 343–352, 2002.

[6] A. Buvanendran, J. S. Kroin, J. M. Kerns, S. N. K. Nagalla, and K. J. Tuman, "Characterization of a new animal model for evaluation of persistent postthoracotomy pain," *Anesthesia and Analgesia*, vol. 99, no. 5, pp. 1453–1460, 2004.

[7] M.-D. C. Julião and G. R. Lauretti, "Low-dose intrathecal clonidine combined with sufentanil as analgesic drugs in abdominal gynecological surgery," *Journal of Clinical Anesthesia*, vol. 12, no. 5, pp. 357–362, 2000.

[8] A. E. Ayad and A. El Masry, "Epidural steroid and clonidine for chronic intractable post-thoracotomy pain: A Pilot Study," *Pain Practice*, vol. 12, no. 1, pp. 7–13, 2012.

[9] L. Manchikanti, V. Singh, K. A. Cash, V. Pampati, and S. Datta, "Preliminary results of a randomized, equivalence trial of fluoroscopic caudal epidural injections in managing chronic low back pain: part 3—Post surgery syndrome," *Pain Physician*, vol. 11, no. 6, pp. 817–831, 2008.

[10] B. Kosharskyy, W. Almonte, N. Shaparin, M. Pappagallo, and H. Smith, "Intravenous infusions in chronic pain management," *Pain Physician*, vol. 16, no. 3, pp. 231–249, 2013.

[11] J. S. Sukhminder, K. Jasbir, A. Vikramjit, G. Sachin, S. Amarjit, and S. S. Parmar, "Comparative evaluation of dexmedetomidine and fentanyl for epidural analgesia in lower limb orthopedic surgeries," *Indian Journal of Anaesthesia*, vol. 5, pp. 365–370, 2011.

[12] I. Saadawy, A. Boker, M. A. Elshahawy et al., "Effect of dexmedetomidine on the characteristics of bupivacaine in a caudal block in pediatrics," *Acta Anaesthesiologica Scandinavica*, vol. 53, no. 2, pp. 251–256, 2009.

[13] I. Grosu and P. Lavand'homme, "Use of dexmedetomidine for pain control," *F1000 Medicine Reports*, vol. 2, no. 1, article 90, 2010.

[14] S. J. S. Bajwa, S. K. Bajwa, J. Kaur et al., "Dexmedetomidine and clonidine in epidural anaesthesia: a comparative evaluation," *Indian Journal of Anaesthesia*, vol. 55, no. 2, pp. 116–121, 2011.

[15] S. J. S. Bajwa, V. Arora, J. Kaur, A. Singh, and S. S. Parmar, "Comparative evaluation of dexmedetomidine and fentanyl for epidural analgesia in lower limb orthopedic surgeries," *Saudi Journal of Anaesthesia*, vol. 5, no. 4, pp. 365–370, 2011.

[16] M. F. Selim, A. M. Elnabtity, and A. M. Hasan, "Comparative evaluation of epidural bupivacaine—dexmedetomidine and bupivacaine-fentanyl on Doppler velocimetry of uterine and umbilical arteries during labour," *Journal of Prenatal Medicine*, vol. 6, no. 3, pp. 47–54, 2012.

[17] A. M. El-Hennawy, A. M. Abd-Elwahab, A. M. Abd-Elmaksoud, H. S. El-Ozairy, and S. R. Boulis, "Addition of clonidine or dexmedetomidine to bupivacaine prolongs caudal analgesia in children," *British Journal of Anaesthesia*, vol. 103, no. 2, pp. 268–274, 2009.

[18] V. G. Anand, A. Thavamani, M. Kannan, and M. J. Bridgit, "Effects of dexmedetomidine added to caudal ropivacaine in paediatric lower abdominal surgeries," *Indian Journal of Anaesthesia*, vol. 55, no. 4, pp. 340–346, 2011.

[19] Q. Xiang, D. Y. Huang, Y. L. Zhao et al., "Caudal dexmedetomidine combined with bupivacaine inhibit the response to hernial sac traction in children undergoing inguinal hernia repair," *British Journal of Anaesthesia*, vol. 110, no. 3, pp. 420–424, 2013.

[20] C. Lee, Y.-D. Kim, and J.-N. Kim, "Antihyperalgesic effects of dexmedetomidine on high-dose remifentanil-induced hyperalgesia," *Korean Journal of Anesthesiology*, vol. 64, no. 4, pp. 301–307, 2013.

[21] G. Jain, P. Bansal, B. Ahmad, D. Singh, and G. Yadav, "Effect of the perioperative infusion of dexmedetomidine on chronic pain after breast surgery," *Indian Journal of Palliative Care*, vol. 18, no. 1, pp. 45–51, 2012.

[22] B. S. Nama Sharanya, D. R. Meenan, and W. T. Fritz, "The use of sub-anesthetic intravenous ketamine and adjuvant dexmedetomidine when treating acute pain from CRPS," *Pain Physician*, vol. 13, no. 4, pp. 365–368, 2010.

[23] S.-S. Li, W.-S. Zhang, J.-L. Yang, Y.-C. Xiong, Y.-Q. Zhang, and H. Xu, "Involvement of protein Kinase B/Akt in analgesic effect of dexmedetomidine on neuropathic pain," *CNS Neuroscience and Therapeutics*, vol. 19, no. 5, pp. 364–366, 2013.

[24] H. S. M. Farghaly, R. B. Abd-Ellatief, M. Z. Moftah, M. G. Mostafa, E. M. Khedr, and H. I. Kotb, "The effects of dexmedetomidine alone and in combination with tramadol or amitriptyline in a neuropathic pain model," *Pain Physician*, vol. 17, no. 2, pp. 187–195, 2014.

[25] P. Lavand'homme and M. De Kock, "The use of intraoperative epidural or spinal analgesia modulates postoperative hyperalgesia and reduces residual pain after major abdominal surgery," *Acta Anaesthesiologica Belgica*, vol. 57, no. 4, pp. 373–379, 2006.

[26] G. R. Lauretti, A. D. M. Rodrigues, J. M. A. Gomes, and M. P. Dos Reis, "Epidural ketamine versus epidural clonidine as therapeutic for refractory neuropathic chronic pain," *Revista Brasileira de Anestesiologia*, vol. 52, no. 1, pp. 34–40, 2002.

21

Ultrasound-Guided Combined Interscalene-Cervical Plexus Block for Surgical Anesthesia in Clavicular Fractures

Onur Balaban,[1] **Turan Cihan Dülgeroğlu**,[2] **and Tayfun Aydın**[1]

[1]*Department of Anesthesiology and Pain Medicine, School of Medicine, Dumlupinar University, Kutahya, Turkey*
[2]*Department of Orthopedic and Trauma Surgery, School of Medicine, Dumlupinar University, Kutahya, Turkey*

Correspondence should be addressed to Onur Balaban; obalabandr@gmail.com

Academic Editor: Michael Frass

Objective. We aim to report our experiences regarding the implementation of the ultrasound-guided combined interscalene-cervical plexus block (CISCB) technique as a sole anesthesia method in clavicular fracture repair surgery. *Materials and Methods*. Charts of patients, who underwent clavicular fracture surgery through this technique, were reviewed retrospectively. We used an in-plane ultrasound-guided single-insertion, double-injection combined interscalene-cervical plexus block technique. During the performance of each block, the block areas were visualized by using a linear transducer, and the needles were advanced by using the in-plane technique. Block success and complication rates were evaluated. *Results and Discussion*. 12 patients underwent clavicular fracture surgery. Surgical regional anesthesia was achieved in 100% of blocks. None of the patients necessitated conversion to general anesthesia during surgery. There were no occurrences of acute complications. *Conclusions*. The ultrasound-guided combined interscalene-cervical plexus block was a successful and effective regional anesthesia method in clavicular fracture repair. Prospective comparative studies would report the superiority of the regional technique over general anesthesia.

1. Introduction

Clavicle fractures account for 35% of injuries to the shoulder girdle and generally occur after blunt traumas. For displaced clavicle fractures with greater than 2 cm of shortening, current recommendation is operative management with open reduction and internal fixation [1, 2].

Clavicle surgery is usually performed under general anesthesia. Any regional anesthesia method for repair of a clavicular fracture has not been described and not commonly performed in current anesthesia practice. Although peripheral nerve blocks are commonly used for a wide variety of surgical procedures on the upper extremity, there are very few reports regarding regional anesthesia for surgery of the clavicle. In the literature, proposed interventional strategies for clavicular fractures include superficial cervical plexus blocks, combined cervical plexus-deep cervical plexus blocks, and interscalene brachial plexus blocks. These techniques are usually used for analgesia of the clavicle [1]. Choosing the optimal nerve block to anesthetize the clavicle requires a thorough understanding of innervation, which remains controversial. The sensory innervation of the clavicle has been attributed to either the cervical or brachial plexus [3, 4].

Ultrasound-guided techniques have enabled the anesthetists to reduce doses of local anesthetic drugs and perform more successful blocks [5, 6]. As local anesthetic doses were reduced with the use of USG and lower doses were administered, combined or multiple blocks have become possible.

In regard to the neuronal anatomy and clinical experience, the combined interscalene-cervical plexus block seems to be an effective block and may be a promising method for sufficient surgical anesthesia in clavicle surgery. We understand from very few case reports that interscalene brachial plexus blocks and combined interscalene-cervical plexus blocks are being used as a single anesthetic modality for surgery of the clavicle in some hospitals [7]. Up to date,

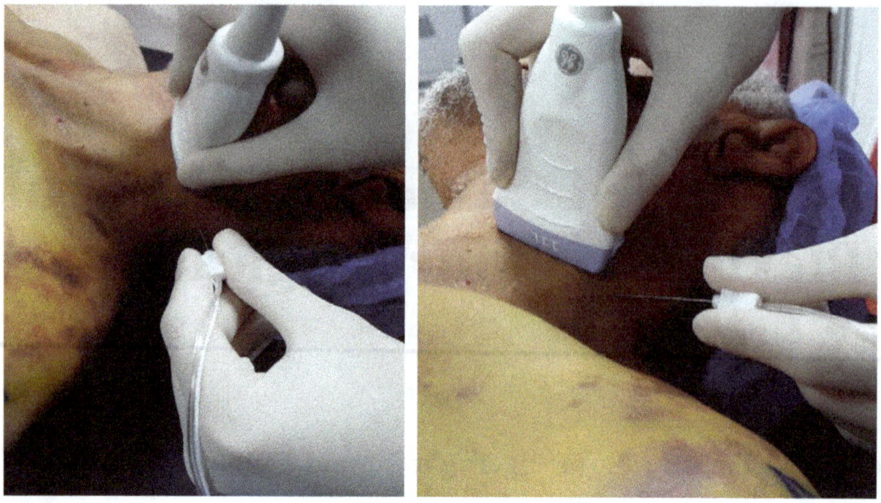

FIGURE 1: Position of the ultrasound transducer and the needle during the performance of blocks.

there is neither a prospective study nor a well-established regional anesthesia method for clavicle surgery.

The objective of our retrospective analysis is to demonstrate that combined interscalene-cervical plexus block is effective and safe as a sole anesthesia method for the patients undergoing clavicle fracture repair. We present a case series of clavicular fractures that were operated under combined interscalene-cervical plexus blocks.

2. Materials and Methods

Patient charts were retrospectively reviewed starting from May 2014. All patients were informed about the treatment, surgery, and anesthesia method before the procedure. Informed consents for the surgery and anesthesia method were obtained. Block success, acute complications as inadvertent arterial puncture, hematoma formation, respiratory distress, Horner's syndrome, pneumothorax, and signs of local anesthetic toxicity were evaluated.

2.1. Anesthesia Method. We define this technique as the in-plane ultrasound-guided single-insertion, double-injection combined interscalene-intermediate cervical plexus block. Cervical plexus blocks combined with interscalene blocks were performed under ultrasound guidance (LOGIQ P5, GE Healthcare, Milwaukee, WI, USA). The skin was prepared using an antiseptic solution, and the transducer was dressed with a sterile cover. A 12-megahertz linear transducer (GE Healthcare, Milwaukee, WI, USA) was used for performing the blocks. The related side of the patient was scanned by ultrasound in a transverse orientation across the neck with the probe marker facing lateral at the level of the interscalene groove (Figure 1). A long axis view of the brachial plexus roots, sternocleidomastoid (SCM) muscle, levator scapula muscle, carotid artery, jugular vein, and anterior and middle scalene muscles was identified (Figure 2).

The blocks were performed using a 5-centimeter block needle (Stimuplex Ultra, Braun, Melsungen, Germany). Initially, an interscalene block was performed under US guidance. The US transducer was placed transversally on the neck at the level of the superior pole of the thyroid cartilage and then slightly aligned laterally where the nerve roots were observed between the anterior and middle scalene muscles at the interscalene groove. The needle insertion site was determined under US guidance as the point where the posterolateral border of the SCM muscle starts. The final target position of the needle was immediately posterior to the space between the C5 and C6 roots (Figure 3). The needle was inserted laterally at the posterior border of the SCM muscle and advanced under US guidance using the in-plane technique. 0.5 ml/kg of the local anesthetic drug (0.5% bupivacaine) was administered under real-time visualization of local anesthetic distribution. After the performance of the interscalene block, the needle was withdrawn and redirected to the cervical plexus. The cervical plexus block was performed as a plane block in the prevertebral fascia posterior to the SCM muscle. The hyperechoic fascia of the SCM muscle on its posterolateral border was identified, and the needle was advanced along the posterior border of the SCM muscle under real-time US guidance to the nerve point of the neck. The needle tip was positioned to inject local anesthetic deep to the SCM muscle along its tapering posterolateral border but superficial to the prevertebral fascia (Figure 4).

At this level, visualization of the nerves can be difficult and cannot sometimes be identified, and it is not necessary to determine nerve structures in the fascial plane. We proceeded to inject to fill the posterior plane of the SCM muscle, where the cervical nerves exist to achieve an effective cervical plexus block and surgical anesthesia. Distribution of the local anesthetic drug was visualized during the procedure (Figures 3 and 4). Half of the total volume of the local anesthetic drug was administered for interscalene blocks, and the remaining half was administered for cervical plexus blocks. Motor blockade was determined by loss of shoulder abduction, and sensory blockade was assessed using the pinprick test at the surgery site. The patient was also checked for pain with mobilization of the arm and palpation of the clavicle by the surgeon. A successful block was defined as one

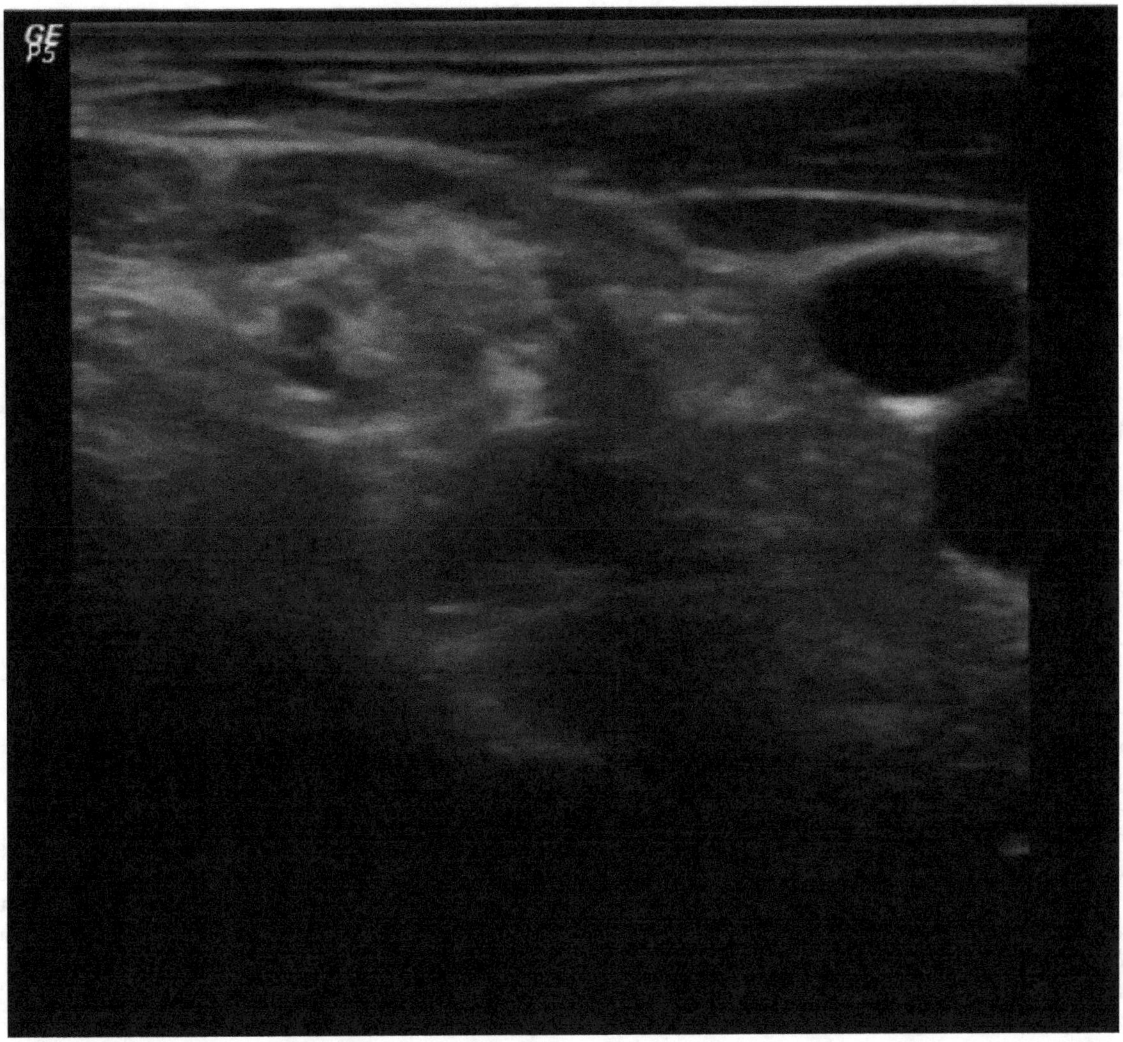

Figure 2: Visualization of the anatomical structures at the midneck level in the transverse plane: sternocleidomastoid muscle, carotid artery, and jugular vein. Brachial plexus can be seen as three hypoechoic nodular structures between the scalene muscles.

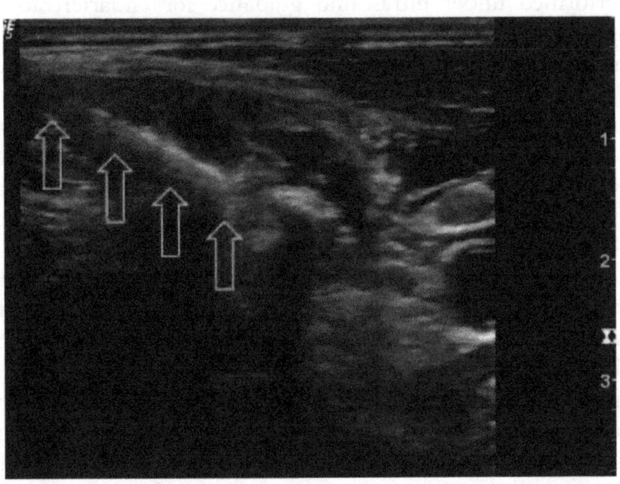

Figure 3: Position of the needle and local anesthetic distribution between the scalene muscles around the nerves in the interscalene region during the performance of the interscalene block. The arrows are showing the body and the tip of the needle.

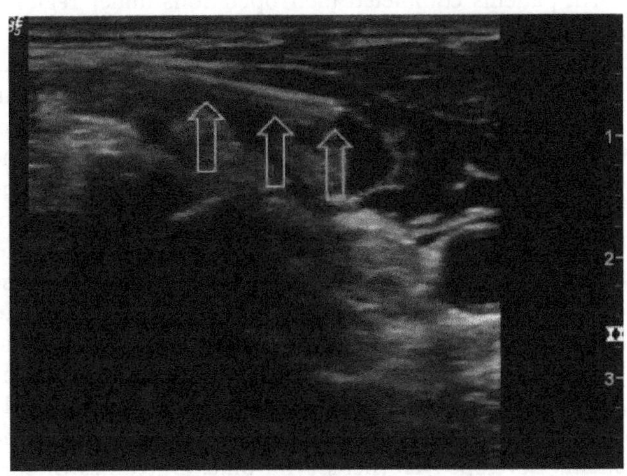

Figure 4: Position of the needle and local anesthetic distribution posterior to the sternocleidomastoid muscle during the performance of the cervical plexus block. The arrows are showing the body and the tip of the needle.

Table 1: Patient characteristics.

	Minimum	Maximum	Mean ± standard deviation
Age (years)	15.00	70.00	34.33 ± 20.11
Height (m)	1.67	1.87	1.74 ± 0.07
Weight (kg)	56.00	85.00	72.33 ± 10.63
BMI (kg/m^2)	17.72	28.73	24.11 ± 4.58

which did not necessitate conversion to general anesthesia. Postoperative analgesia was achieved by intravenous tramadol when necessary. As this procedure also affects the phrenic nerve, it was not performed on those with coexisting cardiac or respiratory disease.

Descriptive statistics of the study are calculated, and the data were analyzed using SPSS Statistics 21.0 program (IBM Corporation, NY, USA). Continuous quantitative data were expressed as number, mean, and standard deviation, and qualitative data were expressed as number and percentage.

3. Results

The patient characteristics are summarized in Table 1. Totally, 12 patients underwent clavicle operation. Eleven patients underwent open reduction and internal fixation of the clavicle fracture (Figure 5). One patient underwent removal of the implant from the clavicle. One of the patients had liver disease, and one patient had diabetes mellitus. Other patients' previous medical history was unremarkable.

The patients were transported to the operating room where standard monitors (electrocardiograph, noninvasive blood pressure, and pulse oximetry) were applied. All blocks were performed in the operating room. Resuscitative measures were present during the performance of blocks and during the operation. All surgeries were performed in supine position.

All patients completed their operations under regional anesthesia, and no patient required conversion to general anesthesia. One of the patients complained of mild pain at the initiation of the surgery. One other patient felt pain with manipulation of the clavicle and required a deeper sedation. 50 micrograms of fentanyl and 50 milligrams of ketamine were administered intravenously to the patients, and the operations continued uneventfully. There was no need of anticholinergic drugs as no side effect of ketamine was observed. We considered these patients as successful because both patients did not need to be intubated and continued to have effective respiration in the remaining course. We did not detect a significant change in blood pressures and heart rates intraoperatively. No surgical complications and early complications related to the blocks occurred. None of the patients developed Horner's syndrome. Outcomes of surgery and anesthesia are summarized in Table 2.

We asked the surgeons about their satisfaction about the anesthesia method. The surgeons' satisfaction was good, and none of them declared negative opinion about the anesthesia method. They were in favor of this method, which may be useful especially for high-risk patients.

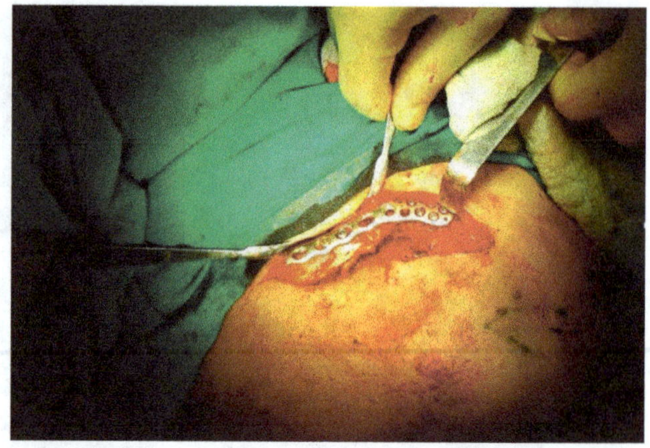

Figure 5: The operation site and clavicular fixation.

Table 2: Outcomes of surgery and anesthesia.

Surgery duration (minutes) (mean ± standard deviation)	73.75 ± 17.02
Acute complications	None
Block success rate (%)	100

4. Discussion

This case series demonstrated that a combined interscalene-intermediate cervical plexus block under ultrasound guidance is feasible in clavicular fracture surgery. Before ultrasound, local anesthetic doses required for successful blocks were substantially high; therefore, the risk for systemic local anesthetic toxicity was high. Advances in the field of ultrasound-guided peripheral nerve blocks have allowed reduction of local anesthetic doses in interscalene blocks [8]. Ultrasound-guided interscalene blocks are performed commonly in our clinic for shoulder surgeries. Cervical plexus blocks are also performed under ultrasound guidance for endarterectomy operations. The idea of using a combination of two blocks was encouraged by and came up after reduction of local anesthetic doses we used to administer to 10–20 milliliters. In consultation with the trauma surgeons, with the guarantee of converting to general anesthesia if surgical pain is felt, we have been offering this method to our patients undergoing clavicular surgery as an alternative to general anesthesia since 2014.

Understanding cervical plexus anatomy, innervation of the clavicle and innervation of the skin over the surgical site is important to establish a regional anesthesia method for clavicular surgery. The ventral rami of the first four cervical spinal nerves constitute the cervical plexus. They are located in front of the C1 to C4 vertebra, deep and posterior to the sternocleidomastoid (SCM) muscle. The plexus gives 4 terminal branches: greater auricular, lesser occipital, supraclavicular, and transverse cervical nerves. They provide sensory innervation to the skin and superficial structures of the anterolateral neck and sections of the ear and shoulder. The branches emerge at the posterior border of the sternocleidomastoid muscle, anterolateral to the levator scapulae and middle scalene muscles at the level of the superior pole of the thyroid cartilage [9, 10].

These nerves enter the skin at the middle of the posterior border of the sternocleidomastoid muscle at the level of C3, a point which lies superior to the locus and was inappropriately termed as Erb's point [11]. Some authors include the fifth cervical nerve to the plexus which contributes to the formation of one of the motor branches of the cervical plexus called the phrenic nerve. Therefore, the cervical plexus can also be defined as a network of nerves formed by the ventral rami of C1–C5 nerves and gives off both motor and sensory branches [12]. The sensory innervation of the clavicle and the overlying skin is not clearly identified and varies depending on the source in the literature between C3 and C6. The supraclavicular, subclavian, and long thoracic/suprascapular nerves, alone or together, may be responsible for pain transmission after clavicular fracture and surgery [1, 13].

Proposed interventional strategies for clavicular fractures include superficial cervical plexus blocks, combined superficial-deep cervical plexus blocks, and interscalene brachial plexus blocks [1]. Cervical plexus blocks are used as a sole anesthesia method in many surgeries such as carotid endarterectomies, dental procedures, submandibular and submental abscess drainage, minimally invasive thyroidectomy, and Zenker's diverticulectomy. Especially in carotid endarterectomies, superficial, intermediate, and deep cervical plexus blocks are widely performed [12, 14, 15]. An ultrasound-guided interscalene block is also a well accepted method in anesthesia practice which is preferred to achieve surgical anesthesia in shoulder surgeries such as arthroscopy, rotator cuff repair, and reductions of shoulder joint dislocations.

Nevertheless, general anesthesia seems to be extensively preferred in clavicular surgery in anesthesia practice. Fear of block failure has been overcome with regularly used regional anesthesia, and an improved block success rate is accomplished with the use of ultrasound-guided blocks. Thereafter, we could be able to change the standard of daily institutional practice of clavicle surgeries performed under general anesthesia to regional anesthesia.

For performance of ultrasound-guided cervical plexus blocks, the aim is to place the needle tip underneath the plexus if visualized. If the plexus is not visualized easily, the needle tip should be placed deep under the SCM muscle, in the plane of the prevertebral fascia [12]. An anatomical study suggests the compartment between the superficial layer and the prevertebral layer of the cervical fascia as a suitable target for cervical plexus blocks. This injection site describes an intermediate cervical plexus block [16]. Anatomically, with superficial blocks, there could be spread of the injectate to structures beneath the deep cervical fascia. This was also observed with real-time US in our study. The superficial cervical space communicates with the deep cervical space, and this may explain the efficacy of the superficial cervical plexus blocks [17].

There is a confusing nomenclature in the articles about cervical plexus blocks. Existing literature indicates that there have been various methods described for the proper injection technique in superficial cervical plexus blocks. The classical technique of superficial cervical plexus blocks was described as subcutaneous injection of the local anesthetic drug, which was found clinically effective for carotid endarterectomy [18]. In some reports, superficial cervical plexus injections have been suggested to be "intradermal" (even more superficial) or to be administered into the body of the sternocleidomastoid muscle. The sub-investing fascia injection might be termed as the "intermediate cervical plexus block" [19]. We preferred the term "intermediate cervical plexus block" which would describe our method correctly as local anesthetic distribution was within the prevertebral fascia in our study.

Ultrasound-guided superficial cervical plexus blocks are found to be successful for treating pain in emergency care settings [9]. Superficial cervical plexus blocks can also be used to provide surgical anesthesia for lymph node biopsy and excision of a thyroid nodule and placement of hemodialysis catheters [20, 21]. Ultrasound-guided bilateral cervical plexus blocks could be performed for postoperative analgesia following thyroid surgeries [22]. In oral and maxillofacial surgical practice and in selected neck surgeries, use of superficial cervical plexus blocks was offered as an alternative to general anesthesia [23, 24].

The combined interscalene-cervical plexus block is a novel method, which was reported in very few cases. Vandepitte et al. used this technique successfully as a primary anesthesia method in a pregnant patient who had a clavicular fracture [7]. They found this method effective for achieving surgical anesthesia. Shanthanna reported two cases of clavicular surgery operated under general anesthesia [25]. The patients were performed superficial cervical plexus block and selective C5 nerve root block under ultrasound guidance, along with general anesthesia. Both patients had an effective regional block and required minimal supplementation of analgesia, both being discharged on the same day.

5. Limitations of the Study

This clinical series is limited by its retrospective nature, and patients were not followed for a postoperative analgesia requirement. This may be a subject of prospective study in the future. As clavicular repair is a rarely performed intervention, the low number of cases was also a limitation. Several measurements were not evaluated such as the number of needle insertion attempts, needle redirections, block performing times, and onset times. Long-term complications were also not evaluated.

6. Conclusions

Our limited experience suggests that the combined interscalene-cervical plexus block is possible as a sole anesthesia method in patients who undergo clavicular fracture surgery. In this case series, regional anesthesia was successful, effective, and well tolerated in all of the patients. This method may be considered as an alternative to general anesthesia. Prospective (randomized) trials are required to determine which constitutes the best option for such operations.

Conflicts of Interest

The authors declare that they have no conflicts of interest.

References

[1] D. Q. Tran, W. Tiyaprasertkul, and A. P. Gonzalez, "Analgesia for clavicular fracture and surgery: a call for evidence," *Regional Anesthesia and Pain Medicine*, vol. 38, no. 6, pp. 539–543, 2013.

[2] P. L. Althausen, S. Shannon, M. Lu et al., "Clinical and financial comparison of operative and nonoperative treatment of displaced clavicle fractures," *Journal of Shoulder and Elbow Surgery*, vol. 22, no. 5, pp. 608–611, 2013.

[3] A. T. Gray, *Atlas of Ultrasound-Guided Regional Anesthesia*, Saunders, Philadelphia, PA, USA, 2nd edition, 2012.

[4] A. Hadzic, *Textbook of Regional Anesthesia and Acute Pain Management*, McGraw-Hill Medical, New York, NY, USA, 2007.

[5] K. Vermeylen, S. Engelen, L. Sermeus et al., "Supraclavicular brachial plexus blocks: review and current practice," *Acta Anaesthesiologica Belgica*, vol. 63, pp. 15–21, 2012.

[6] J. M. Neal, R. Brull, J. L. Horn et al., "The Second American Society of Regional Anesthesia and Pain Medicine evidence-based medicine assessment of ultrasound-guided regional anesthesia: executive summary," *Regional Anesthesia and Pain Medicine*, vol. 41, no. 2, pp. 181–194, 2016.

[7] C. Vandepitte, M. Latmore, E. O'Murchu et al., "Combined interscalene-superficial cervical plexus blocks for surgical repair of a clavicular fracture in a 15-week pregnant woman," *International Journal of Obstetric Anesthesia*, vol. 23, no. 2, pp. 194-195, 2014.

[8] P. Gautier, C. Vandepitte, C. Ramquet et al., "The minimum effective anesthetic volume of 0.75% ropivacaine in ultrasound-guided interscalene brachial plexus block," *Anesthesia and Analgesia*, vol. 113, no. 4, pp. 951–955, 2011.

[9] A. Andrew, M. D. Herring, B. Michael et al., "The ultrasound-guided superficial cervical plexus block for anesthesia and analgesia in emergency care settings," *American Journal of Emergency Medicine*, vol. 30, no. 7, pp. 1263–1267, 2012.

[10] J. H. Lee, K. L. Cheng, Y. J. Choi et al., "High-resolution imaging of neural anatomy and pathology of the neck," *Korean Journal of Radiology*, vol. 18, no. 1, pp. 180–193, 2017.

[11] P. Soeding and N. Eizenberg, "Review article: anatomical considerations for ultrasound guidance for regional anesthesia of the neck and upper limb," *Canadian Journal of Anesthesia*, vol. 56, no. 7, pp. 518–533, 2009.

[12] A. Hadzic, *Hadzic's Peripheral Nerve Blocks and Anatomy for Ultrasound Guided Regional Anesthesia*, McGraw-Hill Medical, New York, NY, USA, 2rd edition, 2012.

[13] D. S. Choi, A. Atchabahian, and A. R. Brown, "Cervical plexus block provides postoperative analgesia after clavicle surgery," *Anesthesia and Analgesia*, vol. 100, no. 5, pp. 1542-1543, 2005.

[14] A. Sait Kavaklı, N. Kavrut Öztürk, R. Umut Ayoğlu et al., "Comparison of combined (deep and superficial) and intermediate cervical plexus block by use of ultrasound guidance for carotid endarterectomy," *Journal of Cardiothoracic and Vascular Anesthesia*, vol. 30, no. 2, pp. 317–322, 2016.

[15] A. Alilet, P. Petit, B. Devaux et al., "Ultrasound-guided intermediate cervical block versus superficial cervical block for carotid artery endarterectomy: the randomized-controlled CERVECHO trial," *Anaesthesia Critical Care and Pain Medicine*, vol. 36, no. 16, pp. 91–95, 2016.

[16] R. Seidel, M. Schulze, K. Zukowski, and A. Wree, "Ultrasound-guided intermediate cervical plexus block. Anatomical study," *Der Anaesthesist*, vol. 64, no. 6, pp. 446–450, 2015.

[17] J. J. Pandit, D. Dutta, and J. F. Morris, "Spread of injectate with superficial cervical plexus block in humans: an anatomical study," *British Journal of Anaesthesia*, vol. 91, no. 5, pp. 733–735, 2003.

[18] R. J. Telford and M. D. Stoneham, "Correct nomenclature of superficial cervical plexus blocks," *British Journal of Anaesthesia*, vol. 92, no. 5, pp. 775-776, 2004.

[19] M. D. Stoneham, D. Stamou, and J. Mason, "Regional anesthesia for carotid endarterectomy," *British Journal of Anaesthesia*, vol. 114, no. 3, pp. 372–383, 2015.

[20] T. Ciftci, H. Daskaya, M. B. Yıldırım et al., "A minimally painful, comfortable, and safe technique for hemodialysis catheter placement in children: superficial cervical plexus block," *Hemodialysis International*, vol. 18, no. 3, pp. 700–704, 2014.

[21] J. D. Tobias, "Cervical plexus block in adolescents," *Journal of Clinical Anesthesia*, vol. 11, no. 7, pp. 606–608, 1999.

[22] Y. Gürkan, Z. Taş, K. Toker et al., "Ultrasound guided bilateral cervical plexus block reduces postoperative opioid consumption following thyroid surgery," *Journal of Clinical Monitoring and Computing*, vol. 29, no. 5, pp. 579–584, 2015.

[23] R. K. Kanthan, "The use of superficial cervical plexus block in oral and maxillofacial surgical practice as an alternative to general anesthesia in selective cases," *Annals of Maxillofacial Surgery*, vol. 6, no. 1, pp. 4–8, 2016.

[24] S. Mukhopadhyay, M. Niyogi, M. Dutta et al., "Bilateral superficial cervical plexus block with or without low-dose intravenous ketamine analgesia: effective, simple, safe, and cheap alternative to conventional general anesthesia for selected neck surgeries," *Local and Regional Anesthesia*, vol. 5, pp. 1–7, 2012.

[25] H. Shanthanna, "Ultrasound guided selective cervical nerve root block and superficial cervical plexus block for surgeries on the clavicle," *Indian Journal of Anaesthesia*, vol. 58, no. 3, pp. 327–329, 2014.

22

A Systematic Review of Postoperative Pain Outcome Measurements Utilised in Regional Anesthesia

E. Pushpanathan,[1] **T. Setty**,[2] **B. Carvalho**,[3] **and P. Sultan**[4]

[1]*Department of Anaesthesia, Guy's and St. Thomas' NHS Foundation Trust, London, UK*
[2]*Department of Anaesthesia, University College Hospitals London NHS Foundation Trust, London, UK*
[3]*Department of Anesthesia, Stanford University School of Medicine, Stanford, CA, USA*
[4]*Department of Anaesthesia, University College Hospitals London NHS Foundation Trust, University College London, London, UK*

Correspondence should be addressed to E. Pushpanathan; ellile@yahoo.com

Academic Editor: Enrico Camporesi

Introduction. Regional anesthesia is a rapidly growing subspecialty. There are few published meta-analyses exploring pain outcome measures utilised in regional anesthesia randomized controlled trials (RCTs), which may be due to heterogeneity in outcomes assessed. This systematic review explores postoperative pain outcomes utilised in regional anesthesia RCTs. *Methods.* A literature search was performed using three databases (Medline, Embase, and CINAHL). Regional anesthesia RCTs with postoperative pain as a primary outcome were included if written in English and published in one of the top 20 impact factor journals between 2005 and 2017. Study quality was assessed using the Cochrane Collaboration's tool for assessing risk of bias. *Results.* From the 31 included articles, 15 different outcome measures in total were used to assess postoperative pain. The most commonly (16/31) used outcome measures were verbal numerical grading of pain out of 10, total opioid consumption, and visual analogue scale 10 cm (VAS). The need for analgesia was used as an outcome measure where studies did not use a pain rating score. Ten studies reported pain scores on activity and 27/31 studies utilised ≥2 pain outcomes. Time of measurement of pain score also varied with a total of 51 different time points used in total. *Conclusion.* Analysis of the articles demonstrated heterogeneity and inconsistency in choice of pain outcome and time of measurement within regional anesthesia studies. Identification of these pain outcomes utilised can help to create a definitive list of core outcomes, which may guide future researchers when designing such studies.

1. Introduction

Regional anesthesia is a rapidly growing subspecialty, with a widening spectrum of applications and uses. Despite growth in this area of research, there have been few published regional anesthesia systematic reviews, meta-analyses, Cochrane reviews, or National Institute for Health and Care Excellence (NICE) guidelines exploring pain outcomes. This may be due to the heterogeneity of outcome variables chosen in regional anesthesia studies, making it difficult to combine and analyse data.

The Cochrane Collaboration, which aims to give the "clinical bottom line" through its reviews, has 39 reviews, which mention regional anesthesia. These reviews commonly cite the outcomes chosen as "incomplete," "poor quality," and "heterogeneous," which impeded the authors' ability to draw meaningful conclusions [1–4]. Additionally, there are four NICE guidelines centered on regional anesthesia [5–8], and of these, only one deals specifically with the use of regional anesthesia to manage surgical or postoperative pain [5].

Identification of outcomes utilised can subsequently help to create a definitive list of core outcomes, which may guide future researchers when designing studies. This systematic review aimed to explore outcomes utilised in regional anesthesia randomized controlled trials (RCTs) to measure postoperative pain.

2. Methods

We have adhered to the Preferred Reporting Items for Systematic Reviews and Meta-Analyses (PRISMA) statement standards in this article [9].

We performed a literature search using three search engines (Medline, Embase, and CINAHL). These databases were searched for RCTs published between 2005 and 2017. The search strategy included manual searching of citations for further relevant articles. The search was initially performed in mid December 2016 and repeated on January 5th 2017. An example of the exact search terms used for each database is included in Appendix A. The review was limited to published English language RCTs exploring regional anesthesia, with a primary outcome of postoperative pain. Articles were included if published between 2005 and 2017, in one of the top 20 impact factor journals (Appendix B, Table 4). Since it was felt that the assessment of pain within the adult population is significantly different to the pediatric and obstetric populations, this review was limited only to adult studies (participants aged 18 years and over).

The selected studies were analysed by two of the authors (E. Pushpanathan and T. Setty). Each study was read and the following data were extracted and tabulated: authors, year of publication, postoperative pain outcome measures utilised, times of postoperative pain assessment, nerve block studied, and personnel collecting the data. The two primary outcomes explored in this systematic review were the type of pain outcome measured and the time of measurement.

The quality of studies included in this systematic review was evaluated using the Cochrane Collaboration's tool for assessing risk of bias [10]. Areas of methodological quality assessed included concealment of allocation, random sequence generation, blinding of the assessors and participants, and accounting for all subjects. Overall quality was graded as low (low risk of bias), high (high risk of bias), or unclear risk of bias for each domain entry [10]. The quality of each study was also assessed using the Jadad score, which examines withdrawals, blinding, and randomization of a study [11], although studies were not excluded on the basis of this assessment. At least two individuals extracted the study data independently utilizing a standardised review protocol and recorded the information on a data spreadsheet. Differences were resolved by reexamination of the original manuscripts and by discussion. The data were then entered into a Microsoft Excel for Mac 2016 spreadsheet (Microsoft Corporation, Redmond, WA) by one of the authors (E. Pushpanathan) and checked by a second investigator (T. Setty).

3. Results

The search identified 407 articles. One author screened the titles and abstracts of these articles, and 308 were excluded. Two authors reviewed the full text of the remaining 99 articles. Of those excluded, 20 were duplicates and 18 were not RCTs. Of the remaining excluded articles, 5 were pediatric studies, 2 were obstetric, 3 were systematic reviews or meta-analyses, 2 were foreign language, 7 did not have postoperative pain as a primary outcome, and 11 were abbreviated studies in supplements so lacked sufficient detail. The results of the literature search are summarised in Figure 1. Thirty-one articles met the inclusion criteria and were included in this systematic review [12–42]. A detailed description of the pain outcomes utilised and timings of measurements in the included studies is provided in Table 1. Table 2 summarises the number of studies utilizing each pain outcome identified from included studies. Median Jadad score of included studies was 3 (range 2–5). The majority of studies demonstrated a low risk of bias in the 7 domains. A summary of risk of bias assessment is provided in Figure 2.

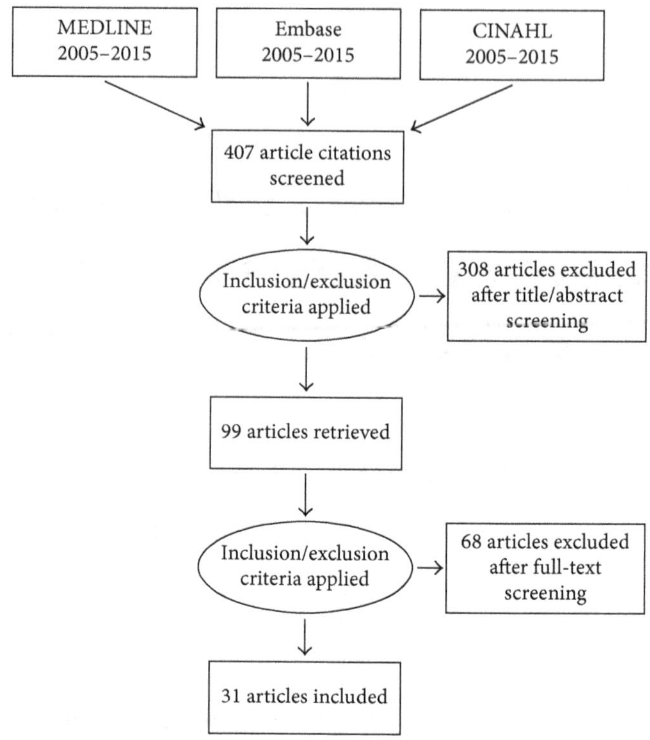

FIGURE 1: Summary of literature search and included studies.

3.1. Postoperative Pain Measurement Tool. Fifteen different outcome measures in total were used in the 31 included studies to assess postoperative pain. The outcome measures utilised in the included studies are summarised in Table 2. The majority of studies (27/31) utilised two or more pain outcomes. The most commonly used outcome measures were numerical grading of pain/numerical reporting scale (NRS) out of 10 (16 studies) [12, 17, 20–24, 27–29, 32–35, 38, 40], opioid consumption (16 studies), and visual analogue scale 10 cm (VAS; 12 studies) [13–16, 25, 26, 31, 36, 37, 39, 41, 42]. Other than reporting total opioid consumption, analgesia usage was also measured with the following outcomes: nonopioid analgesic requirement [14, 16, 32, 33, 36], total supplementary analgesic requirement [34, 35], and cumulative opioid consumption [26, 37]. Other pain outcome measures utilised included: time to first episode of pain [22, 33] and first analgesia or opioid request [18, 28–30, 35–37]. If a study did not use a scoring system to rate pain, the need for analgesia was utilised instead as an outcome measure. There was an evident understanding

Table 1: Summary of measurement timings of pain outcomes utilised in included studies.

Author/year	Country of study	Measurement tool	Time measured	Nerve block
Ambrosoli et al. [12]	Not stated	NRS (not stated; 0–10)	4 hours post-op Upon discharge	Sciatic nerve catheter
		NRS at rest (0–10)	24 hours 48 hours	
		NRS on activity (0–10)	24 hours 48 hours	
		Number of occasions sleep was disturbed by pain	24 hours 48 hours	
Andersen et al. [13]	Denmark	Worst pain during knee movement	On day of surgery	Saphenous nerve block
		VAS (10 cm) at rest		
		Time from surgery to VAS score 3 (not stated)	Hours	
		Sleep disturbance due to pain (yes/no)	D1 post-op D2 post-op D3 post-op	
		Total opioid consumption	48 hours	
Bengisun et al. [39]	Turkey	VAS (10 cm; not stated)	2 hours post-op 4 hours post-op 6 hours post-op 12 hours post-op 24 hours post-op	Interscalene block
Bharti et al. [14]	India	VAS (10 cm; not stated)	Every 30 min for 2 hours Every 1 hour for 6 hours Every 2 hours for 12 hours 24 hours post-op	Supraclavicular brachial plexus block
		Total analgesic requirement (opiate and nonopiate)	24 hours post-op	
Boussofara et al. [15]	Tunisia	VAS (10 cm; not stated)	Every 15 min post-op whilst in PACU	Spinal anaesthetic block
		Total opioid consumption	Whilst in PACU	
Capdevilla et al. [16]	France	VAS (10 cm; not stated)	10 min post-op 1 hour post-op 4 hours post-op 12 hours post-op AM D1 post-op during physiotx AM D2 post-op during physiotx AM D3 post-op during physiotx AM D4 post-op during physiotx	Interscalene and popliteal infusions
		Total analgesic consumption (nonopiate)	Over 72 hours	
Choi et al. [17]	Canada	NRS on activity (0–10)	AM D2 post-op	Femoral nerve block continuous versus single
		Total opioid consumption	48 hours	
		NRS at rest (0–10)	AM D1 post-op	
		NRS on activity (0–10)	D1 post-op	
		Worst NRS (0–10)	D1 post-op	
		NRS (0–10; not stated)	4.5 months post-op	
Diakomi et al. [18]	Greece	Time to first IV opioid request (hours)	No. of hours	Fascia iliaca block
		Total opioid consumption	Over first 24 hours	
Elkassabany et al. [19]	USA	Pain scores (type of pain score not stated)	Before physiotherapy	Femoral nerve block versus adductor canal block
		Pain scores (type of pain score not stated)	After physiotherapy	
		Pain scores (APS-POQ-R)	At 24 hours	
		Total opioid consumption	AM D1 post-op AM D2 post-op	
Fredrickson et al. [20]	New Zealand	NRS (not stated; 0–10)	Emergence Worst in 24 hours on movement Worst in 24 hours at rest Worst in second 24 hours on movement Worst in second 24 hours at rest	Interscalene catheters

Table 1: Continued.

Author/year	Country of study	Measurement tool	Time measured	Nerve block
Fritsch et al. [21]	Austria	NRS at rest (0–10)	4 hours post-op	Interscalene brachial plexus block
			6 hours post-op	
			8 hours post-op	
			10 hours post-op	
			12 hours post-op	
			14 hours post-op	
		NRS on activity (0–10)	4 hours post-op	
			6 hours post-op	
			8 hours post-op	
			10 hours post-op	
			12 hours post-op	
			14 hours post-op	
Hamdani et al. [38]	Switzerland	Average pain score (NRS; 0–10) (not stated)	Over first 24 hours	Continuous interscalene
		Average pain score (NRS; 0–10) (not stated)	Over first 48 hours	
		Total opioid consumption	Over first 24 hours	
		Total opioid consumption	Over first 48 hours	
		Maximum pain score (NRS; 0–10) (not stated)	Over first 24 hours	
		Maximum pain score (NRS; 0–10) (not stated)	Over first 48 hours	
Karthikeyan et al. [37]	India	VAS (10 cm) (not stated)	Admission to PACU	Bilateral cervical plexus block
			2 hours post-op	
			4 hours post-op	
			6 hours post-op	
			8 hours post-op	
			16 hours post-op	
			24 hours post-op	
		Time to first analgesic request	Min	
		Total analgesic consumption (opioid consumption)	24 hours post-op	
Kim et al. [42]	Republic of Korea	VAS (10 cm; not stated)	1 hour post-op	Serratus-intercostal plane block and intermediate cervical plexus block versus control
			3 hours post-op	
			6 hours post-op	
			9 hours post-op	
			24 hours post-op	
Kulhari et al. [36]	Not stated	Time to first rescue analgesia	After administration of block	Pectoral nerve block versus thoracic paravertebral block
		Total analgesic consumption (opioid consumption)	24 hours post-op	
		VAS (10 cm; not stated)	0 hours post-op	
			0.5 hours post-op	
			1 hour post-op	
			2 hours post-op	
			4 hours post-op	
			6 hours post-op	
			8 hours post-op	
			12 hours post-op	
			24 hours post-op	
Moura et al. [35]	Brazil	NRS (not stated; 0–10)	T0 (after recovering consciousness)	Femoral nerve block
			1 hour post-op	
			2 hours post-op	
		Total dose of supplementary analgesia (opioid and nonopioid)	First 2 hours	
		Time to first analgesic supplementation		
Nagafuchi et al. [34]	Japan	NRS (not stated; 0–10)	Exiting operating room	Femoral nerve block-sciatic nerve block versus femoral nerve block-LIA
			3 hours post-op	
			12 hours post-op	
			24 hours post-op	
		Total dose of diclofenac		

Table 1: Continued.

Author/year	Country of study	Measurement tool	Time measured	Nerve block
Salviz et al. [33]	USA	Time to first pain Analgesic consumption (opioid) Maximum NRS (not stated; 0–10)	Hours D1 post-op D2 post-op D3 post-op D4 post-op D5 post-op D6 post-op D7 post-op D1 post-op D2 post-op D3 post-op D4 post-op D5 post-op D6 post-op D7 post-op	Interscalene brachial plexus block
Sawhney et al. [32]	Canada	NRS on activity (0–10) NRS at rest and with knee bending (0–10) NRS on activity (0–10) NRS at rest and with knee bending (0–10) Analgesic consumption (opioid and nonopioid) per day	D1 post-op D1 post-op D2 post-op D2 post-op	Combined adductor canal block with periarticular infiltration versus adductor canal nerve block
Sato et al. [31]	Japan	VAS (10 cm) at rest Morphine consumption	At rest just after surgery 6 hours after surgery AM D1 post-op PM D1 post-op AM D2 post-op PM D2 post-op Over first 48 hours	Sciatic and femoral continuous versus single shot
Siddiqui et al. [41]	USA	VAS (10 cm) at rest	Every 5 min first hour 4 hours post-op 8 hours post-op 16 hours post-op 20 hours post-op 24 hours post-op 28 hours post-op 32 hours post-op 36 hours post-op	Lumbar plexus block
Sindjelic et al. [30]	Serbia	Time to first analgesic request Total opioid consumption	Min 24 hours post-op	Cervical plexus block
Schoenmakers et al. [29]	Netherlands	Time to first analgesic request NRS at rest (0–10) NRS on activity (0–10)	Min Immediately post-op 24 hours Immediately post-op 24 hours	Popliteal continuous
Subramanyam et al. [28]	Canada	NRS (not stated; 0–10)	30 min post-op 60 min post-op 90 min post-op	Supraclavicular brachial plexus block
Stundner et al. [27]	Austria	Time to first analgesic request NRS at rest (0–10) NRS on activity (0–10)	Min Baseline before ISB Immediately post-op 6 hours post-op worst pain 8 hours post-op worst pain 10 hours post-op worst pain 12 hours post-op worst pain 14 hours post-op worst pain AM D1 post-op worst pain Baseline before ISB Immediately post-op 6 hours post-op worst pain 8 hours post-op worst pain 10 hours post-op worst pain 12 hours post-op worst pain 14 hours post-op worst pain AM D1 post-op worst pain	Interscalene brachial plexus block

Table 1: Continued.

Author/year	Country of study	Measurement tool	Time measured	Nerve block
Thybo et al. [26]	Denmark	VAS (10 cm) during 30° hip flexion	4 hours post-op (T4) at T0 (pts able to move toes but before SAB worn off)	Lateral cutaneous femoral nerve block
		Pain at rest VAS (10 cm) and during 30° hip flexion	T0	
		Pain at rest VAS (10 cm) and during 30° hip flexion	T1 (after T0)	
		Pain at rest VAS (10 cm) and during 30° hip flexion	T2 (after T0)	
		Pain at rest VAS (10 cm) and during 30° hip flexion	T4 (after T0)	
		Pain at rest VAS (10 cm) and during 30° hip flexion	T8 (after T0)	
		Pain at rest VAS (10 cm) and during 30° hip flexion	T12 (after T0)	
		Pain at rest VAS (10 cm) and during 30° hip flexion	T24 (after T0)	
		Cumulative oxycodone consumption	0–24 hours post-op	
Wegener et al. [25]	Netherlands	WOMAC score	At rest at 3 months On mobilising at 3 months At rest 12 months On mobilising at 12 months	Sciatic nerve block
		VAS (10 cm)	At rest 3 months On mobilising at 3 months At rest 12 months On mobilising at 12 months	
		Oxford knee score (inc. pain)		
Wegener et al. [24]	Netherlands	NRS at rest (0–10)	AM D1 post-op PM D1 post-op AM D2 post-op PM D2 post-op AM D3 post-op PM D3 post-op	Sciatic and femoral continuous versus single
		NRS on mobilisation (0–10)	AM D1 post-op PM D1 post-op AM D2 post-op PM D2 post-op AM D3 post-op PM D3 post-op	
		Total morphine consumption	D0 post-op D1 post-op D2 post-op D3 post-op	
Wongyingsinn et al. [23]	Canada	NRS at rest (0–10)	24 hours post-op 48 hours post-op 72 hours post-op	Thoracic epidural block
		NRS on walking (0–10)	24 hours post-op 48 hours post-op 72 hours post-op	
		NRS on coughing (0–10)	24 hours post-op 48 hours post-op 72 hours post-op	
YaDeau et al. [40]	USA	NRS at rest (0–10)	30 min post-op 1 hour post-op 2 hours post-op 3 hour post-op 4 hours post-op 24 hours post-op	Lumbar plexus block
		NRS on movement (0–10)	30 min post-op 1 hour post-op 2 hours post-op 3 hour post-op 4 hours post-op 24 hours post-op	

Table 1: Continued.

Author/year	Country of study	Measurement tool	Time measured	Nerve block
Zhai et al. [22]	Not stated	NRS at rest (0–10) Worst NRS (0–10) Time of first shoulder pain	Before block Right before discharge from PACU 4 hours after block 8 hours after block 24 hours after block 24 hours after block	Interscalene brachial plexus block

D0 post-op = Day 0 postoperatively; D1 post-op = Day 1 postoperatively; D2 post-op = Day 2 postoperatively; D3 post-op = Day 3 postoperatively; D4 post-op = Day 4 postoperatively; D5 post-op = Day 5 postoperatively; D6 post-op = Day 6 postoperatively; D7 post-op = Day 7 postoperatively; min- = minutes; NRS = numeric (verbal) rating scale (0 = no pain to 10 = worst imaginable pain); VAS = visual analogue scale (0 mm = no pain to 100 mm = worst imaginable pain); APS-POQ-R = American Pain Society Patient Outcome Questionnaire Revised; WOMAC score = Western Ontario and McMaster Universities Osteoarthritis Index (5 pain questions included) OA specific; Oxford Knee Score 12-item knee questionnaire on pain; for measurement tool, "not stated" = whether pain score recorded at rest or on movement not stated in methods.

Table 2: Summary of pain outcomes reported in included studies.

Pain outcome	No. of studies utilising outcome	Studies
VAS	11	Andersen et al. [13]; Bengisun et al. [39]; Bharti et al. [14]; Boussofara et al. [15]; Capdevilla et al. [16]; Karthikeyan et al. [37]; Kim et al. [42]; Kulhari et al. [36]; Sato et al. [31]; Siddiqui et al. [41]; Wegener et al. [25]
VAS on a specified activity	1	Thybo et al. [26]
Time to VAS 3 cm	1	Andersen et al. [13]
NRS at rest	10	Ambrosoli et al. [12]; Choi et al. [17]; Fritsch et al. [21]; Sawhney et al. [32]; Schoenmakers et al. [29]; Stundner et al. [27]; Wegener et al. [24]; Wongyingsinn et al. [23]; YaDeau et al. [40]; Subramanyam et al. [28]
NRS on activity	9	Ambrosoli et al. [12]; Choi et al. [17]; Fritsch et al. [21]; Sawhney et al. [32]; Schoenmakers et al. [29]; Stundner et al. [27]; Wegener et al. [24]; Wongyingsinn et al. [23]; YaDeau et al. [40]
Maximum NRS score	3	Hamdani et al. [38]; Salviz et al. [33]; Zhai et al. [22]
Average NRS	1	Hamdani et al. [38]
Analgesic consumption	7	Bharti et al. [14]; Capdevilla et al. [16]; Kulhari et al. [36]; Moura et al. [35]; Nagafuchi et al. [34]; Salviz et al. [33]; Sawhney et al. [32]
Opioid consumption	16	Andersen et al. [13]; Bharti et al. [14]; Boussofara et al. [15]; Choi et al. [17]; Diakomi et al. [18]; Elkassabany et al. [19]; Hamdani et al. [38]; Karthikeyan et al. [37]; Kulhari et al. [36]; Moura et al. [35]; Salviz et al. [33]; Sawhney et al. [32]; Sato et al. [31]; Sindjelic et al. [30]; Thybo et al. [26]; Wegener et al. [24]
Time to 1st pain	2	Salviz et al. [33]; Zhai et al. [22]
Time to 1st analgesic request	6	Karthikeyan et al. [37]; Kulhari et al. [36]; Moura et al. [35]; Schoenmakers et al. [29]; Sindjelic et al. [30]; Subramanyam et al. [28]
Time to 1st opioid request	1	Diakomi et al. [18]
Sleep disturbance	2	Ambrosoli et al. [12]; Andersen et al. [13]
WOMAC	1	Wegener et al. [25]
APS-POQ-R	1	Elkassabany et al. [19]

NRS = numerical reported score (verbal; out of 10); VAS = visual analogue scale; APS-POQ-R = American Pain Society Patient Outcome Questionnaire; WOMAC = Western Ontario and McMaster Universities Osteoarthritis Index.

amongst the selected studies that pain may be worse on movement with separate pain scores (NRS or VAS) taken on activity in 10 of the included studies (Table 2). In the studies that utilised a scoring system to measure pain, there were two groups; those that reported scores at individual time points [12, 14–16, 19, 21, 23–26, 28, 29, 31, 32, 34–37, 39–42] and studies that recorded the worst (or maximum) pain score during the study period [17, 20, 22, 27, 33]. Average pain scores were reported in only one study [38].

3.2. Time of Measurement. Time of measurement of pain outcomes also varied with a total of 51 different time points utilised in the 31 studies (Table 1). The time points ranged from immediately following surgery [20, 26, 27, 29, 31, 34, 37, 41] to 12 months postoperatively [25]. Intervals between measurements ranged from every 5 minutes [41] to 6 months [25]. Twenty-two out of 31 of the studies (71%) only evaluated pain over the first 24 hours postoperatively [12, 14, 16, 17, 19, 20, 22–24, 26, 27, 29, 31–34, 36, 38–42].

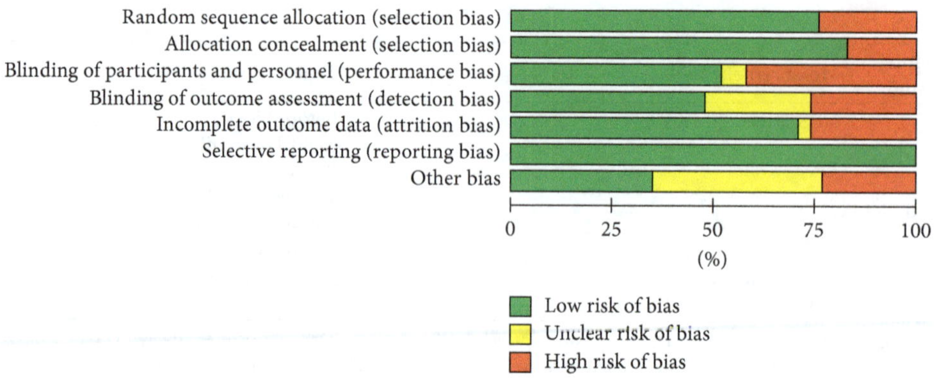

FIGURE 2: Risk of bias assessment in included studies.

TABLE 3: Summary of regional techniques investigated in included studies.

Blocks studied	Number of studies	Studies
Supraclavicular	2	Subramanyam et al. [28]; Bharti et al. [14]
Interscalene	5	Bengisun et al. [39]; Fritsch et al. [21]; Salviz et al. [33]; Stundner et al. [27]; Zhai et al. [22]
Pectoral	1	Kulhari et al. [36]
Serratus-intercostal	1	Kim et al. [42]
Fascia iliaca	1	Diakomi et al. [18]
Femoral	6	Sato et al. [31]; Wegener et al. [24]; Choi et al. [17]; Thybo et al. [26]; Nagafuchi et al. [34]; Elkassabany et al. [19]
Sciatic	4	Sato et al. [31]; Wegener et al. [25]; Wegener et al. [24]; Moura et al. [35]
Adductor	1	Sawhney et al. [32]
Saphenous	1	Andersen et al. [13]
Cervical plexus	2	Sindjelic et al. [30]; Karthikeyan et al. [37]
Lumbar plexus	2	YaDeau et al. [40]; Siddiqui et al. [41]
Thoracic epidural	1	Wongyingsinn et al. [23]
Spinal	1	Boussofara et al. [15]
Interscalene catheter	3	Hamdani et al. [38]; Capdevilla et al. [16]; Fredrickson et al. [20]
Popliteal catheter	2	Capdevilla et al. [16]; Schoenmakers et al. [29]
Sciatic catheter	1	Ambrosoli et al. [12]

3.3. Nerve Blocks Studied. A variety of nerve blocks were studied (16 in total), which are summarised in Table 3 and may indicate which blocks were seen as important over the study period. Six studies explored continuous infusions [12, 16, 20, 23, 29, 38] with either peripheral nerve or epidural infusions. The remaining studies evaluated single-shot peripheral nerve blocks.

3.4. Personnel Collecting Data. Twelve out of the 31 included studies (39%) used an independent or blinded assessor or independent assessment (i.e., postal survey) to assess patients' pain [12, 14, 17, 19, 22, 25–27, 33, 34, 36, 42].

3.5. Acute Pain Studies. All but two of the included studies focused on acute pain outcomes. Choi et al. assessed pain outcomes of acute and chronic pain [17] NRS at 4.5 months postoperatively and Wegener et al. [25] looked at the WOMAC (Western Ontario and McMaster Universities Osteoarthritis Index) score and VAS at two different time points (3 months and 12 months).

4. Discussion

This systematic review demonstrates that postoperative pain in regional anesthesia RCTs is reported inconsistently. The 31 studies included in this review utilised 15 different types of postoperative pain outcomes, measured at 51 different time points. Therefore at present, there appears to be multiple analyses of different nerve blocks in different centers using different acute pain outcome measures.

Heterogeneity in pain outcomes chosen in the included studies was high. One of the difficulties in deciding which pain outcomes to study in regional anesthesia trials is that there is no reliable method of *objectively* measuring postoperative pain [43]. Physiological parameters, such as heart rate and skin conductance, appear to correlate poorly with pain levels [44, 45]. Instead, pain is often measured by patient-reported intensity, surrogate measures such as the use of supplemental analgesia, or measures of the impact of pain on functioning including the following: sleep, coughing, or ability to perform activities of daily living. Each of these assessment strategies has strengths and limitations, which are demonstrated in this review by the majority of studies using two or more outcome measures to assess pain.

The visual analogue scale (VAS) is a widely used tool to assess postoperative pain. It is considered by some to be more sensitive to fine changes in pain score than numerical scales and four point scales [46]. It also has been shown to demonstrate generally high usability and acceptance; however, elderly patients have been found to not engage with this tool as well as younger patients, since lengthy explanations may be necessary and inconsistent marking along the line has previously been reported [47]. The NRS is another widely used tool to measure pain. Both VAS and NRS are one-dimensional pain tools that are easy to measure and largely reproducible, and thus it may explain why these are often chosen in preference to lengthier multidimensional tools, such as the McGill Pain Questionnaire. Since NRS is a verbal tool, requiring no writing or marking (in contrast to VAS), and is simple to perform by clinical and research team members [43], it should perhaps be considered as an ideal core outcome rather than VAS in studies involving elderly age groups.

Total opioid consumption over the study period (excluding daily and cumulative opioid consumption) was another popular outcome choice, which was utilised in 12 of the 31 studies reporting postoperative pain in this review. This outcome can be interpreted in different ways. A higher total opioid consumption value over a study period is presumed to indicate a higher pain state, necessitating requirement for supplemental opioid-based analgesia. Total opioid consumption could also reflect average pain scores (either NRS or VAS), with higher scores indicating greater opioid requirement. The psychological factors involved in patients requesting additional analgesia warrant further consideration. This involves evaluation of anticipated pain outcome with and without further analgesia, and in order for the request to be made, the patient must feel the treatment of pain outweighs the potential risk of side effects from the drug. This has been shown to be a key decision-making factor when patients are in pain [48]. Total opioid consumption as an outcome may therefore result in patients with different pain states, intensities, and satisfaction levels with analgesia being inappropriately grouped together.

Regional anesthesia is gaining popularity, partly due to improvements in safety and success attributed to ultrasound-guided techniques [49]. The Sprint National Anaesthesia Project (SNAP-1) examined patient-reported outcomes related to satisfaction with anesthesia [50]. Anxiety was found to be the worst part of the perioperative experience. With regard to anesthesia, specific reasons for dissatisfaction: thirst, drowsiness, pain at the surgical site, and hoarseness, were found to be among the most troubling for patients. Regional anesthesia (as a whole) was found to be associated with a reduced burden of side effects. It is unclear what level of pain correlates to adequate patient satisfaction in this population. Nine studies included in this systematic review utilised outcomes consisting of a variant of determinant of effective block duration such as time to first pain or time to first analgesic/opioid request. This suggests that some researchers value the importance of duration of patient being pain-free or experiencing a low enough pain level not to require additional analgesia. However, it should also be noted that a prolonged, dense block may not be in the patients' best interests and may be associated with worse patient satisfaction in this population.

Adequate assessment of pain, using validated tools appropriate to the population or individual, is an essential prerequisite of successful pain management. It has been shown in many countries that inadequate pain assessment is common, with resultant failings in management of pain [51]. Although our review may prove helpful to clinicians and researchers in the future, by summarizing some of the available measures, there are still unanswered questions in this field. In order to assimilate multiple studies with meta-analysis and to derive meaningful clinical conclusions, this review highlights the need for the formulation of a minimum set of outcomes that can be used in future regional anesthesia studies. Use of such a "core set of outcomes" would allow for comparison of outcomes from studies. The COMET or (Core Outcome Measures in Effectiveness Trials) group is a United Kingdom initiative set up in 2010 in response to disjointed outcome measures in clinical research as a whole [52]. Their aim is to standardize outcomes and provide a database from which researchers can access existing outcome sets to design future trials. Specific analysis into the subset of patients undergoing regional anesthesia requires further research. The perspective of patients of the correct demographic ("key stakeholders") must be considered when deciding core outcomes for postoperative pain assessment in regional anesthesia. This would require exploration of what patients expect following regional anesthesia, including pain expectations following surgery performed with regional anesthesia.

The core outcome set for chronic pain studies may help researchers decide which outcomes to utilize in future regional anesthesia pain studies. A core outcome set of six outcomes for chronic pain was formalised in 2005 by the Initiative on Methods, Measurement, and Pain Assessment in Clinical Trials (IMMPACT) group [53]. This group formalised outcomes to be used for physical functioning, emotional functioning, participant rating for improvement and satisfaction, symptoms and adverse events, and participant disposition, as well as for the assessment of pain. With regards to pain, recommendations included an 11 point 0–10 scale, usage of rescue analgesics, and categorical scale if the patient was unable to use a verbal scale. This systematic review has shown that the IMMPACT recommended pain outcomes for chronic pain are also the most commonly used in the acute pain setting in regional anesthesia RCTs. The 2005 IMMPACT recommendations, which are primarily for improving clinical trial methodology of chronic pain treatments, do not seem to have made any impact on outcomes in regional anesthesia efficacy studies. This may be because the pain outcomes considered clinically important in recovery following elective surgery are different to those important in patients with chronic pain. Acute pain can be reliably assessed, both at rest (important for comfort) and during movement (important for function and risk of postoperative complications), with one-dimensional tools such as NRS or VAS. Chronic pain assessment however and its impact on physical, emotional, and social functions require multidimensional qualitative tools and health-related quality of life instruments [51]. For example, it should be noted that while VAS was found to be one of the most commonly utilised acute pain outcomes identified in this review, it was omitted as an assessment for chronic pain outcomes.

When deciding what should be a "core outcome set," one must consider if there is an *implied* core set or if there are outcomes that are chosen more commonly among regional anesthesia studies. Until a core outcome set for regional anesthesia pain studies has been formulated, researchers may wish to consider utilizing the most commonly used outcomes identified in this review in order to allow for comparisons between existing data in the literature. It should however be noted that this assumes that the most commonly used outcomes represent what clinicians and researchers believe to be the most important. Based on frequency of utilization, this review suggests that the core outcomes for regional studies exploring acute pain should include NRS (verbal out of 10) at rest, NRS on activity, VAS at rest, total opioid consumption over the study period, analgesic consumption, and time to first analgesic request. The most commonly utilised time points of pain outcome data measurement in the descending order of frequency were 24, 4, 6, 12, and 48 hours postoperatively.

This review does have some limitations. Restricting included RCTs to English language studies may have reduced the number of clinically useful studies analysed. Additionally, the restriction to the top 20 impact factor journals may not reflect the outcome measures utilised in the majority of regional anesthesia studies. This did however serve as a marker of study quality and peer review, which we felt was required in this review. However, there are always risks inherent in limiting groups to be studied. The year of publication of included studies is important to note, and established blocks such as femoral nerve blocks may have already been extensively studied prior to 2005. Use of ultrasound guidance may have made some small differences to pain assessment outcome choice and the debate surrounding adductor canal versus femoral nerve block may continue; however, 2005 to 2017 is a relatively short period of time for major changes in clinical practice to have occurred. We limited the search to articles published over this 12-year period as our intention was to provide the reader with information regarding regional anesthesia studies that would be most relevant to current practice. Finally, although we have attempted to locate all relevant articles by using a robust search methodology, it is possible that with a review of this size, some relevant articles may have been missed. Furthermore, since these studies explore different peripheral nerve and plexus blocks, this may make it more difficult to derive an implied core outcome set from the included group of studies. We appreciate that different surgeries have different temporal pain profiles. Some surgeries for example may peak in pain immediately after surgery, whereas others may have pain that peaks when the nerve block wears off or during days following surgery. However, despite the apparent heterogeneity among the included studies, the vast majority of the RCTs included utilised generic outcomes and only one study used a scoring system specific to the type of surgery performed (the Western Ontario and McMasters Universities Osteoarthritis Index) [25, 54].

In summary, this robust review of the postoperative pain outcomes used in regional anesthesia RCTs between 2005 and 2017 demonstrates significant heterogeneity in choice of outcomes and times of measurements utilised. These findings represent a starting point for further work into developing a core outcome set for future regional anesthesia studies.

Appendix

A: Literature Search Terms

The basic components of the search were as follows:

> Postoperative pain (ti.ab) AND regional anaesthesia (ti.ab) AND randomised controlled trial (ti.ab) AND top 20 impact factor journals (j.n.) [limited to 2005–2017]

These were the search terms used in OpenAthens to formulate the final search:

(1) EMBASE, Medline, CINAHL; (((postoperative pain adj4 pain*) OR (post-operative adj4 pain*) OR post-operative-pain* OR (post* NEAR pain*) OR (post-operative adj4 analgesi*) OR (post-operative adj4 analgesi*) OR (post-operative adj4 analgesi*))) ti.ab

(2) EMBASE, Medline, CINAHAL; (((post-surgical adj4 pain*) OR ("post-surgical" adj4 pain*) OR (post-surgery adj4 pain*))) ti.ab

(3) EMBASE, Medline, CINAHL; ((("pain-relief after surgery") OR ("pain following surg") OR ("pain control after"))) ti.ab

(4) EMBASE, Medline, CINAHL; ((("post surg*" OR post-surg*) AND (pain* OR discomfort))) ti.ab

(5) EMBASE, Medline, CINAHL; (((pain* adj4 "after surg$") OR (pain* adj4 "follow* operat") OR (pain* adj4 "follow* surg*"))) ti.ab

(6) EMBASE, Medline, CINAHL; (((analgesi* adj4 "after surg*") OR (analgesi* adj4 "after operat*") OR (analgesi* adj4 "follow* operat*") OR (analgesi* adj4 "follow* surg*"))) ti.ab

(7) 1 OR 2 OR 3 OR 4 OR 5 OR 6

(8) "An?esthesia, Conduction" ti.ab

(9) "An?esthesia, Spinal" ti.ab

(10) "Analgesi, Epidural" ti.ab

(11) "An?esthesia, Epidural" ti.ab

(12) "An?esthesia, Caudal" ti.ab

(13) "Nerve Block" ti.ab

(14) "regional an?esthesia" ti.ab

(15) "conduction an?esthesia" ti.ab

(16) "spinal block" ti.ab

(17) "Epidural block" ti.ab

(18) "epidural an?esthesia" ti.ab

Table 4

Rank		Impact factor
1	Anesthesiology	5.879
2	Pain	5.213
3	British Journal of Anaesthesia	4.853
4	Pain physician	3.542
5	Anesthesia and Analgesia	3.472
6	Anaesthesia	3.382
7	Regional Anaesthesia and Pain management	3.089
8	Journal of Neurosurgical Anaesthesia	2.99
9	European Journal of Anaesthesia	2.942
10	European Journal of Pain	2.928
11	Canadian Journal of Anesthesia	2.527
12	Clinical Journal of Pain	2.527
13	Pain Practice	2.361
14	Acta Anaesthesia Scandinavia	2.322
15	Minerva Anesthesiology	2.134
16	Journal of Clinical Monitoring and Computing	1.985
17	Current Opinion Anesthesiology	1.979
18	*Pediatric Anesthesia	1.85
19	*International Journal of Obstetric Anesthesia	1.598
20	Journal of Cardiothoracic and Vascular Anaesthesia	1.463
21	BMC Anesthesiology	1.375
22	Anaesthesia and Intensive Care	1.296

*These journals cover obstetric and pediatric anesthesia; hence, they were not used in this study (owing to the inclusion criteria of general adult population).

(19) "plexus block" ti.ab

(20) (plexus AND block) ti.ab

(21) (bier AND block) ti.ab

(22) 8 OR 9 OR 10 OR 11 OR 12 OR 13 OR 14 OR 15 OR 16 OR 17 OR 18 OR 19 OR 20 OR 21

(23) ("randomi?ed controlled trial") OR ("randomi?ed trial") OR ("controlled trial") ti.ab

(24) EMBASE, Medline, CINAHL; ("anesthesiology" OR "pain" OR "british journal of anaesthesia" OR "pain physician"OR "anesthesia and analgesia" OR "anaesthesia" OR "regional anesthesia and pain medicine" OR "journal of neurosurgical anesthesia" OR "european journal of anaesthesia" OR "european journal of pain" OR "canadian journal of anesthesia" OR "clinical journal of pain" OR "pain practice" OR "acta anaesthesia scandinavia" OR "Minerva anesthesiology" OR "journal of clinical monitoring and computing" OR "current opinion anesthesiology" OR "journal of cardiothoracic and vascular anaesthesia" OR "BMC anesthesiology").jn

(25) 7 AND 22 AND 23 AND 24 [Limit to: Publication Year 2005–2017]

B: Top Impact Factor Journal List

These are the current impact factors of all the top international anesthesia journals as of 21st October 2015 [55] and were used as limiting functions in the literature review.

Conflicts of Interest

No study-related external funding or competing interests declared.

Authors' Contributions

All authors are responsible for data collection and data analysis and wrote the manuscript.

References

[1] A. Atchabahian, G. Schwartz, C. Hall, C. Lajam, and M. Andreae, *Regional Analgesia for Improvement of Long-Term Functional Outcome after Elective Large Joint Replacement*, The Cochrane Collaboration, London, UK, 2015.

[2] M. Andreae and D. Andreae, *Local Anaesthetics and Regional Anaesthesia for Preventing Chronic Pain after Surgery*, The Cochrane Collaboration, London, UK, 2012.

[3] M. Parker, H. Handoll, and R. Griffiths, *Anaesthesia for Hip Fracture in Adults*, The Cochrane Collaboration, London, UK, 2004.

[4] B. Afolabi and E. A. Foluso, *Regional versus General Anaesthesia for Caesarean Section*, The Cochrane Collaboration, London, UK, 2012.

[5] NICE, *Ultrasound-Guided Regional Nerve Block (ipg285)*, National Institute of Clinical Excellence Guidance, London, UK, 2009.

[6] NICE, *Hip Fracture: Managment*, National Institute of Clinical Excellence Guidance, London, UK, 2011.

[7] NICE, *Hip Fracture in Adults qs16*, National Institute of Clinical Excellence Guidance, London, UK, 2012.

[8] NICE, *Fractures (Non-Complex): Assessment and Managment (ng38)*, National Institute of Clinical Excellence Guidance, London, UK, 2016.

[9] A. Liberati, D. G. Altman, J. Tetzlaff et al., "The PRISMA statement for reporting systematic reviews and meta-analyses of studies that evaluate healthcare interventions: explanation and elaboration," *British Medical Journal*, vol. 339, no. 1, p. b2700, 2009.

[10] J. P. T. Higgins, D. G. Altman, and J. A. C. Sterne, *Chapter 8: Assessing Risk of Bias in Included Studies*, John Wiley & Sons Ltd., London, UK, 2011.

[11] A. R. Jadad, R. A. Moore, D. Carroll et al., "Assessing the quality of reports of randomized clinical trials: is blinding necessary?," *Controlled Clinical Trials*, vol. 17, no. 1, pp. 1–12, 1996.

[12] A. L. Ambrosoli, L. Guzzeti, M. Chiaranda, S. Cuffari, M. Gemma, and G. Cappelleri, "A randomised controlled trial comparing two popliteal nerve catheter tip positions for postoperative analgesia after day-case hallux valgus repair," *Anaesthesia*, vol. 71, no. 11, pp. 1317–1323, 2016.

[13] H. Andersen, J. Gym, L. Moller, B. Christensen, and D. Zaric, "Continuous saphenous nerve block as supplement to single dose local infiltration analgesia for postoperative pain management after total knee arthroplasty," *Regional Anaesthesia and Pain Medicine*, vol. 38, no. 2, pp. 106–111, 2013.

[14] N. Bharti, D. K. Sardana, and I. Bala, "The analgesic efficacy of dexmedetomidine as an adjunct to local anesthetics in supraclavicular brachial plexus block: a randomized, controlled trial," *Anesthesia and Analgesia*, vol. 121, no. 6, pp. 1655–1660, 2015.

[15] M. Boussofara, M. Carles, M. Raucoules-Aime, M. R. Sellam, and J. L. Horn, "Effects of intrathecal midazolam on post-operative analgesia when added to a bupivicaine-clonidine

mixture," *Regional Anaesthesia and Pain Medicine*, vol. 31, no. 6, pp. 501–505, 2006.

[16] X. Capdevilla, C. Dadure, S. Bringuier et al., "Effect of patient controlled perineural analgesia on rehabilitation and pain after ambulatory orthopaedic surgery: a multicentre randomized trial," *Anesthesiology*, vol. 105, no. 3, pp. 566–573, 2006.

[17] S. Choi, T. O'Hare, J. Gollish et al., "Optimizing pain and rehabilitation after knee arthroplasty: a two-center, randomized trial," *Anesthesia and Analgesia*, vol. 123, no. 5, pp. 1316–1324, 2016.

[18] M. Diakomi, M. Papaioannou, A. Mela, E. Kouskoni, and A. Makris, "Preoperative fascia iliaca compartment block for positioning patients with hip fractures for central nervous blockade: a randomized trial," *Regional Anaesthesia and Pain Medicine*, vol. 39, no. 5, pp. 394–398, 2014.

[19] N. M. Elkassabany, S. Antosh, M. Ahmed et al., "The risk of falls after total knee arthroplasty with the use of a femoral nerve block versus an adductor canal block: a double-blinded randomized controlled study," *Anesthesia & Analgesia*, vol. 122, no. 5, pp. 1696–1703, 2016.

[20] M. J. Fredrickson, C. M. Ball, and A. J. Dalgleish, "Posterior versus anterolateral approach interscalene catheter placement: a prospective randomized trial," *Regional Anaesthesia and Pain Medicine*, vol. 36, no. 2, pp. 125–133, 2011.

[21] G. Fritsch, T. Danninger, K. Allerberger, A. Tsodikov, and T. K. Felder, "Dexmedetomidine added to ropivicaine extends the duration of interscalene brachial plexus blocks for elective shoulder surgery when compared with ropivicaine alone: a single-centre, prospective, triple-blind, randomized controlled trial," *Regional Anaesthesia and Pain Medicine*, vol. 39, no. 1, pp. 37–47, 2014.

[22] W. Zhai, X. Wang, Y. Rong, M. Li, and H. Wang, "Effects of a fixed low-dose ropivicaine with different volume and concentrations on interscalene brachial plexus block: a randomized controlled trial," *BMC Anesthesiology*, vol. 16, no. 1, p. 80, 2015.

[23] M. Wongyingsinn, G. Baldini, P. Charlebois, S. Liberman, B. Stein, and F. Carli, "Intravenous lidocaine versus thoracic epidural analgesia: a randomized controlled trial in patients undergoing laparoscopic colorectal surgery using an enhanced recovery program," *Regional Anaesthesia and Pain Medicine*, vol. 36, no. 3, pp. 241–248, 2011.

[24] J. T. Wegener, B. Van Ooij, C. Van Dijk et al., "Value of single-injection or continuous sciactic nerve block in addition to a continuous femoral nerve block in patients undergoing total knee arthroplasty: a prospective, randomized, controlled trial," *Regional Anaesthesia and Pain Medicine*, vol. 36, no. 5, pp. 481–488, 2011.

[25] J. T. Wegener, B. Van, C. Van, S. A. Karayeva, and M. W. Hollman, "Long-term pain and functional disability after total knee arthroplasty with and without single-injection or continuous sciatic nerve block in addition to continuous femoral nerve block: a prospective, 1 year follow-up of a randomized controlled trial," *Regional Anaesthesia and Pain Medicine*, vol. 38, no. 1, pp. 1098–7339, 2013.

[26] K. H. Thybo, H. Schmidt, and D. Hagi-Pedersen, "Effect of lateral femoral cutaneous nerve block on pain after total hip arthroplasty: a randomised, blinded, placebo-controlled trial," *BMC Anesthesiology*, vol. 16, no. 1, p. 21, 2016.

[27] O. Stundner, M. Meissnitzer, C. M. Brummett et al., "Comparison of tissue distribution, phrenic nerve involvement, and epidural spread in standard vs low-volume ultrasound-guided interscalene plexus block using contrast magnetic resonance imaging: a randomized, controlled trial," *British Journal of Anaesthesia*, vol. 116, no. 3, pp. 405–412, 2016.

[28] R. Subramanyam, V. Vaishnave, V. W. Chan, D. Brown-Shreves, and R. Brull, "Lateral versus medial needle approach for ultrasound-guided supraclavicular block: a randomized controlled trial," *Regional Anaesthesia and Pain Medicine*, vol. 36, no. 4, pp. 387–392, 2011.

[29] K. Schoenmakers, M. Fenten, J. Louwerens, J. Scheffer, and R. Stiensra, "The effects of adding epinephrine to ropivicain for popliteal nerve block on the duration of postoperative analgesia: a randomized controlled trial," *BMC Anesthesiology*, vol. 15, no. 1, pp. 1471–2253, 2015.

[30] R. Sindjelic, G. Vlajkovic, L. Davidovic, D. Markovic, and D. Markovic, "The addition of fentanyl to local anesthetics affects the quality and duration of the cervical plexus block: a randomized, controlled trial," *Anesthesia and Analgesia*, vol. 111, no. 1, pp. 234–237, 2010.

[31] K. Sato, T. Adachi, N. Shirai, and N. Naoi, "Continuous versus single injection sciatic nerve block added to continuous femoral nerve block for analgesia after total knee arthroplasty: a prospective, randomised, double-blind study," *Regional Anaesthesia and Pain Medicine*, vol. 39, no. 3, pp. 225–229, 2014.

[32] M. Sawhney, H. Mehdian, B. Kashin et al., "Pain after unilateral total knee arthroplasty: a prospective randomized controlled trial examining the analgesic effectiveness of a combined adductor canal peripheral nerve block with periarticular infiltration versus adductor canal nerve block alone versus periarticular infiltration alone," *Anesthesia and Analgesia*, vol. 122, no. 6, pp. 2040–2046, 2016.

[33] E. Salviz, D. Xu, A. Frulla et al., "Continuous interscalene block in patients having outpatient rotator cuff repair surgery: a prospective randomized trial," *Anesthesia and Analgesia*, vol. 117, no. 6, pp. 1485–1492, 2013.

[34] M. Nagafuchi, T. Sato, T. Sakuma et al., "Femoral nerve block-sciatic nerve block vs. femoral nerve block-local infiltration analgesis for total knee arthroplasty: a randomized controlled trial," *BMC Anesthesiology*, vol. 15, no. 1, p. 182, 2015.

[35] E. C. Moura, C. A. de Oliveira Honda, R. C. Bringel, C. Leal Pda, J. Filho Gde, and R. K. Sakata, "Minimum effective concentration of bupivicaine in ultrasound-guided femoral nerve block after arthroscopic knee meniscectomy: a randomized, double-blind, controlled trial," *Pain Physician*, vol. 19, no. 1, pp. E79–E86, 2016.

[36] S. Kulhari, N. Bharti, I. Bala, S. Arora, and G. Singh, "Efficacy of pectoral nerve block versus thoracic paravertebral block for postoperative analgesia after radical mastectomy: a randomized controlled trial," *British Journal of Anaesthesia*, vol. 117, no. 3, pp. 382–386, 2016.

[37] V. S. Karthikeyan, S. C. Sistla, A. S. Badhe et al., "Randomized controlled trial on the efficacy of bilateral superficial cervical plexus block in thyroidectomy," *Pain Practice*, vol. 13, no. 7, pp. 539–546, 2013.

[38] M. Hamdani, O. Chassot, and R. Fournier, "Ultrasound-guided continuous interscalene block: the influence of local anesthetic background delivery method on postoperative analgesia after shoulder surgery: a randomized trial," *Regional Anaesthesia and Pain Medicine*, vol. 39, no. 5, pp. 387–393, 2014.

[39] Z. K. Bengisun, P. Ekmekci, B. Akan, A. Korotlu, and F. Tuzuner, "The effect of adding dexmedetomidine to levobupivicaine for interscalene block for postoperative pain managment after arthroscopic shoulder surgery," *Clinical Journal of Pain*, vol. 30, no. 12, pp. 1057–1061, 2014.

[40] J. T. YaDeau, T. Tedore, E. Goytizolo et al., "Lumbar plexus blockade reduces pain after hip arthroscopy: a prospective randomized controlled trial," *Anesthesia and Analgesia*, vol. 115, no. 4, pp. 968–972, 2012.
[41] Z. Siddiqui, M. Cepeda, W. Denman, R. Schumann, and D. Carr, "Continuous lumbar plexus block provided improved analgesia with fewer side effects compared with systemic opioids after hip arthroplasty: a randomized controlled trial," *Regional Anaesthesia and Pain Medicine*, vol. 32, no. 5, pp. 393–398, 2007.
[42] J. S. Kim, J. Lee, E. Y. Soh et al., "Analgesic effects of ultrasound-guided serratus-intercostal plane block and ultrasound-guided intermediate cervical plexus block after single-incision transaxillary robotic thyroidectomy: a prospective, randomized, controlled trial," *Regional Anesthesia and Pain Medicine*, vol. 41, no. 5, pp. 584–588, 2016.
[43] J. Younger, R. McCue, and S. Mackey, "Pain outcomes: A brief review of the instruments and techniques," *Current Pain and Headache Reports*, vol. 13, no. 1, pp. 39–43, 2009.
[44] P. Bossart, D. Fosnocht, and E. Swanson, "Changes in heart rate do not correlate with changes in pain intensity in emergency department patients," *Journal of Emergency Medicine*, vol. 32, no. 1, pp. 19–22, 2007.
[45] D. Harrison, S. Boyce, and P. Loughnan, "Skin conductance as a measure of pain and stress in hospitalised infants," *Early Human Developement*, vol. 82, no. 9, pp. 603–608, 2006.
[46] R. A. Seymour, "The use of pain scales in assessing the efficacy of analgesics in post-operative dental pain," *European Journal of Clinical Pharmacology*, vol. 23, no. 5, pp. 441–444, 1982.
[47] M. A. Williams, M. T. Oberst, B. C. Bjorklund, H. A. Kruse, and S. A. Coggon, "Response formats in questionnaires used with older adults," in *Proceedings of the 12th Annual Midwest Nursing Research Society Conference*, Wichita, KS, USA, December 1988.
[48] T. J. Gan, D. A. Lubarsky, E. M. Flood et al., "Patient preferences for acute pain treatment," *British Journal of Anaesthesia*, vol. 92, no. 5, pp. 681–688, 2004.
[49] F. Mirza and A. R. Brown, "Ultrasound-guided regional anesthesia for procedures of the upper extremity," *Anesthesiology Research and Practice*, vol. 2011, Article ID 579824, 6 pages, 2011.
[50] E. Walker, M. Bell, T. M. Cook, M. P. Grocott, and S. R. Moonesinghe, "Patient reported outcome of adult perioperative anaesthesia in the United Kingdom: a cross-sectional observational study," *British Journal of Anaesthesia*, vol. 117, no. 6, pp. 758–766, 2016.
[51] H. Breivik, P. Borchgrevink, S. Allen et al., "Assessment of pain," *British Journal of Anaesthesia*, vol. 101, no. 1, pp. 17–24, 2008.
[52] "Core outcome measures in effectiveness trials initiative," September 2015, http://www.comet-initiative.org/about/overview.
[53] R. Dworkin, D. Turk, J. Farrar et al., "Core outcome measure for chronic pain clinical trials: IMMPACT recommendations," *Pain*, vol. 113, no. 1, pp. 9–19, 2005.
[54] N. Bellamy, J. Campbell, J. Stevens, L. Pilcher, C. Stewart, and Z. Mahmood, "Validation study of a computerized version of the Western Ontario and McMaster Universities VA3.0 Osteoarthritis Index," *Journal of Rheumatology*, vol. 24, no. 12, pp. 2413–2415, 1997.
[55] M. Wang, J. P. Smith, R. Choy et al., "Impact factor list 2014," July 2018, http://www.citefactor.org/journal-impact-factor-list-2014.html.

23

Effects of Addition of Systemic Tramadol or Adjunct Tramadol to Lidocaine used for Intravenous Regional Anesthesia in Patients undergoing Hand Surgery

Abdulkadir Yektaş, Funda Gümüş, Abdulhalim Karayel, and Ayşin Alagöl

Anesthesiology and Reanimation Clinic, Bagcilar Training and Research Hospital, 34218 Istanbul, Turkey

Correspondence should be addressed to Abdulkadir Yektaş; akyektas722000@yahoo.co.uk

Academic Editor: Kouichiro Minami

Intravenous regional anesthesia (IVRA) is used in outpatient hand surgery as an easily applicable and cost-effective technique with clinical advantages. The present study aimed to investigate the effects of addition of systemic tramadol or adjunct tramadol to lidocaine for IVRA in patients undergoing hand surgery. American Society of Anesthesiologists (ASA) I-II patients ($n = 60$) who underwent hand surgery were included. For this purpose, only lidocaine (LDC), lidocaine+adjunct tramadol (LDC+TRA group), or lidocaine+systemic tramadol (LDC+SysTRA group) was administered to the patients for IVRA and the groups were compared in terms of onset and recovery time of sensory and motor blocks, quality of anesthesia, and the degree of intraoperative and postoperative pain. The onset time of sensorial block was significantly shorter in the LDC+TRA group than that in the LDC+SysTRA group. The motor block recovery time was significantly shorter in the LDC+SysTRA group than that in the LDC+TRA and LDC groups. Administration of tramadol as an adjunct showed some clinical benefits by providing a shorter onset time of sensory and motor block, decreasing pain and analgesic requirement, and improving intraoperative conditions during IVRA. It was determined that systemic tramadol administration had no superiority.

1. Introduction

Intravenous regional anesthesia (IVRA) is used in outpatient hand surgery as an easily applicable and cost-effective technique with clinical advantages and it is an ideal anesthetic method particularly for short lasting procedures [1]. Although IVRA has a history more than a century old, it has regained importance in the recent years as an effective and safe technique [2]. Nevertheless, IVRA has some disadvantages including anesthetic toxicity, slow-onset, poor muscle relaxation, tourniquet pain, and minimal postoperative pain relief [3]. Providing an ideal anesthesia by overcoming these disadvantages is possible with the addition of some adjunct agents to local anesthetics. These adjunct agents, which are added to the local anesthetics to provide improved block efficacy, decreased tourniquet pain, or prolonged duration of postdeflation analgesia in patients receiving IVRA, include opioids (fentanyl, meperidine, morphine, and sufentanil), tramadol, nonsteroidal anti-inflammatory drugs (NSAIDs; ketorolac, tenoxicam, and acetyl-salicylate), clonidine, and muscle relaxants (atracurium, pancuronium, and mivacurium) [3].

Tramadol, one of the adjunct agents used in IVRA, is a synthetic analgesic and has opioid and nonopioid characteristics. As compared to other opioids, tramadol is advantageous as it has lower side effects and abuse potential [4]. Tramadol has been demonstrated to have local anesthetic effect when administered via intradermal [5] and intravenous [6] routes. In an experimental study conducted on rats, tramadol was shown to block nociception and motor function *in vivo* similar to local anesthetics [7]. Addition of tramadol to mepivacaine has been demonstrated to prolong the duration of brachial plexus block without causing any side effect in patients undergoing forearm and hand surgery [8]. It has been determined that addition of tramadol as an adjunct to bupivacaine for supraclavicular brachial plexus block provides a faster onset of sensorial and motor block and a longer duration of motor block [9].

In light of the abovementioned information, the present study aimed to investigate the effects of addition of tramadol to lidocaine for IVRA in patients undergoing hand surgery. For this purpose, only lidocaine, lidocaine+adjunct tramadol, or lidocaine+systemic tramadol was administered to the patients for IVRA and the groups were compared in terms of onset and recovery times of sensory and motor blocks, quality of anesthesia, and the degree of intraoperative and postoperative pain.

2. Methods

2.1. Patients. The present study included American Society of Anesthesiologists (ASA) I-II patients ($n = 60$) who were planned to undergo hand surgery. Patients with Raynaud's disease, those with sickle-cell anemia, and those receiving any drug for history of allergy were excluded. Approval of the ethics committee and informed consents of the patients were obtained for the study.

According to a computer-generated randomization list, the patients were divided into three groups, containing 20 subjects in each. In the first group (LDC+TRA group), IVRA was performed with 3 mg/kg lidocaine (10% lidocaine, Aritmal, Biosel, Turkey) plus 50 mg tramadol, which were administered after diluting with saline to 40 mL. While performing IVRA, 30 mL saline was simultaneously administered to the systemic circulation. In the second group (LDC+SysTRA group), IVRA was performed with 3 mg/kg lidocaine, which was diluted with saline to 40 mL. While performing IVRA, 50 mg tramadol diluted with saline to 30 mL was simultaneously administered to the systemic circulation. In the third group (LDC group), IVRA was performed with 3 mg/kg lidocaine, which was diluted with saline to 40 mL. While performing IVRA, 30 mL saline was simultaneously administered to the systemic circulation. All solutions were prepared by resident anesthesiologists, who were blinded to the study, using identical injectors.

2.2. Surgical Procedure. The patients received premedication 45 min before the surgery with intramuscular 0.07 mg/kg midazolam and 0.01 mg/kg atropine. Two intravenous cannulas, one into the vein in the dorsal aspect of the hand that would undergo surgery and the other into the vein in the dorsal aspect of the opposite hand, were inserted for crystalloid infusion. The arm that would undergo surgery was elevated for 2 min and Esmarch's bandage was used to control blood flow. A double pneumatic tourniquet was placed around the upper arm and the proximal cuff was inflated to 250 mmHg. The absence of radial artery pulse in the arm isolated from the circulation was confirmed by the disappearance of pulse oximeter waves in the index finger of the same hand. The solutions, which were preprepared according to the groups defined above, were injected to the patients for over 90 s by an anesthesiologist blinded to the contents of drugs.

After the injection, the sensorial block was assessed every 30 s until the initiation of surgery by pinprick test using 22-gauge needle on the radial, ulnar, and median nerve stimulation areas of the hand and of the anterior surface of the arm. Motor function was checked by asking the patient to bring the wrist and finger to extension and flexion and the time of complete motor block was recorded when spontaneous movement was impossible. The time elapsing from the injection of the study drug until the sensorial block was provided in all stimulation areas was recorded as the onset time of sensorial block. Likewise, the time elapsing from the injection of the study drug until achieving the complete motor block was recorded as the onset time of motor block. After achieving complete motor block and sensorial block, the distal tourniquet was inflated to 250 mmHg, the proximal tourniquet was deflated, and the surgical procedure was initiated. Mean arterial pressure (MAP), oxygen saturation (SpO_2), and heart rate (HR) were monitored during the surgery, before and after tourniquet application, and until disappearance of anesthesia after deflating the tourniquet.

Pain level of the patients was assessed by 10 cm visual analogue scale (VAS; 0: no pain; 10: worst pain imaginable). VAS scores were recorded before and after tourniquet application as well as at 5th, 10th, 15th, 20th, 30th, 40th, and 50th min during the surgery. If the patient had a VAS score of >4 and if required, 1 μg/kg fentanyl was administered for analgesia and the dosage and time were recorded.

The tourniquet was not deflated earlier than 30 min and it was not inflated more than 2 h. Tourniquet deflation after the surgery was performed by periodic deflation technique. The time of sensorial recovery was recorded (the time elapsing from the deflation of tourniquet to the highest pain felt by the patient via pinprick test performed every 30 s in all stimulation areas). The time of motor block recovery (time elapsing from the deflation of tourniquet to the spontaneous movement of the fingers) was also recorded.

The patients were monitored in the postoperative care unit for the first 2 h and then in the observation room for 24 h by anesthesiologists who were blinded to the study. MAP, HR, and SpO_2 monitoring and VAS measurement were performed at the postoperative 1st, 2nd, 4th, 6th, 12th, and 24th h. The patients with a VAS score of >4 were given 75 mg diclofenac sodium via intramuscular route. Analgesia requirement was recorded as duration and dosage.

The patients were monitored for intraoperative and postoperative complications. In the event of hypotension (systolic arterial pressure < 90 mmHg or a decrease of more than 50 mmHg from the normal value) during the surgery, 5 mg intravenous ephedrine was administered. In case of bradycardia (HR < 50/min), 0.5 mg intravenous atropine was administered. Intravenous 4 mg ondansetron was administered for nausea and vomiting and oxygen was supplied via a facial mask when SpO_2 decreased by more than 91%.

An anesthesiologist and a surgeon, who were blinded to the content of study drug, assessed the quality of anesthesia at the end of surgery as follows: 4: excellent, patient not complaining; 3: good, patient complaining a little, no need for supplemental analgesic; 2: moderate, patient complaining,

Table 1: General characteristics of the patients.

	Groups			
	LDC+TRA $n = 20$	LDC+SysTRA $n = 20$	LDC $n = 20$	p
Age, year	36.55 ± 11.82	41.65 ± 12.47	44.1 ± 13.09	0.063
Gender				
Male	9 (45.0)	14 (70.0)	13 (65.0)	0.233
Female	11 (55.0)	6 (30.0)	7 (35.0)	
Body weight, kg	74.25 ± 15.78	78.6 ± 14.01	77 ± 16.52	0.594
Height, cm	167.95 ± 11.76	172.9 ± 10.7	169.8 ± 10.63	0.605
ASA				
I	15 (75.0)	17 (85.0)	15 (75.0)	0.675
II	5 (25.0)	3 (15.0)	5 (25.0)	
Type of surgery				
Carpal tunnel	5 (25.0)	7 (35.0)	8 (40.0)	0.592
Guyon's channel	6 (30.0)	6 (30.0)	6 (30.0)	1.000
Tendon repair	8 (40.0)	7 (35.0)	6 (30.0)	0.803
Duration of surgery, min	27 (20–40)	25 (20–32.5)	25 (20–33)	0.912
Tourniquet time, min	38 (32.5–55)	42 (36.5–47)	35 (30–43.5)	0.104

ASA, American Society of Anesthesiologists.
Values are presented as mean ± standard deviation, number (%), or median (Q1–Q3).

need for supplemental analgesic; 1: failed, need for general anesthesia.

2.3. Statistical Analysis. The Predictive Analytics Software (PASW) version 18.0 for Windows program (SPSS Inc., Chicago, IL, USA) was used for statistical analysis. Descriptive statistics were expressed as number and percentage for categorical variables and as mean, standard deviation, median, the 25th percentile (Q1: the first quartile), and the 75th percentile (Q3: the third quartile) for numerical variables. For numerical variables, independent multiple group comparisons were performed by Kruskal-Wallis test for nonnormally distributed data and by t-test for normally distributed data. Mann-Whitney U test with Bonferroni correction was used for subgroup analysis of nonnormally distributed numerical variables. For multiple group comparisons of categorical variables, Chi-square test statistics were used in case the assumption of Chi-square test was met, whereas Fisher's exact test was used in case the assumption of Chi-square test was not met. A p value of <0.05 was considered statistically significant.

With the assumption that the difference in the VAS score at the 5th min between the two surgical techniques is 1 and the expected standard deviation for two groups is 0.9, it was estimated to include 20 patients in the groups for which the least difference was expected. The statistical significance level was calculated as 0.015 owing to the presence of 3 groups and with the prediction that repeated measurement analysis would be performed assuming that the Bonferroni correction would be used. The power of the present study was 80% with these calculations.

3. Results

General characteristics of the patients are summarized in Table 1. No difference was determined among the groups in terms of age, gender, body weight, height, ASA level, type and duration of surgery, and tourniquet time.

A significant difference was determined among the groups in terms of onset time of sensorial block and recovery time of motor block. The onset time of sensorial block was significantly shorter in the LDC+TRA group than in the LDC+SysTRA group. The motor block recovery time was significantly shorter in the LDC+SysTRA group than in the LDC+TRA and LDC groups (Table 2).

The changes in VAS scores in time are illustrated in Figure 1. The VAS scores were observed to be generally lower in the LDC+TRA group. There were significant differences among the groups in terms of VAS scores measured after tourniquet application and at the postoperative 24th h (Table 3).

The patients' need for fentanyl and diclofenac as well as quality of anesthesia, which was assessed by the anesthesiologist and the surgeon, is demonstrated in Table 4. Although it was not found to be significant, the number of patients in need of intraoperative fentanyl and postoperative diclofenac was lower in the LDC+TRA group and the score of the quality of anesthesia was higher in the LDC+TRA and LDC+SysTRA groups.

In the LDC+TRA group, intraoperative adverse events were hypotension ($n = 2$), bradycardia ($n = 3$), nausea ($n = 1$), and shivering ($n = 1$) and postoperative adverse events were nausea ($n = 1$), tinnitus ($n = 1$), and vertigo

TABLE 2: Onset and recovery times for sensorial block and motor block.

	Groups			
	LDC+TRA $n = 20$	LDC+SysTRA $n = 20$	LDC $n = 20$	p
SB onset time, s	115 (60–124)[b]	180 (120–205)[a]	120 (80–180)	**0.015**
SB recovery time, s	120 (60–180)	89.5 (60–90)	90 (84–120)	0.071
MB onset time, s	120 (90–211.5)	210 (180–245)	210 (180–240)	0.166
MB recovery time, s	120 (69.5–180)[b]	30 (30–60)[ac]	115 (75–170)[b]	**<0.001**

SB, sensorial block; MB, motor block.
Values are presented as median (Q1–Q3).
[a]Different from the LDC+TRA group; [b]different from the LDC+SysTRA group; [c]different from the LDC group ($p < 0.017$ with Bonferroni correction).

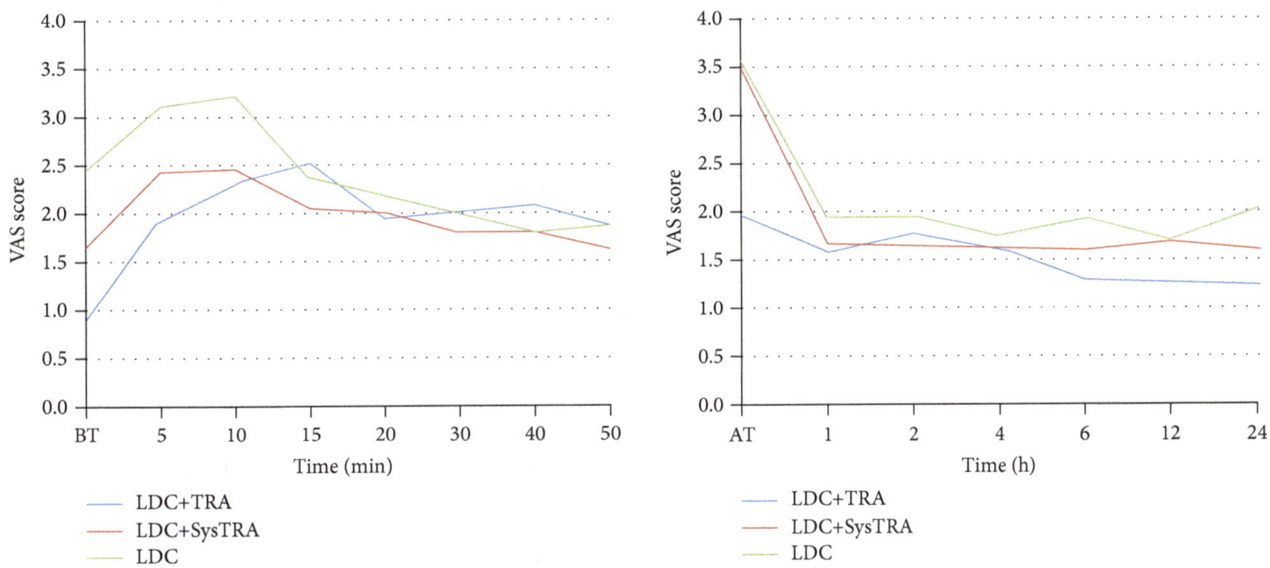

FIGURE 1: Change in visual analogue scale (VAS) scores in time. BT, before tourniquet; AT, after tourniquet.

($n = 2$). The only postoperative adverse event was vertigo in 1 patient in LDC+SysTRA group. Postoperative shivering ($n = 1$) and metallic taste ($n = 1$) were observed in the LDC group.

4. Discussion

Reducing pain and need for analgesics by enhancing the quality of anesthesia is one of the main goals in patients undergoing IVRA. For this purpose, clinical studies have been performed by adding various agents such as dexamethasone [10], midazolam [11], diltiazem [12], dexmedetomidine [13], paracetamol [14], lornoxicam [15, 16], nitroglycerine [17], magnesium [18], and ketamine [19], to the local anesthetic solution and the search for the agent that would provide the most appropriate outcome with the least side effect is ongoing. In the present study, the effects of addition of tramadol to lidocaine were evaluated. In addition, the effects of addition of adjunct or systemic tramadol to lidocaine were compared.

In the present study, the absence of difference among the three patient groups in terms of demographic characteristics such as age, gender, body weight, and height, as well as ASA level, type and duration of surgery, and tourniquet time suggested that the groups were comparable in terms of other parameters. Onset times of sensorial and motor blocks were found to be shorter in the group that received tramadol as an adjunct in IVRA application than in the other two groups; however, the difference was significant only between the LDC+TRA and LDC+SysTRA groups in terms of onset time of sensorial block. In general, VAS scores tended to be lower when tramadol was added to lidocaine. However, statistical significance was determined after tourniquet application and at the postoperative 24th h. With regard to need for analgesics, the number of patients in need of intraoperative fentanyl and postoperative diclofenac was lower in the LDC+TRA group and the scores of quality of anesthesia were higher in the two groups that received tramadol than in the group that received only lidocaine; however, the differences were not statistically significant.

In the literature, studies on the addition of tramadol to lidocaine during IVRA have reported different results. Acalovschi et al. [20] conducted a study in voluntary medical students ($n = 60$) and concluded that a solution including 100 mg tramadol alone had no local anesthetic effect for IVRA. Nevertheless, when administered together

TABLE 3: Visual analogue scale scores at different times.

Measuring time	Groups LDC+TRA $n = 20$	LDC+SysTRA $n = 20$	LDC $n = 20$	p
Before tourniquet	1 (1-1)	1 (1-1)	1 (1–3.5)	0.058
After tourniquet	1.5 (0–4)[bc]	4 (2–5)[a]	3 (2–5.5)[a]	**0.041**
Intraoperative 5th min	1.5 (0.5–3)	2 (1.5–3)	3 (1.5–4.5)	0.103
Intraoperative 10th min	2 (0–4)	2 (2-3)	2 (2–5)	0.409
Intraoperative 15th min	2 (0–3.5)	2 (1.5–2)	2 (2-3)	0.761
Intraoperative 20th min	2 (0.5–2)	2 (2-2)	2 (2-2)	0.895
Intraoperative 30th min	2 (0.5–2)	2 (2-2)	2 (2-2)	0.852
Intraoperative 40th min	2 (1-2)	2 (2-2)	2 (2-2)	0.984
Intraoperative 50th min	2 (0.5–2)	2 (1.5–2)	2 (2-2)	0.739
Postoperative 1st h	2 (0–2)	2 (1.5–2)	2 (2-2)	0.387
Postoperative 2nd h	2 (0.5–2)	2 (1.5–2)	2 (2-2)	0.434
Postoperative 4th h	2 (1-2)	2 (1.5–2)	2 (2-2)	0.692
Postoperative 6th h	2 (0.5–2)	2 (1.5–2)	2 (2-2)	0.092
Postoperative 12th h	1.5 (0.5–2)	2 (2-2)	2 (2-2)	0.081
Postoperative 24th h	1.5 (0.5–2)[c]	2 (1.5–2)	2 (2-2)[a]	**0.025**

Values are presented as median (Q1–Q3).
[a]Different from the LDC+TRA group; [b]different from the LDC+SysTRA group; [c]different from the LDC group ($p < 0.017$ with Bonferroni correction).

TABLE 4: Patients' need for analgesics and evaluation of quality of anesthesia.

	Groups LDC+TRA $n = 20$	LDC+SysTRA $n = 20$	LDC $n = 20$	p
Fentanyl				
Patients in need	6 (30.0)	12 (60.0)	13 (65.0)	0.057
Time of initial need, min	0 (0–5)	5 (0–7.5)	5 (0–10)	0.265
Intraoperative consumption, μg	0 (0–62.5)	50 (0–75)	50 (0–75)	0.142
Diclofenac sodium				
Patients in need	15 (75.0)	18 (90.0)	20 (100.0)	0.055
Time of initial need, min	24 (1.5–420)	360 (120–420)	360 (240–360)	0.071
Total consumption, mg	75 (37.5–150)	75 (75-75)	75 (75-75)	0.801
Score of the quality of anesthesia				
Assessed by the anesthesiologist	4 (3-4)	4 (3-4)	3.5 (2.5–4)	0.334
Assessed by the surgeon	4 (3.5–4)	4 (3-4)	3.5 (2–4)	0.201

Values are presented as median (Q1–Q3) or number (%).

with lidocaine, tramadol modifies its effect and shortens the onset time of sensory block in IVRA. Aslan et al. [21] investigated the effect of addition of morphine or tramadol (1.5 mg/kg) to lidocaine for IVRA in 90 patients undergoing hand and forearm surgery. They concluded that the addition of morphine or tramadol to lidocaine enhanced the levels of sensorial block and postoperative analgesia with no effect on tourniquet pain, quality of motor block, duration of analgesia, and analgesic consumption. Alayurt et al. [22] conducted a study in 60 patients undergoing hand surgery and reported that the addition of 100 mg tramadol to lidocaine for IVRA increased the quality of anesthesia, reduced the onset of the sensory block, delayed the onset time of tourniquet pain, and decreased the intraoperative consumption of opioid; however, it had no effect on the postoperative pain. Langlois et al. [23] investigated the effect of addition of 100 mg tramadol to lidocaine for IVRA in 30 patients undergoing carpal tunnel decompression. They reported that pain scales and analgesic request did not differ at any of the time periods studied; accordingly, efficacy of tramadol and lidocaine combination was concluded not to be higher than lidocaine alone. In their study on 54 patients undergoing upper limb surgery, Tan et al. [24] reported that the addition of 50 mg tramadol to lidocaine for IVRA appeared to be helpful in enhancing the quality of anesthesia and observed that higher number of patients had faster onset of sensory and motor block in the group that received tramadol, although the difference was not significant. Moreover, the pain score 30 min after tourniquet inflation and after changing over to the distal tourniquet was significantly lower in the lidocaine+tramadol group than in the group that received lidocaine alone. The reason for different results obtained in different studies may be the heterogeneous patient groups as well as different tramadol doses used in the studies. In their study on 60 ASA I-II patients who were planned to undergo hand surgery, Siddiqui et al. [25] compared the effects of addition of two different doses of tramadol (50 mg versus 100 mg) to lidocaine. They reported that tramadol 100 mg shortened the onset of sensory block, increased the tourniquet tolerance, and improved the perioperative analgesia and thereby concluded that addition of tramadol 100 mg to lidocaine is useful for IVRA.

In their review, Flamer and Peng [26] compared the local anesthetics and adjunct substances used for IVRA in terms of intraoperative efficacy and postoperative outcomes and reported an acceleration in the onset of sensory block, tourniquet tolerance but inconsistent postoperative benefits, and increased risk of minor side effects with the use of tramadol. It has been reported that intravenous tramadol administration reduces postoperative pain and shivering [27]. In the present study, postoperative shivering was observed in 1 patient and metallic taste was observed in 1 patient in the group that received only lidocaine. In the group that received tramadol as an adjunct, hypotension ($n = 2$), bradycardia ($n = 3$), nausea ($n = 1$), and shivering ($n = 1$) were noted intraoperatively, whereas nausea ($n = 1$), tinnitus ($n = 1$), and vertigo ($n = 2$) were observed postoperatively. In the group that received systemic tramadol, only one patient developed postoperative vertigo.

In conclusion, administration of tramadol as an adjunct showed some clinical benefits by providing a shorter onset time of sensory and motor block, decreasing pain and analgesic requirement, and improving intraoperative conditions during IVRA. The visual analogue scale scores were observed to be generally lower in the LDC+TRA group, and the score of the quality of anesthesia was higher in the LDC+TRA and LDC+SysTRA groups.

Disclosure

Abdulkadir Yektaş is the archival author and attests to the integrity of the original data and the analysis reported in the present paper. Funda Gümüş, Abdulhalim Karayel, and Ayşin Alagöl attest to the integrity of the original data and the analysis reported in the present paper.

Competing Interests

The authors reported no competing interests regarding the publication of this paper.

Authors' Contributions

Abdulkadir Yektaş, Funda Gümüş, and Abdulhalim Karayel had contributed to the design and conduct of the study, data collection and analysis, and preparation of the paper. Ayşin Alagöl had contributed to the data collection and analysis and preparation of the paper.

References

[1] V. W. S. Chan, P. W. H. Peng, Z. Kaszas et al., "A comparative study of general anesthesia, intravenous regional anesthesia, and axillary block for outpatient hand surgery: clinical outcome and cost analysis," *Anesthesia and Analgesia*, vol. 93, no. 5, pp. 1181–1184, 2001.

[2] A. dos Reis Jr., "Intravenous regional anesthesia—first century (1908–2008). Beggining, development, and current status," *Revista Brasileira de Anestesiologia*, vol. 58, no. 3, pp. 299–321, 2008 (Portuguese).

[3] A. Choyce and P. Peng, "A systematic review of adjuncts for intravenous regional anesthesia for surgical procedures," *Canadian Journal of Anesthesia*, vol. 49, no. 1, pp. 32–45, 2002.

[4] M. Vazzana, T. Andreani, J. Fangueiro et al., "Tramadol hydrochloride: pharmacokinetics, pharmacodynamics, adverse side effects, co-administration of drugs and new drug delivery systems," *Biomedicine and Pharmacotherapy*, vol. 70, pp. 234–238, 2015.

[5] W.-W. Pang, M. S. Mok, D.-P. Chang, and M.-H. Huang, "Local anesthetic effect of tramadol, metoclopramide, and lidocaine following intradermal injection," *Regional Anesthesia and Pain Medicine*, vol. 23, no. 6, pp. 580–583, 1998.

[6] W.-W. Pang, P.-Y. Huang, D.-P. Chang, and M.-H. Huang, "The peripheral analgesic effect of tramadol in reducing propofol injection pain: a comparison with lidocaine," *Regional Anesthesia and Pain Medicine*, vol. 24, no. 3, pp. 246–249, 1999.

[7] A. M. Sousa, H. A. Ashmawi, L. S. Costa, I. P. Posso, and A. Slullitel, "Percutaneous sciatic nerve block with tramadol induces analgesia and motor blockade in two animal pain models," *Brazilian Journal of Medical and Biological Research*, vol. 45, no. 2, pp. 147–152, 2012.

[8] S. Kapral, G. Gollmann, B. Waltl et al., "Tramadol added to mepivacaine prolongs the duration of an axillary brachial plexus blockade," *Anesthesia and Analgesia*, vol. 88, no. 4, pp. 853–856, 1999.

[9] V. Nagpal, S. Rana, J. Singh, and S. K. Chaudhary, "Comparative study of systemically and perineurally administered tramadol as an adjunct for supraclavicular brachial plexus block," *Journal of Anaesthesiology Clinical Pharmacology*, vol. 31, no. 2, pp. 191–195, 2015.

[10] Z. Bigat, N. Boztug, N. Hadimioglu, N. Cete, N. Coskunfirat, and E. Ertok, "Does dexamethasone improve the quality of intravenous regional anesthesia and analgesia? A randomized, controlled clinical study," *Anesthesia and Analgesia*, vol. 102, no. 2, pp. 605–609, 2006.

[11] P. Kashefi, K. Montazeri, A. Honarmand, M. Safavi, and H. M. Hosseini, "The analgesic effect of midazolam when added to lidocaine for intravenous regional anaesthesia," *Journal of Research in Medical Sciences*, vol. 16, no. 9, pp. 1139–1148, 2011.

[12] P. Khanna, V. K. Mohan, and R. A. Sunder, "Efficacy of diltiazem as an adjunct to lignocaine in intravenous regional anesthesia," *Saudi Journal of Anaesthesia*, vol. 7, no. 3, pp. 305–309, 2013.

[13] D. Memiş, A. Turan, B. Karamanlioğlu, Z. Pamukçu, and I. Kurt, "Adding dexmedetomidine to lidocaine for intravenous regional anesthesia," *Anesthesia and Analgesia*, vol. 98, no. 3, pp. 835–840, 2004.

[14] H. Sen, Y. Kulahci, E. Bicerer, S. Ozkan, G. Dagl, and A. Turan, "The analgesic effect of paracetamol when added to lidocaine for intravenous regional anesthesia," *Anesthesia and Analgesia*, vol. 109, no. 4, pp. 1327–1330, 2009.

[15] S. Sen, B. Ugur, O. N. Aydin, M. Ogurlu, E. Gezer, and O. Savk, "The analgesic effect of lornoxicam when added to lidocaine for intravenous regional anaesthesia," *British Journal of Anaesthesia*, vol. 97, no. 3, pp. 408–413, 2006.

[16] N. Sertoz, N. Kocaoglu, and H. Ö. Ayanoğlu, "Comparison of lornoxicam and fentanyl when added to lidocaine in intravenous regional anesthesia," *Brazilian Journal of Anesthesiology*, vol. 63, no. 4, pp. 311–316, 2013.

[17] S. Sen, B. Ugur, O. N. Aydin, M. Ogurlu, F. Gursoy, and O. Savk, "The analgesic effect of nitroglycerin added to lidocaine on intravenous regional anesthesia," *Anesthesia and Analgesia*, vol. 102, no. 3, pp. 916–920, 2006.

[18] A. Turan, D. Memiş, B. Karamanlioğlu, T. Güler, and Z. Pamukçu, "Intravenous regional anesthesia using lidocaine and magnesium," *Anesthesia and Analgesia*, vol. 100, no. 4, pp. 1189–1192, 2005.

[19] C. M. Viscomi, A. Friend, C. Parker, T. Murphy, and M. Yarnell, "Ketamine as an adjuvant in lidocaine intravenous regional anesthesia: a randomized, double-blind, systemic control trial," *Regional Anesthesia and Pain Medicine*, vol. 34, no. 2, pp. 130–133, 2009.

[20] I. Acalovschi, T. Cristea, S. Margarit, and R. Gavrus, "Tramadol added to lidocaine for intravenous regional anesthesia," *Anesthesia and Analgesia*, vol. 92, no. 1, pp. 209–214, 2001.

[21] B. Aslan, S. Izdeş, E. Kesimci, T. Gümüs, and O. Kanbak, "Comparison of the effects of lidocaine, lidocaine plus tramadol and lidocaine plus morphine for intravenous regional anesthesia," *Agri*, vol. 21, no. 1, pp. 22–28, 2009.

[22] S. Alayurt, D. Memis, and Z. Pamukcu, "The addition of sufentanil, tramadol or clonidine to lignocaine for intravenous regional anaesthesia," *Anaesthesia and Intensive Care*, vol. 32, no. 1, pp. 22–27, 2004.

[23] G. Langlois, J.-P. Estèbe, M. E. Gentili, L. Kerdilès, P. Mouilleron, and C. Ecoffey, "The addition of tramadol to lidocaine does not reduce tourniquet and postoperative pain during iv regional anesthesia," *Canadian Journal of Anesthesia*, vol. 49, no. 2, pp. 165–168, 2002.

[24] S. M. Tan, L. L. Pay, and S. T. Chan, "Intravenous regional anaesthesia using lignocaine and tramadol," *Annals of the Academy of Medicine Singapore*, vol. 30, no. 5, pp. 516–519, 2001.

[25] A. K. Siddiqui, H. A. Mowafi, A. M. Al-Ghamdi, S. A. Ismail, and H. A. AbuZeid, "Tramadol as an adjuvant to intravenous regional anesthesia with lignocaine," *Saudi Medical Journal*, vol. 29, no. 8, pp. 1151–1155, 2008.

[26] D. Flamer and P. W. H. Peng, "Intravenous regional anesthesia: a review of common local anesthetic options and the use of opioids and muscle relaxants as adjuncts," *Local and Regional Anesthesia*, vol. 4, no. 1, pp. 57–76, 2011.

[27] S. Grond and A. Sablotzki, "Clinical pharmacology of tramadol," *Clinical Pharmacokinetics*, vol. 43, no. 13, pp. 879–923, 2004.

24

Does the use of Nitroglycerin Patch Improve Local Anaesthetic Effects in Bier's Block?

Ahmed Said Elgebaly

Department of Anesthesia and Postsurgical Intensive Care, Faculty of Medicine, Tanta University, Tanta, Egypt

Correspondence should be addressed to Ahmed Said Elgebaly; elgebaly_13@hotmail.com

Academic Editor: Michael Frass

Aim. The aim of the study was to assess the nitroglycerin patch as a new additive to Bier's block and its impact on the effects and dose of lidocaine. *Methods.* Forty patients of each sex belonging to ASA I or II underwent elective tendon repair surgeries of the forearm and hand. The patients were divided into two equal groups as follows: Group C received only lidocaine (1.5 mg/kg, 0.25%) and Group N received lidocaine (1.5 mg/kg, 0.25%) + 5 mg transcutaneous nitroglycerin patch. Onset and recovery times for sensory and motor block, visual analogue scale (VAS) scores for bandage pain, postoperative VAS score, analgesic requirements, patients' satisfaction, and surgeons' opinion were recorded. *Results.* Sensory block onset time was shorter in Group N (3.80 ± 1.0) than that in Group C (5.72 ± 1.46), and motor block onset time was shorter in Group N (10.72 ± 1.93) than that in Group C (13.56 ± 1.26). Sensory block recovery time was prolonged in Group N (10.56 ± 1.12) than Group C (6.88 ± 1.45), recovery time of motor block was prolonged in Group N (13.04 ± 1.57) than Group C (11.96 ± 1.72). Bandage pain had lower VAS scores in Group N. Postoperative VAS scores showed significant differences between both groups at the following points of measurement: 30 minutes, 1 hour, and 4 hours after bandage deflation. Postoperative analgesic effect was the longest in Group N (187.20 ± 60.79 min) than Group C (51.60 ± 25.28 min). Patients' satisfaction and surgeons' opinion were better in Group N than Group C. *Conclusion.* Supplementation of Bier's block with transcutaneous nitroglycerin patch reduces the lidocaine dose, the sensory and motor block onset times, VAS scores, and analgesic consumption intra- and postoperatively. Length of the block recovery times for the sensory and motor effects, duration of postoperative analgesic effect, and the first time to analgesic requirement improved the quality of Bier's block with better patients' satisfaction and surgeons' opinion and had no adverse effects.

1. Introduction

Bier's block is a technique that is mostly used for providing anaesthesia and analgesia during the operation. Using additives with lidocaine may provide satisfactory anaesthesia and prolong the duration of postoperative analgesia [1].

Intravenous regional anaesthesia (IVRA) which was firstly described by August Bier in 1902 [2] is used successfully as a sole technique for upper limb surgeries [3]. It is a reliable, simple, cost-effective, and widely accepted technique of regional anaesthesia [1].

Disadvantages of Bier's block include the potential for local anaesthetic toxicity, emergence of pain following removal of the bandage (within three to five minutes), and lack of postoperative analgesia [4, 5]. Several adjuncts have been used including narcotics, nonsteroidal anti-inflammatory drugs (NSAIDs), muscle relaxants, α_2 agonists, and neostigmine [6].

Nitroglycerin (NTG) and nitric oxide generator contained in transcutaneous nitroglycerin help the distribution and absorption of local anaesthetic agents to neuron and trunks by vasodilatation [7, 8]. The aim of the present study was to evaluate whether the supplementation of 5 mg nitroglycerin patch to low-dose lidocaine will improve the overall Bier's block effect either intra- or postoperatively as primary outcomes and analgesic requirements, patients' satisfaction, and surgeons' opinion as secondary outcomes.

2. Materials and Methods

After obtaining the approval from the native Ethics and Research Committee, written informed consent from all the study participants was obtained. A double-blind prospective randomized study enrolled 40 ASA physical status I or II patients of each sex, aged ≥18 years and undergoing elective tendon repair surgeries of the forearm. Patients who refused; patients with Reynauld's disease, sickle-cell disease, crush injuries, and swelling or skin infection at the site of injection; and patients with a history of allergy to nitroglycerin or lidocaine and surgeries >60 minutes or <30 minutes were excluded from the study.

After history taking, complete clinical examination and laboratory investigations, monitoring of the patient with noninvasive blood pressure (NIBP), ECG, and peripheral oxygen saturation was performed. A peripheral venous line with 20-Gauge cannula was inserted in the contralateral hand for crystalloid infusion.

Randomization by use of sealed envelopes and allocation of patients to two equal groups were done as follows:

Group C (control group): 40 cc of 1.5 mg/kg of 0.25% lidocaine diluted in normal saline (0.9% NaCl) was used for administering Bier's block. Empty nitroglycerin patch was applied on the ventral aspect of the proximal forearm of the operative arm 2 hours preoperatively.

Group N (lidocaine and transdermal nitroglycerin patch group): 40 cc of 1.5 mg/kg of 0.25% lidocaine diluted in normal saline (0.9% NaCl) with application of 5 mg of transcutaneous nitroglycerin patch was used for administering Bier's block. Nitroglycerin patch was applied on the ventral aspect of the proximal forearm of the operative arm 2 hours preoperatively. Another peripheral venous line with 22-Gauge cannula was inserted in the dorsum of the operative hand (as distal as possible) for injection of the study drugs.

A double pneumatic bandage was placed on the upper arm with generous layers of cotton padding on the operative side ensuring that no wrinkles are formed and the bandage edges do not touch the skin, and then it was exsanguinated by 2-minute elevation and wrapping with an Esmarch bandage.

Before lidocaine was injected, circulatory isolation of the arm was verified by inspection, absence of radial pulse, and loss of pulse oximetry tracing in the ipsilateral index finger, and then the lidocaine solution was injected by inflation to a minimum of 250 mmHg for bandage lying at the proximal site.

Block onset was estimated after ten minutes of local anaesthetic administration. Distal bandage was inflated up to 250 mmHg after fifteen minutes, and the proximal bandage was deflated after taking out transdermal nitroglycerin patch. If no block occurs up to 15 minutes, the patient was excluded and replaced with another matched one. Deflation of cuff was not done until thirty minutes after lidocaine injection passed because systemic toxicity of lidocaine may occur and was not inflated for more than one and a half hours.

Assessment of demographic data, duration of surgery, sensory and motor block onset and recovery times, onset time of bandage pain and number of patients complaining from it, and intraoperative and 24-hour postoperative analgesic requirements was performed. Postoperative VAS score and first time of analgesic requirement were recorded.

Patients' satisfaction was obtained by asking the patient to rate the operative conditions according to the following numerical scale: 0 = unsuccessful, 1 = poor, 2 = moderate (pain required supplemental analgesia), 3 = good (minor pain with no need of supplemental analgesia), and 4 = excellent (no pain). Also surgeons' opinion was also obtained. As surgeons were blind to randomization of the patients, they rate the conditions of the operation with regard to movement of limb or bleeding, and the scores were as follows: 4 = excellent, 3 = good, 2 = acceptable, 1 = poor, and 0 = unsuccessful. Complications such as CNS (circum oral numbness, headache, convulsions, or coma) or CVS (bradycardia, arrhythmia, or hypotension) were recorded.

2.1. Statistical Analysis. IBM SPSS software package version 20.0 was used for analysis of the collected data. Mean ± standard deviation (SD) was used to express the quantitative data. Frequency and percentage were used to express the qualitative data. When comparing between two means, the independent-samples *t*-test of significance was used. In order to compare proportions between two qualitative parameters, chi-square (χ^2) test of significance was used.

3. Results

Age, sex, weight, ASA physical status, duration, and type of surgery showed insignificant difference with regard to comparable demographic data (Table 1).

Sensory block onset time was shorter in Group N (3.80 ± 1.0) than Group C (5.72 ± 1.46), and motor block onset time was shorter in Group N (10.72 ± 1.93) than Group C (13.56 ± 1.26). Sensory block recovery time was prolonged in Group N (10.56 ± 1.12) than Group C (6.88 ± 1.45), and recovery of motor block time in Group N was prolonged (13.04 ± 1.57) than Group C (11.96 ± 1.72) (Table 2).

VAS scores for bandage pain showed significant differences between the two groups at the following points of measurement: 10, 15, 20, and 30 minutes after tourniquet inflation. Also, there was a significant difference in the number of patients complained of bandage pain between the two groups: in Group C, 52% of patients complained of bandage pain, whereas in Group N, only 24% of patients complained of bandage pain. The onset time of bandage pain was longer in Group N (29.17 ± 2.04 min) than Group C (21.54 ± 3.15 min) (Table 3).

Postoperative VAS scores showed significant differences between the two groups at the following points of measurement: 30 minutes, 1 hour, and 4 hours after bandage deflation, with lower VAS scores in Group N (1.36 ± 0.81, 1.92 ± 0.40) (Table 4). Postoperative analgesic effect was longer in Group N (187.20 ± 60.79 min) than Group C (51.60 ± 25.28 min). Postoperative analgesic requirement was the lowest in Group N (33.60 ± 9.95 mg) (Table 5) (Figure 1).

Table 1: Demographic data.

	Group C ($n = 20$)	Group N ($n = 20$)	P value
Age (years)	31.28 ± 9.91	28.36 ± 9.31	0.637
Sex (%)			0.951
M	60	64	
F	40	36	
Weight (kg)	72.24 ± 12.53	68.40 ± 9.97	0.202
ASA (%)			1.000
I	84	88	
II	16	12	
Duration of surgery (min)	44.92 ± 8.30	45.48 ± 8.16	0.980

Data are represented as mean ± SD; yr: year; kg: kilogram; min: minute; M: male; F: female.

Table 2: Sensory and motor block onset and recovery times.

	Group C ($n = 20$)	Group N ($n = 20$)	P value
Sensory block onset time (min)	5.72 ± 1.46	3.80 ± 1.0	<0.001*
Motor block onset time (min)	13.56 ± 1.26	10.72 ± 1.93	<0.001*
Sensory block recovery time (min)	6.88 ± 1.45	10.56 ± 1.12	<0.001*
Motor block recovery time (min)	11.96 ± 1.72	13.04 ± 1.57	<0.001*

Data are represented as mean ± SD; *statistically significant at $P < 0.05$.

Table 3: VAS scores for tourniquet pain.

	Group C ($n = 20$)	Group N ($n = 20$)	P value
5 min	0.68 ± 0.69	0.52 ± 0.59	0.065
10 min	1.44 ± 0.77	0.68 ± 0.63	<0.001*
15 min	2.24 ± 0.52	1.04 ± 0.35	<0.001*
20 min	3.28 ± 0.79	1.44 ± 0.58	<0.001*
25 min	2.68 ± 0.69	2.12 ± 0.78	<0.001*
30 min	2.44 ± 0.58	2.96 ± 0.61	0.001*
End of surgery	2.24 ± 0.44	2.52 ± 0.51	0.099

Data are represented as mean ± SD; *statistically significant at $P < 0.05$; min: minutes.

Table 4: Postoperative VAS score.

	Group C ($n = 20$)	Group N ($n = 20$)	P value
30 min	2.96 ± 1.06	1.36 ± 0.81	<0.001*
1 hr	2.96 ± 1.02	1.92 ± 0.40	<0.001*
2 hr	2.08 ± 0.64	2.56 ± 1.42	0.243
4 hr	2.16 ± 0.47	3.12 ± 1.05	<0.001*
6 hr	2.0 ± 0.29	2.0 ± 0.50	0.918
8 hr	2.08 ± 0.49	2.20 ± 0.41	0.698
12 hr	1.68 ± 1.46	1.88 ± 0.60	0.439
16 hr	1.44 ± 1.29	1.76 ± 0.83	0.189
20 hr	0.76 ± 1.09	0.76 ± 1.16	0.593
24 hr	0.44 ± 0.77	0.44 ± 0.71	0.254

Data are represented as mean ± SD; *statistically significant at $P < 0.05$; hr: hours.

Table 5: Analgesic requirements.

P value	Group C ($n = 20$)	Group N ($n = 20$)	P value
Intraoperative (pethidine 0.5 mg/kg)	39.23 ± 6.07	31.67 ± 5.16	0.002*
Postoperative (ketorolac 30 mg)	40.80 ± 14.70	33.60 ± 9.95	0.013*

Data are represented as mean ± SD; *statistically significant at $P < 0.05$; mg: milligram; kg: kilogram.

In the present study, the patients' satisfaction about the operation and the surgeons' opinion about the operative conditions were better in Group N than Group C.

No adverse effects or complications were seen in this study. No evidence of central nervous system complications (such as circum oral numbness, headache, convulsions, or coma) or cardiac complications (such as arrhythmias, hypotension, or bradycardia) was seen after lidocaine administration, before and during the surgery, and after release of the bandage.

4. Discussion

Our study results showed that the addition of 5 mg transcutaneous nitroglycerin patch as adjuvant to Bier's block reduced the lidocaine dose to 1.5 mg/kg of 0.25% lidocaine; reduced the onset times of sensory and motor block, VAS scores, and analgesic consumption; prolonged the sensory and motor block recovery times and the duration of postoperative analgesic effect of Bier's block; delayed the first time to analgesic requirement; and improved the quality of Bier's block with no adverse effects.

The mechanism of action of nitroglycerin seems to be augmented by the direct potent vasodilatory effect that allows distribution of lidocaine to nerves that is mainly dose-dependent [9]. Several studies explained the pain-relieving mechanism of nitroglycerin [10, 11]. Nitroglycerin produces its analgesic effect by metabolization in the cell to nitric oxide, which causes an increase in the intracellular concentration of cyclic guanosine monophosphate, which produces pain modulation in the nervous systems (central and peripheral). Topical application of nitroglycerin generators also induces analgesia and anti-inflammatory effects by blocking the neurogenic component of inflammatory edema and hyperalgesia [12].

The first study on adding nitroglycerin to lidocaine to Bier's block for hand and forearm surgery was performed by Sen et al. [13] who studied the effect of adding nitroglycerin to lidocaine to Bier's block on 30 patients undergoing hand surgery in two groups: Group C, $n = 15$, as the control group which received 3 mg/kg of lidocaine diluted with saline, a total dose of 40 mL, and Group NTG, $n = 15$, as the nitroglycerin group in which patients received an additional 200 μg of nitroglycerin.

In agreement with our results, Sen et al. [13] proved that there was hemodynamic stability in the perioperative period, shortened onset time of sensory and motor blocks, higher VAS scores of bandage pain with prolonged sensory block recovery time, and improved quality of anaesthesia in the nitroglycerin group, whereas VAS scores were lower in the nitroglycerin group in the postoperative period. First analgesic

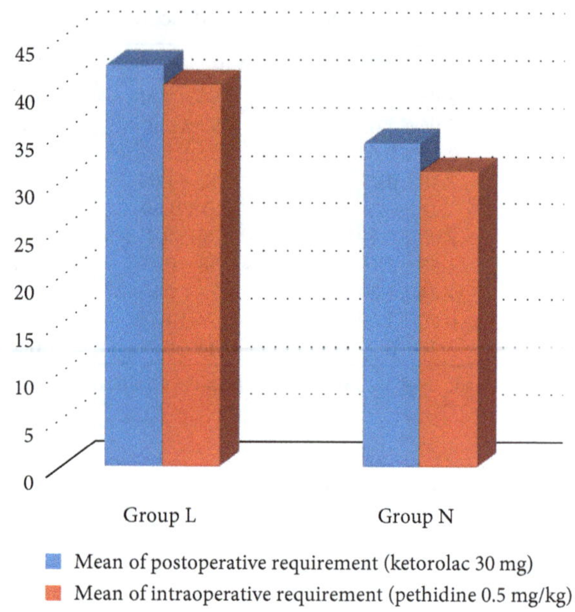

FIGURE 1: Intra- and postoperative analgesic requirements for both groups.

requirement time was longer in the nitroglycerin group than in Group C. In the nitroglycerin group, requirements for analgesia postoperative were significantly smaller.

Similar results were obtained by various other authors. Cakmak et al. [5] studied 60 patients undergoing elective hand, wrist, and forearm surgery procedures distributed into three groups: Group L: lidocaine group whichreceived 3 mg/kg of 2% lidocaine to a total volume of 40 mL and was diluted with saline; Group LL: lidocaine and lornoxicam group which received 3 mg/kg of 2% lidocaine to a total volume of 40 mL and was diluted with saline and also 8 mg of lornoxicam was added to the solution; and Group LL-N: lidocaine with lornoxicam and transdermal nitroglycerin group in which nitroglycerin patch 5 mg was applied to the surgical site and received 3 mg/kg of 2% lidocaine diluted with saline to a total volume of 40 mL and also 8 mg of lornoxicam was added to the solution, and they found shortened sensory and motor block onset times and prolonged sensory and motor block recovery times in the group which contained the nitroglycerin patch and lidocaine with lornoxicam than the lidocaine-alone group.

Previous researches did not study the patients' satisfaction, surgeons' opinion, and adverse effects or complications. In the present study, we focused on these parameters and found that the patients' satisfaction about the operation and surgeons' opinion of the operative conditions were better in Group N than Group C with no adverse effects or complications seen in this study.

Contrary to Cakmak et al. [5], although we used the transcutaneous nitroglycerin as they did, in our study we got the same results with low lidocaine concentration (40 cc of 1.5 mg/kg of 0.25% lidocaine diluted in normal saline (0.9% NaCl) was used for administering Bier's block). Low lidocaine concentration was the primary and effective cause for decreased resulted adverse effects and complications intra- and postoperatively and increased patients' satisfaction and surgeons' opinion in our study.

Also, Asadi and Mehri [14] studied the analgesic effect of nitroglycerin when added to lidocaine for Bier's block on 40 patients scheduled for elective forearm and hand surgery and agreed our results by reporting shorter sensory block onset time and delay in sensory block recovery time after bandage release in the nitroglycerin group with shorter motor block onset time and delay in recovery time after bandage release in the first group; the frequency of opioid injections was significantly lower in those who administered lidocaine and nitroglycerin.

Elmetwaly et al. [6] studied the effect of adding ketamine or nitroglycerin to lidocaine for Bier's block on seventy-five patients undergoing hand surgery and found that, in the control group, the starting four hours postoperatively, the VAS scores were higher compared with the other study groups. Also, Cakmak et al. [5] noted and agreed these results by approving that, in Group C, the starting four hours postoperatively, the VAS scores were higher in comparison to other groups.

5. Study Limitations and Recommendations

The major limitation of the present study was the current small sample size since we were able to enroll only 40 patients. More studies with high and sufficient sample sizes are required to confirm these results. We recommend further larger studies to determine the effect of different doses of lidocaine and nitroglycerin and other additives that can affect Bier's block conditions.

6. Conclusion

From the results of the present study, we conclude that, the addition of 5 mg of transcutaneous nitroglycerin patch as supplementation to 1.5 mg/kg of 0.25% lidocaine for Bier's block reduced the dose of lidocaine, sensory and motor block onset times, VAS scores, and analgesic consumption. Length of the sensory and motor block recovery times, the duration of postoperative analgesic effect, and the first time to analgesic requirement improved the quality of Bier's block with better patients' satisfaction and surgeons' opinion and had no side effects.

Conflicts of Interest

The author declares that there are no conflicts of interest.

References

[1] S. M. Marashi, A. Yazdanifard, G. Shoeibi, H. Bakhshandeh, and P. Yazdanifard, "The analgesic effect of intravenous neostigmine and transdermal nitroglycerin added to lidocaine on intravenous regional anesthesia (bier's block): a randomized, controlled study in hand surgery," *International Journal of Pharmacology*, vol. 4, no. 3, pp. 218–222, 2008.

[2] B. Gupta, R. K. Verma, S. Kumar, and G. Chaudhary, "Comparison of analgesic efficacy of dexmedetomidine and midazolam as adjuncts to lignocaine for intravenous regional

anesthesia," *Anesthesia: Essays and Researches*, vol. 11, no. 1, pp. 62–66, 2017.

[3] R. N. Verma, S. Hasnain, D. K. Sreevastava, and T. V. S. P. Murthy, "Anesthetic management of forearm fractures using a combination of haematoma block and intravenous regional anesthesia," *Medical Journal Armed Forces India*, vol. 72, no. 3, pp. 247–252, 2016.

[4] A. A. Jafarian, F. Imani, R. Salehi, F. N. Mazaher, and F. Moini, "Simple arm tourniquet as an adjunct to double-cuff tourniquet in intravenous regional anesthesia," *Anesthesiology and Pain Medicine*, vol. 6, no. 3, p. e29316, 2016.

[5] B. M. Cakmak, G. Cakmak, E. Akpek, G. Arslan, and M. S. Sahin, "Peri- and postanalgesic properties of lidokain, lornoxicam, and nitroglycerine combination at intravenous regional anesthesia," *BioMed Research International*, vol. 2014, Article ID 737109, 7 pages, 2014.

[6] K. F. Elmetwaly, N. A. Hegazy, A. A. Aboelseoud, and A. A. Alshaer, "Does the use of ketamine or nitroglycerin as an adjuvant to lidocaine improve the quality of intravenous regional anesthesia?," *Saudi Journal of Anaesthesia*, vol. 4, no. 2, pp. 55–62, 2010.

[7] L. Glantz, G. Godovic, M. Lekar, M. Kramer, and L. A. Eidelman, "Efficacy of transdermal nitroglycerin combined with etodolac for the treatment of chronic post-thoracotomy pain: an open-label prospective clinical trial," *Journal of Pain and Symptom Management*, vol. 27, no. 3, pp. 277–281, 2004.

[8] G. R. Lauretti, M. V. Perez, M. P. ReIs, and N. L. PereIra, "Double-blind evaluation of transdermal nitroglycerine as adjuvant to oral morphine for cancer pain management," *Journal of Clinical Anesthesia*, vol. 14, no. 2, pp. 83–86, 2002.

[9] L. L. Jorge, C. C. Feres, and V. E. Teles, "Topical preparations for pain relief: efficacy and patient adherence," *Journal of Pain Research*, vol. 4, pp. 11–24, 2010.

[10] G. R. Lauretti, I. C. Lima, M. P. Reis, W. A. Prado, and N. L. Pereira, "Oral ketamine and transdermal nitroglycerin as analgesic adjuncts to oral morphine therapy for cancer pain management," *Anesthesiology*, vol. 90, no. 6, pp. 1528–1533, 1999.

[11] S. Hashimoto and A. Kobayashi, "Clinical pharmacokinetics and pharmacodynamics of glyceryl trinitrate and its metabolites," *Clinical Pharmacokinetics*, vol. 42, no. 3, pp. 205–221, 2003.

[12] J. F. Butterworth, D. C. Mackey, J. D. Wasnick, J. F. Butterworth, D. C. Mackey, and J. D. Wasnick, *Morgan & Mikhail's Clinical Anesthesiology*, Vol. 15, McGraw-Hill, New York, NY, USA, 5th edition, 2013.

[13] S. Sen, B. Ugur, O. N. Aydin, M. Ogurlu, F. Gursoy, and O. Savk, "The analgesic effect of nitroglycerin added to lidocaine on intravenous regional anesthesia," *Anesthesia & Analgesia*, vol. 102, no. 3, pp. 916–920, 2006.

[14] H. K. Asadi and D. Mehri, "The analgesic effect of nitroglycerin added to lidocaine on quality of intravenous regional anesthesia in patients undergoing elective forearm and hand surgery," *Acta Cirurgica Brasileira*, vol. 28, no. 1, pp. 19–25, 2013.

25

The Effect of Prophylactic Dexmedetomidine on Hemodynamic Disturbances to Double-Lumen Endotracheal Intubation

Tanyong Pipanmekaporn,[1,2] Yodying Punjasawadwong,[2] Somrat Charuluxananan,[3] Worawut Lapisatepun,[2] and Pavena Bunburaphong[3]

[1] *Clinical Epidemiology Program, Faculty of Medicine, Chiang Mai University, Chiang Mai 50200, Thailand*
[2] *Department of Anesthesiology, Faculty of Medicine, Chiang Mai University, Chiang Mai 50200, Thailand*
[3] *Department of Anesthesiology, Faculty of Medicine, Chulalongkorn University, Bangkok 10330, Thailand*

Correspondence should be addressed to Tanyong Pipanmekaporn; tanyong24@gmail.com

Academic Editor: Peter Andrews

The purpose of this study was to determine the effect of dexmedetomidine on hemodynamic responses to DLT intubation compared to placebo and to assess the adverse effects related to dexmedetomidine. Sixty patients were randomly allocated to receive 0.7 μg/kg dexmedetomidine ($n = 30$) or normal saline ($n = 30$) 10 minutes before general anesthesia. Systolic blood pressure (SBP), diastolic blood pressure (DBP), mean arterial pressure (MAP), heart rate (HR), and rate pressure product (RPP) between groups were recorded. During intubation and 10 minutes afterward (T1-T10), the mean SBP, DBP, MAP, HR, and RPP in the control group were significantly higher than those in the dexmedetomidine group throughout the study period except at T1. The mean differences of SBP, DBP, MAP, HR, and RPP were significantly higher in the control group, with the value of 15.2 mmHg, 10.5 mmHg, 14 mmHg, 10.5 beats per minute, and 2,462.8 mmHg min^{-1}. Four patients in the dexmedetomidine group and 1 patient in the control group developed hypotension, while 2 patients in the dexmedetomidine group had bradycardia. Prophylactic dexmedetomidine can attenuate the hemodynamic responses to laryngoscopy and DLT intubation with minimal adverse effects. This trial is registered with ClinicalTrials.gov NCT01289769.

1. Introduction

A double-lumen endotracheal tube (DLT) is a device frequently used in thoracic surgery. It effectively provides lung separation and facilitates changing from two- to one-lung ventilation [1]. A previous study found that both laryngoscopy and DLT intubation could stimulate significant hemodynamic responses and increase the plasma concentration of catecholamines [2]. Although these hemodynamic responses including tachycardia and hypertension are transient, they can be harmful to patients with hypertension, myocardial ischemia, or cerebrovascular disease [3, 4]. The supplement of an inhaled anesthetic agent during anesthetic induction and intubation using a nondepolarizing muscle relaxant is a normal practice at our hospital. However, we observe that this practice is found ineffective to attenuate the hemodynamic responses to intubation and rescue treatment is frequently required. Therefore, some measures should be added in order to optimize this condition.

Several drugs have been used to attenuate the hemodynamic responses to laryngoscopy and DLT intubation. Dexmedetomidine, a highly selective $\alpha 2$ receptor agonist, produces sedative, analgesic, and central sympatholytic effects. It reduces norepinephrine release at the neuroeffector junction, inhibits neurotransmission of sympathetic nerves, and decreases plasma catecholamines, which results in a slight

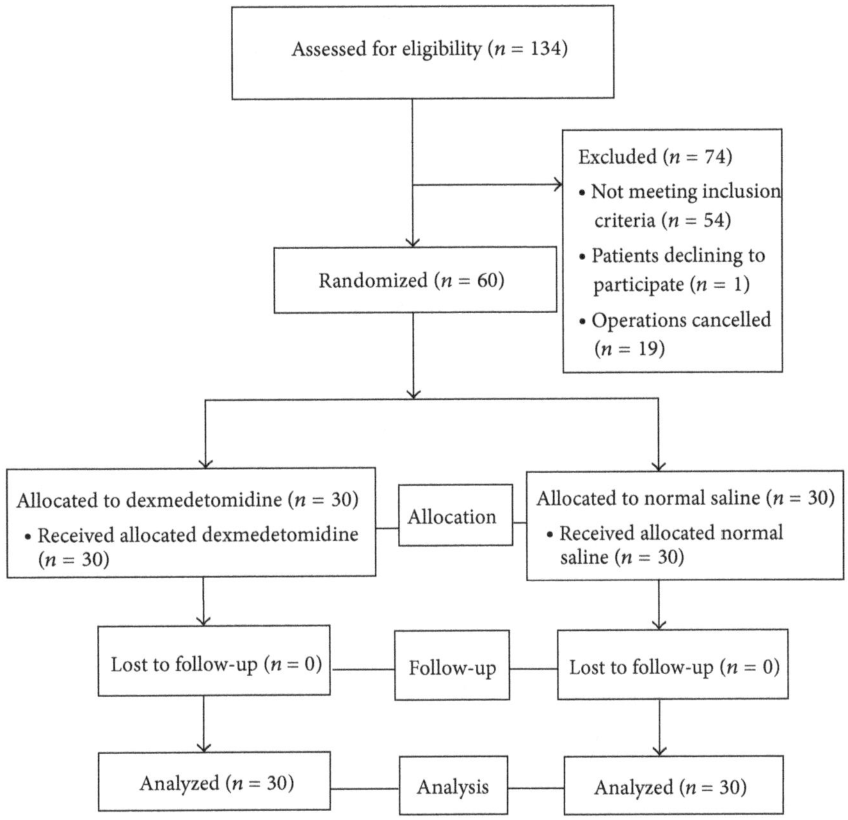

FIGURE 1: The Consolidated Standards of Reporting Trials flow diagram of the study.

decrease in blood pressure and lowering of the heart rate [5, 6]. On the other hand, dexmedetomidine can also increase SBP, the effect mediated by peripheral $\alpha 2$ receptor agonism at the vascular smooth muscle. This effect is associated with a higher dose of dexmedetomidine or rapid drug administration [7]. Dexmedetomidine has been used to attenuate the hemodynamic responses to single-lumen endotracheal tube intubation [8–12]; however, its effect on the hemodynamic responses during DLT intubation has not been investigated. The purpose of the present study is to determine the effect of dexmedetomidine on the hemodynamic responses to DLT intubation compared to placebo and to assess the adverse effects related to dexmedetomidine.

2. Methods

After approval from the institutional review board and written informed consent were obtained, 60 patients with the American Society of Anesthesiologists (ASA) physical status I-III, aged 18–65 years, undergoing scheduled thoracic surgery between March and December 2011 were enrolled in the study. Exclusion criteria were preoperative arrhythmias, bradycardia (heart rate < 50 beats per minute), second- or third-degree atrioventricular block, tachycardia (heart rate > 100 beats per minute), coronary artery disease, previous cerebrovascular accident, poorly controlled hypertension, renal or liver impairment and suspected difficult intubation. All patients had 0.2 mg/kg of diazepam orally two hours before surgery. In the operating theater the following monitoring was established: noninvasive blood pressure monitoring, electrocardiography (ECG) using the three-lead electrode system, peripheral oxygen saturation, and radial artery catheterization with a 20 G catheter. Patients were randomly allocated into two groups: the dexmedetomidine group and the control group, using a block of four randomizations with each randomized number concealed in a sealed, opaque envelope which would be opened after radial artery catheterization. The dexmedetomidine group received dexmedetomidine, 0.7 μg/kg in 0.9% NaCl 20 mL, while the control group received 0.9% NaCl 20 mL. Both the dexmedetomidine solution and 0.9% NaCl were prepared by a nurse who was not involved in the study so that the investigators would be unaware of the group identity. The designated solution was infused over 10 minutes before the induction of anesthesia. Propofol 2.5 mg/kg and fentanyl 1 μg/kg were given followed by rocuronium 0.6 mg/kg to facilitate endotracheal intubation. Anesthesia was maintained with 1% vaporizer setting of concentration of sevoflurane until tracheal intubation. Four minutes later, the laryngoscopy and endotracheal intubation were performed using a 39 Fr, 37 Fr, or 35 Fr endobronchial tube as recommended by Slinger and Campos [13]. All intubation attempts were performed by the same anesthesiologist (TP). Hemodynamic parameters (systolic blood pressure (SBP), diastolic blood pressure (DBP), mean arterial pressure (MAP), heart rate (HR), and rate pressure product (RPP, SBP × HR)) were recorded at baseline, just before intubation,

Table 1: Patient characteristics and operative data.

Variables	Dexmedetomidine group (n = 30)	Control group (n = 30)
Age (yr)	48.0 ± 19.4	47.8 ± 15.1
Sex		
Female	12 (40)	17 (57)
Male	18 (60)	13 (43)
ASA		
I	11 (37)	8 (27)
II-III	19 (63)	22 (73)
Body mass index (kg/m^2)	21.2 ± 3.3	20.8 ± 3.3
Concurrent disease		
Hypertension	10 (33)	6 (20)
Diabetes mellitus	3 (10)	1 (3)
Duration of anesthesia (minutes)	172 ± 80	154 ± 68
Duration of surgery (minutes)	142.3 ± 80.4	121.3 ± 67.5
Type of operation		
Thoracoscopy	11 (37)	18 (60)
Thoracotomy	19 (63)	12 (40)
Extent of surgery		
Explorative thoracotomy	9 (31)	11 (39)
Wedge resection	5 (17)	6 (21)
Lobectomy	15 (52)	10 (36)
Pneumonectomy	0	1 (4)
Baseline hemodynamic variables		
SBP (mmHg)	141.6 ± 19.7	136.1 ± 18.9
DBP (mmHg)	78.9 ± 9.6	74.8 ± 12.4
MAP (mmHg)	101.9 ± 12.2	95.9 ± 14.9
HR (beats per minute)	78.4 ± 17.1	81.2 ± 16.7
RPP (mmHg min^{-1})	11,094.0 ± 2,571.2	10,931.7 ± 2,381.8
Intubation time (seconds)	19.8 ± 6.9	20.7 ± 8.7

Data are presented as mean ± SD or number (%).
ASA: The American Society of Anesthesiologists, SBP: systolic blood pressure, DBP: diastolic blood pressure, MAP: mean arterial pressure, HR: heart rate, RPP: rate pressure product.

during intubation, and every minute after intubation for 10 minutes. Recording of parameters including intubation time (time from applying a laryngoscopy to tracheal cuff inflation) was done by another nurse who was not involved in the study. The incidences of hypotension (a decrease in SBP > 25% of baseline or SBP < 90 mmHg) and bradycardia (a decrease in HR > 25% of baseline or HR < 50 beats per minute) were also noted. Rescue medication was comprised of ephedrine 3 mg increments for hypotension (SBP < 90 mmHg for 60 seconds), nicardipine 0.5 mg increments for hypertension (SBP > 200 mmHg or DBP > 120 mmHg for 60 seconds) [2, 14, 15], and atropine 0.3 mg increments for bradycardia (HR < 50 beats per minute). The flow diagram of the study, recommended by the Consolidated Standards of Reporting Trials, is presented in Figure 1.

The primary endpoint of this study was to determine the differences of hemodynamic parameters between groups. The secondary endpoint was the adverse effects of dexmedetomidine such as hypotension, hypertension, bradycardia, or airway obstruction during study drug administration. Based on our pilot study, a sample size of 24 patients per group was required to detect a 25% change of MAP between groups with a power of 90% at the 5% significant level. However, we decided to recruit 30 patients per group to compensate for 20% of dropouts. All statistical analysis was performed using Stata software (version 11.0, College station, TX, USA). Data were presented as mean ± SD for continuous data and number and percent for categorical data. The Shapiro-Wilk test was used to determine normal distribution of data. Statistical analyses were performed using Fisher's exact probability test, unpaired t-test, or the Mann-Whitney U tests as appropriate. If the difference of the hemodynamic parameters between groups is marginally insignificant, a multi-level mixed model would be analyzed. The multilevel mixed model was used to investigate the effects of group, time, and individuals. The number needed to treat (NNT) was calculated to demonstrate the efficacy of dexmedetomidine administration and defined as numbers of patients needed to be treated to prevent one episode of an increase in MAP more than 25% after intubation compared to baseline value.

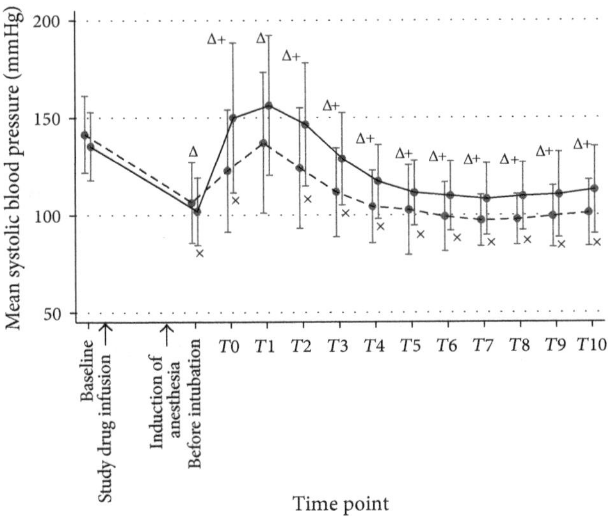

FIGURE 2: A line graph demonstrated the mean SBP and their standard deviation comparing groups at different time points. Baseline refers to the point of time before the study drug is administered. Before intubation refers the point of time after anesthetic induction just before DLT intubation. T0 is the period during intubation. T1–T10 refer the points of time as minutes after intubation. SBP: systolic blood pressure. ^{+}P value < 0.05 compared between groups. $^{\Delta}P$ value < 0.05, significant difference compared with baseline in the control group. $^{\times}P$ value < 0.05, significant difference compared with baseline in the dexmedetomidine group.

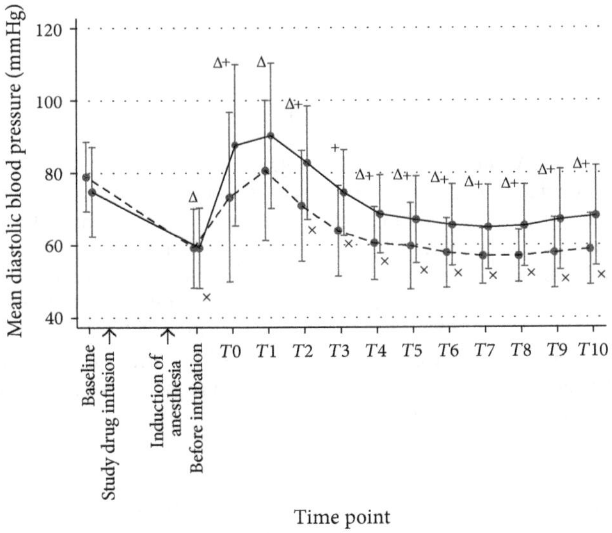

FIGURE 3: A line graph demonstrated the mean DBP and their standard deviation comparing groups at different time points. Baseline refers to the point of time before the study drug is administered. Before intubation refers the point of time after anesthetic induction just before DLT intubation. T0 is the period during intubation. T1–T10 refer the points of time as minutes after intubation. DBP: diastolic blood pressure. ^{+}P value < 0.05 compared between groups. $^{\Delta}P$ value < 0.05, significant difference compared with baseline in the control group. $^{\times}P$ value < 0.05, significant difference compared with baseline in the dexmedetomidine group.

A P value lower than 0.05 was considered to be statistically significant. Statistical analysis was based on the intention to treat.

3. Results

Sixty patients were randomized and completed the study. Patient characteristics, baseline hemodynamic variables, and intubation time were comparable between both groups (Table 1). Before intubation, mean SBP, DBP, MAP, and RPP in both groups were not significantly different; however, mean HR in the dexmedetomidine group was significantly lower than that of the control group ($P < 0.05$). During DLT intubation (T0) and 10 minutes afterward (T1–T10), the mean SBP, DBP, MAP, HR, and RPP in the control group were significantly higher than those of the dexmedetomidine group throughout the study period except T1, in which the blood pressures (BP) were not statistically different (Figures 2, 3, 4, and 5). A maximal increase of mean HR was observed at T0 in the control group, while a maximal increase of the mean HR in the dexmedetomidine group occurred at T1. Meanwhile, the mean differences of SBP, DBP, MAP, HR, and RPP were significantly higher in the control group between baseline, before intubation, during intubation, and T1–T10 after being adjusted for age, gender, ASA, concurrent disease, intubation time, baseline hemodynamic variables, and intubation attempts ($P < 0.001$) as shown in Table 2. In the dexmedetomidine group, the mean SBP, DBP, and MAP decreased significantly from the baseline before intubation, during intubation, and all through 10 minutes afterward except at T1 ($P < 0.05$). The mean SBP before intubation was 106.5 ± 20.7 mmHg, while the lowest mean SBP was observed at T7 (97.2 ± 13.2 mmHg). Significant decreases of mean HR from the baseline were before intubation and from T6 to T10, with the lowest mean value of 67.3 ± 13.1 beats per minute before intubation ($P < 0.05$). The mean values of SBP, DBP, MAP, HR, and RPP at different time points in both groups were presented in Table 3. Table 4 shows the incidences of adverse effects during and after intubation, which were not significantly different between groups. Four patients in the dexmedetomidine group and 1 patient in the control group developed hypotension, all of whom but 1 in the dexmedetomidine group required rescue medications. No patient in the control group had bradycardia. In the dexmedetomidine group, 2 patients had bradycardia and only 1 patient required treatment. All patients who received rescue medications responded very well to treatment. There was no episode of respiratory obstruction observed during administration of the study drug. NNT to prevent an increase of MAP more than 25% of baseline for dexmedetomidine was 10 (95% CI: 3.4–10.6). All patients were able to be extubated after the operation.

4. Discussion

An inhaled anesthetic agent is commonly used in combination with an intravenous anesthetic agent before a nondepolarizing muscle relaxant reaches its onset. In our practice, 1% concentration of sevoflurane may be sufficient to prevent

TABLE 2: The multivariate mean difference of systolic blood pressure, diastolic blood pressure, mean arterial pressure, and heart rate by treatment group adjusted for multiple variables†.

	Difference*	P value	95% CI
Systolic blood pressure (mmHg)	15.2	<0.001	6.9–23.6
Diastolic blood pressure (mmHg)	10.5	<0.001	5.6–15.3
Mean arterial pressure (mmHg)	14.0	<0.001	7.4–20.6
Heart rate (beats per minute)	10.5	<0.001	6.2–14.8
Rate pressure product (mmHg min^{-1})	2, 462.8	<0.001	1, 415.7–3, 510.0

The mean difference of each hemodynamic variable was estimated from hemodynamic change between baseline, before intubation, during intubation, and T1–T10.
†Adjusted for age, gender, ASA classification, preexisting hypertension, baseline hemodynamic variables, intubation time, and intubation attempts.
*Placebo group-treatment group.

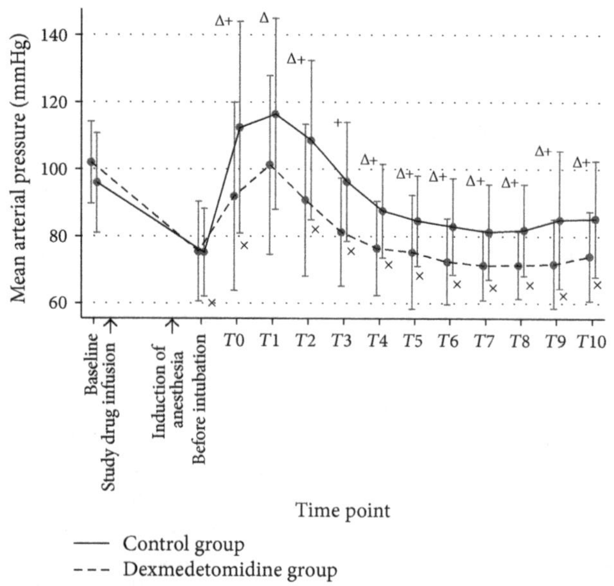

FIGURE 4: A line graph demonstrated the mean MAP and their standard deviation comparing groups at different time points. Baseline refers to the point of time before the study drug is administered. Before intubation refers the point of time after anesthetic induction just before DLT intubation. T0 is the period during intubation. T1–T10 refer the points of time as minutes after intubation. MAP: mean arterial pressure. ^{+}P value < 0.05 compared between groups. $^{\Delta}P$ value < 0.05, significant difference compared with baseline in the control group. $^{\times}P$ value < 0.05, significant difference compared with baseline in the dexmedetomidine group.

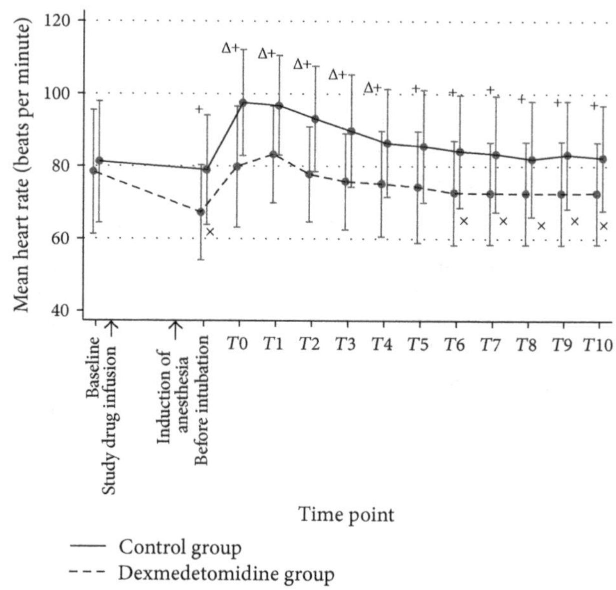

FIGURE 5: A line graph demonstrated the mean HR and their standard deviation comparing groups at different time points. Baseline refers to the point of time before the study drug is administered. Before intubation refers the point of time after anesthetic induction just before DLT intubation. T0 is the period during intubation. T1–T10 refer the points of time as minutes after intubation. HR: heart rate. ^{+}P value < 0.05 compared between groups. $^{\Delta}P$ value < 0.05, significant difference compared with baseline in the control group. $^{\times}P$ value < 0.05, significant difference compared with baseline in the dexmedetomidine group.

awareness during induction of anesthesia [16]; however, this concentration does not effectively attenuate the hemodynamic responses to intubation. This study found that the mean SBP, DBP, MAP, HR, and RPP in the control group were significantly higher than those of the dexmedetomidine group all through 10 minutes after DLT intubation, except mean SBP, DBP, and MAP between groups at T1. Corresponding to a previous study, this study showed that maximal increases of blood pressure and heart rate occurred 1 to 2 minutes after DLT intubation in the control group and returned to baseline within 5 minutes [2]. Thompson et al. showed that an increase of hemodynamic responses after DLT intubation in patients with an adequate depth of anesthesia was associated with an increase of the plasma level of norepinephrine [2]. In addition, previous studies reported that RPP was one of the major determinants of myocardial oxygen consumption and RPP > 20,000 mm Hg min^{-1} could precipitate angina pectoris [17]. Four patients (13%) in the control group and 1 patient (3%) in the dexmedetomidine group had an RPP of more than 20,000 mm Hg min^{-1}, which could increase the risk of myocardial ischemia [17, 18]. The effect of dexmedetomidine on lowering SBP, HR, and RPP could decrease the myocardial oxygen requirement and may be advantageous for patients at risk of coronary artery disease [19]. Moreover, the effect of dexmedetomidine in the controlling of blood pressure and heart rate during intubation may be beneficial in patients with preexisting hypertension or risk of stroke [20].

TABLE 3: Mean systolic blood pressure, diastolic blood pressure, mean arterial pressure, heart rate, and rate pressure product in dexmedetomidine and control groups at baseline, during and after intubation.

(a)

Time	SBP (mmHg) Dex group (n = 30)	SBP (mmHg) Control group (n = 30)	P value	DBP (mmHg) Dex group (n = 30)	DBP (mmHg) Control group (n = 30)	P value	MAP (mmHg) Dex group (n = 30)	MAP (mmHg) Control group (n = 30)	P value
Baseline	141.6 ± 19.7	135.4 ± 17.6	0.204	79.0 ± 9.6	74.8 ± 12.4	0.151	102 ± 12.2	95.9 ± 14.9	0.092
Before intubation	106.5 ± 20.7#	101.9 ± 17.2#	0.360	59.2 ± 10.9#	59.2 ± 11.1#	0.991	75.5 ± 14.9#	75.2 ± 13.1#	0.934
T0	122.8 ± 31.3#	149.4 ± 37.3#	0.004*	73.3 ± 23.4	87.4 ± 21.8#	0.009*	91.9 ± 28.1#	111.2 ± 29.6#	0.012*
T1	137.2 ± 36.1	153.4 ± 31.3#	0.068	80.7 ± 19.3	88.9 ± 18.5#	0.099	101.3 ± 26.6	114.4 ± 26.1#	0.058
T2	124.1 ± 30.9#	143.9 ± 28.5#	0.012*	70.9 ± 15.3#	82.2 ± 14.9#	0.005*	90.8 ± 22.6#	107.1 ± 21.9#	0.006*
T3	111.8 ± 22.8#	127.3 ± 21.0#	0.008*	63.9 ± 12.5#	74.2 ± 11.4	0.002*	81.3 ± 16.1#	95.2 ± 16.6	<0.001*
T4	104.4 ± 22.8#	116.0 ± 16.6#	0.013*	60.5 ± 10.1#	68.4 ± 10.4#	0.004*	76.5 ± 14.0#	86.9 ± 12.6#	0.002*
T5	102.7 ± 23.0#	111.3 ± 16.5#	0.017*	59.7 ± 12.0#	66.6 ± 11.2#	0.025*	75.3 ± 17.0#	84.1 ± 12.8#	0.008*
T6	99.2 ± 17.6#	109.1 ± 16.7#	0.028*	57.9 ± 9.6#	65.8 ± 11.5#	0.006*	72.5 ± 12.8#	82.4 ± 13.7#	0.005*
T7	97.2 ± 13.2#	107.1 ± 16.4#	0.012*	56.9 ± 7.7#	65.0 ± 11.8#	0.003*	71.4 ± 10.4#	81.1 ± 13.9#	0.003*
T8	97.7 ± 12.9#	109.4 ± 17.0#	0.003*	57.0 ± 7.2#	65.8 ± 11.7#	<0.001*	71.5 ± 10.0#	82.2 ± 13.9#	0.001*
T9	99.4 ± 15.6#	109.1 ± 19.1#	0.035*	57.9 ± 9.7#	66.6 ± 12.9#	0.005*	71.8 ± 13.3#	81.1 ± 13.9#	0.003*
T10	101.1 ± 17.0#	112.2 ± 20.9#	0.028*	58.8 ± 9.8#	67.9 ± 13.5#	0.004*	74.1 ± 10.0#	84.7 ± 16.3#	0.008*

(b)

Time	HR (beat per minute) Dex group (n = 30)	HR (beat per minute) Control group (n = 30)	P value	RPP ($mmHg\ min^{-1}$) Dex group (n = 30)	RPP ($mmHg\ min^{-1}$) Control group (n = 30)	P value
Baseline	78.4 ± 17.1	81.2 ± 16.7	0.529	11, 094.1 ± 502.3	10, 9317 ± 434.8	0.808
Before intubation	67.3 ± 13.1#	78.9 ± 15.1	0.002*	7, 174.6 ± 2, 050.3#	8, 034.5 ± 2, 001.2#	0.106
T0	79.9 ± 16.7	97.5 ± 14.6#	<0.001*	10, 011.1 ± 4, 242.7	14, 855.0 ± 5, 259.0#	<0.001*
T1	83.3 ± 13.4	96.8 ± 13.7#	<0.001*	11, 612.6 ± 4, 342.8	15, 246.7 ± 4, 372.6#	0.003*
T2	77.8 ± 13.1	93.1 ± 14.5#	0.001*	9, 791.1 ± 3, 678.7#	13, 682.6 ± 3, 708.2#	<0.001*
T3	75.8 ± 13.2	89.8 ± 15.5#	<0.001*	8, 561.6 ± 2, 758.6#	11, 571.8 ± 2, 940.7	<0.001*
T4	75.2 ± 14.6	86.4 ± 14.9#	0.004*	7, 963.7 ± 2, 751.3#	10, 091.2 ± 2, 253.7	0.002*
T5	74.3 ± 15.4	85.6 ± 15.5	0.007*	7, 798.3 ± 3, 228.5#	9, 530.6 ± 2, 313.2#	0.020*
T6	72.7 ± 14.4#	84.1 ± 15.6	0.005*	7, 291.7 ± 2, 353.6#	9, 232.4 ± 2, 290.3#	0.002*
T7	72.6 ± 14.1#	83.4 ± 16.0	0.007*	7, 109.1 ± 1, 960.8#	8, 992.1 ± 2, 239.0#	0.001*
T8	72.6 ± 14.2#	82.0 ± 15.9	0.018*	7, 131.9 ± 1, 865.2#	8, 979.1 ± 2, 207.4#	<0.001*
T9	72.6 ± 14.3#	83.2 ± 14.8	0.007*	7, 260.9 ± 2, 005.5#	9, 195.8 ± 2, 449.2#	0.001*
T10	72.6 ± 14.1#	82.3 ± 14.5	0.011*	7, 395.6 ± 2, 107.0#	9, 292.2 ± 2, 422.4#	0.002*

Data are presented as mean ± SD. Dex group: dexmedetomidine group. SBP: systolic blood pressure. DBP: diastolic blood pressure. MAP: mean arterial pressure. HR: heart rate. RPP: rate pressure product. Baseline refers to the point of time before the study drug is administered. Before intubation refers to the point of time after anesthetic induction just before intubation. T0 is the period during intubation. T1–10 refer to minutes after intubation. * P value < 0.05 compared between groups. # P value < 0.05 compared to baseline values.

Table 4: Incidence of adverse effects during and after intubation.

Events	Dexmedetomidine group ($n = 30$)	Control group ($n = 30$)	P value
Hypotension			
SBP < 90 mmHg	4 (13%)	1 (3%)	0.313
Hypertension			
SBP > 200 mmHg	1 (3%)	4 (13%)	0.171
Bradycardia			
(HR < 50 beats per minute)	2 (7%)	0	0.496

Data are presented as number (%). SBP: systolic blood pressure, HR: heart rate.

Various dosages of preoperative dexmedetomidine ranging from 0.5 to 2 μg/kg have been investigated to attenuate the sympathoadrenal and hemodynamic responses following single-lumen endotracheal tube intubation [8, 10, 12, 21]. A randomized controlled trial study demonstrated that the use of 0.5 μg/kg of dexmedetomidine could decrease the HR and MAP at the 10th minute after intubation compared to placebo in patients undergoing general surgery [22]. However, the HR seemed to be inadequately attenuated few minutes after intubation as observed from the result of the former study. Moreover, the investigators did not compare hemodynamic parameters between groups at that time interval in their study. The use of 1 μg/kg of dexmedetomidine in patients undergoing general surgery could lower both HR and MAP more effectively than the use of fentanyl alone 1, 3, and 5 minutes after intubation and reduce the requirement of intraoperative fentanyl and isoflurane [12]. The administration of 2 μg/kg of dexmedetomidine lowered SBP, DBP, and HR significantly compared to a placebo and reduced the intraoperative isoflurane requirement [21]. During our pilot study, the investigator began with 1 μg/kg of dexmedetomidine infusion over 10 minutes and we found that some patients developed severe hypotension and bradycardia after the induction of general anesthesia and intubation. Therefore, we decided to decrease dose of dexmedetomidine to 0.7 μg/kg in order to minimize its adverse effects.

In the dexmedetomidine group, mean HR and RPP were significantly lower than those in the control group all through 10 minutes after intubation. Maximal increases of blood pressures in the dexmedetomidine group occurred at T1 and they were not significantly different from those in the control group. However, these differences were marginally insignificant. In addition, we observed that some patients had exaggerated hemodynamic responses during and after intubation. The analysis of average mean difference between groups at different time points is may be inappropriate in this situation. Therefore, the multilevel mixed model analysis was then used to evaluate the differences of hemodynamic parameters between groups throughout the study period. The results showed that mean differences adjusted for multiple variables of SBP, DBP, and MAP were significantly higher in the control group than those of the dexmedetomidine group over 10 minutes after intubation. However, dexmedetomidine at dose of more than 0.7 μg/kg may be required in order to ensure the complete abolishment of hemodynamic responses at T1.

Hypotension and bradycardia are common adverse hemodynamic effects in patients receiving dexmedetomidine as a result of decreasing the central sympathetic nervous activity or preserving the baroreceptor reflex [7]. In the present study, only a few patients had significant hypotension and bradycardia during or after dexmedetomidine administration and responded well to rescue medications. Hypotension and bradycardia occur frequently in patients receiving an initial loading dose of dexmedetomidine especially with rapid administration and also in those with concurrent negative chronotropic medications [19]. Previous studies reported that the undesirable effects of dexmedetomidine were dose related. Basar et al. reported that the incidence of bradycardia after a single dose of 0.5 μg/kg of dexmedetomidine was about 5% [8], while a study of Sulaiman et al. showed development of hypotension or bradycardia with a similar dosage of dexmedetomidine [22]. The incidence of hypotension occurred by about 20% with the use of 1 μg/kg of dexmedetomidine in patients undergoing coronary artery bypass graft surgery [11]. Nevertheless, transient tachycardia, hypertension, and oxygen desaturation were observed after the use of 1 μg/kg of dexmedetomidine in the study of Bajwa et al. [12]. A randomized controlled trial investigated the effect of 2 μg/kg of dexmedetomidine and placebo on anesthetic requirement and perioperative hemodynamic stability. The former study reported that the incidences of intraoperative hypotension, bradycardia, and partial airway obstruction were 20%, 24%, and 12%, respectively. In addition, 56% of patients in the dexmedetomidine group developed bradycardia in the postanesthesia care unit and subsequently had a significantly longer stay in the postanesthesia care unit compared to the placebo group [21]. In this study, although we did not observe any adverse event during the use of 0.7 μg/kg of dexmedetomidine in the pilot study, hypotension (13%) and bradycardia (7%) were observed after intubation in the main study. However, we could not detect any difference in adverse effects between groups.

There were a few limitations of this study. First, we did not measure the plasma concentration of catecholamines. Therefore, we could not demonstrate the effectiveness of this dosage of dexmedetomidine in decreasing the sympathetic nervous system activity. Second, in this study, we could not confirm the anesthesia depth in both groups due to lack of facility. Inadequate depth of anesthesia can, to some extent, increase the hemodynamic responses to intubation.

5. Conclusion

Prophylactic dexmedetomidine can attenuate the hemodynamic responses to laryngoscopy and DLT intubation with minimal adverse effects. This application may be useful to patients who are at risk of cardiovascular complications related to severe hypertension and tachycardia after DLT intubation.

Conflict of Interests

The authors declare that they have no conflict of interests.

Acknowledgments

This work was supported by Faculty of Medicine Research Fund, Chiang Mai University, Chiang Mai, Thailand. The authors would like to thank Professor Dr. Jayanton Patumanond, Clinical Epidemiology and Medical Statistics, Faculty of Medicine, Chiang Mai University for his support, for the analysis of this study.

References

[1] S. V. Chhangani, "Ventilation techniques for 1-lung anesthesia," *Seminars in Anesthesia Perioperative Medicine and Pain*, vol. 21, no. 3, pp. 196–203, 2002.

[2] J. P. Thompson, K. J. West, and A. J. Hill, "The cardiovascular responses to double lumen endobronchial intubation and the effect of esmolol," *Anaesthesia*, vol. 52, no. 8, pp. 790–794, 1997.

[3] E. J. Fox, G. S. Sklar, C. H. Hill, R. Villanueva, and B. D. King, "Complications related to the pressor response to endotracheal intubation," *Anesthesiology*, vol. 47, no. 6, pp. 524–525, 1977.

[4] W. L. Roy, G. Edelist, and B. Gilbert, "Myocardial ischemia during non-cardiac surgical procedures in patients with coronary-artery disease," *Anesthesiology*, vol. 51, no. 5, pp. 393–397, 1979.

[5] B. C. Bloor, D. S. Ward, J. P. Belleville, and M. Maze, "Effects of intravenous dexmedetomidine in humans: II. Hemodynamic changes," *Anesthesiology*, vol. 77, no. 6, pp. 1134–1142, 1992.

[6] Z. P. Khan, C. N. Ferguson, and R. M. Jones, "Alpha-2 and imidazoline receptor agonists. Their pharmacology and therapeutic role," *Anaesthesia*, vol. 54, no. 2, pp. 146–165, 1999.

[7] A. Arcangeli, C. D'Alò, and R. Gaspari, "Dexmedetomidine use in general anaesthesia," *Current Drug Targets*, vol. 10, no. 8, pp. 687–695, 2009.

[8] H. Basar, S. Akpinar, N. Doganci et al., "The effects of preanesthetic, single-dose dexmedetomidine on induction, hemodynamic, and cardiovascular parameters," *Journal of Clinical Anesthesia*, vol. 20, no. 6, pp. 431–436, 2008.

[9] K. Dogru, T. Arik, K. Yildiz, C. Bicer, H. Madenoglu, and A. Boyaci, "The effectiveness of intramuscular dexmedetomidine on hemodynamic responses during tracheal intubation and anesthesia induction of hypertensive patients: a randomized, double-blind, placebo-controlled study," *Current Therapeutic Research*, vol. 68, no. 5, pp. 292–302, 2007.

[10] T. Kunisawa, O. Nagata, M. Nagashima et al., "Dexmedetomidine suppresses the decrease in blood pressure during anesthetic induction and blunts the cardiovascular response to tracheal intubation," *Journal of Clinical Anesthesia*, vol. 21, no. 3, pp. 194–199, 2009.

[11] F. Menda, Ö. Köner, M. Sayin, H. Türe, P. Imer, and B. Aykaç, "Dexmedetomidine as an adjunct to anesthetic induction to attenuate hemodynamic response to endotracheal intubation in patients undergoing fast-track CABG," *Annals of Cardiac Anaesthesia*, vol. 13, no. 1, pp. 16–21, 2010.

[12] S. J. Bajwa, J. Kaur, A. Singh, S. Gupta, V. Sharma, and A. Panda, "Attenuation of pressor response and dose sparing of opioids and anaesthetics with pre-operative dexmedetomidine," *Indian Journal of Anaesthesia*, vol. 56, no. 2, pp. 123–128, 2012.

[13] P. D. Slinger and J. H. Campos, "Anesthesia for thoracic surgery," in *Miller 's Anesthesia*, R. D. Miller, L. I. Eriksson, L. A. Fleisher, J. P. Wiener-Kronish, and W. Young, Eds., pp. 1819–1887, Elsevier, Churchill Livingstone, Philadelphia, Pa, USA, 7th edition, 2010.

[14] S. Sugiura, S. Seki, K. Hidaka, M. Masuoka, and H. Tsuchida, "The hemodynamic effects of landiolol, an ultra-short-acting β1-selective blocker, on endotracheal intubation in patients with and without hypertension," *Anesthesia & Analgesia*, vol. 104, no. 1, pp. 124–129, 2007.

[15] A. Maguire, J. P. Thompson, C. Guest, P. J. Sadler, J. W. Strupish, and K. J. West, "Comparison of the effects of intravenous alfentanil and esmolol on the cardiovascular response to double-lumen endobronchial intubation," *Anaesthesia*, vol. 56, no. 4, pp. 319–325, 2001.

[16] M. S. Avidan, L. Zhang, B. A. Burnside et al., "Anesthesia awareness and the bispectral index," *The New England Journal of Medicine*, vol. 358, no. 11, pp. 1097–1108, 2008.

[17] B. F. Robinson, "Relation of heart rate and systolic blood pressure to the onset of pain in angina pectoris," *Circulation*, vol. 35, no. 6, pp. 1073–1083, 1967.

[18] D. V. Cokkinos and E. M. Voridis, "Constancy of pressure rate product in pacing induced angina pectoris," *British Heart Journal*, vol. 38, no. 1, pp. 39–42, 1976.

[19] J. D. Tobias, "Dexmedetomidine: applications in pediatric critical care and pediatric anesthesiology," *Pediatric Critical Care Medicine*, vol. 8, no. 2, pp. 115–131, 2007.

[20] A. L. Kovac, "Controlling the hemodynamic response to laryngoscopy and endotracheal intubation," *Journal of Clinical Anesthesia*, vol. 8, no. 1, pp. 63–79, 1996.

[21] C. J. Lawrence and S. De Lange, "Effects of a single pre-operative dexmedetomidine dose on isoflurane requirements and perioperative haemodynamic stability," *Anaesthesia*, vol. 52, no. 8, pp. 736–744, 1997.

[22] S. Sulaiman, R. B. Karthekeyan, M. Vakamudi, A. S. Sundar, H. Ravullapalli, and R. Gandham, "The effects of dexmedetomidine on attenuation of stress response to endotracheal intubation in patients undergoing elective off-pump coronary artery bypass grafting," *Annals of Cardiac Anaesthesia*, vol. 15, no. 1, pp. 39–43, 2012.

26

Comparison of Spinal Block Levels between Laboring and Nonlaboring Parturients using Combined Spinal Epidural Technique with Intrathecal Plain Bupivacaine

Yu-Ying Tang,[1] Jie Zhou,[2] Xiao-Hui Ren,[3] and Xue-Mei Lin[1]

[1] *Department of Anesthesiology, West China Second Hospital, Sichuan University, Sichuan, Chengdu 610041, China*
[2] *Department of Anesthesiology, Perioperative and Pain Medicine, Brigham and Women's Hospital, Harvard Medical School, 75 Francis Street, Boston, MA 02115, USA*
[3] *Department of Anesthesiology, Median Area of Maternal and Child Care Service Center, Sichuan, Neijiang 641000, China*

Correspondence should be addressed to Xue-Mei Lin, hxfeymz@sohu.com

Academic Editor: Takashi Nishino

Background. It was suggested that labor may influence the spread of intrathecal bupivacaine using combined spinal epidural (CSE) technique. However, no previous studies investigated this proposition. We designed this study to investigate the spinal block characteristics of plain bupivacaine between nonlaboring and laboring parturients using CSE technique. *Methods.* Twenty-five nonlaboring (Group NL) and twenty-five laboring parturients (Group L) undergoing cesarean delivery were enrolled. Following identification of the epidural space at the L3-4 interspace, plain bupivacaine 10 mg was administered intrathecally using CSE technique. The level of sensory block, degree of motor block, and hemodynamic changes were assessed. *Results.* The baseline systolic blood pressure (SBP) and the maximal decrease of SBP in Group L were significantly higher than those in Group NL ($P = 0.002$ and $P = 0.03$, resp.). The median sensory level tested by cold stimulation was T6 for Group NL and T5 for Group L ($P = 0.46$). The median sensory level tested by pinprick was T7 for both groups ($P = 0.35$). The degree of motor block was comparable between the two groups ($P = 0.85$). *Conclusion.* We did not detect significant differences in the sensory block levels between laboring and nonlaboring parturients using CSE technique with intrathecal plain bupivacaine.

1. Introduction

Combined spinal epidural (CSE) anesthesia is commonly used for cesarean delivery. It has been suggested that nonlaboring parturients have a higher sensory block level than those in labor during CSE anesthesia [1]. This proposition was derived from combining two independent randomized studies on spinal block levels designed separately for laboring and nonlaboring parturients [2, 3]. There was a 5-dermatome level difference between nonlaboring (C6) [2] and laboring (T3) [3] parturients using 10 mg hyperbaric bupivacaine with CSE technique. However, there has been no previous study examining the effect of labor on the level of the subarachnoid block during CSE. The effect of CSE technique on the spinal block level of hyperbaric bupivacaine in nonlaboring parturients was not consistent. Horstman et al. reported that sensory block level was at T3 with CSE in nonlaboring parturients using 20% higher dose of hyperbaric bupivacaine [4]. We speculate that baricity of the hyperbaric bupivacaine used by Ithnin et al. could be a confounding factor, because the block level could be easily manipulated with the positioning of the parturients when hyperbaric local anesthetic was used. The effect of labor on the spread of local anesthetics may be better examined by using plain or isobaric agents which hold the least gravity-generated flow dynamics in cerebrospinal fluid (CSF). This study was therefore designed to compare the spinal block characteristics between the laboring and nonlaboring parturients using plain bupivacaine injected intrathecally with the needle-through-needle CSE technique.

2. Methods

This research was conducted at the West China Second Hospital of Sichuan University, Chengdu, Sichuan Province, China. With median two-segment dermatome blockade level difference to be clinically significant and variability (interquartile range) of two dermatomes in sensory block, 20 parturients in each group were required in each group to address a 2-segment difference with a power of 0.9 and a level of significance of 5%.

Following the institutional research ethics board (IRB) approval and written informed consents, we enrolled two groups of parturients with 25 in each group. Group NL were 25 nonlaboring parturients undergoing elective cesarean delivery, and Group L were 25 parturients in spontaneous active labor (having regular uterine contractions and cervical dilation greater than 3 cm) undergoing cesarean delivery for failure to progress. All parturients were between 20 and 40 years of age, ASA physical status I-II with a singleton pregnancy at greater than 36 weeks gestation, and received a lower segment transverse incision for cesarean delivery. The decision for cesarean delivery was made by the obstetric team, independent of the study investigators. Exclusion criteria included parturient refusal, having received any analgesic treatment, any contraindication to CSE or general anesthesia, height less than 150 cm or greater than 175 cm, body weight greater than 100 kg, obstetric and/or medical comorbidities such as preeclampsia, any cardiac, renal, neurologic, or other systemic diseases, unilateral block, or maximal pinprick sensory block level below T10 at 20 min postspinal injection.

Each parturient was preloaded with 500 mL of lactated Ringer's solution intravenously (IV). On arrival in the operation room, baseline vital signs were recorded and the initial severity of labor pain for a laboring parturient was assessed on a 10 cm visual analog scale (VAS) before CSE anesthesia was placed. The degree of cervical dilations for laboring parturient was also recorded.

One anesthesiologist performed all CSE procedures following previously published methodology [2, 3]. With the parturient in the right lateral decubitus position, epidural space was identified at the L3-4 interspace with a 17-gauge Tuohy needle using the loss of resistance to air technique. The L3-4 interspace was identified by the line connecting the iliac crests to cross the spine. The volume of air used was limited to no more than 2 mL. Using the needle-through-needle technique, a 25-gauge Whitacre spinal needle (BD Durasafe) was advanced via the epidural needle with the orifice facing cephalad direction. When cerebrospinal fluid was detected, 10 mg plain bupivacaine (2 mL of 0.5% w/v bupivacaine), which was the same as the previously published studies by Ithnin and Lim et al. [2, 3], was injected over 10 seconds without barbotage or aspiration. Immediately after intrathecal injection, the epidural needle was removed without inserting an epidural catheter. All parturients were promptly placed in a supine position with left uterine displacement.

A second anesthesiologist recorded vital signs at two-minute intervals for 20 minutes. IV phenylephrine 100 μg was administrated for a decrease in systolic blood pressure (SBP) to less than 90 mmHg or a 30% reduction in SBP and was repeated as necessary. Bradycardia with less than 50 beats per minute was treated with IV atropine 0.3 mg. Sensory level of the block was assessed bilaterally at two-minute intervals using alcohol swab (sensory blockade level to cold) and 25-gauge hypodermic needle (sensory blockade level to pinprick) in the cephalad direction. The degree of motor blockade was evaluated bilaterally using the modified Bromage scale [5]. The peak sensory and motor blockade and the amount of time taken to achieve it were compared. Other side effects such as shivering, nausea, and vomiting were recorded.

Skin incisions were made 20 minutes after intrathecal injection. Prior to delivery of the fetuses, any reaction to surgical stimulation (including any verbal complaint of pain or withdrawal of extremities to pinprick) was supplemented with IV ketamine at a dose of 0.5 mg/kg each time until adequate anesthesia was achieved. After childbirth, midazolam 0.03 mg/kg was administrated to all parturients, and IV pethidine 0.5 mg/kg each time was also utilized according to parturient's reaction to ensure adequate anesthesia. General anesthesia was reserved as a back-up plan. Time intervals from skin incision to uterine incision, from uterine incision to fetus delivery, and surgical time were collected. The Apgar scores and parturients' satisfaction with anesthesia care were recorded. All parturients were followed for three days postoperatively.

2.1. Statistical Analysis. Statistical analysis was performed using SPSS Version 13.0 software. One-sample Kolmogorov-Smirnov test was applied to analyze the distribution of the data. Student's unpaired t-test was used to examine the differences of quantitative data between groups. The Mann-Whitney U test was performed to analyze the ordered variables, such as median sensory levels, VAS scores, modified Bromage scores, and those skewed quantitative data. The incidences of hypotension, shivering, and nausea/vomiting between the two groups were compared with Fisher's exact test. The correlations between sensory blockade level and cervical dilation or labor pain scores were analyzed with Spearman's rank correlation. A P value <0.05 was considered statistically significant.

3. Results

All 50 parturients enrolled completed the study. No technical difficulty or inadvertent dural puncture was encountered. Demographical data including age, weight, height, and gestation weeks were presented in Table 1.

All parturients had similar bilateral sensory block level, and all the peak pinprick sensory block levels were above T10. Median peak dermatomal sensory block level to pinprick and cold sensation and the time taken to achieve it in 20 min after spinal injection were comparable between the two study groups (Table 2).

Spearman's correlation coefficients were 0.07 and −0.44, respectively, for sensory blockade level to pinprick in relation

Table 1: Demographical data.

Demographical data	Group NL (n = 25)	Group L (n = 25)	P value
Age (years old)	30.3 (5.1)	29.7 (5.2)	0.52
Weight (kg)	68.3 (8.3)	64.7 (4.5)	0.07
Height (cm)	158.6 (5.1)	155.9 (4.5)	0.05
Gestational age (wk)	38.4 (1.3)	37.4 (1.4)	0.02
Initial cervical dilatation (cm)	0	6.7 (2.2)	<0.001
Initial VAS score of labor pain	0	7 (6–8)	<0.001
Baseline SBP (mmHg)	116.6 (11.5)	131.8 (6.1)	0.002
Time period from skin incision to uterine incision (minutes)	4.9 (1.5)	5.4 (1.1)	0.13
Time period from uterine incision to delivery (seconds)	57.3 (9.2)	56.8 (13.0)	0.06
Duration of operation (minutes)	48.0 (9.5)	52.3 (10.0)	0.54
Apgar score at 1 minute	10 (9-10)	10 (8–10)	0.32
Apgar score at 5 minutes	10 (10-10)	10 (9-10)	0.20

Results are expressed as the mean (SD) or the median (interquartile range), as appropriate.

Table 2: Block characteristics 20 minutes after intrathecal injection.

Block characteristics	Group NL (n = 25)	Group L (n = 25)	P value
Median sensory blockade level to cold	T6 (T4–T6)[a]	T5 (T4–T6)[a]	0.46
Time to achieve cold blockade level (minutes)	10.9 (2.1)[b]	10.7 (2.3)[b]	0.83
Median sensory blockade level to pinprick	T7 (T6–T8)[a]	T7 (T7-T8)[a]	0.35
Time to achieve pinprick blockade level (minutes)	11.2 (2.2)[b]	10.5 (2.6)[b]	0.36
Motor block grade	3 (3-4)[a]	3 (3-4)[a]	0.85
Time to achieve motor block (minutes)	8.0 (2.5)[b]	7.7 (2.6)[b]	0.42
Phenylephrine (μg)	0 (0–100)[a]	0 (0-0)[a]	>0.99
Maximal decrease of SBP (mmHg)	23.2 (13.2)[b]	34.6 (9.2)[b]	0.03
Hypotension	8 (32%)[c]	5 (20%)[c]	0.52
Shivering	5 (20%)[c]	12 (48%)[c]	0.07
Nausea and vomiting	3 (12%)[c]	1 (4%)[c]	0.61

[a]Results are expressed as the median (interquartile range); [b]results are expressed as the mean (SD); [c]results are expressed as the number of parturients (percent).

with cervical dilation and labor pain scores (P = 0.81 and P = 0.10, resp.). In addition, Spearman's correlation coefficients for sensory blockade level to cold in relation with cervical dilation and labor pain scores were 0.22 and 0.17, respectively (P = 0.43 and P = 0.54, resp.). During surgery, there were separately 14 nonlaboring parturients and 8 laboring parturients required rescue analgesic (P = 0.15). The median rescue ketamine dosage was 30 mg (IR: 0–50 mg) for nonlaboring parturients and 0 mg (IR: 0–40 mg) for laboring parturients (P = 0.21). The median rescue pethidine dosage was 30 mg (IR: 0–40 mg) for nonlaboring parturients and 0 mg (IR: 0–40 mg) for laboring parturients (P = 0.19). No conversion to general anesthesia was warranted.

With regard to hemodynamic variables, the baseline SBP and the maximal decrease of SBP significantly higherwere observed in the laboring group (P = 0.002 and P = 0.03, resp., Tables 1 and 2). No difference was found in the incidence of hypotension or the phenylephrine dosage between the two groups (Table 2). None of the parturients developed significant bradycardia. All parturients were satisfied with the anesthesia care. No incidence of postdural puncture headache or other neurological complications was noted postoperatively.

4. Discussion

Ithnin et al. attributed the significantly higher block level in nonlaboring parturients with CSE technique to the neutralization of the negative pressure of the epidural space and reduction of the dural sac volume [2]. Researchers from the same institution also concluded that labor-induced variable increase of epidural pressure countered the above effects [3]. Combining the aforementioned two studies, Macarthur suggested that CSE might generate higher block level in nonlaboring parturients [1]. However, we demonstrated that there was no statistical difference in the level of sensory blockade to either pinprick or cold between laboring and nonlaboring parturients with CSE technique. Neither did the block level relate to cervical dilation nor did the severity of labor pain. Within the same line of out findings, Horstman et al. confirmed that, compared to simple spinal technique, the change of epidural pressure from CSE technique was negligible to cause significant change of intrathecal anesthetic spread [4]. We believe that with the relatively fixed size and low compliance nature of the skeletal spinal canal, physiological labor contraction would only generate hydraulic pressure evenly transmitted along the spinal dural sac, leaving little fluid dynamic alteration to the intrathecally administered local anesthetics. This was also confirmed by Dubelmanand Forbes who found that vigorous coughing had no influence on the cephalad spread of spinal anesthesia [6].

With the same CSE technique, the median peak sensory level in the present study achieved was no higher than T5, while previous studies using same amount of hyperbaric bupivacaine reported a median peak sensory level between C6 [2] and T3 [3] on nonlaboring and laboring parturients, respectively. The only difference among the above three studies was the baricity of bupivacaine. It has been widely accepted that, under the influence of gravity, hyperbaric anesthetic solutions injected into spinal space at the L3-4 level (the peak of lumbar lordosis) are more likely to spread into and halt at the lower thoracic region (the nadir of thoracic kyphosis). Hirabayashi et al. demonstrated flattening of both lumbar lordosis and thoracic kyphosis during later stages of pregnancy using magnetic resonance imaging in

Japanese women [7]. Interestingly, both the present study and the studies by Ithnin and Lim et al. were conducted on Asian parturients. We believe that the flattening of the curvatures of the spinal column, especially the disappearing of the upward slope in the high thoracic spine, could enhance the cephalad spread of intrathecally administered hyperbaric anesthesia solutions, leading to the unusually high blockade reported by Ithnin et al. Such effect was eliminated by using plain bupivacaine solution when block level was much less affected by curvatures of the spine and body position. We are not certain if these anatomic changes were specific to Asian parturients, as previous studies on western parturient showed that baricity had no differences in subarachnoid spread of bupivacaine, in which bupivacaine was used at higher dose or combined with opioids [8, 9].

Hypotension during spinal anesthesia primarily results from decreased systemic vascular resistance after blockade of preganglionic sympathetic fibers, and patients with a higher sympathetic drive are more prone to develop hypotension [10]. So, a laboring parturient with spinal anesthesia would be more prone to hypotension than a nonlaboring parturient because both epinephrine and norepinephrine levels are increased during labor [11]. In this study, we also found a greater decrease of SBP in laboring parturients. However, the compensation of the autologous transfusion with uterine contractions [12] and higher baseline SBP of laboring parturients resulted in similar incidence of hypotension or the phenylephrine dosage.

The choice of the dose of bupivacaine (10 mg) in the present study was based on previous studies [2, 3], which provided comparability among the studies. The median sensory blockade to pinprick was lagged at T7 in this study, which could not provide an absolute pain-free situation for parturients during cesarean operation. However, the inadequate blockade level was easily rectified by ketamine and pethidine as stated in the materials section; no significant adverse effect on the clinical outcome of parturient and neonate was noticed. Followups of parturients were satisfactory.

Selection bias was one of the concerns that could not be excluded completely from this study because of the nonrandomized design. Laboring parturients were shorter in height (2.7 cm difference in average) and lighter in weight (3.6 kg difference in average) than those of nonlaboring parturients, which might in part explain the reason for their failure to progress resulting in cesarean delivery. However, it has been demonstrated that height, weight, and bodymass index did not influence the spread of sensory blockade after subarachnoidal injection of bupivacaine [13, 14]. The obese and nonobese parturients also had a similar effective dose of intrathecal bupivacaine for cesarean delivery [15]. Of course, a carefully designed randomized controlled trial would eliminate these possible confounding factors. Although the gestational age had a significant difference between two groups, all parturients we enrolled had pregnancy greater than 36 weeks. To avoid the potential interference in judgment of level of sensory loss, laboring parturients who had received analgesics prior to cesarean delivery were excluded from this study.

In conclusion, our study could not demonstrate difference in the block level of spinal anesthesia between the laboring and nonlaboring parturients using plain bupivacaine injected with the CSE technique.

Authors' Contribution

Y.-Y. Tang and J. Zhou contributed equally to this work and should be considered co-first authors.

References

[1] A. J. Macarthur, "Gerard W. Ostheimer "What's new in obstetric anesthesia" lecture," *Anesthesiology*, vol. 108, no. 5, pp. 777–785, 2008.

[2] F. Ithnin, Y. Lim, A. T. Sia, and C. E. Ocampo, "Combined spinal epidural causes higher level of block than equivalent single-shot spinal anesthesia in elective cesarean patients," *Anesthesia and Analgesia*, vol. 102, no. 2, pp. 577–580, 2006.

[3] Y. Lim, W. Teoh, and A. T. Sia, "Combined spinal epidural does not cause a higher sensory block than single shot spinal technique for cesarean delivery in laboring women," *Anesthesia and Analgesia*, vol. 103, no. 6, pp. 1540–1542, 2006.

[4] D. J. Horstman, E. T. Riley, and B. Carvalho, "A randomized trial of maximum cephalad sensory blockade with single-shot spinal compared with combined spinal-epidural techniques for cesarean delivery," *Anesthesia and Analgesia*, vol. 108, no. 1, pp. 240–245, 2009.

[5] T. W. Breen, T. Shapiro, B. Glass, D. Foster-Payne, and N. E. Oriol, "Epidural anesthesia for labor in an ambulatory patient," *Anesthesia and Analgesia*, vol. 77, no. 5, pp. 919–924, 1993.

[6] A. M. Dubelman and A. R. Forbes, "Does cough increase the spread of subarachnoid anesthesia?" *Anesthesia and Analgesia*, vol. 58, no. 4, pp. 306–308, 1979.

[7] Y. Hirabayashi, R. Shimizu, H. Fukuda, K. Saitoh, and M. Furuse, "Anatomical configuration of the spinal column in the supine position. II. Comparison of pregnant and mon-pregnant women," *British Journal of Anaesthesia*, vol. 75, no. 1, pp. 6–8, 1995.

[8] I. F. Russell and E. L. O. Holmqvist, "Subarachnoid analgesia for Caesarean section. A double-blind comparison of plain and hyperbaric 0.5% bupivacaine," *British Journal of Anaesthesia*, vol. 59, no. 3, pp. 347–353, 1987.

[9] M. G. Richardson, H. V. Collins, and R. N. Wissler, "Intrathecal hypobaric versus hyperbaric bupivacaine with morphine for cesarean section," *Anesthesia and Analgesia*, vol. 87, no. 2, pp. 336–340, 1998.

[10] R. M. Lewinsky and S. Riskin-Mashiah, "Autonomic imbalance in preeclampsia: evidence for increased sympathetic tone in response to the supine-pressor test," *Obstetrics and Gynecology*, vol. 91, no. 6, pp. 935–939, 1998.

[11] M. Cascio, B. Pygon, C. Bernett, and S. Ramanathan, "Labour analgesia with intrathecal fentanyl decreases maternal stress," *Canadian Journal of Anaesthesia*, vol. 44, no. 6, pp. 605–609, 1997.

[12] R. V. Brizgys, P. A. Dailey, S. M. Shnider, D. M. Kotelko, and G. Levinson, "The incidence and neonatal effects of maternal hypotension during epidural anesthesia for cesarean section," *Anesthesiology*, vol. 67, no. 5, pp. 782–786, 1987.

[13] N. P. Ekeløf, E. Jensen, J. Poulsen, and P. Reinstrup, "Weight gain during pregnancy does not influence the spread of spinal

analgesia in the term parturient," *Acta Anaesthesiologica Scandinavica*, vol. 41, no. 7, pp. 884–887, 1997.
[14] M. C. Norris, "Patient variables and the subarachnoid spread of hyperbaric bupivacaine in the term parturient," *Anesthesiology*, vol. 72, no. 3, pp. 478–482, 1990.
[15] B. Carvalho, J. Collins, D. R. Drover, L. Atkinson Ralls, and E. T. Riley, "ED50 and ED95 of intrathecal bupivacaine in morbidly obese patients undergoing cesarean delivery," *Anesthesiology*, vol. 114, no. 3, pp. 529–535, 2011.

27

Procedural Complications of Spinal Anaesthesia in the Obese Patient

Manuel Wenk,[1] Christian Weiss,[2] Michael Möllmann,[3] and Daniel Matthias Pöpping[1]

[1] *Department of Anesthesiology, Intensive Care and Pain Medicine, University Hospital Muenster, Albert-Schweitzer Campus 1, A1, 48149 Muenster, Germany*
[2] *Medical School, University of Muenster, 48149 Muenster, Germany*
[3] *Department of Anesthesiology and Intensive Care, St. Franziskus Hospital, 48145 Muenster, Germany*

Correspondence should be addressed to Manuel Wenk, manuelwenk@uni-muenster.de

Academic Editor: Michael R. Frass

Background. Complications of spinal anaesthesia (SpA) range between 1 and 17%. Habitus and operator experience may play a pivotal role, but only sparse data is available to substantiate this claim. *Methods.* 161 patients were prospectively enrolled. Data such as spread of block, duration of puncture, number of trials, any complication, operator experience, haemodynamic parameters, was recorded and anatomical patient habitus assessed. *Results.* Data from 154 patients were analyzed. Success rate of SpA in the group of young trainees was 72% versus 100% in the group of consultants. Trainees succeeded in patients with a normal habitus in 83.3% of cases versus 41.3% when patients had a difficult anatomy ($P = 0.02$). SpA in obese patients (BMI ≥ 32) was associated with a significantly longer duration of puncture, an increased failure ratio when performed by trainees (almost 50%), and an increased number of bloody punctures. *Discussion.* Habitus plays a pivotal role for SpA efficiency. In patients with obscured landmarks, failure ratio in unexperienced operators is high. Hence, patient prescreening as well as adequate choice of operators may be beneficial for the success rate of SpA and contribute to less complications and better patient and trainee satisfaction.

1. Background

Ever since the introduction of spinal anaesthesia more than a century ago, complications have been part of the technique; failed or insufficient block, headaches, nausea, vomiting, and pain around the injection site are common minor complications [1, 2]. The technique of spinal anaesthesia (SpA) is considered a basic skill, however, one that first has to be mastered. According to literature, the incidence of failed or partially failed SpA ranges between 0.5 and 17% [3–5]. The incidence of postdural puncture headaches (PDPHs) ranges between 0,7 and 11% based on the type of needle used [6, 7], and transient neurologic syndromes can still be observed after SpA with an incidence of 0–7% [8].

As with many other procedures in medicine, intuition suggests that procedure-specific experience of the operator should be beneficial and reduce complications. However, there is only sparse data available to demonstrate that this is the case for SpA [9, 10].

Furthermore, with an increasing number of severely obese patients in western society, anesthesiologists are—more than ever—faced with patients where the individual habitus causes a challenge to perform a seemingly simple basic skill like SpA because it relies on identifiable anatomical structures termed "landmarks." These can be completely obscured in the obese patient [11, 12].

The aim of this study was to evaluate the impact of the individual patient habitus on the success rate of SpA and the incidence of immediate complications related to SpA in the context of operator experience.

2. Methods

After approval from the Ethics Committee of the Medical Faculty of the University of Muenster (protocol 2009-459-f-S), 161 patients planned for elective orthopedic or vascular surgical procedures of the lower limb under SpA were enrolled in the study. Informed consent was obtained from each patient.

Operators were divided into two groups ($n = 5$/each group). Group T were anesthetic trainees with ≤1 year experience in anaesthesia and group C anesthetists with ≥5-year experience in anaesthesia and >150 previously performed SpA as well as ongoing regular exposure to SpA.

Exclusion criteria were as follows:

(i) <18 or >90 years of age,

(ii) coagulation disorders or any combination of the following: INR > 1.5, aPTT > 40 sec, thrombocytes < 100.000 per microliter blood,

(iii) neurological disorders,

(iv) sepsis or severe infection or local infection around the typical injection site,

(v) known allergies to local anesthetics, and

(vi) American Society of Anesthesiologists Score (ASA) ≥ IV.

Besides demographic data, we recorded the following characteristics: number of puncture trials, change of spinal segment, bleeding from the introducer or the spinal needle, duration of procedure, paresthesias during puncture, spread of sensory and motor block, failed or partially failed SpA as well as hemodynamic changes in blood pressure and heart rate. A relevant hypotensive episode was defined as a systolic blood pressure <85 mmHg or a decrease in systolic pressure >30% below the initial systolic blood pressure.

An anaesthesiologist with >20-year experience as an anesthetic consultant assessed each patients' spinal anatomy based on palpation as well as X-rays, when available. Patients were divided into an "easy" and a "difficult habitus for SpA" group. The habitus was considered "difficult" when no spinous processes were palpable at the L3–L5 level and above, which could be used as landmarks to guide the operator to identify a midline. Furthermore, in patients with lumbar scoliosis and subsequent longitudinal rotation of the spinous processes towards the concave side as identified by X-ray, the habitus was considered "difficult."

All patients were attached to standard monitoring (noninvasive blood pressure, electrocardiogram, and peripheral oxygen saturation). An intravenous access was established, and an infusion of 1000 mL of a balanced electrolyte solution (Sterofundin-ISO, B.Braun, Melsungen, Germany) was started. Patients were then turned into a lateral position, and after usual sterile preparations SpA was performed with a 25-gauge pencil point spinal needle (PenPoint, B.Braun, Melsungen, Germany). A standard introducer needle was used to facilitate spinal needle puncture. Once a free flow of cerebrospinal fluid (CSF) was obtained, the color of CSF was compared against a color scale measuring the amount of blood in CSF.

Local anesthetics used were isobaric bupivacaine 0.5% (3 mL) for endoprosthetic surgery or isobaric ropivacaine 0.5% (2.5–4 mL) for all other procedures. If the surgical procedure was expected to be of longer duration, 0.1 mg morphine was additionally injected into the subarachnoid space.

Table 1: Demographic data.

Age (years)	64.9 ± 15.0
Sex ratio (male/female)	64/90
Height (cm)	170 ± 9.7
Weight (kg)	79 ± 16.1
Body mass index (kg/m^2)	27.2 ± 4.9
BMI ≤ 24.9 (n)	52
BMI ≤ 29.9 (n)	53
BMI ≤ 34.9 (n)	38
BMI ≤ 39.9 (n)	9
BMI ≥ 40 (n)	2
ASA I (n)	42
ASA II (n)	87
ASA III (n)	25

Statistical analysis was performed using SPSS Statistics 18.0 (SPSS Inc., Chicago, IL, USA). Categorical variables are expressed as frequency and percentage, whereas continuous variables are represented as means with standard deviation or as median and interquartile range (25th percentile; 75th percentile). Before statistical testing, each continuous variable was analysed exploratively for its normal distribution using Kolmogorov-Smirnov test. The Mann-Whitney test was then applied for comparison of nonparametric variables between the two study groups. The nonparametric patients' baseline characteristics were assessed using the Kruskal-Wallis test. Friedman's signed rank test was used to compare the nonparametric time-dependent variables and the chi-square test for comparison of categorical variables.

Differences were considered as statistically significant at $P < 0.05$.

3. Results

161 patients were enrolled in the study. 7 patients were excluded due to changes in the treatment plan. Complete data sets of 154 patients were subsequently analyzed.

Demographic data of all patients is displayed in Table 1.

Overall success rate of SpA in the group of young trainees was 72% versus 100% in the group of consultants. 51 (35%) patients were rated to have a "difficult" anatomy/habitus. Trainees succeeded to perform SpA in patients with an easy habitus in 83.3% of cases versus 52.4% when patients had a difficult anatomy ($P = 0.005$). When trainees failed a SpA, an operator from group C took over, and they were successful in 100% of the cases hence all patients enrolled in the study had the planned surgical procedure done under SpA.

Table 2 lists specific complications encountered in both operator groups and the two patient groups. Obese patients with a BMI ≥ 32 were significantly higher at risk to experience complications during SpA. Duration of puncture was longer, trainees failed SpA in almost half the cases, and there were significantly more bloody punctures and a higher incidence of paresthesias. Furthermore, even consultants

TABLE 2: Incidences of immediate complications for patients with "easy" and "difficult" habitus and the respective operator experience.

	Easy habitus			Difficult habitus		
	Trainees ($n = 46$)	Consultants ($n = 57$)	P	Trainees ($n = 21$)	Consultants ($n = 30$)	P
Duration of puncture (sec)	117 ± 80	63 ± 48	0.001*	154 ± 89	102 ± 91	n.s.
Success on first puncture	19 (41.3%)	48 (84.1%)	0.002*	2 (9.5%)	11 (36.7%)	0.03*
Failed SpA	6 (13.0%)	0	0.01*	10 (47.6%)	0	0.0003*
Insufficient spread of SpA	2 (4.3%)	1 (1.6%)	n.s.	1 (4.8%)	1 (3.3%)	n.s.
Segment change	7 (15.2%)	3 (5.2%)	0.05	8 (38.1%)	12 (40%)	n.s.
Blood in introducer needle	5 (10.9%)	5 (8.8%)	n.s.	8 (38.1%)	9 (45%)	n.s.
Blood in CSF	4 (8.7%)	1 (1.6%)	n.s.	3 (14.3%)	5 (16.7%)	n.s.

Values indicate total number of patients and percentage. Column P displays the respective P values where *indicates significance ($P < 0.05$) and n.s.: not significant.

TABLE 3: Incidences of complications on day one postoperatively and respective operator experience.

Trainees	Consultants	P	Difficult anatomy	Easy anatomy	P	
Transient neurological syndrome (%)	2.2	1.1	n.s.	1.1	2.0	n.s.
Pain at insertion site (%)	4.4	9.5	n.s.	10.0	6.7	n.s.
Urinary retention (%)	0	0	n.s.	0	0	n.s.
PONV (%)	11.1	10.5	n.s.	14.0	8.9	n.s.

Values indicate total number of patients and percentage. n.s.: not significant.

required 3 or more punctures to perform successful SpA in 42.5% of the patients with a BMI ≥ 32.

The height of the achieved sensory and motor block was not related to weight or BMI of the patient.

Consultants caused less paraesthesias when performing SpA as compared to trainees; however, the difference was not statistically significant ($P = 0.31$). Patients that were rated to have a difficult habitus had significantly more paresthesias during puncture than patients with identifiable landmarks (13.2 versus 2%; $P = 0.005$). Furthermore, patients with a difficult habitus had significantly more pain during the procedure than patient with an easy habitus (11.3 versus 1.9%; $P = 0.02$).

Isobaric bupivacaine 0.5% in equipotent doses caused significantly more hypotensive episodes after intrathecal injection as compared to isobaric ropivacaine 0.5% (21 (25%) versus 2 (3.1%); $P = 0.0002$). There was no significant difference in hypotensive episodes between patients with a BMI < 30 versus ≥30 ($P = 0.05$).

Bradycardia with a heart rate of 45 beats per minute or below was observed in 9 (6%) patients and was not significantly related to the local anaesthetic used but was significantly correlated with the level of puncture.

Interestingly, patients who required 4 or more punctures to place a successful SpA had a significantly greater drop in blood pressure.

On day one postoperatively, two patients (1.3%) showed typical features of a transient neurologic syndrome, 6 patients (3.9%) reported difficulties passing urine during the first 12 hours, but no patient required bladder catheterization. 15 patients (9.7%) had one or more episodes of PONV (Table 3).

No major complications such as severe hemodynamic disturbances, cardiac arrest, cauda equina syndrome, or permanent neurologic complications were observed.

4. Discussion

Spinal anaesthesia has an excellent safety record in terms of major complications. However, there is a significant number of minor complications that—each on its own—may cause unpleasant sequelae for the patient [3, 4, 13]. The majority of complications are associated with the procedure itself. Insufficient or failed SpA ranges from 0 to 17% and bloody punctures as well as significant hypotension are not uncommon [3, 9]. The current study shows that the overall failure rate of SpA is comparable to previously published data. We have shown that success and failure rate appears to be directly dependent on the operator's experience and the individual patient habitus. Trainees failed significantly more attempts to perform SpA, had more difficulties placing SpA in patients with obscured landmarks, and had significantly more bloody punctures, and the procedure duration was significantly longer as compared to experienced specialists. It has been shown previously that SpA is a complex procedure that is more difficult to master than, for example, endotracheal intubation [14]. Furthermore, it has been estimated that the experience of around 100 performed SpA is required to achieve a 90% success rate [15]. Our data shows that young trainees had a success rate of 84% in patients with a normal anatomy, indicating that some trainees have probably mastered the technique while others were still on the ascending part of the learning curve. However, this picture changes completely when patients present with obscured landmarks or difficult anatomy. Trainees, who were able to perform SpA successfully in anatomically "easy" patients, suddenly faced a failure rate of 52% in those patients with a difficult habitus, significantly different to "easy" patients. Consultants were able to place a SpA even in the difficult patients but in 42.5% of cases, 3 or more punctures were required to position the spinal needle in the correct location. To our knowledge, this is the first study that specifically investigated the role of the individual patient habitus by rating landmarks and other anatomical features. Part of educating trainees is to accept that they do have a higher failure rate [16, 17], and it is the responsibility of the relevant societies to define what is an acceptable failure rate for which procedure [18]. Based on our findings we postulate that an experienced anesthesiologist should anatomically rate all patients who are about to receive SpA and if the habitus is considered to be difficult, young trainees should probably not perform SpA to avoid frustration and build a more solid foundation based on successfully performed punctures rather than failing every second attempt. However, from our data, it appears that young trainees do have a higher failure rate, but they do not cause significantly more complications. Hence exposure to the difficult patient is relatively safe, once a solid foundation of the technique has been established. We recommend that the level of supervision should be adequate to avoid that the operator's success or fail rate in these patients is significantly lower than in experienced operators. Multiple attempts by young trainees as well as experienced operators lead to a more significant reaction of hemodynamic parameters. Blood pressures dropped significantly more in patients where multiple attempts were necessary. We offer two possible explanations. Firstly, multiple attempts may lead to the operator changing spinal segments, and the direction is usually upwards thus causing more sympathetic block. Secondly, multiple attempts may cause stress and enhance anxiety in the patient hence causing disturbances of the autonomous sympathetic regulation. Last but not least, avoiding multiple attempts may also affect patient satisfaction, but we have not investigated that matter.

As a training tool for young trainees as well as a tool to use in the anatomically challenging patient, the introduction of ultrasound-guided SpA may be worthwhile to consider. Some studies have shown increased success rates when ultrasound is used in patients with obscured landmarks or difficult anatomy [19–21]. However, this might involve teaching both SpA and the use of an ultrasound machine to trainees at the same time, which may be an even bigger challenge. Furthermore, similar to current discussions on the comprehensive use of ultrasound for central venous catheter placement, it needs to be discussed whether trainees should in general learn to perform landmark techniques before they add ultrasound or vice versa.

Our study has limitations. Firstly, patients were not randomized to experienced or unexperienced operators but were consecutively allocated to operators available. Secondly, operators could not be blinded to patient habitus for obvious reasons. However, operators were blinded to the assessment of the anatomical structures and the subsequent grading.

Since trainees were on the ascending part of the learning curve during the study period, repeated exposure to performing SpA itself may have influenced their individual performance and subsequently the results. Furthermore, our study was not powered to comment on incidences of rare major complications such as severe hemodynamic disturbances, cardiac arrest, cauda equina syndrome, or permanent neurologic complications since this was never the aim of this study.

5. Conclusion

Albeit a relatively safe technique, SpA has its problems and pitfalls, and our study has shown that increased operator-experience results in a higher success rate of SpA. Furthermore, the individual patient's habitus plays a pivotal role when trainees are involved in performing SpA. Even for experienced anesthesiologists this group of patients has its challenges, but the failure rate of SpA is still very low. We conclude that careful patient selection and prescreening as well as adequate choice of operators is beneficial for the success rate of SpA and may contribute to less complications, greater safety, better patient, and trainee satisfaction.

References

[1] A. Bier, "Versuche über Cocainisirung des Rückenmarkes," *Deutsche Zeitschrift für Chirurgie*, vol. 51, no. 3-4, pp. 361–369, 1899.

[2] H. F. W. Wulf, "The centennial of spinal anesthesia," *Anesthesiology*, vol. 89, no. 2, pp. 500–506, 1998.

[3] P. D. W. Fettes, J. R. Jansson, and J. A. W. Wildsmith, "Failed spinal anaesthesia: mechanisms, management, and prevention," *British Journal of Anaesthesia*, vol. 102, no. 6, pp. 739–748, 2009.

[4] B. L. Sng, Y. Lim, and A. T. H. Sia, "An observational prospective cohort study of incidence and characteristics of failed spinal anaesthesia for caesarean section," *International Journal of Obstetric Anesthesia*, vol. 18, no. 3, pp. 237–241, 2009.

[5] P. J. Tarkkila, "Incidence and causes of failed spinal anesthetics in a university hospital: a prospective study," *Regional Anesthesia*, vol. 16, no. 1, pp. 48–51, 1991.

[6] E. J. Krommendijk, R. Verheijen, B. Van Dijk, E. M. Spoelder, M. J. M. Gielen, and J. J. De Lange, "The PENCAN 25-gauge needle: a new pencil-point needle for spinal anesthesia tested in 1,193 patients," *Regional Anesthesia and Pain Medicine*, vol. 24, no. 1, pp. 43–50, 1999.

[7] D. K. Turnbull and D. B. Shepherd, "Post-dural puncture headache: pathogenesis, prevention and treatment," *British Journal of Anaesthesia*, vol. 91, no. 5, pp. 718–729, 2003.

[8] D. Zaric and N. L. Pace, "Transient neurologic symptoms (TNS) following spinal anaesthesia with lidocaine versus other local anaesthetics," *Cochrane Database of Systematic Reviews*, no. 2, Article ID CD003006, 2009.

[9] P. Sirivararom, T. Virankabutra, N. Hungsawanich, P. Premsamran, and W. Sriraj, "The Thai Anesthesia Incidents Monitoring Study (Thai AIMS) of adverse events after spinal anesthesia: an analysis of 1,996 incident reports," *Journal of the Medical Association of Thailand*, vol. 92, no. 8, pp. 1033–1039, 2009.

[10] S. T. Vilming, H. Schrader, and I. Monstad, "Post-lumbar-puncture headache: the significance of body posture. A controlled study of 300 patients.," *Cephalalgia*, vol. 8, no. 2, pp. 75–78, 1988.

[11] "Adiposity in the first half of life," in *Abstracts of the 27th Annual Meeting of the German Society for Obesity Research*, vol. 4, supplement 2, pp. 1–40, Obes Facts, Bochum, Germany, October 2011.

[12] C. R. Broadbent, W. B. Maxwell, R. Ferrie, D. J. Wilson, M. Gawne-Cain, and R. Russell, "Ability of anaesthetists to identify a marked lumbar interspace," *Anaesthesia*, vol. 55, no. 11, pp. 1122–1126, 2000.

[13] H. Hyderally, "Complications of spinal anesthesia," *Mount Sinai Journal of Medicine*, vol. 69, no. 1-2, pp. 55–56, 2002.

[14] S. Charuluxananan, O. Kyokong, W. Somboonviboon, and S. Pothimamaka, "Learning manual skills in spinal anesthesia and orotracheal intubation: is there any recommended number of cases for anesthesia residency training program?" *Journal of the Medical Association of Thailand*, vol. 84, supplement 1, pp. S251–S255, 2001.

[15] C. Konrad, G. Schüpfer, M. Wietlisbach, and H. Gerber, "Learning manual skills in anesthesiology: is there a recommended number of cases for anesthetic procedures?" *Anesthesia and Analgesia*, vol. 86, no. 3, pp. 635–639, 1998.

[16] I. G. Kestin, "A statistical approach to measuring the competence of anaesthetic trainees at practical procedures," *British Journal of Anaesthesia*, vol. 75, no. 6, pp. 805–809, 1995.

[17] J. Sivaprakasam and M. Purva, "CUSUM analysis to assess competence: what failure rate is acceptable?" *Clinical Teacher*, vol. 7, no. 4, pp. 257–261, 2010.

[18] A. F. Smith and J. D. Greaves, "Beyond competence: defining and promoting excellence in anaesthesia," *Anaesthesia*, vol. 65, no. 2, pp. 184–191, 2010.

[19] K. J. Chin, V. W. S. Chan, R. Ramlogan, and A. Perlas, "Real-time ultrasound-guided spinal anesthesia in patients with a challenging spinal anatomy: two case reports," *Acta Anaesthesiologica Scandinavica*, vol. 54, no. 2, pp. 252–255, 2010.

[20] K. J. Chin, A. J. R. Macfarlane, V. Chan, and R. Brull, "The use of ultrasound to facilitate spinal anesthesia in a patient with previous lumbar laminectomy and fusion: a case report," *Journal of Clinical Ultrasound*, vol. 37, no. 8, pp. 482–485, 2009.

[21] M. A. Peterson and J. Abele, "Bedside ultrasound for difficult lumbar puncture," *Journal of Emergency Medicine*, vol. 28, no. 2, pp. 197–200, 2005.

28

Effect of Ondansetron on the Occurrence of Hypotension and on Neonatal Parameters during Spinal Anesthesia for Elective Caesarean Section

Walid Trabelsi, Chihebeddine Romdhani, Haythem Elaskri, Walid Sammoud, Mohamed Bensalah, Iheb Labbene, and Mustapha Ferjani

Department of Anesthesia and Intensive Care Unit, Tunisian Military Hospital, 1008 Tunis, Tunisia

Correspondence should be addressed to Walid Trabelsi; walid_trabelsi2009@yahoo.fr

Academic Editor: Steven K. Howard

To prevent hypotension during spinal anesthesia for caesarean section, we assessed IV ondansetron of invasive maternal hemodynamic and fetal gazometric parameters.

1. Introduction

Spinal anesthesia has become the gold standard anesthetic technique for elective caesarean section. It is a simple, fast performed, powerful, and reliable technique. The main problem is hypotension associated with a decrease in cardiac output and uteroplacental flow which may induce fetal morbidity [1]. It is therefore crucial to prevent and/or to treat it quickly and effectively.

The spinal anesthesia for cesarean indeed requires a sensory block until T5, which always leads to an extended sympathetic block and hypotension occurs in 55% to 90% of cases, despite the partial left lateral decubitus (with the objective of limiting the aortocaval compression caused by the gravid uterus).

The main treatment is the vascular filling with crystalloid or starches and use of vasopressors. However, many studies [2–5] showed that it was inefficient and a recent review found that no intervention reliably prevents hypotension during spinal anesthesia for caesarean section [6].

The physiopathological mechanism involved in the occurrence of hypotension is systemic vascular resistance and central venous pressure from sympathetic block with vasodilation [7–11]. Bradycardia can occur from shift in cardiac autonomic balance toward the parasympathetic system, from activation of left ventricular mechanoreceptors from a sudden decrease in left ventricular volume (Bezold-Jarisch reflex) (BJR).

Pharmacological and animal studies [12] suggest that 5-HT (serotonin) may be an important factor associated with inducing the BJR and this effect can be blocked at the 5-HT3 receptor [13].

Based on these considerations, this randomized, controlled, double-blind study was performed to investigate the use of intravenous ondansetron for prophylaxis of hypotension after spinal anesthesia in parturients scheduled for elective caesarean section and its consequences on newborns' parameters.

2. Material and Methods

After local ethics committee approval (provided by Tunisian Military Hospital Ethics Committee, Tunis, Tunisia), recording in the Australian New Zealand Clinical Trials Registry with an assigned number of ACTRN12613000036718, and written informed consent, ASA physical status class I primipare parturients undergoing elective caesarean section at term were enrolled in this prospective, randomized, controlled, double-blinded study.

Exclusion criteria were emesis gravidarum, contraindication to spinal anesthesia (patient refusal, unstable hemodynamic, and coagulation abnormalities), chronic hypertension or preeclampsia, morbid obesity, and/or any study drugs allergy.

Patients were randomized (during preanesthetic consultation) to one of 2 groups using a random sequence (https://www.random.org/): group O received intravenously 4 mg ondansetron in 10 mL saline, 5 minutes before spinal puncture, and the control group received 10 mL of saline in the same way and same timing.

On arrival to the operating room, standard monitoring was applied and an arterial catheter was placed into the radial artery after infiltration of lidocaine (10–20 mg). Baseline (t_0) measurements of noncalibrated invasive SAP, DAP, MAP, and HR were recorded.

Stroke volume (SV), cardiac output (CO), systemic vascular resistance (SVR), and other estimated variables based on continuous arterial waveform analysis system (dP/dt max, cardiac cycle efficiency (CCE) and pulse pressure variation (PPV)) were recorded, using MOSTCARE (MOSTCARE; Vytech Health, France). This new low-invasive method is capable of deriving CO from the analysis of arterial pulse wave (pulse contour method (PCM)) and allows beat-by-beat hemodynamic parameters' determination using an uncalibrated PCM named pressure recording analytical method (PRAM).

Then, a fast infusion of 10 mL/kg of saline solution was completed approximately 5 minutes before anesthesia.

The anesthesiologist in charge of the patient and performing anesthesia was blind to patient's group like all other involved personnel except for the nurse preparing the syringe and injecting the solution according to random table made using Internet-free LOGICIEL (https://www.random.org/).

With patients in the sitting position, spinal anesthesia was performed at the L2-L3 or L3-L4 with a 25 G Whitacre needle (VYGON, France), and, 5 minutes after the administration of ondansetron/placebo solution, patients received 2 mL of a hyperbaric 5 mg/mL bupivacaine solution (Bupivacaine, UNIMED Tunisie) and 0.5 mL of a 5 μg/mL sufentanil solution.

Parturients were placed in a supine position immediately after the injections were completed. A left lateral tilt was applied by default to all parturients and a sensory block was assessed according to loss of pinprick sensation (25 G hypodermic needle) every 5 minutes for 15 minutes, beyond which parturients were excluded if sensory level was below T6. Surgery started as soon as the T6 dermatome was anesthetized; patients who failed to reach at least this level were excluded from the study, and general anesthesia was then administered at the attending anesthesiologist's discretion.

All hemodynamic parameters were recorded every 2 minutes to 20 minutes and then every 5 minutes until skin closure.

Hypotension, defined as a decrease from baseline values of ≥20% in systolic arterial pressure or SAP < 80 mmHg, was treated by an infusion of crystalloids (100 mL) and ephedrine bolus (6 mg) until restoration of baseline values. Ephedrine was chosen because of local unavailability of phenylephrine.

Table 1: Demographic characteristics.

	Group O (n = 40)	Group S n = 40	P
Age (years)	33 ± 4	33 ± 4	0.883
Weight (kg)	79 ± 11	77 ± 10	0.447
HR (bpm)	90 ± 13	92 ± 11	0.642
SAP (mm Hg)	124 ± 10	126 ± 11	0.456
DAP (mm Hg)	80 ± 10	80 ± 11	0.984
MAP (mm Hg)	95 ± 9	94 ± 10	0.417
Weight of newborns (gr)	3443 ± 650	3372 ± 431	0.567

HR: heart rate, SAP: systolic arterial pressure, DAP: diastolic arterial pressure, and MAP: mean arterial pressure.

Bradycardia, defined as a 30% drop in HR or ≤45 bpm, was also treated with fluids and ephedrine up to 25 mg; if bradycardia did not resolve within 30 seconds of treatment, IV atropine 0.5 mg was given every 30 seconds until resolution. We took note of total dose of atropine and ephedrine needed.

Clinical manifestations (retching or vomiting) and/or any requests for antiemetic medication (until end of surgery) were considered as episodes of nausea-vomiting.

An investigator who was not involved with intraoperative care performed a blood gas analysis of the umbilical artery immediately after clamping of the umbilical fetal blood lactate and pH. Apgar score was at 1, 3, 5, and 10 minutes (as recommended in our institution) and newborn weight was also noted.

After delivery, patients were advised to request analgesics as soon as significant pain developed in the operated area, with a subjective numerical rating scale (NRS) score > 3 out of 10. They were prescribed IV paracetamol 1000 mg four times daily starting from their report of pain; nefopam 20 mg intravenously was then available on request every 6 h and was infused slowly over 20 minutes.

3. Sample Size Calculation and Statistical Analysis

Sahoo et al. [14] found that the MAP in placebo group was 82.2 ± 10.5 mmHg. With an alpha error of 5% and power of 80% and assuming a 10% decrease in the MAP, we estimated that 26 patients would be needed in each group. Therefore 80 patients were included (40 patients in each group).

Statistical Analysis. We compared categorical data, between the groups, using Pearson's χ^2 test. Categorical data was described by count (percentages). We evaluated the data distribution using the Kolmogorov-Smirnov test. We used one-way analysis of variance for normally distributed continuous variables. We compared groups using Kruskall-Wallis test for nonnormally distributed continuous variables (pairwise comparison was performed by Mann-Whitney U test). Continuous variables were expressed as mean and standard deviation (SD) or median and interquartile range, depending on the normality distribution of the data. A P value of less

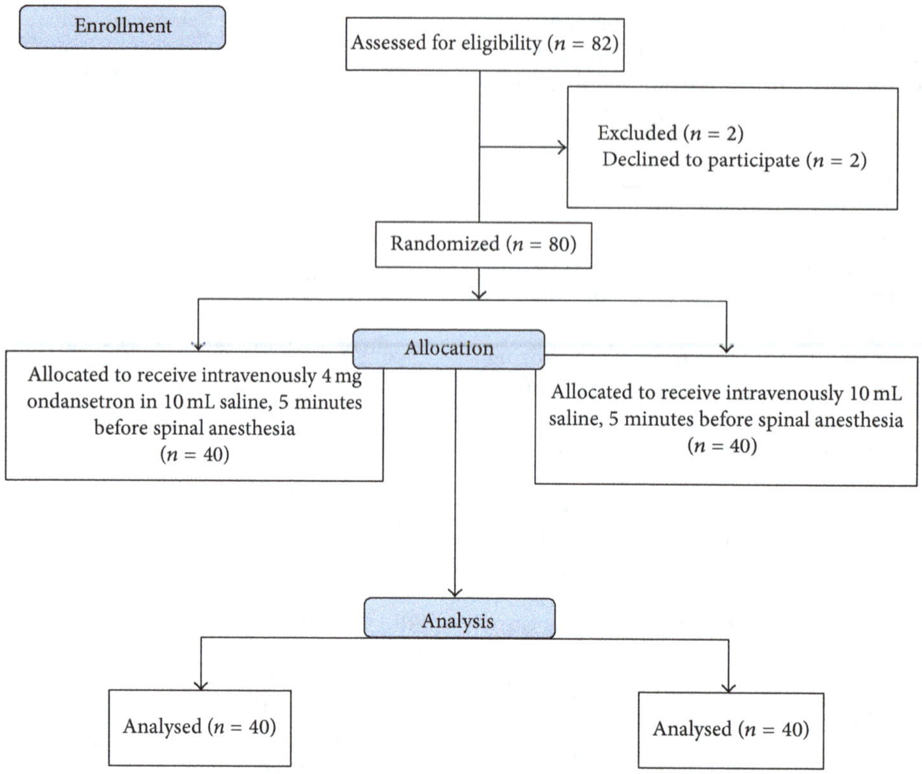

FIGURE 1: Flowchart of parturients enrolled in the study.

than 0.05 was considered significant. All statistics were done using R v.2.15.1 (R Development Core Team 2012).

4. Results

The flowchart of patients consented and recruited is shown in Figure 1. There were no significant differences between groups in terms of parturients physical characteristics and newborns' weight (Table 1).

SAP, DAP, and MAP were higher in group O than in group S between the 4th and 10th minutes and no difference was found until the 60th minute (Figures 2, 3, and 4, resp.).

Fewer patients in the O group experienced hypotension as compared to those in the S group: 15 (37.5%) and 31 (77.5%) ($P < 0.001$). Thus, the average consumption of ephedrine intraoperatively was 5.10 ± 7.78 mg in group O while it was 12.90 ± 9.24 mg in group S with a significant difference ($P <$ 0001).

HRs were similar in both groups and bradycardia was observed in 6 patients in group O (15%), whereas it was more frequent in the S group (15 cases, 37.5%) with a significant difference ($P = 0.022$). Atropine consumption of in group S was 0.12 ± 0.22 mg. Yet, no atropine was required in group O.

Hemodynamic parameters recorded with MOSTCARE were as below. dP/dt MAX in group O was significantly higher ($P < 0.001$) than that in group S only until the 12th minute (Figure 6(a)). In addition, Cce was stable in group O while it decreased up to 40% from baseline to the 10th minute in group S (Figure 6(b)).

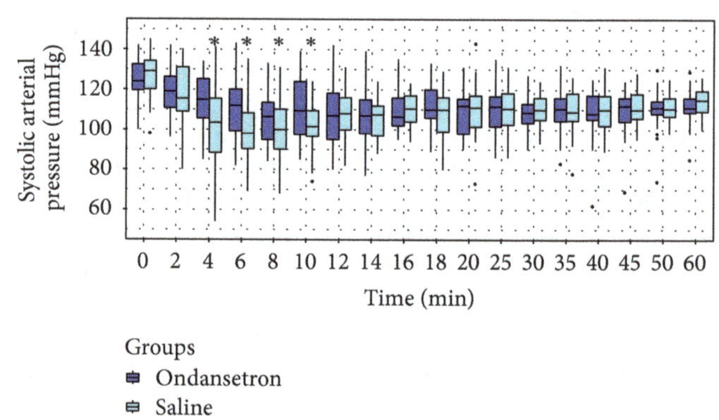

FIGURE 2: Trends of systolic blood pressure (SAP). * < 0.05.

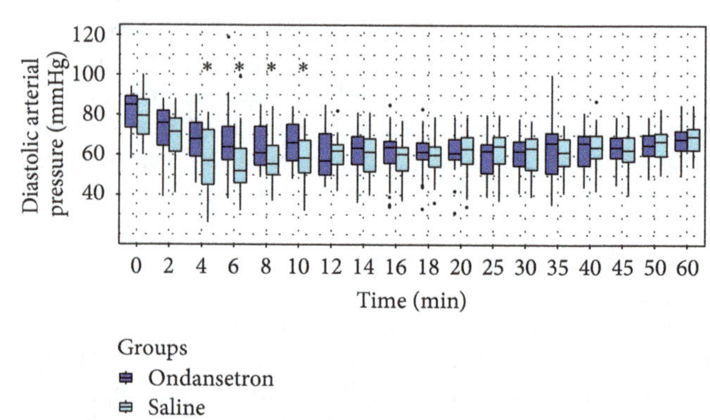

FIGURE 3: Trends of diastolic blood pressure (DAP). * < 0.05.

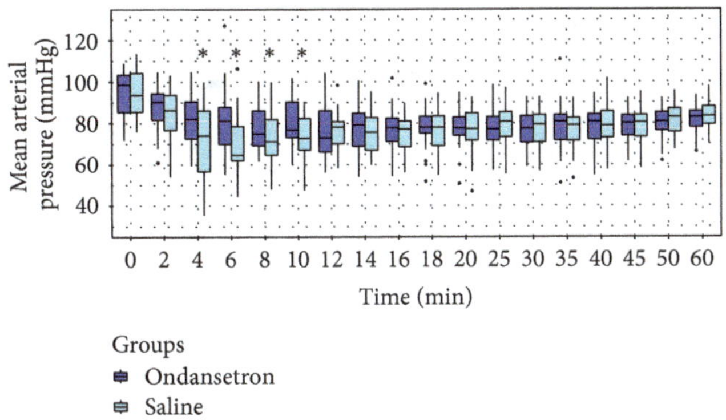

Figure 4: Trends of mean blood pressure (MAP). * < 0.05.

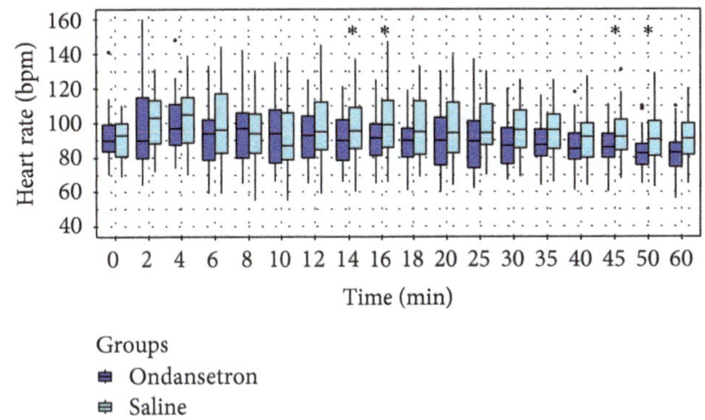

Figure 5: Trends of heart rate (HR). * < 0.05.

Both groups showed comparable small decrease in the CO not exceeding 28% between the second and the 12th minutes (Figure 6(c)). On the other hand, parturients in group S showed a major decrease in SV from baseline to the 12th minute (not observed in group O) (Figure 6(d)).

PPV was more pronounced in group S between the third and the 12th minutes (peak variation of 22% at the 6th minute). This variation did not exceed 9% in group O (Figure 6(e)).

Concerning afterload, SVR decreased more significantly in group S from the 5th minute to the 8th minute, and then no differences were noted between both groups (Figure 6(f)).

Fewer patients in group O experienced nausea and vomiting as compared to those in group S: 9 (22.5%) and 25 (62.5%), respectively ($P < 0.001$).

Apgar scores in group O were higher than those in group S until the fifth minute after birth (Figure 7). In addition, lactate of newborns whose mothers belonged to group O was lower than newborns whose mothers belonged to group S (2.09 ± 0.552 versus 3.22 ± 1.158, resp.; $P < 0.001$). Also noted is that pH of blood from the umbilical artery was closer to physiologic ranges in group O than in group S (7.38 ± 0.045 versus 7.35 ± 0.047, resp.; $P = 0.01$).

5. Discussion

Ondansetron was shown to attenuate arterial blood pressure drop due to spinal anesthesia in general surgery population in a study by Owczuk et al. [13] and in obstetrical population in a study by Sahoo et al. [14] (Figure 5). However, it was not shown to decrease this risk in obstetrical population in study of Ortiz-Gómez et al. [15]. A larger randomized controlled trial was performed here in order to further test the hypothesis that prophylactic ondansetron (5 mg) decreased the incidence of maternal hypotension following spinal anesthesia for elective caesarean section. Possible reasons include the specific population, sample size, study design, and anesthetic technique.

Our study compared ondansetron 5 mg ($n = 40$) with placebo ($n = 40$), Owczuk et al. [13] compared ondansetron 8 mg ($n = 35$) with placebo ($n = 36$), and Sahoo et al. [14] compared ondansetron 4 mg ($n = 24$) with placebo ($n = 24$) while Ortiz-Gómez et al.'s [15] study included three doses of ondansetron (2, 4, and 8 mg versus placebo).

Owczuk et al. [13] studied a general surgical population while Sahoo et al. [14] and Ortiz-Gómez et al. [15] studied obstetric patients undergoing caesarean delivery.

We consider the anesthetic technique the most important factor that might account for the difference between the studies.

Each of the three studies used a different dose of hyperbaric bupivacaine: we and Sahoo et al. [14] used 10 mg and Owczuk et al. [13] used 20 mg. In contrast, Ortiz-Gómez et al. [15] personalised each dose (mean dose of 9.7 ± 0.4 mg in the placebo group and 9.6 ± 0.3 mg in each of the ondansetron groups) to finally obtain doses which are slightly smaller than the 10 mg we used. This was interesting and may avoid over- or underdosing in women at the upper or lower extremes of height.

Differences in the design of the three studies should be noted. The first is the definition of hypotension. Owczuk et al. [13] did not supply a definition while Sahoo et al. [14] used a SBP < 90 mmHg or DBP < 60 mmHg. On the other hand, we (as well as Ortiz-Gómez et al. [15]) used the criteria outlined in the Cochrane review of hypotension in obstetrics [6].

Another difference is that Sahoo et al. administered intravenous fentanyl if the patient felt pain and tramadol or promethazine to treat adverse effects. These medications could modify blood pressure either directly or indirectly, possibly through a central mechanism.

Also, we routinely use intrathecal opioids to improve the quality of spinal anesthesia. This makes a direct comparison with the findings of Sahoo et al. [14] (but not with Ortiz-Gómez et al. [15] who used intrathecal fentanyl) difficult as the mechanism of action of ondansetron may be central and therefore affected by intrathecal opioids. Finally, we (as well as Ortiz-Gómez et al. [15]) did not use other supplemental analgesia and if required, those women were to be eliminated from the study.

Neither we nor Sahoo et al. [14] have reported their oxytocin protocol after umbilical cord clamping. This is important to explain results because of side effects which could affect maternal haemodynamics. Only Ortiz-Gómez et al. [15] have detailed oxytocin injection. They used low doses of (1 U), followed by an infusion of 2.5 U/h. Ours differ largely

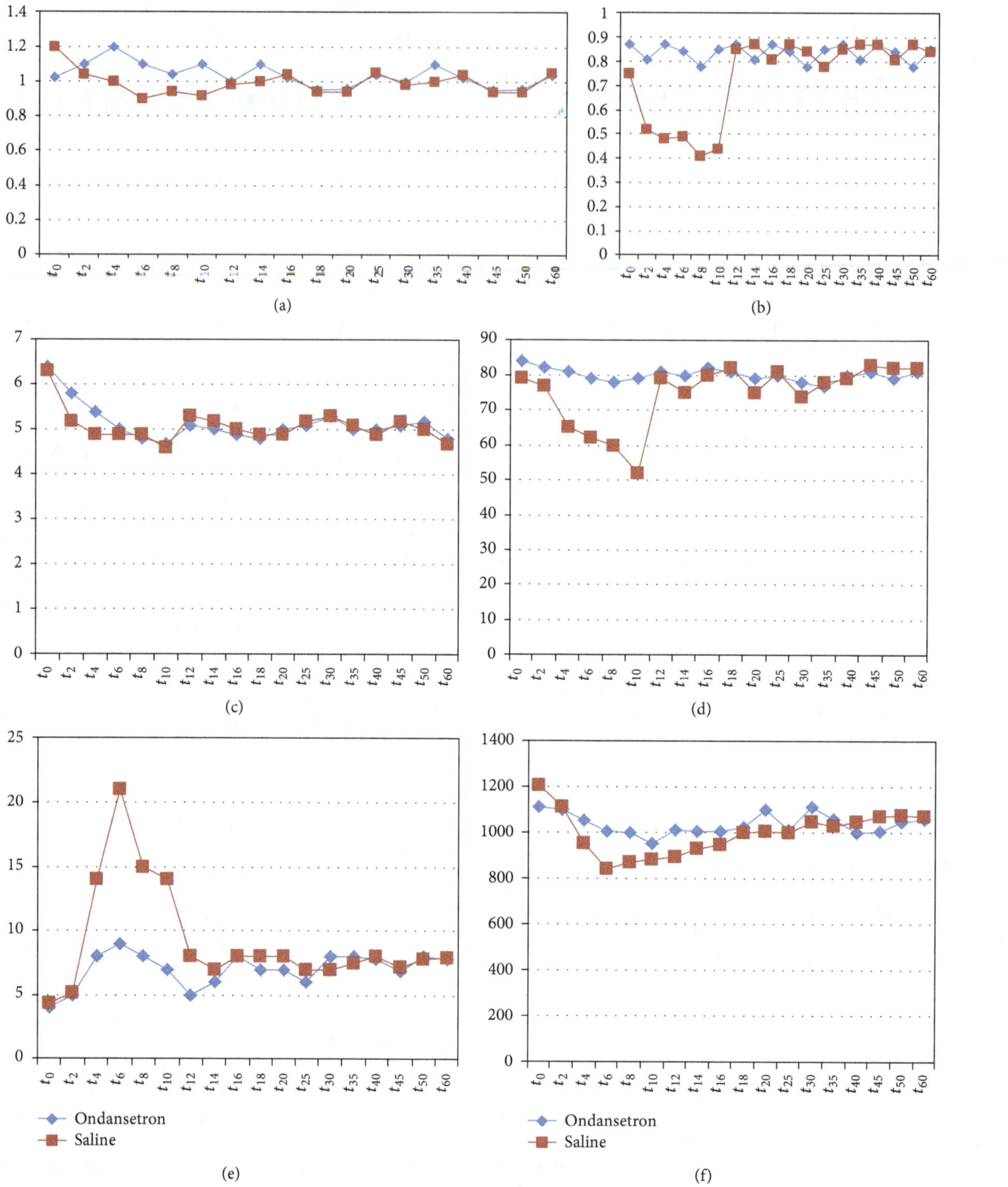

FIGURE 6: (a) Trends of mean dP/dt MAX. (b) Trends of mean cardiac cycle efficiency (CCE). (c) Trends of cardiac output (L·min^{-1}). (d) Trends of mean stroke volume (mL·min^{-1}). (e) Trends of mean pulse pressure variation. (f) Trends of mean systemic vascular resistance (dynes·s·cm^{-5}). t: time in minutes.

from this protocol. In fact we use bolus of 5 U in 5 minutes followed by an infusion of 2.5 U/h.

In conclusion, our results and those from Ortiz-Gómez et al., although methodologically close, differ because of different hypotension's management (type of loading fluids, type of vasopressor, and oxytocin protocol). This is sometimes due to economic constraints. For example, the unique vasopressor we have in our country is ephedrine (does not reflect current best practice) known to be associated with fetal acidosis [16, 17].

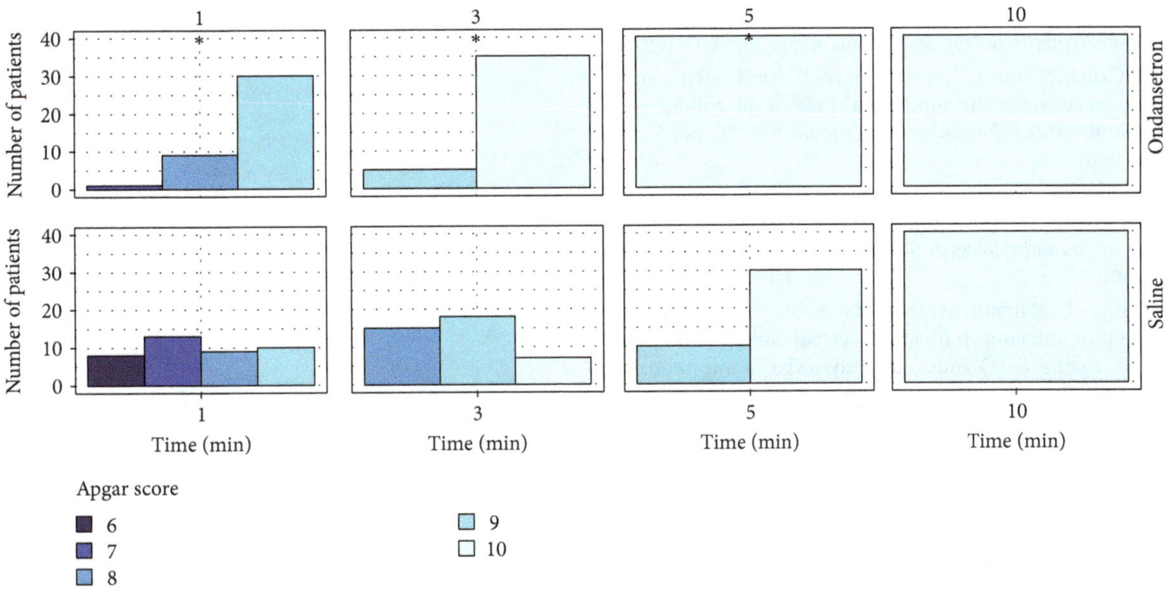

FIGURE 7: Apgar score of newborns during 1, 3, 5, and 10 minutes after birth. ∗ < 0.05.

The strength of our study lies in two subjects. The first is "minimally invasive" hemodynamic parameter monitoring to try to explain the mechanism of action of ondansetron. We know that the use of the MOSTCARE device (which is not yet validated in obstetric parturients) is not excessive (compared to transesophageal echocardiography) for this indication and it took a long time for the local ethics committee to give its agreement for this study. Echocardiography would have been an alternative but unavailability led us to choose MOSTCARE.

It seems that ondansetron may act at cardiac level (enhancing contractility and efficiency) and also at vascular level (stable SVR) via vascular and/or medullar specific receptors. Studies including more invasive haemodynamic technique (i.e., Swan-Ganz catheter) could be helpful.

The second is the neonatal parameters, and we showed that ondansetron can be helpful to improve metabolic and vital parameters of newborns, in any case, under our skies.

6. Conclusion

Our study showed that prophylactic ondansetron had a significant effect on the incidence of hypotension in healthy parturients undergoing spinal anaesthesia with bupivacaine and sufentanil for elective caesarean delivery.

Conflict of Interests

All authors have no commercial or financial interests in the products or companies described in this paper.

Acknowledgment

Financial support was only provided by departmental and institutional (Tunisian Military Hospital) funding.

References

[1] F. J. Mercier, M.-P. Bonnet, A. de la Dorie et al., "Spinal anaesthesia for caesarean section: fluid loading, vasopressors and hypotension," *Annales Francaises d'Anesthesie et de Reanimation*, vol. 26, no. 7-8, pp. 688–693, 2007.

[2] C. C. Rout, D. A. Rocke, J. Levin, E. Gouws, and D. Reddy, "A reevaluation of the role of crystalloid preload in the prevention of hypotension associated with spinal anesthesia for elective cesarean section," *Anesthesiology*, vol. 79, no. 2, pp. 262–269, 1993.

[3] R. Jackson, J. A. Reid, and J. Thorburn, "Volume preloading is not essential to prevent spinal-induced hypotension at caesarean section," *British Journal of Anaesthesia*, vol. 75, no. 3, pp. 262–265, 1995.

[4] S. W. Husaini and I. F. Russell, "Volume preload: lack of effect in the prevention of spinal-induced hypotension at caesarean section," *International Journal of Obstetric Anesthesia*, vol. 7, no. 2, pp. 76–81, 1998.

[5] P. J. Morgan, S. H. Halpern, and J. Tarshis, "The effects of an increase of central blood volume before spinal anesthesia for cesarean delivery: a qualitative systematic review," *Anesthesia & Analgesia*, vol. 92, no. 4, pp. 997–1005, 2001.

[6] R. S. Emmett, A. M. Cyna, M. Andrew, and S. W. Simmons, "Techniques for preventing hypotension during spinal anaesthesia for caesarean section," *Cochrane Database of Systematic Reviews*, no. 3, Article ID CD002251, 2002.

[7] G. A. Rooke, P. R. Freund, and A. F. Jacobson, "Hemodynamic response and change in organ blood volume during spinal anesthesia in elderly men with cardiac disease," *Anesthesia and Analgesia*, vol. 85, no. 1, pp. 99–105, 1997.

[8] J. Butterworth, "Physiology of spinal anesthesia: what are the implications for management?" *Regional Anesthesia and Pain Medicine*, vol. 23, no. 4, pp. 370–373, 1998.

[9] R. F. Brooker, J. F. Butterworth IV, D. W. Kitzman, J. M. Berman, H. I. Kashtan, and A. C. McKinley, "Treatment of hypotension after hyperbaric tetracaine spinal anesthesia: a randomized,

double-blind, cross-over comparison of phenylephrine and epinephrine," *Anesthesiology*, vol. 86, no. 4, pp. 797–805, 1997.

[10] L. A. H. Critchley and F. Conway, "Hypotension during subarachnoid anaesthesia: haemodynamic effects of colloid and metaraminol," *British Journal of Anaesthesia*, vol. 76, no. 5, pp. 734–736, 1996.

[11] R. Z. Løvstad, G. Granhus, and S. Hetland, "Bradycardia and asystolic cardiac arrest during spinal anaesthesia: a report of five cases," *Acta Anaesthesiologica Scandinavica*, vol. 44, no. 1, pp. 48–52, 2000.

[12] M. Yamano, T. Kamato, A. Nishida et al., "Serotonin (5-HT)3-receptor antagonism of 4,5,6,7-tetrahydrobenzimidazole derivatives against S-HT-induced bradycardia in anesthetized rats," *Japanese Journal of Pharmacology*, vol. 65, no. 3, pp. 241–248, 1994.

[13] R. Owczuk, W. Wenski, A. Polak-Krzeminska et al., "Ondansetron given intravenously attenuates arterial blood pressure drop due to spinal anesthesia: a double-blind, placebo-controlled study," *Regional Anesthesia and Pain Medicine*, vol. 33, no. 4, pp. 332–339, 2008.

[14] T. Sahoo, C. SenDasgupta, A. Goswami, and A. Hazra, "Reduction in spinal-induced hypotension with ondansetron in parturients undergoing caesarean section: a double-blind randomised, placebo-controlled study," *International Journal of Obstetric Anesthesia*, vol. 21, no. 1, pp. 24–28, 2012.

[15] J. R. Ortiz-Gómez, F. J. Palacio-Abizanda, F. Morillas-Ramirez, I. Fornet-Ruiz, A. Lorenzo-Jiménez, and M. L. Bermejo-Albares, "The effect of intravenous ondansetron on maternal haemodynamics during elective caesarean delivery under spinal anaesthesia: a double-blind, randomised, placebo-controlled trial," *International Journal of Obstetric Anesthesia*, vol. 23, no. 2, pp. 138–143, 2014.

[16] W. D. Ngan Kee, K. S. Khaw, P. E. Tan, F. F. Ng, and M. K. Karmakar, "Placental transfer and fetal metabolic effects of phenylephrine and ephedrine during spinal anesthesia for cesarean delivery," *Anesthesiology*, vol. 111, no. 3, pp. 506–512, 2009.

[17] A. S. Habib, "A review of the impact of phenylephrine administration on maternal hemodynamics and maternal and neonatal outcomes in women undergoing cesarean delivery under spinal anesthesia," *Anesthesia and Analgesia*, vol. 114, no. 2, pp. 377–390, 2012.

Permissions

All chapters in this book were first published in ARP, by Hindawi Publishing Corporation; hereby published with permission under the Creative Commons Attribution License or equivalent. Every chapter published in this book has been scrutinized by our experts. Their significance has been extensively debated. The topics covered herein carry significant findings which will fuel the growth of the discipline. They may even be implemented as practical applications or may be referred to as a beginning point for another development.

The contributors of this book come from diverse backgrounds, making this book a truly international effort. This book will bring forth new frontiers with its revolutionizing research information and detailed analysis of the nascent developments around the world.

We would like to thank all the contributing authors for lending their expertise to make the book truly unique. They have played a crucial role in the development of this book. Without their invaluable contributions this book wouldn't have been possible. They have made vital efforts to compile up to date information on the varied aspects of this subject to make this book a valuable addition to the collection of many professionals and students.

This book was conceptualized with the vision of imparting up-to-date information and advanced data in this field. To ensure the same, a matchless editorial board was set up. Every individual on the board went through rigorous rounds of assessment to prove their worth. After which they invested a large part of their time researching and compiling the most relevant data for our readers.

The editorial board has been involved in producing this book since its inception. They have spent rigorous hours researching and exploring the diverse topics which have resulted in the successful publishing of this book. They have passed on their knowledge of decades through this book. To expedite this challenging task, the publisher supported the team at every step. A small team of assistant editors was also appointed to further simplify the editing procedure and attain best results for the readers.

Apart from the editorial board, the designing team has also invested a significant amount of their time in understanding the subject and creating the most relevant covers. They scrutinized every image to scout for the most suitable representation of the subject and create an appropriate cover for the book.

The publishing team has been an ardent support to the editorial, designing and production team. Their endless efforts to recruit the best for this project, has resulted in the accomplishment of this book. They are a veteran in the field of academics and their pool of knowledge is as vast as their experience in printing. Their expertise and guidance has proved useful at every step. Their uncompromising quality standards have made this book an exceptional effort. Their encouragement from time to time has been an inspiration for everyone.

The publisher and the editorial board hope that this book will prove to be a valuable piece of knowledge for researchers, students, practitioners and scholars across the globe.

List of Contributors

Sarah Ciechanowicz and Vinod Patil
Department of Anaesthesia, BHR University Hospitals NHS Trust, Romford, London RM7 0AG, UK

Edward A. Shipton
Department of Anaesthesia, University of Otago, Christchurch 8042, New Zealand

Hironori Tsuchiya
Department of Dental Basic Education, Asahi University School of Dentistry, 1851 Hozumi, Mizuho, Gifu 501-0296, Japan

Maki Mizogami
Department of Anesthesiology and Reanimatology, University of Fukui Faculty of Medical Sciences, 23-3 Matsuokashimoaizuki, Eiheiji-cho, Yoshida-gun, Fukui 910-1193, Japan

Maria Bauer
Department of Outcomes Research, Cleveland Clinic, Cleveland, OH 44195, USA

Ehab Farag
Department of Outcomes Research, Cleveland Clinic, Cleveland, OH 44195, USA
Anesthesiology Institute, Cleveland Clinic, Cleveland, OH 44195, USA

John E. George III and John Seif
Anesthesiology Institute, Cleveland Clinic, Cleveland, OH 44195, USA

Nicholas C. K. Lam, Matthew Charles, Codruta Soneru, Jennifer Dillow and Francisco Jaime
Department of Anesthesiology & Critical Care Medicine, University of New Mexico, Albuquerque, NM 87131, USA

Timothy R. Petersen
Department of Anesthesiology & Critical Care Medicine, University of New Mexico, Albuquerque, NM 87131, USA
Department of Anthropology, University of New Mexico, Albuquerque, NM 87131, USA

Deana Mercer
Department of Orthopaedics & Rehabilitation, University of New Mexico, Albuquerque, NM 87131, USA

Edward R. Mariano
Department of Anesthesiology, Perioperative and Pain Medicine, Stanford University School of Medicine, Stanford, CA, USA
Anesthesiology and Perioperative Care Service, Veterans Affairs Palo Alto Health Care System, 3801 Miranda Avenue (112A), Palo Alto, CA 94304, USA

Dominic Hegarty
Department of Anaesthesia and Intensive Care, Cork University Hospital, Cork, Ireland
Department of Pharmacology and Therapeutics, University College Cork, Clinical Sciences Building, Cork, Ireland

P. H. Conroy
Department of Anaesthesia, Adelaide and Meath National Children's Hospital, Tallaght, Dublin, Ireland

C. Luyet
Universitätsklinik für Anästhesiologie und Schmerztherapie, Inselspital, Bern University Hospital, 3010 Bern, Switzerland

C. J. McCartney and P. G. McHardy
Department of Anesthesia, Sunnybrook Health Sciences Centre, Room M3-200, 2075 Bayview Avenue, Toronto, ON, Canada M4N 3M5

Nathaniel H. Greene, Benjamin G. Cobb and Christopher D. Kent
Department of Anesthesiology and Pain Medicine, University ofWashington School of Medicine, Seattle,WA 98195, USA

Ken F. Linnau
Department of Radiology, University ofWashington School of Medicine, Seattle,WA 98195, USA

Edward A. Shipton
Department of Anaesthesia, University of Otago, Christchurch 8042, New Zealand

Jośe Aguirre and Alain Borgeat
Division of Anesthesiology, Balgrist University Hospital, 8008 Zurich, Switzerland

Alicia Del Moral and Irina Cobo
Department of Anesthesiology, General University Hospital of Valencia, 46014 Valencia, Spain

Stephan Blumenthal
Department of Anesthesiology, Triemli Hospital, 8063 Zurich, Switzerland

Anirban Chattopadhyay
Lilavati Hospital & Research Center, Mumbai 400050, India

Souvik Maitra and Suvadeep Sen
Department of Anaesthesiology and Intensive Care, AIIMS, New Delhi 110029, India

Sulagna Bhattacharjee, Amitava Layek and Sugata Pal
Department of Anaesthesiology, IPGME&R and SSKM Hospital, Kolkata 700020, India

Kakali Ghosh
Department of Cardiac Anaesthesiology, IPGME&R and SSKMHospital, Kolkata 700020, India

Mark J. Young
Department of Anesthesiology, Critical Care and Pain Medicine, Massachusetts General Hospital Boston, MA 02114, USA

Vicki E. Modest and Sadeq A. Quraishi
Department of Anesthesiology, Critical Care and Pain Medicine, Massachusetts General Hospital Boston, MA 02114, USA
Harvard Medical School, Boston, MA 02115, USA

Andrew W. Gorlin
Department of Anesthesiology, Perioperative and Pain Medicine, Brigham and Women's Hospital Boston, MA 02115, USA

Clifford Bowens Jr. and Ramprasad Sripada
Department of Anesthesiology, Vanderbilt University School of Medicine, 1301 Medical Center Drive 4648 The Vanderbilt Clinic, Nashville, TN 37232-5614, USA

Jagdeep Sharma
Senior Resident, Dept. of Anaesthesia & Intensive Care, Govt. Medical College & Hospital, Sector-32, Chandigarh, India

Ruchi Gupta and Anita Kumari
Professor, Dept. of Anaesthesia & Intensive Care, Shri Guru Ram Das Institute of Medical Sciences and Research, Vallah, Amritsar, India

Lakshmi Mahajan
Assistant Professor, Dept. of Anaesthesia & Intensive Care, Shri Guru Ram Das Institute of Medical Sciences and Research, Vallah, Amritsar, India

Jasveer Singh
Associate Professor, Dept. of Anaesthesia & Intensive Care, Govt. Medical College & Hospital, Sector-32, Chandigarh, India

Ashwin Sankar
Department of Anesthesia, University of Toronto, Toronto, ON, Canada

Minou Behboudi and Richard Brull
Department of Anesthesia and Pain Management, Toronto Western Hospital, University Health Network, Toronto, ON, Canada

Faraj W. Abdallah
Department of Anesthesia and Keenan Research Centre, Li Ka Shing Knowledge Institute, St. Michael's Hospital, Toronto, ON, Canada

Alan Macfarlane
Department of Anaesthesia, Glasgow Royal Infirmary, Glasgow, UK
Department of Anaesthesia, Critical Care and Pain Medicine, University of Glasgow, Glasgow, UK

Seid Adem Ahemed, Zewditu Abdissa Denu, Habtamu Getinet Kassahun and Demeke Yilikal Fentie
Department of Anesthesia, College of Medicine and Health Sciences, University of Gondar, Gondar, Ethiopia

Giorgio Capogna, Emanuele Capogna and Angelica Del Vecchio
European School of Obstetric Anesthesia (EESOA), Maternal Neonatal Simulation Centre, Roma, Italy

Alessandra Coccoluto
European School of Obstetric Anesthesia (EESOA), Maternal Neonatal Simulation Centre, Roma, Italy
Policlinico Casilino Hospital, Roma, Italy

Riyadh Firdaus, Besthadi Sukmono, Annemarie Chrysantia Melati and Berial Dewin Marzaini
Department of Anesthesiology and Intensive Care, Cipto Mangunkusumo National Central Hospital and Faculty of Medicine, Universitas Indonesia, Jakarta 10430, Indonesia

Manuel Wenk, Christina Massoth and Daniel M. Pöpping
Department of Anesthesiology, Intensive Care and Pain Medicine, University Hospital Muenster, Muenster, Germany

Michael Möllmann
Department of Anesthesiology and Intensive Care, St. Franziskus Hospital, Muenster, Germany

Ashraf Eskandr and Sadik Abdel Maseeh
Department of Anaesthesia, ICU and Pain Therapy, Faculty of Medicine, Menoufiya University, Shibin El-Koom 32518, Egypt

Onur Balaban and Tayfun Aydın
Department of Anesthesiology and Pain Medicine, School of Medicine, Dumlupinar University, Kutahya, Turkey

Turan Cihan Dülgeroğlu
Department of Orthopedic and Trauma Surgery, School of Medicine, Dumlupinar University, Kutahya, Turkey

E. Pushpanathan
Department of Anaesthesia, Guy's and St. omas' NHS Foundation Trust, London, UK

T. Setty
Department of Anaesthesia, University College Hospitals London NHS Foundation Trust, London, UK

B. Carvalho
Department of Anesthesia, Stanford University School of Medicine, Stanford, CA, USA

P. Sultan
Department of Anaesthesia, University College Hospitals London NHS Foundation Trust, University College London, London, UK

Abdulhalim Karayel
Anesthesiology and Reanimation Clinic, Bagcilar Training and Research Hospital, 34218 Istanbul, Turkey

Ahmed Said Elgebaly
Department of Anesthesia and Postsurgical Intensive Care, Faculty of Medicine, Tanta University, Tanta, Egypt

Somrat Charuluxananan and Pavena Bunburaphong
Department of Anesthesiology, Faculty of Medicine, Chulalongkorn University, Bangkok 10330, Thailand

Tanyong Pipanmekaporn
Clinical Epidemiology Program, Faculty of Medicine, Chiang Mai University, Chiang Mai 50200, Thailand
Department of Anesthesiology, Faculty of Medicine, Chiang Mai University, Chiang Mai 50200, Thailand

Yodying Punjasawadwong and Worawut Lapisatepun
Department of Anesthesiology, Faculty of Medicine, Chiang Mai University, Chiang Mai 50200, Thailand

Yu-Ying Tang and Xue-Mei Lin
Department of Anesthesiology, West China Second Hospital, Sichuan University, Sichuan, Chengdu 610041, China

Jie Zhou
Department of Anesthesiology, Perioperative and Pain Medicine, Brigham and Women's Hospital, Harvard Medical School, 75 Francis Street, Boston, MA 02115, USA

Xiao-Hui Ren
Department of Anesthesiology, Median Area of Maternal and Child Care Service Center, Sichuan, Neijiang 641000, China

Manuel Wenk and Daniel Matthias Pöpping
Department of Anesthesiology, Intensive Care and Pain Medicine, University Hospital Muenster, Albert-Schweitzer Campus 1, A1, 48149 Muenster, Germany

Christian Weiss
Medical School, University of Muenster, 48149 Muenster, Germany

Michael Möllmann
Department of Anesthesiology and Intensive Care, St. Franziskus Hospital, 48145 Muenster, Germany

Walid Trabelsi, Chihebeddine Romdhani, Haythem Elaskri, Walid Sammoud, Mohamed Bensalah, Iheb Labbene and Mustapha Ferjani
Department of Anesthesia and Intensive Care Unit, Tunisian Military Hospital, 1008 Tunis, Tunisia

Index

www.ingramcontent.com/pod-product-compliance
Lightning Source LLC
LaVergne TN
LVHW060540210926
848485LV00005B/1234